Wilson Fox

An atlas of pathological anatomy of the lungs

Wilson Fox

An atlas of pathological anatomy of the lungs

ISBN/EAN: 9783742831927

Manufactured in Europe, USA, Canada, Australia, Japa

Cover: Foto ©Lupo / pixelio.de

Manufactured and distributed by brebook publishing software (www.brebook.com)

Wilson Fox

An atlas of pathological anatomy of the lungs

AN ATLAS

OF THE

PATHOLOGICAL ANATOMY

OF

THE LUNGS

BY THE LATE

WILSON FOX, M.D., F.R.S.

FELLOW OF THE ROYAL COLLEGE OF PHYSICIANS
PHYSICIAN IN ORDINARY TO HER MAJESTY THE QUEEN
PHYSICIAN TO HIS ROYAL HIGHNESS THE DUKE OF EDINBURGH
HOLME PROFESSOR OF CLINICAL MEDICINE IN UNIVERSITY COLLEGE
PHYSICIAN TO UNIVERSITY COLLEGE HOSPITAL

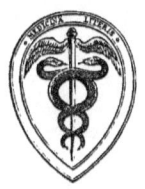

LONDON
J. & A. CHURCHILL
11 NEW BURLINGTON STREET
1888

PREFACE.

Dr. WILSON FOX left, at his death, the manuscript and other materials for two works, which had occupied him during many years. The works are a 'Treatise on Diseases of the Lungs' and an 'Atlas of the Pathological Anatomy of the Lungs.' It was the Author's intention that the two should be published together. Unfortunately the manuscript, although complete in extent, had not received the final revision necessary to fit it for the press, and the character of the works is such that the revision requires a considerable amount of time. The two works, although related, are essentially independent. Hence it seems unjustifiable to delay the appearance of the smaller of the two, the Atlas, while the larger work is being prepared for the press. The Atlas is therefore published first.

It was the wish of the Author that, in the event of his death, the manuscript should be prepared for the press by a personal friend—who has attempted, so far as regards the present work, to carry out, to the best of his ability, the wishes of one for whom he had a profound regard and warm affection.

The following pages are substantially as their Author left them. The only alterations are such verbal changes as were absolutely necessary. Certain additions have, however, been made, viz. the summary at the head of each case and the description of the coloured plates. The description of the microscopical plates was complete, but, apparently, the plan of the work had not included any separate account of the coloured plates, for which, it was intended, the history of the cases should suffice. The absence of such description would, however, have lessened the utility of the work, especially to the student. Accordingly a short account of each figure has been prepared, chiefly from the history of the case illustrated. Various references have also been added in the hope of facilitating the use of the work.

Much pains have been taken to secure accuracy, but the task has been one of great difficulty. The plates had undergone many alterations during the progress of the work. Figures had been changed, new plates introduced, and the corresponding changes in the text had not always been made. In some instances the precise figure referred to could only be ascertained by internal evidence. Another difficulty was met with in the descriptions of some of the microscopical plates. These had apparently been written from the preparations themselves, as well as from the figures, and the reference letters, in some instances, had evidently been added to and altered in view of an intended revision of the descriptions. In many cases rectification has been practicable; in a few it has been thought better to leave the discrepancy with this explanation of its origin.

W. R. G.

LONDON: *July*, 1888.

CONTENTS.

INTRODUCTION. ON THE ULTIMATE STRUCTURE OF THE LUNGS, 1. Arrangement of the bronchi, 1; infundibula, 3; acini and lobules, 6. Structure of the bronchial tubes, 7; of the alveolar passages and alveoli, 9; the epithelium, 10; capillaries, 11; lymphatics, 11.

ACUTE PNEUMONIA, 15. Stage of engorgement, 15; of red hepatisation, 16; of grey hepatisation, 17; of suppuration, 18. Serous, œdematous, and ichorous pneumonia, 18. Microscopic appearances—exudation, 18; cell-elements, 19; source of the corpuscles, 21; transition to grey and suppurative stages, 22.

ACUTE CATARRHAL PNEUMONIA OR BRONCHO-PNEUMONIA, 22. Characters of the lobular form, 23; distinction from collapse, 23; distribution, 24; confluence to 'pseudo-lobar' form, 24. Conditions of bronchi, 24. Associated collapse, 25; secondary inflammation and 'splenisation,' 25. Affection of pleura, 26. Associated emphysema, 26.
Histology, 27; origin of cells, 28; micro-organisms, 29; changes in bronchi, 29, and around them, 30. Suppuration, 31. Secondary forms; in diphtheria, 32; variola, 32. Caseation, 32. Classification and terminology, 33. Artificial broncho-pneumonia, 35.
Catarrhal pneumonia in the adult, 35; in old age, 36.

OTHER FORMS OF ACUTE PNEUMONIA, 39. Use of the term 'catarrhal,' 39. Infective pneumonia, 38. 'Desquamative pneumonia,' 39.

HYPOSTATIC OR CONGESTIVE PNEUMONIA, 30. Seat, 40; appearances, 40; mechanism, 40; affection of pleura, 41.

ACUTE INTERSTITIAL PNEUMONIA, 42. Case illustrated, 42; mechanism of production, 43.

CHRONIC PNEUMONIA, CHRONIC INTERSTITIAL PNEUMONIA, 44. Passage of acute pneumonia into a chronic stage, 44. Chronic red hepatisation, 46. Fibroid induration, 47. Fibroid changes due to compression, 47, to collapse, 48. Use of the term 'interstitial pneumonia,' 48. Dilatation of the bronchi in fibroid lungs, 49; pneumonic changes secondary to bronchial dilatation, 50. Chronic ulcerative pneumonia, 50.

BROWN INDURATION, 51. Microscopic changes, 52.

DISEASES CAUSED BY INHALATION OF DUST, 53. Aspect of lung, 53; source of pigment, 54. Microscopic changes, 54. Relation to tubercle, 55. Cavities, 56. Affection of the glands, 56.

COLLAPSE OF THE LUNG, 56. Congenital atelectasis, 57. Collapse from obstruction of the bronchi, 57. Collapse from pressure, 58.

PULMONARY EMBOLISM, 58. The hæmorrhagic infarct, 58; mechanism of the hæmorrhage, 59. Embolic pneumonia, 60.

GANGRENE OF THE LUNG, 61; diffuse, 61; circumscribed, 61; from embolism, 62; traumatic form, 62.

PHTHISIS, 63. Morbid appearances. Granulations—Grey granulations, 63; changes, 64. Soft opaque white granulations, 65. Larger opaque white granulations, 65. Yellow granulations, 65. Indurated granulations, 66. Infiltrations.—Red hepatisation, 66. Grey infiltration, 67. Gelatinous infiltration, 68. Caseous infiltration, 69. Induration, various forms, 70; of granulations, 70; diffuse, 71; dilatation of bronchi, 71. Cavities,—mode of origin, 72; changes, 74; composite and sinuous, 74; encapsuling and cicatrisation, 75; cretification of contents, 77; origin of calcareous masses, 78. Gangrene, 78. Changes in bronchi, 78; relation to tubercle, 79; peribronchitis, 79; ulceration, 80; dilatation, 80; contents, 81; contraction and obliteration, 83.
Histology of the granulations.—In acute tuberculosis, 83. Grey granulations, 83. Granulations containing giant-cells, 85. Description of giant-cells, 86; nuclei, 86; origin, 87; theories discussed, 88. Pseudo-giant cells, 90. Site of the giant-cells, 90. Structure of granulations containing them, 91. Changes in giant-cells, 91; their relation to tubercle, 92. Epithelial granulations, 93. Soft amorphous or caseous granulations, 94. Granulations in ordinary phthisis, 94. Caseous granulations and nodules, 94. Indurated granulations and nodules, 96. Seat and origin of the granulation, 99; peribronchial relations, 99; bronchial tubercle, 100; perivascular relations, 101; alveolar granulations, 102; interstitial granulations, 104.
Histology of infiltrations and caseation, 104. Red hepatisation, 104. Gelatinous infiltration, 104. Grey infiltration, 105; distension of alveoli, 106; diffuse thickening of alveolar walls, 106; origin and nature of the growth, 108. Destructive changes in granulations and infiltrations, 109. Caseation, 109; fatty and hyaline degeneration, 110; the influence of arrest of circulation, 112. Characters of the process in various forms of granulations in acute tuberculosis, 114; in ordinary phthisis, 115; the diffuse caseations of phthisis, 117. Acute softening, 118. Genuine suppurative changes, 119. Mechanism of the softening of caseous matter, 120. Diffuse induration, 121.

SYPHILITIC DISEASES OF THE LUNG, 122. Gummata, 122; distinction of small forms from tubercle, 123. Syphilitic pneumonia, 124; lobular form, 126. Syphilitic indurations, 128. Changes in lymphatics, 129. Microscopic appearances of gummata, 129; of syphilitic pneumonia, 131. Syphilitic phthisis, 132.

CANCER OF THE LUNG, 133. Varieties, 134. Infiltrating form, 134. Mode of growth, 135. Epithelioma, 135; squamous, 136; cylindrical, 137.

THE ARTIFICIAL PRODUCTION OF TUBERCLE, 139. Specificity of infection, 139; modes of inoculation, 139

viii   CONTENTS

Inoculation as a test, 140. Identity of bovine and human tuberculosis, 140; of their bacilli, 141. Micro-organisms of tubercle, 142; specificity of the bacillus, 142. Results of inoculation, 142. Variety of animals susceptible, 144. Changes observed after inoculation —in the eye, 144; in the peritoneum, 146; beneath the skin, 147; into the veins, 148. Changes in the lymphatic glands, 149; in the spleen, 150; in the lung, 150, granulations, 152, perivascular and peri-bronchial growth, 152, alveolar growth, 153, diffuse infiltrations, 154. Changes in the intestines, 154; in the liver, 155; in the kidney, 156. Identity of the inoculated and human disease, 156.

CASES.

	PAGE		PAGE
1. Acute Pneumonia; Grey Hepatisation; *Joseph Kirk*, æt. 46	158	27. Indurating and Caseating Tubercular Pneumonia; *J. Overall*, æt. 38	196
2. Pneumonia, suppuration (Carswell)	158	28. Indurating Tubercular Pneumonia; *William Smith*, æt. 40	199
3. Chronic Pneumonia, Syphilis; *Elizabeth Hawkins*, æt. 55	159	29. Indurating Tubercular Pneumonia; Laryngeal Tubercle; *James Brown*, æt. 44	201
4. Acute Broncho-pneumonia; *John Tanner*, æt. 1	160	30. Chronic Phthisis, Indurating Tuberculosis; *Mary Ann Carr*, æt. 36	203
5. Acute ulcerating and suppurating Pneumonia, *Sarah Brown*, æt. 31	161	31. Tubercular Induration and Pneumonia; *John Lack*, æt. 45	205
6. Acute Tubercle; *John H. Polley*, æt. 6	163	32. Chronic Induration of Lungs; *William Atwood*, æt. 66	207
7. Acute Tubercle; *Alfred Coombes*, æt. 18	165	33. Indurated and Pigmented Tuberculisation; *W. H. Coppin*, æt. 80	208
8. Suppuration of Glands, Tuberculosis; *Sarah Shimmick*, æt. 8	167	34. Chronic Phthisis; Tubercular Induration; *H. Cox*, æt. 27	210
9. Acute Tuberculisation, Caseation of Glands; *Alfred Vick*, æt. 26	168	35. Indurating Tuberculisation; *Caroline Roberts*, æt. 26	212
10. Tuberculosis, Pleurisy; *George Unwin*, æt. 49	170	36. Indurating Tuberculisation; *Emma Mears*, æt. 15	213
11. Tuberculosis, Tubercular Peritonitis; *George Beale*, æt. 45	172	37. Indurating Tuberculisation; *Alfred Schofield*, æt. 27	215
12. Acute Tubercular Pneumonia; *Catherine Price*, æt. 33	173	38. Potter's Phthisis; *Charles Barlow*, æt. 56	216
13. Diabetic Phthisis; *Alfred Broom*, æt. 19	175	38a. Potter's Phthisis "	217
14. Diabetic Phthisis; " "	176	39. Miner's Phthisis (Greenhow) "	218
15. Tuberculisation and Tubercular Pneumonia; *William Scarrow*, æt. 20	176	40. Disease of Lungs in Copper Miner, ib.	219
16. Acute Tubercular Pneumonia; *William Henshaw*, æt. 20	177	41. Disease of Lung in Flax-dresser, ib.	219
17. Acute Destructive Pneumonia; *T. Ellsom*, æt. 42	179	42. Siderosis Pulmonum (Zenker)	220
18. Tubercular Suppurating Pneumonia; *John Brodrick*, æt. 43	181	43. Pulmonary Induration in Heart-disease; *William Thomas*, æt. 10	222
19. Chronic Indurating and Caseating Tubercular Pneumonia; *Walter Griffin*, æt. 41	183	44. Emphysema of Lung (Carswell)	223
20. Caseating Tubercular Pneumonia; *John Thomas*, æt. 39	186	45. Secondary Cancer of Lung; *Harriet Parsons*, æt. 28	224
21. Chronic Phthisis, Pneumonic Infiltration; *Gowling*	187	46. Cancerous Infiltration of Lung	225
22. Acute Caseating Tubercular Pneumonia; *T. Gardiner*, æt. 28	187	47. Secondary Cancer of Lung, Columnar Epithelioma; *Phœbe Leather*, æt. 50	225
23. Caseating Tubercular Pneumonia; *Jane Lloyd*, æt. 27	190	48. Sarcoma of Lung; *Mary Fisher*, æt. 60	226
24. Acute Phthisis; Caseating Tubercular Pneumonia; *Margaret Hall*, æt. 23	191	49. Pulmonary Embolism; *William Rowe*, æt. 25	227
25. Chronic Phthisis; Indurating Tubercular Pneumonia; *Mary Corney*, æt. 17	193	50. Syphilitic Growth in Infant's Lung (Lebert)	228
26. Chronic Phthisis; Indurating Tuberculisation; *Esther Heath*, æt. 36	194	51. Syphilitic Growths in Cerebellum and Lungs, *W. D.*, æt. 68	229
		52. Syphilis (?) Pneumonia (Greenfield)	229
		53. Syphilitic Disease of Brain and Lung; *Sarah Hanner*, æt. 48	230

ALPHABETICAL LIST OF CASES 231
DESCRIPTION OF PLATES:
 § A. Coloured Plates (I. to XXIV.) 232
 § B. Microscopical Plates (XXV. to XLV.) 249
INDEX OF AUTHORS REFERRED TO 279
GENERAL INDEX 284

INTRODUCTION.

ON THE ULTIMATE STRUCTURE OF THE LUNGS.

As a comprehension of the pulmonary structure is essential to a clear understanding of the processes involved in embolism, lobular pneumonia, and tubercle, I believe that this will be facilitated if I append a short description of the most recently expressed views on the subject. The following account contains no original matter, and for it I am chiefly indebted to Eilhard Schulze's article in Stricker's 'Handbuch der Lehre von der Geweben,' to Kölliker's 'Gewebelehre' and his more recent investigations in the 'Verhandlungen der Med. Gesellschaft zu Würzburg,' N.F. xvi. 1881, and also to Todd and Bowman's 'Physiological Anatomy;' Waters, 'The Anatomy of the Human Lung'; Klein, 'Atlas of Histology,' and 'Anatomy of the Lymphatic System'; Küttner's articles in Virchow's 'Archiv,' vols. lxvi. and lxxiii., Rossignol, 'Structure Intime du Poumon'; 'Adriani, 'Diss. de Subtiliore Pulmonum Structura,' and Schäfer's article in Quain and Sharpey's 'Anatomy.' I have thought it best to omit the references to the extensive bibliography on this subject, which will be found in the authors referred to.

The lungs essentially form a glandular structure of the racemose type for the excretion of carbonic acid, and are constituted by the subdivision of the ducts or bronchial tubes, terminating in a series of expansions into cavities resembling the terminal acini of a gland. These are collected into lobules and lobes, defined and surrounded by connective tissue; the whole being contained in a capsule which, on its external surface, is covered by an endothelium of the lymphatic type—the pleura. The gland thus constituted is supplied abundantly with blood-vessels and lymphatics and also with nerves.

The Bronchi within the Lung.—After entering the lung the larger tubes undergo a series of dichotomous and sometimes trichotomous divisions, giving off also smaller branches until they are reduced to a size of $\frac{1}{6}$ to $\frac{1}{8}$ inch (four millimetres) in diameter. The dichotomous division of the main tubes then ceases, but a series of branches are given off at an acute angle, alternating in a spiral form around the tubes. These branches again divide dichotomously at right angles to one another, but without anastomosing, until they attain the size of $\frac{1}{20}$ of an inch, and this continued rectangular branching gives to the whole structure a peculiar intricacy.

The tubes generally are straight until the final series of dichotomous branchings is attained. These latter are, however, often curved.[1] The openings of the larger tubes from their tubes of origin are more or less oval, but they become circular in the smaller tubes and appear (as was observed by Rossignol) as if cut with a punch (Waters). After a variable number of divisions (from five to eight), the terminal bronchus is attained, this being, as already stated, from $\frac{1}{20}$ to $\frac{1}{30}$ of an inch in diameter. At this point, which is situated about $\frac{1}{8}$ of an inch from the surface of the lung (Rainey[2]), the structure (to be hereafter described) and the configuration of the tube alter. A slight enlargement commonly appears in it, and the tube is continued into a series of passages which constitute the proper respiratory structure of the lung.

---

[1] See Rossignol's figure (Fig. 1); also Waters, *The Anatomy of the Human Lung*, p. 111.

[2] Within the lung the larger interlobular septa stand in this respect in the same relation to the terminations of the bronchi as the pleural surface, and the infundibula and alveoli in which the bronchi terminate rest upon these septa in the same manner as they do upon the pleura.

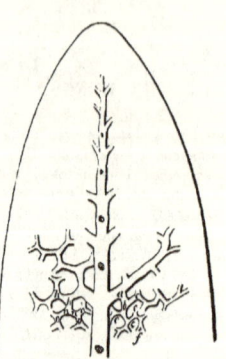

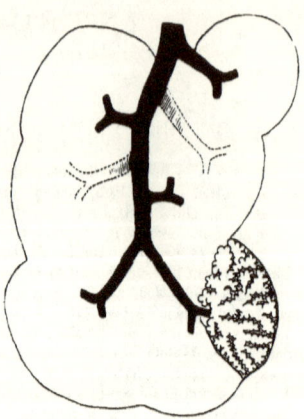

Fig. 1.—From Rossignol. Showing the ramification of an intralobular bronchus in a conical lobule. 'A branch of the second order, a, passing off at right angles, affords at its origin a branch, b, of the third order. It is elbowed to give off a third, c, and similarly, five, six, or eight successive branches are furnished, continuing its primary deviation amid these bends, towards the surface of the lobules. . . . Each of the divisions of the third order produces in a short course several branches of the fourth order, and terminates in a bifurcation at an acute angle. It is ordinarily at the extremity of the divisions of the fourth order that the tubes of the reunion of the infundibula ('alveolar passages' of Schulze) occur, but the ramifications may be pushed yet farther. In the dichotomous or trichotomous type of division (shown on the left), a branch of the second order ends, after a short course, and without lateral branches, in two or three tubes which come off from the same place hh, and present a similar division into tubules of the fourth order nn, which furnish other branches of the fifth order oo, and so on.'—Rossignol, p. 27.

Fig. 2.—From Rindfleisch. 'An exact copy of a lobule, ⅔ of an inch in length by ½ of an inch in width. A "corrosions preparation," produced by injection of the bronchus with gum and glycerine, and soaking in alcohol acidulated with hydrochloric acid. It is seen that the bronchus entering the root has, by a series of six branchings, produced seven smaller bronchioles, each of which passes into two short bronchioles of the smallest calibre. The smallest bronchioles open directly into a group of 3 to 5 branching alveolar passages. These collectively form the equivalent of an acinus of an acinose gland, and must be termed "pulmonary acini." The pulmonary acinus is a much more constant unity of the lung-structure than the lobule—at least in respect of size. Two of them may be sufficient to form a lobule. The lobule here represented contains fourteen such acini, but some may consist of 20 to 30 acini. The lobule may, however, be a more important structural element, with its pathological relations, because it is determined by the branching of the pulmonary "vessels" and the distribution of the interstitial (interlobular) connective tissue. Embolisms, infarcts, and abscesses are therefore limited by the lobules.' Rindfleisch proceeds to state that tubercle tends to form at the spot where the bronchiole divides into the alveolar passages, a view which I have not been able to confirm.—*Lehrb. der Path. Gewebelehre*, p. 134.

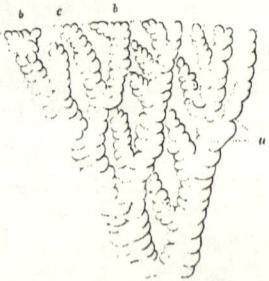

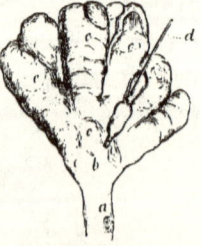

Fig. 3.—From Addison, *Phil. Trans.* 1842. 'Intralobular bronchial ramifications, partly inflated and highly magnified. a, cul-de-sac terminations lying against the lateral inflations of adjacent branches; b, b, c, the multilocular culs-de-sac at the surface of a lobule.'

Fig. 4.—From Waters. 'A terminal bronchial tube with a group of air-sacs connected with it ("lobuleite")—human. a, The terminal bronchial tube; b, the dilated extremity of the terminal bronchial tube; ccc, individual air-sacs. At d, a bristle is seen passed into an air-sac; one end is seen opening into the common cavity in which the bronchial tube terminates. At c and c (above b) are seen the openings of other sacs which lie beneath those which are exposed; six sacs are seen converging to the common centre. The markings in the air-sacs denote the boundaries of the alveoli.' Waters' *Anatomy Human Lung*, p. 136.

STRUCTURE OF THE LUNGS

These passages, termed by Rossignol 'tubes of reunion of the infundibula,' by Addison 'intralobular bronchial ramifications,' by Rainey 'intercellular passages,' by Todd 'lobular passages,' by Schulze 'alveolar passages,' and by Klein 'alveolar ducts'—a term which appears the most appropriate of any yet chosen—divide into a limited number of secondary branches, and then, expanding towards their termination, form a series of funnel-shaped bodies, the infundibula of Rossignol, or, as termed by Waters, 'air-sacs,' in which the tubes thus dilated end at the surface of the lung in alveolated extremities.

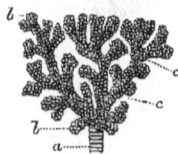

FIG. 5.—From Schulze. 'System of alveolar passages with the infundibula from the lung of an ape (cercopithecus) filled with mercury. *a*, Terminal branch of bronchus; *bb*, infundibula; *cc*, alveolar passages. × 10 diam.—Schulze, Stricker's *Handbuch*, p. 465.

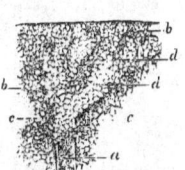

FIG. 6.—From Schulze. 'Section from the lung of a cat, filled with alcohol and hardened. *a*, terminal branch of bronchus; *bb*, infundibula; *cc*, transverse sections of alveolar passages; *dd*, longitudinal sections of alveolar passages. × 12 diam.—Schulze, Stricker's *Handbuch*, p. 465.

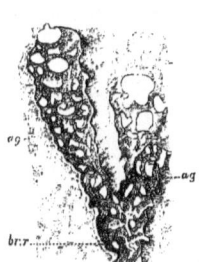

FIG. 7.—From Kölliker. 'A respiratory bronchiole, *br,r,* and two alveolar passages, *ag*, from the dog. × 85 diam.' Kölliker, *Verhand. Phys. Med. Gesellsch. zu Würzburg*, N.F. vol. xvi.

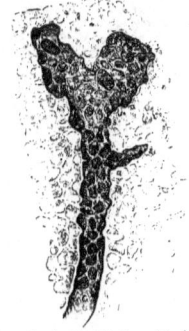

FIG. 8.—From Rossignol. 'Section of the lung of a dog. The terminal passages are opened to the infundibula. In the section of the bronchus are seen parietal alveoli and the orifices of numerous infundibula.'

These infundibula open on all sides into a series of imperfect cavities, divided by septa and forming a honeycombed structure, the 'alveoli' of Rossignol, the 'air-cells and air-vesicles' of other writers. Each infundibulum ends in a group of three or more of these, and similar sacs open laterally on all sides of the alveolar ducts and infundibula from their commencement to their termination. Hence, when a section is made across the lung near the pleural surface, a series of cavities is seen which are the truncated ends of the infundibula, each terminating in a group of vesicles. The passages widen from the point at which they leave the terminal bronchus, and finally end in the blind alveolated extremity, already described, at the pleural surface, and their shape is, as Rossignol stated, that of an inverted funnel ('infundibulum') or cone with its base at the surface of the lung.

Schulze states the diameter of the alveolar passages in the adult to be from $\frac{1}{60}$ to $\frac{1}{120}$ of an inch. Todd and Bowman give them from $\frac{1}{100}$ to $\frac{1}{200}$; Kölliker from $\frac{1}{70}$ to $\frac{1}{115}$. Rossignol gives the following measurements of the infundibula: in a man ætat. 40, orifices from $\frac{1}{50}$ inch to $\frac{1}{70}$ inch,

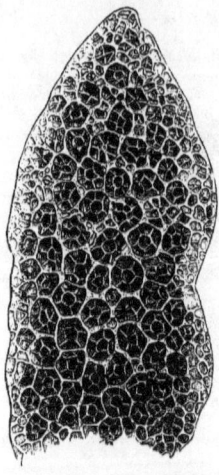

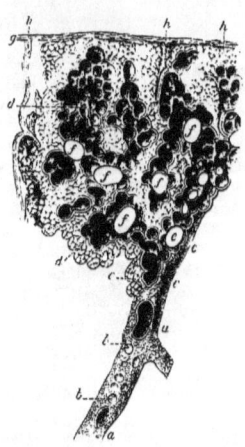

FIG. 9. From Rossignol. 'Thin section from pleural surface, considerably magnified. At the borders are seen only isolated alveoli. At the centre, where it is thicker, it is seen that all the alveoli are enclosed in infundibula, or rise from the floor of them like so many terminal cells. The spaces or septa which separate these infundibula are marked by more or less distinct depressions, which are the origin of as many alveoli. The latter rest on the external walls of the subpleural infundibula, and are also enclosed in infundibula, as may be seen in a section somewhat thicker than that here figured.'

FIG. 10.—From Küttner. 'Preparation from an adult dog, lung injected with nitrate of silver and gelatine. a, Terminal bronchus with solitary lateral alveoli, b; c, opened alveolar passages; d, opened infundibula, i.e. alveolar groupings ("*alveolen complex*"). The points and lines, and the sections of the "intercalary" cells ("*Schaltzellen*") and interstitial lines between the epithelium (*Kittleisten*)—these, for the sake of distinctness, are only figured on the convex surfaces of the alveoli; e, opening of an alveolar passage; f, openings of laterally branching infundibula; g, pleura; h, bands of connective tissue proceeding from the pleura and separating the single lobulettes.'—Stereoscopic view. × 90 diam. Küttner, Virchow's *Archiv*, vol. lxvi.

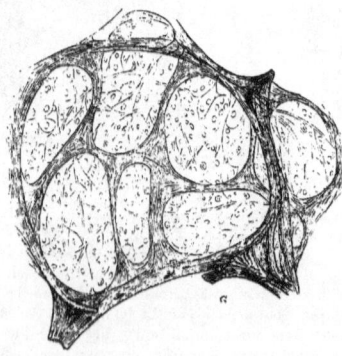

FIG. 11.—From Schulze. Section through a laterally-placed infundibulum. From a human adult lung, filled with alcohol acidulated with acetic acid, and hardened. Opening from the alveolar passage into the infundibulum; the upper border is partly removed by the section; a, non-striated muscular fibres with nuclei × 80 diam.'—Schulze. Stricker's *Handbuch*.

STRUCTURE OF THE LUNGS

base from $\frac{1}{50}$ inch to $\frac{1}{37}$ inch; in a child ætat. 3, orifice, $\frac{1}{500}$ inch to $\frac{1}{100}$ inch, base $\frac{1}{125}$ inch to $\frac{1}{50}$ inch; in a man ætat. 75, orifice $\frac{1}{75}$ inch to $\frac{1}{50}$ inch, base $\frac{1}{37}$ inch to $\frac{1}{18}$ inch.

For a calf he gives the following series: lobular branch (i.e. where it enters the lobule at its origin) $\frac{1}{70}$ inch, first branch $\frac{1}{87}$; second branch $\frac{1}{60}$, third branch $\frac{1}{50}$, fourth branch $\frac{1}{50}$. Tubes of reunion of infundibula $\frac{1}{60}$, orifices of infundibula $\frac{1}{75}$, base of infundibula $\frac{1}{50}$, pulmonary alveoli $\frac{1}{100}$ inch.

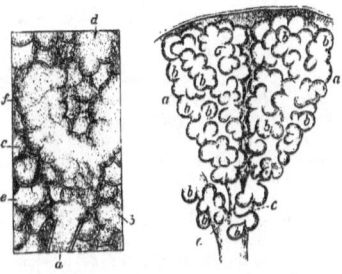

FIG. 12.—From Harting. 'A thin section of the dried lung of a man, at the distance of about a centimetre from the surface. The air-passages are filled with uncoloured transparent white wax. The capillaries can scarcely be distinguished with this low power.
'(a) Bronchus, in which two layers of elastic fibres can still be distinguished.
'(b) Parietal alveoli on the same branch, which have externally a nodular aspect.
'(c) The site of bifurcation of this branch, where it passes into two infundibula divided longitudinally. One of these, f, is seen entire, and in its middle are seen the septa of the parietal alveoli resting on the infundibulum.
'(d) An infundibulum, cut across, with many lateral alveoli.
'(e) Another infundibulum, cut transversely, with fewer alveoli. × 80 diam.'—Adriani, *Diss. de Subtiliore Pulm. Structura.*

FIG. 13.—From Kölliker. 'Half-diagrammatic figure of two smallest "lobulettes," aa, with the 'air-cells,' bb, and the smallest bronchial tubes, cc. From newly-born child. × 25 diam.'—Kölliker, *Microscopische Anatomie,* ii. 309.

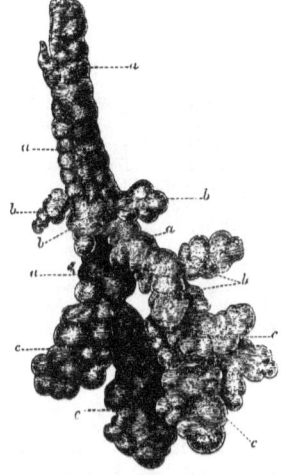

FIG. 14.—From Küttner. A preparation by 'corrosion' (see fig. 2) from an adult human being. a, Alveolar passages; b, smaller laterally-placed infundibula; c, terminal infundibula. Stereoscopic view. × 90 diam.—Küttner, Virchow's *Archiv,* vol. lxvi.

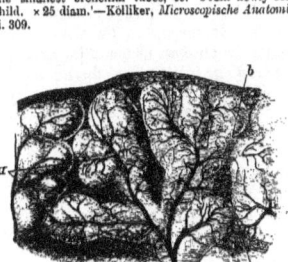

FIG. 15.—From Küttner. Lung injected from the pulmonary artery after closure of the capillaries by means of nitrate of silver injected into the bronchi. The bronchi filled with gelatine; pleural surface. The pulmonary artery divides into as many branches as there are infundibula. Stereoscopic figure × 42 diam.—Küttner, Virchow's *Archiv,* vol. lxxiii.

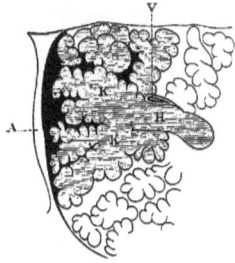

FIG. 16.—From Charcot. 'A pulmonary acinus injected with wax from a newly-born infant. H, Bronchiole; V, branch of pulmonary artery; KK, alveolar ducts; A, interlobular space.'—Charcot, *Progrès Médical* vol. v. 1877, p. 604.

Dr. Waters gives for adults—ultimate bronchial tube $\frac{1}{20}$, $\frac{1}{70}$, $\frac{1}{100}$ inch, its terminal dilatation $\frac{1}{15}$ to $\frac{1}{10}$, 'air-sacs' (infundibula) $\frac{1}{75}$, $\frac{1}{60}$, $\frac{1}{25}$ inch. For infants under one year, terminal bronchial tube $\frac{1}{80}$, $\frac{1}{100}$, $\frac{1}{120}$ inch, its terminal dilatation $\frac{1}{30}$ to $\frac{1}{15}$ inch, 'air-sacs' $\frac{1}{50}$, $\frac{1}{70}$, $\frac{1}{120}$, $\frac{1}{150}$ inch.

Infundibula, Acini, and Lobules.—It will be seen from the foregoing description that each terminal bronchus ends in a series of structures, the infundibula, which represent the final acini of a racemose gland, and are independent of those derived from the corresponding terminations of adjacent terminal bronchi. The ultimate ramifications of each terminal bronchus form therefore, as Rossignol remarked, small lobules within the larger lobules, but having no direct communication with those surrounding them except through the tubes which open into them. This is seen by the preceding figures.

Each 'infundibulum' is thus the representative of an ultimate 'acinus,' while the final distribution of the terminal bronchial tube consists of a group of these infundibula, which unite in part, by means of the alveolar passages, within the ultimate lobule which they compose, and which finally converge to the terminal bronchial tube.

Each infundibulum is separated from those surrounding it by a zone of inter-infundibular fibrous tissue; a similar arrangement surrounds each group of these, and in this capsule are contained vessels, nerves, and lymphatics.

It has been proposed by Rindfleisch, instead of regarding each infundibulum as an 'acinus,' to apply this term to the whole group of infundibula proceeding from the terminal bronchial tube, and to regard it as the 'unit' of pulmonary structure, and in this he has been followed by M. Charcot (*see* Figs. 2 and 16). Kölliker and Sharpey, however, regard the infundibulum of Rossignol as the ultimate pulmonary lobule. There appears to be a certain advantage in recognising the special form assumed by the final distribution of the terminal bronchus in a group of alveolar passages and infundibula by a term (acinus) which signifies the change in anatomical structure which occurs at this point. It has also the utility of distinguishing this group of ultimate 'lobules' from the larger 'lobule,' with which they may otherwise be confounded.

This larger lobule (fig. 2.) represents, as Rindfleisch has stated, the distribution of a single bronchial tube, the 'intralobular bronchus,' which, at the point of entrance into the 'lobule,' acquires certain anatomical peculiarities both in structure and size, being on an average $\frac{1}{15}$ of an inch in diameter, but varying from this to $\frac{1}{10}$ and $\frac{1}{20}$ of an inch (Sappey). The branches of this constitute the larger composite lobule. This bronchus is, however, only terminal in the sense that each such lobule contains only one chief bronchus, which by subdivision gives rise to the *true terminal* bronchi, viz. the bronchi which end in a dilatation from which pass the alveolar ducts proceeding to the infundibula.

Dr. Waters felt the need of distinguishing the group of structures thus found at the extremity of each terminal bronchus, and proposed for it the name of 'lobulette,' which is synonymous in this sense with the term of 'acinus' proposed by Rindfleisch. Etymologically the term 'acinus' is both indefinite and arbitrary,[1] but being already in use for the ultimate lobule of the liver (though in this organ it is rather defined by its relations to the portal and hepatic veins than to the duct) it has acquired a certain significance which enables it to be applied to the lung.

In this sense the 'acinus,' like the 'infundibula' of which it is composed, is pear-shaped or conical, with its base at the periphery, and tapering inwards to the terminal bronchus from which it springs.

The lobule, in the wider sense, consists of an indefinite number of 'acini.' It is bounded by a zone of interlobular fibrous tissue which separates it from adjacent lobules.

The intralobular bronchus, and its ramifications within the lobule (which may be from three to four or more in number before the terminal bronchi are reached), are enclosed in a sheath of fibrous

---

[1] It must be remarked that the vagueness of this term induced the late Dr. Sharpey—whose extreme accuracy has impressed so many who regret his loss—to propose that it should be altogether abandoned. It was apparently first used by Malpighi to signify the ultimate lobule of the liver (*De Gland. Structura*, iii. 18). It appears even originally to have been used indefinitely for a bunch of grapes, a single grape, and also the stone of a grape; and, like many figurative terms, is incapable now of exact definition. It is only in its parallel with the lobule of the liver that it is capable of being applied to the lung. In the liver there is not the same confusion of terms between ultimate lobules and groups of lobules as in the lung. Dr. Waters' term of 'lobulette' expresses the difference, but as in the liver the meaning of the term acinus is fully understood, it appears in this sense capable of extension to the lung.

STRUCTURE OF THE LUNGS

tissue; closely adjacent to them, and enclosed in the same sheath, are the terminal branches of the pulmonary artery as well as branches of the bronchial artery and lymphatics. The veins follow a separate course, and for the most part, together with the lymphatics, are found in the perilobular (or interlobular) fibrous tissue.

The divisions between the larger lobules are usually distinctly marked on the surface of the lung, forming spaces of $\frac{1}{4}$ to $\frac{1}{2}$ an inch, or even of 1 inch, across. Those of the 'acini' (the true lobules) are less apparent; their base is from $\frac{1}{14}$ to $\frac{1}{12}$ and $\frac{1}{7}$ inch (Kölliker).

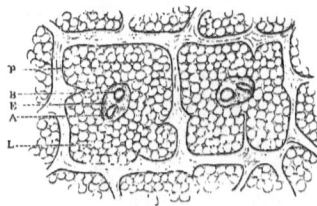

FIG. 17.—From Joffroy. Diagrammatic section (transverse) of two lobules at the level of their root. Each lobule bounded by the perilobular connective tissue, contains in its centre the bronchus and the pulmonary artery surrounded by intralobular connective tissue. A, Pulmonary artery; B, bronchus; E, intralobular connective tissue (peribronchial and perivascular tissue which contains lymphatics); P, perilobular connective tissue; L, pulmonary alveoli.—Joffroy, *Différentes Formes de la Broncho-Pneumonie*, Paris 1880, p. 10.

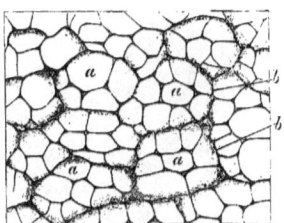

FIG. 18.—From Harting. 'External surface of lung of cow, filled with wax. *aaa*, alveoli; *bb*, borders of the smallest "lobulettes" or infundibula.' ×30 diam.—Harting, from Adriani, *loc. cit.*, ii. 311.

Structure of the bronchial tubes.—Each tube is surrounded by a sheath of loose fibrous tissue in which, as already stated, are lymphatic vessels, and which also contains small masses of lymphatic tissue.

The true bronchial tubes, until attaining a size of $\frac{1}{15}$ of an inch, are composed of four layers (*see* Fig. 19).

(*a*) A fibrous layer of tough fibroid tissue, arranged in long bundles, between which are also some circular bundles, and a few elastic fibres. Embedded among these fibres are cartilages, which at first form half-rings, arranged around the whole circumference of the larger tubes, but gradually becoming smaller and more scattered as the tubes diminish in size, until in the smaller ones they are only isolated plates, and they disappear in those of $\frac{1}{15}$ to $\frac{1}{18}$ of an inch in diameter. The cells in these cartilages have a peculiar arrangement: those under the surface are flat and lie parallel to the surface, but those in the deeper layers are arranged in rows at right angles to the surface. The mucous glands of the larger bronchi penetrate from the interior to this outer fibrous layer, but they disappear simultaneously with the cartilages.

(*b*) The muscular coat lies within the fibrous layer, and is composed of circular bundles of striated muscles, crossing one another so as to form an almost continuous coat; it varies from $\frac{1}{50}$ to $\frac{1}{300}$ of an inch in thickness (the latter in tubes of $\frac{1}{15}$ of an inch in diameter.—Schulze).

(*c*) Within this lies a layer of elastic fibres, disposed in bundles running longitudinally and prominent on the inner surface; they are held together by a fine fibroid tissue which also is disposed longitudinally.

A fine basement-membrane bounds this layer. It consists of a single layer of large flattened endothelial cells (Debose, quoted by Klein; the existence of these cells is, however, denied by Kölliker).

(*d*) The epithelial layer (fig. 20) consists of cylindrical ciliated epithelium, between which are chalice or goblet cells.' It has been asserted by Schulze and numerous other observers that the epithelium consists only of a single layer of these cells, but Kölliker's observations on the human lung in a recent state have convinced him that there are in reality three layers :—(*a*) Immediately on the mucosa a series of basal cells of irregularly cylindrical shape. (*b*) Immediately above this is a layer of supplementary cells of variable form, from spindle-shaped to cylindrical, and above these are the ciliated cells with goblet cells between.[1]

Beneath the epithelial layer mucous glands (Fig. 19, *d' d'*) pass into the wall of the tube extending to the cartilages of the outer fibrous layer. They are racemose—their orifice is lined with a cylindrical epithelium; their branches are lined with mucous cells or granular epithelial cells.

In bronchi that have diminished to $\frac{1}{25}$ of an inch in diameter, at which size the tubes usually enter the lobules, the structure varies from that before described. They contain neither cartilages nor mucous glands. These outer fibroid layers have become of extreme tenuity, and finally almost disappear. The muscular layer also becomes limited to single circular bands, crossed by longitudinal

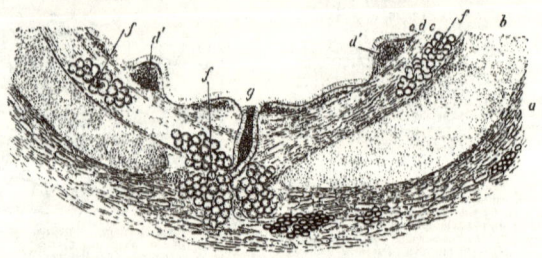

FIG. 19.—From Schulze. Part of a transverse section of a bronchial tube (human) $\frac{1}{3}$ of an inch in diameter. *a*, Capsule with wide spaces and accumulation of fat. *f*; *b*, cartilage; *c*, muscular layer; *d*, inner fibroid layer with elastic fibres in bundles; *e*, epithelial layer; *d' d'*, mucous glands, the duct of one of them is seen at *g*.—Schulze, Stricker's *Handbuch*. × 30 diam.

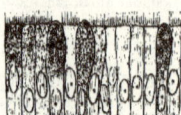

FIG. 20.—From Schulze. Epithelium of a bronchial tube of a dog, $\frac{1}{8}$ of an inch in diameter, showing the cylindrical ciliated cells and chalice cells. × 320 diam.—Schulze, Stricker's *Handbuch*.

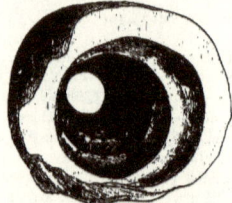

FIG. 21.—Spiral arrangement of the air-cells, from Dr. Edward Smith, *Consumption*, 1862, p. 168.

elastic bundles continued from those above. The goblet cells disappear and the epithelial cells also become shorter, and losing their cilia become flat cubical cells of $\frac{1}{2500}$ to $\frac{1}{3500}$ of an inch (Küttner), passing into small, flat pavement-cells. At this point they are termed 'respiratory bronchioles' (Kölliker, see Fig. 7), on account of alveoli proceeding from them, and also because even while one side of the tube may still possess cubical cells, on the other side may be found a respiratory epithelium, viz. flat plates of the same nature as those lining the alveoli mingled with small pavement-cells measuring $\frac{1}{2500}$ to $\frac{1}{7500}$ inch in diameter, which form groups of twenty to fifty in number. These are continued into the alveolar passages, gradually diminishing in number, and giving place to the larger plates or scales which characterise the alveolar lining. These measure $\frac{1}{1250}$ to $\frac{1}{830}$ of an inch, according to Kölliker, who terms them the 'respiratory epithelium.' He believes that these terminations of the bronchioles take part in the true respiratory function, the more so as they are in part supplied by capillaries of the pulmonary artery.

[1] Kölliker, *Verhand. Phys. med. Gesellschaft zu Würzburg*, N.F. xxvi. 1881.

STRUCTURE OF THE LUNGS

At the end of the terminal bronchus, and even before the alveolar passages commence, a few alveoli open into the cavity of the tubes (see Figs. 4, 7 and 8).

The Alveolar Passages and Alveoli.—The alveolar passages and infundibula are chiefly composed of unstriped muscular fibres arranged circularly, and supported by a delicate fibroid tissue mingled with elastic fibres which the late Dr. Edward Smith stated to be arranged in a spiral form. In the delicate fibrous tissue are seen branched cells of the lymph-canalicular system (Klein).

The walls of the alveolar passages are, however, interrupted in all directions by the openings of the alveoli, so that they scarcely form a continuous membrane, but mainly consist of the boundaries of these openings and in part of these septa (Schulze). The alveoli are both lateral and terminal, and from fifteen to twenty are found in the course of each passage (Rossignol). A few, with well-defined openings, are found in the walls of the terminal bronchial tubes. Those in connection with the infundibula are more irregularly placed, and form rather projections from the interior; the infundibulum thus differs from a gland-duct giving off terminal acini, and resembles, as Kölliker remarked, a pear-shaped sac with sacculated walls. The junction of the alveoli with the passage is, however, commonly marked by a circle of muscular fibres and by a thickening of the elastic fibres. *See* Fig. 11 (Schulze).

The walls of the air-vesicles consist of a delicate membrane, crossed by a network of elastic fibres. Muscular fibres from the alveolar passages and infundibula pass also for a short distance into them (Klein).[1] In this membrane are ovoid nuclei (Schulze), and also stellate anastomosing cells of the lymph-canalicular system (Klein). The septa between the alveoli proceeding from any single infundibulum are imperfect, and many alveoli communicate before opening into the alveolar passage (Kölliker). Some, arising from adjacent passages, also appear to communicate, but those belonging to different 'acini' seem for the most part to be devoid of all communication with one another, being separated by fine bundles of interlobular (or interacinose) fibrous tissue. The septa between the terminal alveoli are less marked and less deep than between those that come off laterally in the course of the alveolar ducts and infundibula.

The alveoli vary considerably in size. Their mean diameter in middle life is about $\frac{1}{130}$ of an inch, but in the non-distended, adult state they vary between $\frac{1}{76}$, $\frac{1}{170}$, and $\frac{1}{300}$ inch (Kölliker); in the newly born child from $\frac{1}{540}$ to $\frac{1}{270}$, and when not distended by inflation, they are very commonly found even smaller in children of from two to five years: I have measured them only $\frac{1}{430}$ of an inch, even when filled with inflammatory products; in old age, they are from $\frac{1}{70}$ to $\frac{1}{47}$ in width, by $\frac{1}{50}$ to $\frac{1}{130}$ in depth (Schulze).[2] Their shape tends to the round form, but by mutual pressure they are often polygonal. Variations in this form are also produced by the relative degrees of their expansion.

The Epithelium of the Alveolar Passages and of the Alveoli presents some remarkable differences and peculiarities. The cells in the passages are described by Küttner as the same small cubical flat epithelium that lines the terminal bronchioles, and are, as already stated, of $\frac{1}{3500}$ to $\frac{1}{7000}$ of an inch in size, but according to Kölliker they are interspersed among the large flat cells already described. Immediately within the alveoli they at once increase in size, and form large cells of squamous epithelium, $\frac{1}{500}$ of an inch (Küttner)—'placoids' (Klein). A few cells of the type of those lining the alveolar passages are scattered between the large ones, but these also become enlarged and flattened during full inspiration (Klein). The cells are united by an interstitial substance in which the smaller cells are imbedded ('intercalary cells'—Küttner).[3] Into this interstitial substance

---

[1] For other references on the muscular fibres of the lung, see Eberth, Virchow's *Archiv*, lxxii.

[2] The following measurements of the alveoli are given by different authors in fractions of an inch. Todd and Bowman, in man, $\frac{1}{100}$ to $\frac{1}{70}$ inch; in the calf $\frac{1}{200}$. Dr. Addison, in man, $\frac{1}{250}$ to $\frac{1}{70}$. Rossignol, fœtus, from 5 to 6 months, $\frac{1}{1200}$ to $\frac{1}{500}$; mean $\frac{1}{600}$; infant at end of intrauterine life, either before or after respiration, $\frac{1}{500}$ to $\frac{1}{100}$; mean $\frac{1}{300}$; children from 1 year to 18 months, $\frac{1}{317}$ to $\frac{1}{110}$; mean $\frac{1}{200}$; children of 3 or 4 years old, $\frac{1}{210}$ to $\frac{1}{100}$; mean $\frac{1}{160}$; children ætat. 5 to 15, $\frac{1}{250}$ to $\frac{1}{126}$; means, $\frac{1}{100}$ to $\frac{1}{100}$; adults ætat. 18 to 30, $\frac{1}{110}$ to $\frac{1}{100}$; means, $\frac{1}{106}$ to $\frac{1}{100}$; adults ætat. 35 to 60, $\frac{1}{120}$ to $\frac{1}{90}$; means, $\frac{1}{100}$ to $\frac{1}{80}$; old people from ætat. 70 to 80, $\frac{1}{80}$ to $\frac{1}{60}$; mean, $\frac{1}{70}$. Dr. Waters gives the measurements for an infant under 1 year—$\frac{1}{410}$, $\frac{1}{151}$, $\frac{1}{500}$, $\frac{1}{500}$ and $\frac{1}{256}$ of an inch; in adults, $\frac{1}{70}$, $\frac{1}{100}$, $\frac{1}{78}$, $\frac{1}{150}$, and $\frac{1}{80}$;

in a woman ætat. 67 without emphysema, $\frac{1}{80}$ to $\frac{1}{200}$. The measurements must evidently vary much with the degree of distension, and Kölliker gives it as his opinion that in medium distension they are one-third more, and in full distension twice as wide as the condition in which they are found after death.

[3] Kölliker (*Verhandl. Phys. Med. Gesellschaft zu Würzburg.* N.F. 1881, vol. xvi.) denies the accuracy of Küttner's interpretation of these small cells placed between the larger plates as being *sui generis* or intercalary cells (Schaltzellen), and regards them as being identical with the smaller pavement-cells of the respiratory bronchioles. He also states that they are only found in great numbers at the borders of the alveoli, proceeding from the respiratory bronchioles, and not on those opening from the alveolar passages and infundibula.

penetrate prolongations of the stellate cells found in the wall beneath the epithelium (Klein; Küttner). There are also found in this interstitial substance, both in the alveoli, infundibula, and alveolar passages, pseudostomata corresponding in character with those found in the serous membranes (Klein).

The smaller cells are more granular than the large ones, and are more commonly found in the interstices between the capillaries, while the flat cells are extended over and closely applied to them (Schulze). It has been held that the larger cells are endothelial, and are the derivatives of the endothelial lining (membrana propria) of the bronchi, but Küttner's researches have shown that

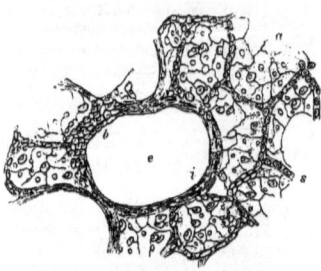

Fig. 22.—From Klein, reduced. From a section through the lung of a cat, stained first with nitrate of silver and then with hæmatoxylin. *a*, alveoli lined with flat, transparent, nucleated cells. Amongst them are small polyhedral nucleated cells more deeply stained; they are especially well shown where the alveolar wall is seen in profile. Between the large flat cells are smaller or larger clear spaces corresponding to pseudostomata. *s*, alveolar septum; *b*, a group of small polyhedral cells continued from the bronchus; *c*, alveolar duct in section; *i*, the circular muscular coat.—Klein, *Atlas of Histology*, pl. xxxvi.

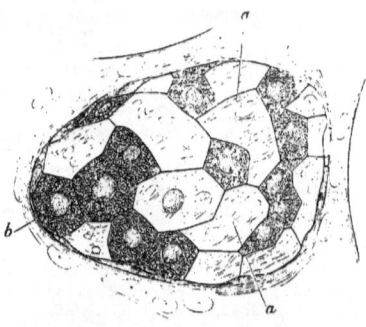

Fig. 23.—From Schulze. Floor of an alveolus; from a section close to the surface, curved parallel to the pleura; from the lung of a child born at eighth month and living two days; treated with nitrate of silver. *a*, large epithelial cells; *b*, granular cells. × 500 diam. Schulze, Stricker's *Handbuch*.

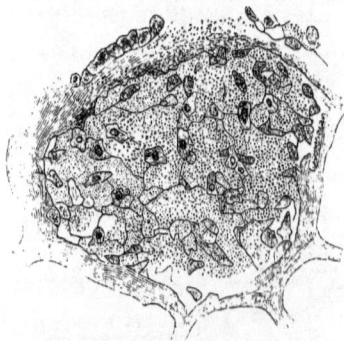

Fig. 24.—From Kölliker. Respiratory epithelium of an alveolus. Large cells, showing indications of division in lines which sometimes proceed from the smaller cells, sometimes from the borders of the large ones, and which indicate that the large cells may be formed from the fusion of the smaller. × 300 diam.—Kölliker, *Verhandl. med. Gesellsch. Würzburg*, N.F. xvi. (This description is taken in part from that of another figure, less adapted for a woodcut.)

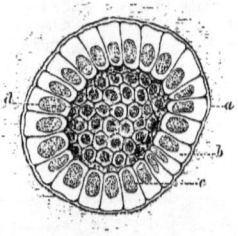

Fig. 25.—From Küttner. Transverse section from the unexpanded termination of a bronchial process or infundibulum (End-Kolben) in an embryo calf. Stained with nitrate of silver and distended with gelatine. *a*, membrana limitans; *b*, cylindrical epithelium; *c*, nuclei; *d*, floor of the cavity with cylindrical epithelium, seen from the surface. × 840 diam.—Küttner, Virchow's *Archiv*, vol.lxvi.

they are derived from the hypoblast, while the membrana propria, belonging as it does to the fibrous structures of these tubes, is derived from the mesoblast of the embryo. Moreover, as Küttner has shown, during the embryonic period and up to the time when the lungs expand, the alveoli are lined by cells identical in character with those of the smallest bronchioles and alveolar passages, and it is the expansion of the vesicles which causes these cells to assume the flattened form which they are found to present during life. In disease also interfering with the expansion of the lungs, as cirrhosis, the alveoli become again lined with a cubical epithelium; while in emphysema, where there is over-distension, the cubical epithelium covering the septa becomes converted into a squamous epithelium (Küttner).

Capillaries of the Infundibula and Alveoli.—The capillaries on the outer side of the infundibula have the surface towards the interior free in the cavity and only covered by the epithelium. Those in the septa between the alveoli project on each side into the cavities and are connected by numerous anastomoses, so as to form a continuous network with very narrow meshes, leaving spaces, which are sometimes only $\frac{1}{2500}$ of an inch, between the vessels where these anastomose between the walls of adjacent alveoli (Stricker), while the capillaries themselves have a diameter of from $\frac{1}{4000}$ to $\frac{1}{3000}$ of an inch (Schulze), or $\frac{1}{2500}$ to $\frac{1}{5000}$ (Quain and Sharpey). The capillaries often

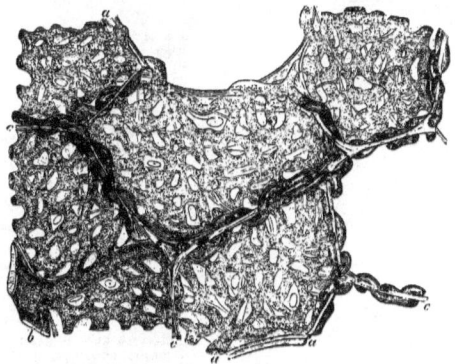

FIG. 26.—From Schulze. Distribution of capillaries in human lung injected from pulmonary artery. *aa*, free borders of the alveoli; *b*, small arterial branch; *cc*, vertical section of alveolar walls.

project into the interior of the alveoli in loops, which are seen most distinctly on the free borders. The capillaries are crossed by the branched cells of the wall of the alveolus, which communicate with the lymph-canalicular system (Klein).

Each terminal twig of the pulmonary artery is distributed over several alveoli, and forms numerous anastomoses with the capillaries of the bronchial artery. The arteries are distributed for the most part in the convex surface of the infundibula, while the veins lie in the depressions between them (*see* Küttner's figure). The larger non-nucleated plates of the epithelium lie in the capillaries, the smaller nucleated cells in their interstices (Kölliker), showing that the former are the true respiratory epithelium.

The Lymphatics of the lungs have been especially described by Klein. Those of the alveolar wall commence with a lymph-canalicular system, containing branched cells and imbedded in a homogeneous ground-substance between and outside the capillaries. The processes of these branched cells penetrate and merge into the interstitial substance between the epithelium (*see* Figs. 27, 28, 32) (Klein), and the lacunae lie in the alveolar walls (Figs. 29, 30).

In the alveoli, lying beneath the pleura, they form a dense plexus, which unites with rootlets from the pleura. Efferent trunks from these pass in some parts to the bronchial glands through the

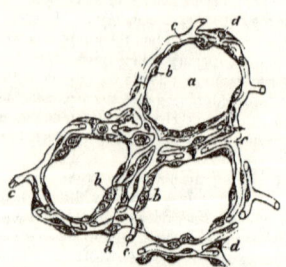

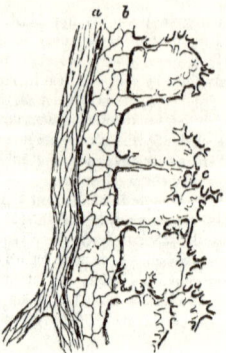

Fig. 27.—From Klein. Transverse section through the lung of a guinea-pig. *a*, alveolar cavity; *b*, lining epithelium; *c*, capillary blood-vessels not represented as numerous as in actual preparation; *d*, interalveolar connective-tissue corpuscles sending processes between the epithelial cells of the alveoli (pseudostomatous tissue). × 220 diam.—Klein, *Anatomy of Lymphatic System*, part ii. pl. iii.

Fig. 29.—From Klein. Section through guinea-pig's lung injected with nitrate of silver. *a*, branch of pulmonary artery; *b*, lymphatic vessels in connection with (*c*) interalveolar lymph-spaces or the lymph-canalicular system.—Klein, *Anatomy of Lymphatic System*, part ii. pl. iii. × 150 diam.

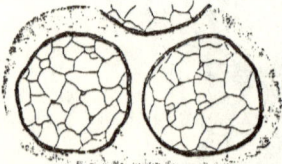

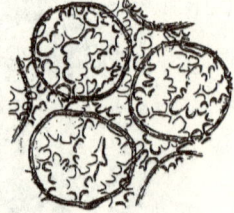

Fig. 28.—From Klein. From the same lung as Figs. 30 and 31, showing the lining epithelium of the alveoli between three small holes—pseudostomatous canals. See Fig. 29.

Fig. 30.—From Klein. From the same lung as Fig. 22, showing the interalveolar lymph-spaces in the surface view. × 150 diam.

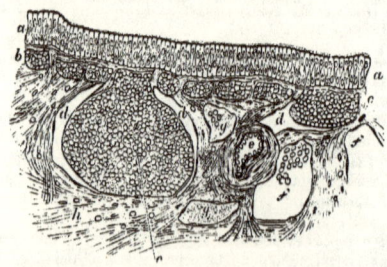

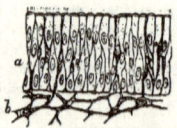

Fig. 31.—From Klein. Longitudinal section through small bronchus of a guinea-pig's lung. *a*, ciliated epithelium; *b*, circular coat of unstriped muscles transversely cut; *c*, lymphatic follicles belonging to wall of lymphatic vessels, *d*; *e*, branch of pulmonary artery; *f*, lymphatic vessels; *g*, the same filled with granulated material (coagulated plasma). In some of the lymphatic vessels, clusters of lymph-corpuscles are to be found.—Klein, *Anatomy of Lymphatic System*, part ii. pl. i.

Fig. 32.—From Klein. Section of epithelium of bronchus of a rabbit. *a*, epithelium with intra-epithelial nucleated cells. Pseudostomatous cells in connection with, *b*, nucleated cells of sub-epithelial connective tissue. Klein, *Anatomy of Lymphatic System*, part ii. pl. iii. × 300 diam.

ligamenta pulmonum; others join the perivascular lymphatics. These perivascular lymphatics have their rootlets in the walls of the alveoli. Some invaginate both the arteries and veins; others 'form a dense plexus of intercommunicating sinuses around the larger branches' (Klein).

The peribronchial lymphatics lie in the outer sheath of the bronchi. They anastomose with the perivascular lymphatics, and communicate with a fine network in the mucosa, beneath which are found small masses of lymphatic tissue (Burdon-Sanderson and Kölliker), and occasionally a diffuse reticular lymphatic growth (Klein). The former are generally surrounded by a dilatation or a lymph-sinus of a peribronchial lymphatic (Klein). These structures are found in the smallest tubules.

Immediately beneath the mucosa of the bronchi are a series of branched, nucleated cells which are in continuity with the tuberculous connective tissue of the mucosa. These penetrate between the epithelial cells and reach the surface by an elongated process (Fig. 32). These inter-epithelial connective-tissue cells are considered by Klein to form a pseudostomatous tissue, and, though not directly communicating with the lymphatics, are yet capable of doing so; and the spaces in which they lie are the canals of communication between the free surface and the interfascicular lymph-spaces surrounding the connective-tissue cells of the mucosa. It is by means of these that solid particles injected into the bronchi reach the lymphatics and glands, and they may be regarded as the rootlets of the lymphatics in the bronchial wall.

PNEUMONIA.

The illustrations of pneumonia here given are the following: Acute Pneumonia (*a*) Red Hepatisation, Plate I.; (*b*) Grey or Suppurative Hepatisation, Plates II. and IV. fig. 4; Congestive Pneumonia (Hypostatic Pneumonia), Plate III.; Broncho-Pneumonia, Plate V.; Chronic Pneumonic Induration, Plates IV. and XLII.; Interlobular Pneumonia, Plate XXIV. fig. 2.

ACUTE PNEUMONIA.

ACUTE STHENIC PNEUMONIA; FIBRINOUS PNEUMONIA (VIRCHOW); *CROUPOUS PNEUMONIA* (ROKITANSKY).

Plates I. II. and IV. fig. 4.[1]

The first stage of the process of acute pneumonia can have been very rarely seen in the primary disease, because death seldom or never takes place until hepatisation has commenced. How rapidly hepatisation may occur is shown by two cases of Jürgensen, one dying within eight, and the other within thirty-four hours from the invasion, in both of which this stage was reached.[2] It is described by various authors and systematic writers as the stage of 'congestion' or 'engorgement,' but I am not acquainted with any case in medical literature in which it is clear that the condition described was really that of simple pneumonia in the first stage (with the exception of a case by Rindfleisch to be presently quoted). It appears to me probable that the descriptions given of this stage are those of parts adjacent to hepatised portions.

I have met with one case (not figured) where the lungs corresponded to the description given of this stage, but I am not certain that death was not due to intense congestive bronchitis, and there is, as far as I am aware, no positive proof attainable that in such a case the morbid process would have developed into the typical disease, acute sthenic pneumonia. The case was that of a boy, aged 12, from whom no history could be obtained, and, owing to the acuteness of the case, no notes were taken during life. He was admitted, with urgent dyspnœa, on the afternoon of October 12, 1868. There was extreme cyanosis, with sugillations on the face, hands, and feet, and the skin was cold. The chest was barrel-shaped, and the heart covered by the lungs. The pulse was weak, and the respiration rapid. The chest was everywhere resonant. Respiration was loud and harsh, especially at bases; expiration was prolonged, and no râles were audible. He was relieved by the application of mustard poultices and by an ether draught, and passed a comparatively quiet night.

---

[1] The Roman numerals in the text refer, in all cases, to the plates.
[2] Jürgensen, *Croupöse Pneumonie*, Tübingen, 1883, p. 216 *et seq.* The appearances in the first case are not fully described. Those in the second are of complete hepatisation, in one part proceeding to suppuration.

On the following morning he had a rigor, passed immediately into a state of collapse, and died within two hours. *Post mortem*, all organs were healthy except the lungs, but the head was gorged with blood. Both lungs were over-distended in their upper portions. Both bases were loaded with blood of a dark colour and with much serosity. There were, in addition, patches of brighter tint, extending through areas of from one to two inches in diameter. Some spots of induration (collapse) were also present.

Stokes has given the most minute account of the 'first' stage, as occurring in the upper parts of lungs in which consolidation existed at the base, in a child dying of an extensive burn, and also in acute phthisis. He describes the pulmonary tissue as being 'drier than usual, not at all engorged, as in Laennec's first stage, and of a bright vermilion colour from intense arterial congestion.' This appearance, however, is more likely to be due to pulmonary over-distension with collateral hyperæmia, and it is doubtful whether the part so changed would have passed into the state of hepatisation.

The stage of 'engorgement,' Laennec's first stage, may be very commonly met with at the margins of hepatised portions, where it is probable that this process is proceeding.[1] Here the lung presents the appearance of intense congestion, almost, if not entirely, identical in character with that seen in the more solidified parts of Pl. III. The lung is of a dull red, and sometimes a purplish colour; it pits to the finger, and tears more readily than natural, but less easily than the consolidated part. It still contains some air, but in a variable degree and less than natural. It is more or less œdematous—the amount of serum varying in inverse ratio to the degree to which hepatisation has advanced—and in it spots and tracts of consolidation can be seen. The fluid expressed is more or less viscous, but this also varies with the degree of hepatisation. This fluid is intensely bloody, but contains, in addition, both large and small cells, of the nature and appearance of those hereafter to be described as found in the air-vesicles. This stage is called by some writers, and notably by Rokitanski, 'splenisation.' Rokitanski states that the pulmonary tissue so affected is diminished in volume, but it has appeared to me that when this is the case, some collapse has simultaneously occurred—a condition common in the neighbourhood of hepatised parts at all ages, and which, in childhood, sometimes constitutes a large proportion of the consolidated area.

Second stage—*Hepatisation* (Pl. I. *from a patient who died on the fifth day*).—In this stage the lung has become absolutely solid from a fibrinous solidified exudation, mingled with extravasated blood in variable proportions. It contains no air, and sinks at once in water. The colour is of a dull brownish-red (not very accurately likened to mahogany), and becomes brighter on exposure. This is often mingled with a fine sprinkling of a greyish-white colour, which, together with the pigment present, often gives it a marbled aspect. The exudation fills and over-distends the vesicles, alveolar passages, bronchioles, and even the smaller bronchi, and thus the lung is enlarged to the full degree of inspiratory expansion and may even retain the impress of the ribs. In some cases the solid exudation may extend to the larger bronchi, and simulate the condition known as 'fibrinous bronchitis.' [2]—*See* Pl. V*a*, fig. 2 (Carswell).

The cut surface of the lung has lost entirely its normal transparency and glistening appearance. It is dull and opaque, and presents, in addition, a granular appearance, which is due to the filling of the air-vesicles with the exudation. Casts of these, together

---

[1] Rindfleisch (*Lehrbuch der path. Gewebelehre*, 5te Auflage, 1878, p. 378) describes a whole lobe as presenting this condition. He does not, however, mention the day of the disease at which death occurred.

[2] Grancher has termed this condition 'Pneumonie Massive,' but it does not appear to me to be necessary to find it a distinctive name. (*Gaz. Méd. de Paris*, 1878, No. 8.)

ACUTE PNEUMONIA

with mouldings of the alveolar passages and bronchioles, may be removed by scraping (Fig. 33). Some serum still exudes on pressure, but it is more opaque and less in quantity than in the prior stage; it is, however, deeply blood-stained. The lung is softened and breaks down readily under the finger, and the fractured surface is more distinctly granular than is that of the section. The vesicular structure of the lung is no longer apparent, but the interlobular tissue and the vessels can still be traced. The latter are frequently obstructed by fibrinous coagula.

The granular character is, I believe, present to a greater or less degree in all cases of true red hepatisation, but in the earlier stages, and at the margins of parts where hepatisation is advancing, it may be less distinct, and the surface may be smooth and glistening. It is less marked in children, owing to the smaller size of the air-vesicles, and the statement is sometimes made that the granular aspect is absent in them. Its apparent absence is, I believe, due to the extent to which collapse is mingled with the pneumonic portions; in these it may usually be perceived, but on a smaller scale, if the section is scraped, and Legendre[1] regarded the granular appearance as sufficient to decide between pneumonia and collapse. In emphysematous lungs this character is often exaggerated. Hasse describes such a lung in which the size of the granules was so greatly increased as to attain that of hemp-seeds. They were of a dull yellow colour and of the consistency of soft butter, and very imperfectly filled small smooth cavities of irregular shape. They were seated in the midst of grey hepatisation, and all transitions could be observed between the granules occupying the dilated and those in the undilated vesicles.[2] In some forms of acute pneumonia, where the exudation is less solid (to which allusion will be made), the granular character is less perfect and the surface may be smooth.

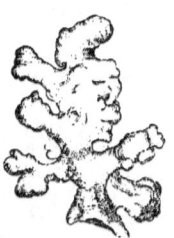

FIG. 33.—Moulded cast of bronchioles, infundibula, and alveoli. From Rokitanski, Path. Anat. vol. iii.

The bronchial mucous membrane is hyperæmic. The contents of the tubes are commonly a viscid, blood-stained mucus. They may, however, be filled with fibrinous exudation. The pleura over the hepatised lung, when the change has reached the surface, is almost always inflamed, although in varying degree. The membrane is always hyperæmic and often ecchymosed, and has lost its transparency. Exudation first appears as a roughening of the surface, and this proceeds to the formation of thick layers, which may become puriform, and may be attended with a variable amount of fluid effusion, either sero-fibrinous or purulent. The costal pleura tends to be secondarily affected.

Third stage—*Grey Hepatisation.*[3] Plate IV. fig. 4.—The stage of 'red hepatisation' just described passes very insensibly into that of 'grey hepatisation.' The bright red colour gradually disappears, often in patches, and the tissue assumes a greyer appearance, sometimes still mingled with red, until in rare instances a uniform dirty-grey is assumed, as in the preparation from which IV. 4 is taken. The granular appearance of the lung is still generally maintained (as in the figure), but this is not always the case, and when much œdema is present—as occurs sometimes in old people, or in others with enfeebled constitutions, or when there is albuminuria—the section may be smooth, and even somewhat glistening, though still devoid of transparency. The softness of the lung has much increased, and it breaks down very readily into a pulp, and yields a thick opaque dirty-grey fluid. In some cases of albuminuria the colour is even paler, and is of a whitish tint, the surface being still granular.[4]

---

[1] Legendre, *Rech. sur quelq. Malad. des Enfance.* 1846, p. 163.
[2] Hasse, *Dis. of the Organs of Circ. and Resp.* Syd. Soc. Trans. 1846, p. 209.
[3] It ought to be noted that Laennec (*Ausc. Médiate,* 2nd ed. p. 101) objected to the term 'grey hepatisation'

as signifying many conditions and as being undistinguishable from suppuration. It appears to me, however, to represent a less advanced stage than that in which suppuration exists.
[4] Lancereaux, *Atlas Anat. Path.* pl. xxviii. fig. 2, and pp. 292 3.

D

Fourth stage—*Suppuration.* Plate II. represents a further stage of the changes which occur in grey hepatisation. This condition is one in which it is not common to find the whole of the affected portion of the lung. The illustration given is from an unpublished drawing by Sir R. Carswell. The colour is of a dirty-greyish yellow, the grey and yellow being intermingled in spots and patches. (Carswell's drawing is of a deeper yellow than I have seen uniformly diffused.) Spots of pus frequently exude from the bronchi, and a dirty-grey fluid escapes abundantly on scraping and on section. The granular character is less marked. The most striking characteristic, in addition to the change of colour, is the extreme softening of the lung, which breaks down at once into a pulp, and this may easily lead to the misapprehension that a complete disorganisation has occurred, amounting to abscess. The formation of abscess is probably a limited condition of complete liquefactive destruction of the alveolar walls during the stage of suppuration. Its characteristic is the limited area in which it occurs.

The variations in the appearance of acute pneumonia depend, as already stated, on the proportion of fibrin in the exudation, and in some cases on the rapid breaking down of the lung. Among these the most prominent are the following.

The *Pneumonia Serosa* of Wunderlich,[1] or *Pneumonie Œdémateuse* of Cruveilhier,[2] has been likened by Traube[3] to a pleural effusion in which the fibrinous element is wanting. It commonly occurs in the presence of general œdema. It may be found in the state of both red and grey hepatisation, and is distinguished by the large amount of serum pervading the pulmonary tissue. The surface is sometimes granular, but in many cases it is smooth and glistening. This state is met with both as an acute primary affection (when it is most common in aged persons) and also in forms of secondary pneumonia. The differences between it and simple œdema have been described by Cruveilhier as the same as those existing between an œdematous and an erysipelatous limb. In the œdematous pneumonia the serosity is yellow, and is a mixture of blood and pus ; the tissue tears with greater facility than in simple œdema. In simple œdema the admixture of pus with the serosity is absent.

The *Ichorous Pneumonia* of Wunderlich constitutes a variety of grey hepatisation, in which the exudation is unusually fluid and the lung breaks down with great facility. It is akin to gangrene, but is not truly gangrenous.

The MICROSCOPIC APPEARANCES in acute pneumonia consist essentially in the filling of the alveoli of the lung with a coagulable exudation in which cells of various forms are imbedded.

The *Exudation* constitutes one of the most marked features of this process, but the proportion which it bears to other products of inflammation varies considerably, more so than might be inferred from the descriptions that are sometimes given.

Cases of pneumonia occasionally occur, presenting the typical features of the acute disease, in which the alveoli are entirely filled with large cells of the epithelial type, and little or no fibrinous exudation is found. Heitler[4] has described a case of this nature. Buhl also[5] has described another, which, however, though lobar in character, and with the clinical aspects already referred to, he still classes with 'desquamative pneumonia' (*see* Phthisis). A coagulable exudation also is sometimes found in catarrhal pneumonia, and in some cases of phthisical pneumonia.[6]

The essential characteristic of this exudation consists in its spontaneous coagulation

---

[1] *Spec. Path. u. Therapie*, vol. iii. abth. ii. n, p. 313 *et seq.*
[2] *Atlas Anat. Path. Corps Humain*, liv. 40, plate 4, p. 6.
[3] *Gesammelte Beiträge*, 948, iii. 811.
[4] Stricker's *Wiener Med. Jahrbücher*, 1874.

[5] *Mittheilungen aus der Path. Institut zu München*, 1878, p. 175.
[6] Sommerbrodt (Virchow's *Archiv*, vol. lv.) produced lobular spots of fibrinous pneumonia by the insertion of perchloride of iron into the lung. Cornil and Ranvier have

into a network of fibres, showing its fibrinous character, a condition which, with the exceptions just alluded to, is rarely found in any other of the inflammations and diseases of the lung (see XXV. 1, 2). It is this peculiarity which caused Rokitansky to term the disease 'croupous'; but this name implies an affinity with the diphtheritic processes, with which, anatomically and clinically, pneumonia has nothing in common.

In diphtheritic exudations in mucous membranes, the epithelium and often the submucous connective tissue are essentially concerned, undergoing changes which cause them to form part of the false membrane, if not of the exudation.[1] Buyer,[2] indeed, has attempted to show that in acute pneumonia the epithelium of the alveoli undergoes similar changes, but his observations have not been confirmed. The large amount of the exudation, and the rapidity of its production, as well as the freedom of the walls of the alveoli from any destructive changes, would further militate against any analogy between the process in pneumonia and that in croup or diphtheria.

It is probable that this exudation is derived from the blood, but whether directly, or indirectly, is still open to question. The causes, also, that determine its production in such a preponderant degree as is occasionally observed in this form of inflammation, have not been fully elucidated. Virchow[3] believed that the connective tissue, from the close relation which it bears to the lymphatic structures, is the source of fibrinous exudations, through a change in the nutritive process. He has further pointed out that the exudation-processes of inflammation have a close affinity to secretions; that fibrinous exudations are at times more or less interchangeable with those in which a material resembling mucin is formed; and further, that all stages of transition, in respect to the qualities of the exudation, may be observed between 'catarrhal' and 'croupous' inflammations.[4] He has lately asserted that the true fibrinous character only appears in the later stages (yellow hepatisation) after the breaking down of the blood-corpuscles.[5] Rindfleisch's figures,[6] however, show that a true fibrinous coagulation occurs in the earliest stage. Buhl considers that when such an exudation occurs on mucous surfaces it is the result of transformation of, or by, epithelial structures. Cohnheim attributes the coagulation to the exit of the corpuscles which afford the fibrogenic element to the blood-plasma,[7] and the degree to which this occurs varies with the nature and with the intensity of the inflammation. But the discussion of this point of general pathology lies beyond the limits of this article.

The next most remarkable point is the freedom of the alveolar walls from any grave participation in the process. The capillaries are greatly distended with blood (see XXV. 4), but the elastic fibres show but little alteration, and no cell-growth or thickening, as a rule, appears among them even in the advanced stages of the disease. Buhl, however, says that pus-corpuscles may be found in the walls in cases of purulent hepatisation,[8] and Rindfleisch describes them in this stage as existing between the capillaries.[9]

Cell-elements in great abundance are found mingled with the exudation in the solidified tissue, even in the stage of red hepatisation, but they vary in character in different cases of the disease. Thus the characters in a case of acute red hepatisation (Pl. I.), dying on the fifth day, are those seen in XXV. 7, but in large areas, they were identical with those shown in fig. 3 of the same plate (pneumonia fatal on the tenth day, and when much of the tissue was in a state of grey hepatisation); in this the cells filling the alveoli have almost entirely the character of pus-cells, but it also (fig. 2) presents cells of another character. Figs. 4, 5, and 6 are from a case of pneumonia dying on the twelfth day, and show cells differing somewhat from each of the foregoing.

---

also observed it after the injection of nitrate of silver. *Manuel Hist. Pathol.* 2nd ed. p. 27.
[1] See Buhl, *Sitzungsbericht der Bayerischen Akademie*, 1863, and *Archiv für Biologie*, 1863, vol. iii.; also Ed. Wagner, *Archiv der Heilkunde*, 1866, vol. viii.; and Otto Weber, Pitha and Billroth's *Handb. der Chirurgie*, p. 330.
[2] *Archiv der Heilkunde.* 1867 and 1868, vols. viii. an l ix.
[3] *Gesammelte Abhandlungen*, 1856, p. 137.

[4] See *Spec. Path. u. Therap.* art. 'Entzündung,' also his *Archiv*, iv. 310.
[5] *Charité-Annalen*, 1875, p. 730.
[6] *Lehrb. Path. Gewebelehre*, p. 870.
[7] *Vorlesungen über Ally. Pathologie*, i. 214.
[8] *Lungenentzündung, Tuberculose und Schwindsucht*, p. 34.
[9] *Lehrb. der path. Gewebelehre*, 1878, p. 289.

The general characters of the cells found in red, and also in part in grey, hepatisation are depicted singly in XXV. 9, A.

§ 1. A very large proportion resemble a, b, c, such as are seen *in situ* in figs. 2, 5, and 7. They are round cells with a single nucleus, more or less finely granular from protein matter. The nucleus often shows a strongly refracting nucleolus. In many parts the preponderating number are like a, viz. cells, measuring from $\frac{1}{2500}$ inch to $\frac{1}{2500}$ inch ; the size of the nucleus being from $\frac{1}{7500}$ inch to $\frac{1}{4500}$ inch. Some of these cells may, however, be as small as $\frac{1}{3800}$, with a nucleus of $\frac{1}{7000}$ inch.

§ 2. Many of these cells undergo pigmentary changes, and they increase in size during the process, until they form large round cells like p and q, and may attain the size of $\frac{1}{1000}$ inch, the nucleus being $\frac{1}{1000}$ inch. The nucleus gradually becomes obscured by the deposit of pigment as in q, in which the obscuration is taking place.

Rindfleisch[1] deduces these pigment-cells from the migration of pigmented cells in the interstitial tissue, but the manner in which the pigment is seen gradually to increase in these round cells (which I am disposed to regard as derivatives of the epithelium) induces me to believe that it results from the transformation of blood-pigment.

Pigmented nuclei measuring $\frac{1}{7000}$ to $\frac{1}{1000}$ inch, either free in the interior of the alveoli (fig. 9, r) or scattered thickly on the walls (r'), may be found in parts. In some places, where there has been a large extravasation of red blood-corpuscles, these may be found shrivelling into crystalline forms, but I have not observed hæmatoidin crystals within the larger cells in cases of acute pneumonia.

§ 3. In a few rare cases, large cells may be found, like s, t, measuring $\frac{1}{1500}$ to $\frac{1}{1200}$ inch, and more or less filled with a large hyaline nucleus. It appears to me probable that this condition is the result of a mucoid change.

§ 4. Large placoids like n, measuring $\frac{1}{1500}$ inch, with a nucleus of $\frac{1}{2800}$, are found in all forms in varying degree. Sometimes they are more or less granular.

§ 5. Cells showing multiple nuclei are very common, and are often seen arranged in groups and masses. They are sometimes round and finely granular, like g. The cells measure from $\frac{1}{2500}$ to $\frac{1}{2000}$ inch, the nuclei from $\frac{1}{5000}$ to $\frac{1}{4000}$; but in some of the cells of this nature the nuclei, lying excentrically, measure only $\frac{1}{14000}$ to $\frac{1}{12000}$. A few cells of a larger size ($\frac{1}{1500}$ inch) m, are also occasionally found with multiple nuclei, the nuclei not being, however, increased proportionally in size, but measuring $\frac{1}{15000}$ inch. In other cases the cells are not round, but of a flattened, epithelioid appearance h ; their measurements are, like the bulk of g, $\frac{1}{2500}$ to $\frac{1}{2000}$ inch.

§ 6. Cells showing a tendency to the division of the nucleus are not uncommon. A frequent type is shown at d, where an elongated nucleus is seen constricted in the middle. These cells measure $\frac{1}{2500}$; the nucleus, $\frac{1}{4500}$ in length (as nearly as can be calculated) by $\frac{1}{7000}$ in width. Other stages of fissiparous division of the nuclei are seen in f, k, l. The cells average $\frac{1}{2000}$, the nuclei from $\frac{1}{7000}$ to $\frac{1}{5000}$ inch.

The origin of these cell-forms still remains a subject of dispute. Since Cohnheim's researches it has been very generally believed that they are entirely deducible from the migration of the white corpuscles of the blood. Apart, however, from the evidence adduced by Stricker[2] and reaffirmed by Buhl,[3] that the earlier view of the production of pus by endogenous multiplication of nuclei is still tenable, it appears to me most probable that no small proportion of them are derived from the epithelium lining the alveoli.

---

[1] *Lehrb. der Path. Gewebelehre*, p. 381. [2] In his *Vorlesung. allg. Pathol.*
[3] *Lungenentzündung, Tuberculose und Schwindsucht.*

Direct evidence of endogenous cell-formation within the epithelial cells has been found by Heitler[1] and by Dreschfeld.[2] It has been again recently studied by Veraguth under the influence of the direct introduction of irritants into the lung. He finds that the larger epithelial cells are desquamated and break down, and form probably part of the fibrinous network. The smaller cells enlarge, and their nuclei multiply, producing still smaller cells, which fill the alveoli. This change precedes the exudation of fibrin, and Veraguth seems to consider that it is almost a necessary antecedent to the latter, which also occurs before the exit of white corpuscles. Later, this exit takes place, and the alveoli become crowded with lymphoid cells.[3]

Feuerstack, on the other hand, denies the breaking down of the larger non-nucleated placoids, though he admits that some are separated and undergo fatty degeneration, but he considers that the smaller nucleated cells of the air-vesicles are abundantly desquamated. He states also that the epithelium is regenerated from the smaller cells, while Cornil and Ranvier assert that this regeneration takes place from lymphatic cells adhering to the wall.[4] Feuerstack further states that all pneumonias contain some fibrinous exudation, and that the acute form is distinguished by the excess of this, which is not, however, derived from the epithelium.[5]

The numbers of free nuclei (XXV. 9 r) found in some specimens might indeed support Lionel Beale's view that they are 'bioplasts,' or masses of germinal matter which have passed through the walls of the blood-vessels. Measuring only $\frac{1}{4000}$ to $\frac{1}{2500}$ of an inch, they are smaller than white corpuscles;[6] but they correspond closely in dimensions to the nuclei of the medium-sized cells (see description of Pl. XXV.), and it appears to me probable that in many instances at least they are set free from the interior of these.

The correctness of Cohnheim's views has been strongly supported by Friedländer's researches on the pneumonia resulting from the division of vagi.[7] He asserts that the alveoli fill with lymphoid cells, beneath which the epithelium may be found intact; but the forms met with in both catarrhal and fibrinous pneumonia appear to show that some changes in the epithelium likewise occur, and it is interesting to observe that, even in human lungs that appear otherwise healthy, accumulations of epithelial-like cells, sometimes with multiple nuclei, have been found within the alveoli by Kölliker, who regards them as the derivatives of the smaller pavement-epithelium.[8] I think it probable that the larger cells (placoids) fig. 9 n, are thrown off unchanged, but that the smaller cells intervening between these, and which probably are destined to supply the places of the larger ones, are the source of the cell-proliferation which ensues. The size of some of the larger cells (c p q m) militates against the idea that they are the derivatives of the white corpuscles, unless these are greatly swollen by imbibition. On the other hand, the dimensions of the nuclei of these are, in many instances, less than those of the white corpuscles which have been said to penetrate within the cells, and thus simulate the multiplication of their nuclei.

That a diapedesis of the red corpuscles takes place is a matter of extreme probability, for the rapidity of resolution is opposed to the assumption that there is any extensive rupture of the capillaries. It is probable also that a similar diapedesis of the white corpuscles occurs, and this may take place to a varying amount in different cases, and probably increases in the later stages. Whether, however, they form the source of the bulk of the cells found in the earlier stages may, I think, be considered somewhat doubtful. Even throughout the whole process of pneumonia, the proportion which these corpuscles

---

[1] Stricker's *Wien. med. Jahrbücher*, 1871.
[2] *Lancet*, 1876, i. 47.
[3] Veraguth, Virchow's *Archiv*, vol. lxxxii.
[4] *Manuel Hist. Path.* 2nd ed. p. 31.
[5] Feuerstack, *Verhalten des Epithels der Lungenalveolen bei der fibrinösen Pneumonie* (Göttinger Diss. 1882).

[6] *Microscopical Journal*, 1864, vol. xii. and the *Microscope in Medicine*, pp. 277-391.
[7] *Untersuchungen über Lungenentzündung*, Berlin, 1873.
[8] *Verhand. phys. med. Gesellschaft zu Würzburg*, N. F. 1861, vol. xvi.

bear to the other cells is part of the larger question of pus-formation, which as yet can hardly be considered to be set entirely at rest.[1]

Red blood-corpuscles are found in large numbers in the exudation (*see* XXV. 6, *b b*). They constitute a prominent feature of the early stages of red hepatisation, and are the cause of the peculiarity of colour in the lung in this stage, and also of the red rusty tinge of the sputa. The amount present varies, however, and in some forms of the disease, which may be appropriately termed 'hæmorrhagic pneumonia,' they are in great excess and constitute a large proportion of the exudation.[2] They lose their hæmatin by exosmosis, and this, imbibed by other adjacent cell-forms, is the chief source of the pigmentation observed. They sometimes also shrivel, and form masses of pigment, which is occasionally crystalline in the alveoli and in the alveolar walls.

The passage from the red hepatisation to the grey and suppurative forms is marked by the redistribution of the hæmatin as just described, and also by a gradual increase of cells resembling pus-cells. A considerable proportion of large cells may still be found within the alveoli, as was the case in the lung shown at IV. 4 (*see* also XXV. 4, 6), and the change in colour is due in great measure to the increase in number of the cells, and also to their fatty degeneration. The exudation softens, and Rindfleisch has stated that it gradually acquires the character of mucin, being precipitated by acetic acid.[3] In this stage resolution occurs, and it is probable that a large proportion of the exudation and of the fattily-degenerated and broken-down cells is removed by absorption, inasmuch as the physical signs of consolidation often disappear with great rapidity, sometimes within twenty-four hours, without any corresponding increase of expectoration. The lung, however, remains softer, more œdematous, and more vascular than natural, with a loss of elasticity.[4]

Inflammation of the lymphatics of the lung is described by Cornil and Ranvier as attending acute pneumonia, and they may be so distended by exudation as to bear considerable resemblance to the pulmonary alveoli.[5]

ACUTE CATARRHAL PNEUMONIA, OR BRONCHO-PNEUMONIA.

'LOBULAR,' 'DISSEMINATED,' OR 'VESICULAR,' PNEUMONIA.

Plate V. figs. 1, 2, and 3.

The anatomical distinction of other forms of pneumonia from the acute fibrinous type is at times a problem of considerable difficulty. By some authors the definition has been made to depend on the character of the exudation, and on the cell-forms found in the interior of the alveoli, but neither of these tests is universally applicable, since fibrinous exudations may occasionally be found in pneumonia, however this has commenced, and the types of cells filling the alveoli are also liable to considerable variation. This question will be discussed later, and it appears desirable, for its more complete elucidation, that

---

[1] See Perls, *Lehrb. allg. Pathol.* 1877.
[2] Cornil and Ranvier, *Manuel Hist. Path.* ii. 114, state that in the pneumonia of the horse, the effusion of blood is so extreme as to resemble pulmonary apoplexy.
[3] *Lehrb. pathol. Gewebelehre*, 1878, p. 391.
[4] I have found this after three weeks has elapsed from the date of resolution.
[5] *Manuel Hist. Path.* 2nd ed. ii. 121.

the simplest type of catarrhal pneumonia should first be considered—viz., that arising from extension of inflammation from the bronchial tubes to the alveoli of the lung.[1] This pneumonia is essentially a lobular, vesicular, or infundibular inflammation; nevertheless, by extension of the process or in consequence of certain special conditions, it may spread over larger areas and even become lobar or 'pseudo-lobar.' It is, in all cases, a secondary process. The pneumonia, instead of being a primary affection of the lung-substance, is a result of bronchitis, whether this is idiopathic or the consequence of an acute febrile disease, such especially as measles and whooping-cough, or affections that have a tendency to implicate the bronchi, such as variola and diphtheria. The lungs in this condition present very varied appearances. These are chiefly due to the co-existence, with the bronchial and alveolar inflammation, of collapse (either pure and simple, or followed by secondary congestion and hepatisation), to emphysema in other portions, and to dilatations of the bronchi.

The islets of lobular pneumonia are those to which attention is now specially directed. These are seen in V. 2 and 3. Fig. 2 is from an unpublished drawing by Sir R. Carswell, to which no further description is appended than 'Pneumonia in Child affected with Measles,' but it admirably represents the appearances often seen in this form of pneumonia. Fig 3 is from *Case 4 (Tanner)*.

The extension of the inflammation to the pulmonary tissue is indicated by spots of consolidation varying in size from a twelfth to a quarter of an inch in diameter, but sometimes only affecting a few vesicles, and possibly even infundibular, so as only to be recognised by the microscope.[2] These spots, in their early stages, are slightly prominent, of a dull red colour, and often finely granular; corresponding very closely in their aspect with that of red hepatisation in the adult. The granular appearance is, however, often indistinct, and these areas can, at first, be distinguished from nodules of lobular collapse only by the impossibility of insufflating them. This lobular collapse indeed sometimes, but not always, forms the first stage of the inflammatory process, in the manner subsequently to be described in detail. A further distinction between pneumonic spots and collapsed lobules is that the former are soft, and easily broken down by pressure. They assume, apparently very quickly, a duller grey or yellowish tint (V. 2), the 'grey hepatisation' of authors. In this stage they are still very slightly prominent, but in this respect different islets may vary. Some are tolerably well-defined, while others fade at their margins into the surrounding tissue. The degree of their prominence depends very much on whether or not adjacent lobules are compressed and collapsed, or whether they still contain air and are congested (*see* XXVI. 1, 2). These islets are incapable of insufflation and sink in water. They tend to become confluent, and then form indistinctly racemose groups; the racemose character is less marked than in tubercle, owing to the absence of induration in the peri-alveolar tissue, and it is chiefly indicated by the irregularity of their outlines.[3]

The islets of genuine vesicular pneumonia are indifferently scattered throughout the lungs, but they are most abundant in the middle and lower lobes. Those that are secondary to the process of collapse, presently to be described, are chiefly met with in the lower

---

[1] It is impossible for any author to enter upon a description of this form of pneumonia without expressing his obligation to the exhaustive description given of it by Barthez and Rilliet in their *Maladies des Enfants* (2nd ed. 1853), to which little of importance has been since added, although valuable and instructive descriptions have been afforded by Bartels (Virch. *Archiv*, vol. xxi.) and by Ziemssen (*Pleuritis und Pneumonie im Kindesalter*, Berlin, 1862.)

[2] Colberg. *Deutsch. Archiv klin. Med.* 1866, vol. ii.

[3] It must here be remarked that many of the cases of broncho-pneumonia in childhood are complicated by tubercle, and this complication involving a growth in the alveolar walls, gives to the islets of such broncho-pneu

lobe and in the anterior part of the left upper lobe. In their later stages they appear capable of softening into a purulent detritus, forming the *grains jaunes* of Barthez and Rilliet, and they may contribute to the formation of the larger purulent spots, the 'vacuoles' of French authors. To both of these appearances, reference will be made later.

The confluence of these spots may give rise to the infiltration of larger areas with pneumonic consolidation—the pseudo-lobar form. From the great rapidity with which consolidation sometimes occurs (as in the cases shown at V. 1 and 4) it is probable that this pseudo-lobar form may also arise independently, and as a more diffuse process, by the direct implication of the pulmonary tissue. Its most common origin, however, is by the development of pneumonic consolidation in portions of collapsed lung, by means of a process hereafter to be described.

The conditions of the bronchi and lung-tissue that accompany acute bronchitis in childhood are, however, manifold, and give rise to much complexity in the appearances observed and to corresponding variations in their description by different authors. The bronchi are intensely inflamed. The mucous membrane is swollen, thickened, and highly congested; punctiform extravasation is observed in numerous places. The whole wall also tends to undergo thickening, so that the cut orifices of the tubes stand out prominently from the surrounding tissue. They are commonly loaded with secretion, sometimes mucoid, but more commonly, in fatal cases, fluid and puriform. The tubes, in some instances, may appear almost filled with this secretion, but in other cases it is scanty and may be almost absent in the smaller branches. In cases of some duration, it becomes thickened and inspissated, filling the tubes, and capable of being expressed in lumps; in some instances, when the smallest tubes are thus obstructed, they may form a network of yellow lines on the cut surface of the collapsed but pale tissue of the lung.[1] The tubes are almost invariably dilated; in those of the third and fourth divisions the dilatation is generally similar and fusiform, but in the smaller bronchi it tends to the globular shape (see V. 3). This dilatation may be so uniformly diffused as to give the whole lung a cribriform aspect, or an appearance as if it contained numerous cavities, and near the surface of the lung the bronchi may have a diameter of two-fifths of an inch (Barthez and Rilliet). In some cases, the globular dilatation contrasts remarkably with the narrowed portion of the tube from which it springs.[2] These globular dilatations may vary in size from a millet-seed to a hemp-seed, or even a filbert, but the larger cavities are usually the result of a more complex process, involving the destruction of the alveolar walls of the terminal infundibula. They are filled with puriform-looking fluid, which escapes on puncture, and they may form prominences on the surface of the lung, which appear yellow through the covering pleura. They are rare in cases dying within the first week, but are common if the disease has lasted for a fortnight or more. It is further to be remarked that this acute dilatation of the bronchi in recent inflammation of the tubes, is much less common in adult life than in childhood. Its greater frequency in the earlier periods of life is probably in part due directly to the intensity with which the inflammation attacks the bronchial walls, in part also to the more yielding character of their tissues, for, as observed by Bartels,[3] there may be a cylindrical dilatation associated with simple thinning of the walls, which are then membranous and transparent. That it is not limited to childhood, but may also be found in more advanced life, will be stated hereafter.

monia a greater degree of prominence than is observed in pure forms of the disease.
[1] Bartels, Virchow's *Archiv*, xxi. 81.
[2] Ziemssen. *Pleuritis und Pneumonie im Kindesalter*.
[3] *Die häutige Bräune*, Deutsch. Arch. klin. Med. 1867, ii. 388.

Collapse of the lung is a very constant accompaniment of the condition, and in addition may lead to pneumonic changes. Its presence and the changes that ensue in parts of the lung thus affected, have been the chief causes of the varying descriptions given by different authorities, and also of the diverse interpretations attached to the appearances observed.

It is first met with at the bases posteriorly, where it forms sunken, wedge-shaped areas, with the base of the wedge at the lower margin of the lung, and the apex extending upwards. These are sunk below the surface, and at first are of a bluish or purple tint. On section, the surface is smooth and glistening, and the interlobular septa are distinct ; in the early stages it is elastic and resists pressure, but it sinks in water. In addition to these characters it is at once distinguished by the fact that its normal aspect is restored on insufflation, although, owing to its containing more blood than the sound lung, this process gives it a brighter colour than the adjacent tissue. Later, it becomes œdematous and pits on pressure, but can still be insufflated.

The collapse is not, however, limited to the bases.. It may also occur at the apices, though these are more commonly the seat of emphysema. Islets and spots may also be found, with the same characters, scattered throughout the lung, and it is very commonly met with at the anterior margin of the left upper lobe where this overlaps the heart.

In the latter situation another appearance is common, which, however, may be found in all cases of collapse of long standing in parts in which pneumonic changes have not occurred. In this condition the lung is hard, resistant, and lobulated. It has, in fact, returned to and assumed the appearance of a racemose gland, resembling the tissue of the pancreas [1] (*see* XXI. 2, from Cruveilhier). The interlobular septa are very prominent and appear thickened, but the lung-tissue is pale, almost white. There is an entire absence of any sign of exudation into the vesicles in many parts, although among them there may be found pneumonic spots and also some vesicles containing air. It appears as if the walls of the vesicles were agglutinated together ; they cannot be inflated without great difficulty, and sometimes cannot be inflated at all, but this is possibly due to the complete closure of the bronchi leading to them. The condition of collapse is very frequently the first stage in the production of subsequent pneumonic processes, although this does not appear to be common in the state of induration last described.

The pneumonia which occurs in collapsed portions is usually of a diffused type, but tends to extend gradually, so that, while some tracts appear consolidated, portions are still capable of insufflation. In some, it occurs through an extension of the condition just described as frequently present in the islets of lobular consolidation—the condition that may be recognised in the collapsed area by the greater prominence of the islets, by their opacity, and by their greyish-yellow or whiter tint. It may apparently occur without the intervention of collapse, though this may be superadded, and may also in some cases possibly precede it.

In many instances it takes place in the manner described by Bartels and Ziemssen. through the medium of an intenser congestion, followed by œdema, which occurs in the collapsed parts. To this the term 'splenisation' is applicable, while the term 'carnisation' more appropriately expresses the firm, resistant, airless condition of simple collapse. In this state of 'splenisation' the lung is gorged with bloody serosity, has lost its elasticity.

---

[1] Sir James Alderson, *Med.-Chir. Trans.* 1830. Fuchs (*Die Bronchitis der Kinder*, 1849) terms this change *Drüsenartige Verhärtung*. Fuchs stated that these parts could be inflated, but I have found this impossible in some cases.

and has become somewhat more friable. It is, however, capable of imperfect sufflation, though in variable degrees. It cannot be regarded as the subject of pneumonic consolidation, for the congestion and œdema observed are probably in great measure mechanical, and due to the impediment to the passage of the blood—an impediment caused both by the state of collapse and also by the absence of the alternate movements of expansion and retraction which largely favour the free circulation in the pulmonary tissue in a state of health. The œdema, and, to a less degree, the congestion, tend to spread beyond the collapsed portions, but the latter may usually be distinguished by the greater depth of colour, and also by the fact that the serosity exuding from the former is mingled with air; such parts, moreover, float in water, though they will often sink after being pressed between the thumb and fingers. The occurrence of inflammation (by the products of which the air-vesicles are again distended) is marked by the sunken portions regaining their normal level. The elevation may have been already in part effected by the changes last noted, but it now occurs to the extent of full expansion. The dark colour of congestion becomes paler; the areas are dull and opaque; the surface feels more solid, but is at the same time more friable, breaking into a pulp under the fingers. The serosity also is clouded and sometimes even milky. The interlobular septa have disappeared. The surface is uniform, and when the process is complete, the section presents an appearance little distinguishable from that of ordinary red hepatisation, except that within it, islets of air-containing tissue are not unfrequently found,[1] that the dilated bronchi and spots of collapse are mingled in the section, and that the tissue tends more rapidly to assume a duller grey colour. A finely granular surface is sometimes seen when the section is scraped, but this is not always apparent (see V. 1).

A point of considerable importance, and one which seems to distinguish inflammatory changes of the air-vesicles from both collapse and splenisation, is that whenever the former reaches the surface in a lobular or in a more diffused area, the pleura becomes implicated in a very large proportion of cases (though not in all). It loses its transparency, presents increased injection, and rapidly becomes covered with a film of false membrane. On the other hand, both in collapse and splenisation, the pleura retains its translucency, though showing the congestion beneath and sometimes sharing in it (as is shown by punctiform ecchymoses) while false membranes are absent. Over bronchial dilatations, there may or may not exist plastic pleurisy.

Hæmorrhagic ecchymoses are very common in some forms of broncho-pneumonia. They are most abundant under the pleura, but are found also in the pulmonary tissue. They occur in measles, whooping-cough, diphtheria, influenza, and also in the pneumonia artificially produced by section of the vagi.[2] In some cases they may form considerable extravasations or infarcts, varying in size from a pea to a hemp-seed or walnut.[3]

Another change attending this process is the rapid production of vesicular emphysema in the non-collapsed and non-hepatised portions. The over-distension of the vesicles sometimes occurs between and around scattered nodules of collapse; it may also sometimes be found in the middle of larger areas, where the emphysema is distinguished by its paler aspect and by its prominence. It occurs also to a marked degree at the apices and throughout the upper lobes, especially at their anterior margins; these lobes are sometimes uniformly distended, and contrast markedly with the collapsed and congested

---

[1] This also occurs, it should be remarked, in the acute lobar pneumonia of childhood.
[2] See Juffroy, Des différentes Formes de la Broncho-pneumonie (Thèse d'agrégation, Paris, 1880); also, Frey, Die Lungenveränderungen nach Lähmung der Nervi Vagi.
[3] Bartels, 'Die häutige Bräune,' Deutsch. Archiv f. klin. Med. 1867, ii. 395.

condition of the bases. Hard nodules of collapse may frequently be found among these emphysematous portions. In some few cases interlobular emphysema occurs from rupture of the vesicles, and is recognised by the bead-like nodules in the septa, whence they commonly extend beneath the pleura and also into the mediastinum.

The concurrence of these conditions—dilated bronchi loaded with pus, inflamed vesicles and nodules, collapsed portions of lung passing into congestion and pneumonic consolidation—gives rise, by the variations they present, to very peculiar appearances. In some cases, groups of dilated bronchi, filled with liquid or inspissated puriform matter, traverse areas of collapse, and may occupy so much of the tissue that the lung, when dried, may present the aspect of a honeycomb;[1] they may also be found in emphysematous portions. Spots of vesicular pneumonia may be found in the emphysematous parts, and also in the firmer lobulated areas of collapse, as well as in the more uniformly 'carnified' parts, and in those in which congestion and œdema have produced the condition of 'splenisation.' On the other hand, emphysema and collapse, though tending to occur in different regions of the lung, may also, as we have seen, be combined.

It must further be remarked that in many cases, even of ten days' or a fortnight's duration, very little may be found after death except the dilated bronchi filled with pus, the '*grains jaunes*,' and extensive areas of collapse and splenisation, and that the small islets of lobular consolidation may be either absent or almost undiscoverable. This apparent absence of these islets of consolidation is sometimes due to their small size, and to their concealment by the œdematous swelling and congestion of the 'splenised' parts; but in not a few cases it would appear as if death were due to the bronchitis and consecutive collapse, without any large extension of the inflammation of the alveolar tissue. In the vast majority of cases, as noticed by Barthez and Rilliet, the affection is bilateral; but the relative degree in which the two lungs may be affected varies considerably. In some there may be lobular pneumonia on one side and lobar on the other; or one may be affected with lobular pneumonia and bronchial dilatation, and the other only with collapse and splenisation.

The Histology of Catarrhal Pneumonia, like its macroscopic anatomy, has been the subject of much dispute. The chief discussion has been on the question whether any true inflammatory changes take place in the lung. Their occurrence was formerly denied, as by Béhier,[2] and even recently by Buhl.[3] The latter has reasserted the opinion expressed by Legendre and Bailly and by Fauvel, and disputed by Barthez and Rilliet,[4] that the purulent fluid found in the vesicles has only gravitated from the bronchi. That this occurs in connection with bronchial dilatation is, I think, highly probable, and I believe that the '*grains jaunes*' and the 'vacuoles' of Barthez and Rilliet owe their origin in great measure to this process, but I believe that microscopic examination is sufficient to prove that inflammatory processes take place within the air-vesicles, and concur in the production of the last-named conditions. The histological appearances of the lung shown in V. 3 (*Case 4, Tanner*), are depicted in XXVI. 1, 2, 3, 4. Magnified by a low power (figs. 2 and 3), the alveoli and the infundibula are seen to be distended with epithelioid and pyoid cells, while their walls are highly injected and filled with red blood-corpuscles, among which some white corpuscles are seen here and there. In the specimens that I have examined, I have not seen a fibrinous exudation within the vesicles, although this has

---

[1] Graily Hewitt, *The Pathology of Hooping Cough*, London, 1855.
[2] Béhier, *Clinique Médicale*, 1864.
[3] Buhl, *Lungenentzündung, &c.* 1872. p. 14.
[4] See *Mal. des Enfants*, i. 418, 419.

been observed by Damaschino in cases of whooping-cough, and also by Balzer, by Rautenberg, and by Cornil and Ranvier.[1] In other parts the infundibula may be seen similarly distended by a mass of cells, mingled with granular detritus, as in XXVI. 1. I believe this to be an infundibulum, on account of its size, $\frac{1}{100}$th of an inch in diameter. It is manifestly distended, and the tissue around is collapsed. Had it been a whole ' acinus,' or ' ultimate lobule,' the diameter would probably have been considerably more. All trace of the alveolar passages has disappeared, except that the mass filling the infundibulum is broken up into separate elongated portions, which might be taken for alveolar passages were they not too small, their average width being only the $\frac{1}{500}$th of an inch. The pulmonary tissue around these distended infundibula may be found collapsed and hyperæmic, as in fig. 1, or groups of terminal alveoli and infundibula may be seen similarly distended with inflammatory products, as in fig. 2.

In some places the breaking down of infundibula could be clearly traced; puriform masses resulted, which probably constitute the *grains jaunes* of Barthez and Rilliet. They present, on a large scale, precisely the appearances seen in fig. 1, except that the alveolar tissue appears to be breaking down into detritus. In parts an infiltration of pyoid-looking cells into the walls of the alveoli and interlobular tissue appeared to precede this change, as described by Lebert.[2] But I have not seen this, under the circumstances, proceed to any material thickening of the alveolar walls; as a rule, these appeared to break down at once, and merge in the inflammatory débris.[3] The process is akin to that observed in bronchial dilatation, and also in the extreme forms of emphysema, with the exception that here the destruction of the pulmonary parenchyma appears to take place acutely, under the influence of the inflammation.

Much discussion has taken place respecting the origin of the cells that fill the alveoli. The appearances actually seen in disease are strongly in favour of their epithelioid origin. This is seen in XXV. 8, and XXVI. 3, 4. The two latter figures especially show various forms of alteration in the epithelial lining. The larger cells are mostly mono-nucleated, and measure the $\frac{1}{3200}$th to the $\frac{1}{2100}$th of an inch, but, mingled with these, as in XXVI. 2, are smaller ones, ranging from $\frac{1}{7000}$th to $\frac{1}{3000}$th of an inch. In some cases, however (XXV. 8) the cells are still more distinctly epithelioid and larger, measuring from $\frac{1}{2000}$ to $\frac{1}{1500}$th of an inch, and multiplication of their nuclei can be distinctly seen. Some alveoli are almost entirely filled with these larger cells, but in others smaller forms predominate; and this may be observed, not only of individual alveoli in the same specimen, but of different cases in general—in some the larger cells and in others the smaller ones are more abundant throughout the affected parts. Friedländer, from his study of the process of inflammation after section of the vagi, expresses the opinion that the epithelium swells and is thrown off, and that the exudation of white corpuscles forms the larger proportion of the cell-growth. In this he has been closely followed by Frey.[4]

The observations already quoted (*see* Acute Pneumonia, p. 21) appear to show that a large part of the cell-products found in the alveoli are of epithelial origin, but that

---

[1] Damaschino, *Des différentes Formes de la Pneumonie Aiguë chez les Enfants*, Paris, 1867; Balzer, *Contribution à l'Etude de la Broncho-pneumonie*, Thèse de Paris, 1878, p. 22; Rautenberg, *Jahrbuch für Kinderheilkunde*, N.F. 1875, viii. 105 *et seq.*; Cornil and Ranvier, *Manuel de l'Histologie Pathologique*, 2nd ed. pp. 99, 107.

[2] See Barthez and Rilliet, i. 419.

[3] As we shall hereafter see, a large infiltration occasionally takes place around the bronchi.

[4] Frey, *Lungenveränderungen nach Lähmungen der Nervi Vagi*, Leipzig, 1877. It may be desirable to recall the fact that Frey's observations appear conclusively to prove that the pneumonia following section of the vagus is essentially a broncho-pneumonia, due to the penetration of the saliva and food into the air-passages.

probably a certain proportion of them, which varies in different cases, is due to the migration of white corpuscles, and that the amount of these may possibly also vary with the intensity of the inflammation, with the degree of injury to the walls of the capillaries, and with the extent to which the epithelial structures have also suffered.[1] The view upheld by Buhl, and by some other writers since Fauvel, that the contents of the vesicles are due to aspiration from the bronchi, is, in the author's opinion, untenable.[2] It is not improbable that in the larger purulent collections (vacuoles), some gravitation does occur, but recent histological research appears to show that a primary change of an inflammatory type takes place within the alveolar cavities.

Another, and very interesting fact, which has been recently established is the existence of masses of micro-organisms in the sheaths of the bronchi and vessels, and also in the alveoli of the lungs (Figs. 34 and 35). These have been found by Buhl, Eberth, and Otto Wyss, in the catarrhal pneumonia accompanying measles, diphtheria, influenza, whooping-cough, variola, and typhoid.[3]

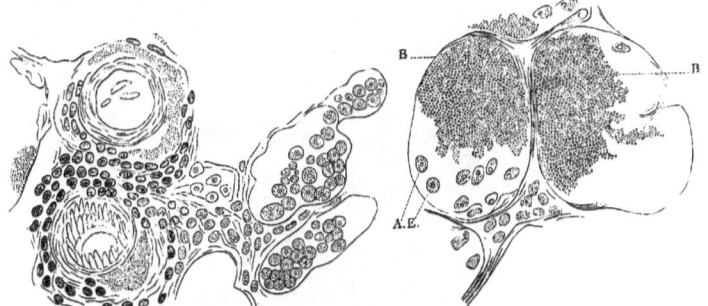

Figs. 34 and 35. Fig. 34, micrococci in peribronchial sheath, and, fig. 35, in interior of alveoli. AE, alveolar epithelium cells; BB, micrococci. (From Otto Wyss.)

Alterations in the Bronchi.—Thickening and infiltration of the walls of the bronchi have been noticed in a large number of cases of broncho-pneumonia. It is, in fact, to this change that their prominence and rigidity are in great measure due. In some cases, as described by Barthez and Rilliet[4] and by Lebert,[5] a zone of suppuration may surround the bronchus. The suppuration may even extend into the bronchi by lateral perforation, and this, in one case, appeared to me to have commenced from the mucous membrane. The infiltration sometimes invades the muscular coat, according to the observations of Balzer. He states, also, that the epithelium is sometimes preserved; but very commonly it is desquamated, and pyoid cells may be observed beneath it.

---

[1] Balzer (art. 'Broncho-pneumonie,' *Dict. de Méd. et de Chirurgie pratiques,* 1880, vol. xxvii. and also *Contribution à l'Etude de la Broncho-pneumonie,* Paris, 1878), has described a proliferation of the epithelium in the 'splenised' tissue. As this often constitutes a first stage of the pneumonic process, his observations can be fully accepted.

[2] Damaschino (*Des différentes Formes de la Pneumonie Aiguë chez les Enfants,* Paris, 1867, p. 31) has observed that in some cases the smaller bronchi may be found filled with pus, while the air-vesicles are crowded with epithelial cells, and he rightly argues that the latter must have originated *in situ*. Bartels also (Die häutige Bräune, *loc. cit.* p. 394) expresses a very strong opinion that the lobular consolidations in diphtheria are not due to simple gravitation from the bronchi, or even to a direct extension of the diphtheritic process. The appearances of the lungs in diphtheria will be described at a subsequent page.

[3] See Otto Wyss, art. 'Katarrhal-Pneumonie,' Gerhardt's *Handbuch der Kinderkrankheiten,* iii. 752.

[4] *Loc. cit.* p. 439.

[5] *Klinik der Brustkrankheiten,* i. 160.

A large share of the changes in broncho-pneumonia has been attributed by Balzer to the peribronchial changes. He appears to lay greater stress on them than on those which I have described as occurring in the terminal vesicles. According to him there is an infiltration of leucocytes into the wall of the bronchus as it traverses the lobule.[1] Outside this is a zone of hepatisation of the pulmonary tissue, surrounding the inflamed bronchus, which constitutes what he terms the 'true peribronchial nodule'; in this the alveoli are filled with products of inflammation, and around this again is the collapsed and congested tissue to which he applies the term splenisation. Balzer thus appears to regard the extension of the inflammation from the bronchi to the lung-tissue as a process of extension by external contiguity,[2] instead of regarding it as an extension by continuity along the inner surface of the true terminal bronchus into the alveolar.

I am still disposed to regard the latter view, which is that hitherto generally adopted, as the correct one. It is perfectly true that in many cases, both in diphtheria, in measles, and also in idiopathic broncho-pneumonia, considerable thickening and infiltration can be seen around the

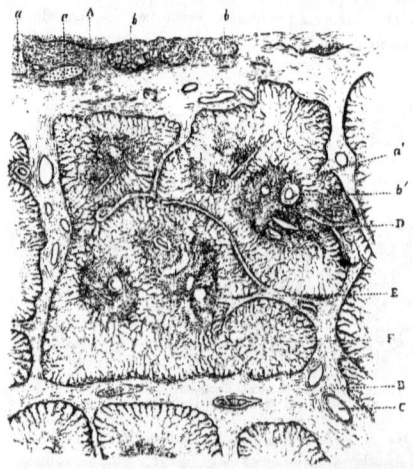

Fig. 36.—A, section of the wall of a medium-sized bronchus; *a a*, cartilages; *b b*, glands; B, thickened perilobular tissue; C, section of vessel; D, lymphatic; E, peri-acinous connective tissue; *a'*, *b'*, a bronchiole and an arteriole in the middle of a peribronchial nodule of hepatisation (several of these are seen in the figure). F, nodules of 'splenisation' (collapse?). (From Balzer.)

smaller bronchi, and also, but to a less degree, around the smaller arteries. In some cases this presents, very distinctly, the character of suppuration. In others it resembles the small-celled growth of tubercle, and in some of those I think it very probable that the process has this signification, since tubercular changes may be excited in predisposed subjects by this form of inflammation. These peribronchial changes also, as observed by Balzer, are usually found in the centre of areas of pneumonic infiltration of the alveoli, and also sometimes in areas of collapse, but I believe that the extension is, in the majority of cases, from the bronchial surfaces, and not by mere contiguity, and that the pulmonary tissue surrounding these inflamed bronchi has been affected

---

[1] Balzer apparently uses the term 'lobule' as a name for the larger compound anatomical element consisting of many acini, for though he describes these peribronchial spaces as 'acineuses,' yet the bronchus does not traverse the 'acinus' in the sense here meant, but the 'acinus' represents the termination of the bronchus in the series of alveolar passages.

[2] See Balzer's *Thesis*, pp. 20, 22, 23. It is true that in this article in the *Dict. de Méd. et Chir. pratiques* (xxvii. 537) he speaks of an extension of the inflammation by continuity, but he appears to apply this rather to 'splenisation' than to the lobular form of pneumonia, to which he applies the term 'lobule peribronchique.'

through its own direct alveolar passages, and not, as a general rule, by lateral extension from the inflamed bronchial sheath. But undoubtedly, the possibility of the latter process must be admitted; it may occur in measles and also in diphtheria.[1] It must also be remarked that over considerable areas affected with pneumonic inflammation, both in the diffuse and also in the lobular forms, these peribronchial nodules are not found, while in some specimens the appearances are almost exclusively those which I have figured in Plate XXVI. showing that the lobular pneumonia is essentially infundibular in its nature and origin.

The larger dilatations of the bronchi, when filled with pus, probably represent the 'vacuoles' of Barthez and Rilliet. More discussion has taken place respecting the nature of the smaller punctiform accumulations of yellow fluid, the *grains jaunes* of these authors, and it is not improbable that they may be due to diverse conditions. In some cases they may possibly be due to purulent accumulations in the ampullar dilatations at the end of the terminal bronchi, especially when, as described by Barthez and Rilliet, they are hard and resistant, contrasting with adjacent islets of red hepatisation, though allowing fluid to escape when pricked, and directly continuous with a bronchus. But in other cases, as described by these authors, where the fluid escapes on pressure by

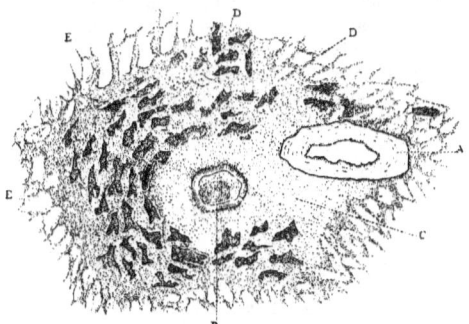

Fig. 37. A, an artery; B, bronchus containing pus, with the epithelium intact; C, thickened peribronchial tissue; DD, zones of hepatisation (alveoli filled with fibrine and with globules of pus); E, tissue in a state of 'splenisation' (collapse?). (From Balzer.)

numerous small openings, it appears more probable that they are due to softening of the infundibula, such as has been already described.

This latter condition may also apparently give rise to *abscesses*, which, again, may have a striking resemblance to the 'vacuoles' of Barthez and Rilliet, and it is not improbable that the former may lead to the latter. This would explain the different descriptions given of vacuoles; some bounded only by the pleura, others surrounded by a wall and by condensed lung-tissue, and, in a third class, forming, as already stated, directly around the bronchi. Abscesses of the first class may rupture into the pleura and give rise to pneumothorax.[2] These variations in appearance account for the different descriptions furnished by different writers of the character of broncho-pneumonia. Thus Gerhardt and Bartels describe little but the collapse, splenisation, and subsequent pneumonic nodules and pneumonic areas; while Barthez and Rilliet describe in addition the yellow nodules and the vacuoles,

[1] See Bartels, 'Ueber die häutige Bräune.' *Deutsch. Archiv klin. Med.* 1867. ii. 423 (case).
[2] Balzer (*Thèse*, p. 36) says that these abscesses always

commence in the peribronchial alveoli, and that they may occupy only the centre of the lobule.

the difference being chiefly due to the acuteness of the process and the character of the disease. The appearances last mentioned, as already stated, are found in greatest frequency and intensity in whooping-cough, but they are also met with after protracted broncho-pneumonia, and after measles when death is delayed.

In *diphtheria* the process is commonly too acute for the production of 'vacuoles,' though they may sometimes be observed.[1] The filling of the bronchial tubes with exudation may be indicated, as Bartels has observed, by leaf-like figures on the surface of the infiltrated lung. In many cases indeed, as this writer's descriptions show, nothing may be found in addition to the changes in the bronchi, beyond extensive emphysema, collapse, splenisation, and islets of lobular pneumonia of a reddish colour. The latter are for the most part confined to the posterior portions of the lungs, affecting the base in a preponderant degree if tracheotomy has not been performed, but they also occur in the upper lobe, while the base is less affected, in cases dying after tracheotomy. In some cases, it has been observed by Balzer that the pulmonary changes are most intensely marked around the hilus, and thence extend in a diminishing degree towards the periphery.

The pneumonia of diphtheria may, as I have seen, assume in the adult a different form, and Sanné remarks that it tends to pass into grey hepatisation with a frequency unusual in the child. In other cases it appears as yellow or whitish nodules, in the midst of collapsed tissue ; these nodules are not sections of the bronchi but islets of vesicular pneumonia. In other places grey or whitish or yellowish spots may be seen dusted on a reddish granular ground of pneumonic hepatisation. In other regions, again, islets of consolidation of the size of a hazel-nut are scattered through the congested tissue. Microscopically, these lungs afford three sets of appearances in the inflamed parts. In addition to the bronchi filled with pus or with amorphous exudation-matter, there are areas where the alveoli are filled with epithelioid cells, and where all stages of the enlargement of these may be seen. In other places, the alveoli are filled with a more amorphous exudation, akin to that seen in the bronchi, and in these gravitation may possibly have occurred, although it is also possible that the appearance in question may be due to breaking down of the cell-forms, and may represent a stage of resolution. Lastly, there are tracts where all cell-forms have disappeared, and a breaking down of the stroma of the lung is taking place by a process analogous to that seen in XXXV. 1 and 5 (*Acute Tubercular Pneumonia*), and which may possibly be a stage in the formation of ' vacuoles ' or of abscess.

In *variola*, I have found nodules of all sizes from a millet-seed to a split pea, soft, reddish, but tending to a yellow tinge in their centres, and in these all forms of epithelial change may be observed within the alveoli. Some are crowded with large epithelial cells, breaking down in the manner that I have already described. Others are filled with pus-corpuscles and pyoid cells, while some nodules are almost exclusively hæmorrhagic. Large tracts may be here and there found of an amorphous exudation, possibly resulting from the breaking down of cells as before described. Peribronchial infiltration may also be found to a very marked degree, and yellow spots consisting of puriform collections in dilated bronchi may also be observed in childhood.[2]

It has been stated by Otto Wyss[3] that one of the most frequent terminations of broncho-pneumonia is in *caseation*. I must take the liberty of expressing a doubt as to

---

[1] Sanné, *Traité de la Diphthérie*, Paris, 1877, p. 89.
[2] Steffen, *Klinik der Kinderkrankheiten*, p. 204. Legendre (*Rech. Malad. de l'Enfance*, 217) described them also in variola in the adult, but, as they were only found in a limited portion of the lung, he considers their presence to have been accidental.
[3] Gerhardt, *Handbuch der Kinderkrankheiten*, iii. 742.

this event in the uncomplicated disease, at any rate so far as regards the pulmonary tissue. It is hardly mentioned by the other earlier authorities on the subject, nor have I seen it apart from tubercle. Wyss states that it is most common in scrofulous and cachectic children, and further adds that tubercle is one of the most common complications of broncho-pneumonia in children—a statement which requires further examination by statistics. I should regard the occurrence of caseation in the lung-tissue, for reasons hereafter to be stated, as an almost certain proof of tubercle in this disease except under the condition mentioned by Buhl,[1] where it may be simulated by micro-organisms. It has been proved, by the observations of Ziemssen, that caseous thickening may occur in the pus contained within the bronchial tubes, but this differs markedly from true caseation of the pulmonary tissue. The latter has also been described by Ziemssen, but likewise only as occurring in scrofulous and cachectic children. Small-celled growths, identical in character with those found in tubercle, may be found in some cases of measles, both in the peribronchial tissue and to a less degree in the alveolar tissue. I am disposed to attribute to these the production of caseous change, although I believe they are probably of a tubercular nature, and that the tubercle arises as a result of the inflammation excited by the measles, probably also as a consequence of an antecedent predisposition.

It remains to say a few words on the classification and terminology employed by some recent writers for the appearances observed in broncho-pneumonia. Barthez and Rilliet, who first systematised our knowledge of this disease, described, in addition to the appearances of collapse, 'carnification' and 'splenisation,' a 'vesicular bronchitis' or 'pneumonia,' and also a 'disseminated' and a 'generalised hepatisation.' These categories appear to include the whole of the essential appearances and modes of origin, inasmuch as the 'vesicular' pneumonia includes the extension of the bronchitis to the infundibula and alveoli, while the other forms may occur in collapsed portions, both lobular and more or less diffuse. Damaschino and Roger [2] have added to these terms that of 'mammillation,' and have applied it chiefly to the vesicular form. It appears to me that this term is better avoided, for the following reasons. In the first place, the appearance of mammillation, as stated by Barthez and Rilliet, is produced both by the bronchioles which are thickened and distended with pus (the *grains jaunes*), and also by the consolidated nodules of hepatisation in the midst of collapsed tissue. In the second place, the islets of vesicular pneumonia are not always so prominent and firm as to justify the designation. Lastly, this appearance of mammillation is often most marked in a condition which is not inflammatory, namely, the extreme degrees of collapse, mingled or not with emphysema; in this the pancreas-like appearance is produced, and to this the application of the term, as designating a form of inflammation, would be both erroneous and misleading. The other appellations of 'pseudo-lobar' and 'lobar' may perhaps be preserved, although their use appears to involve no material advantage, and the multiplication of terms without special significance is, as far as possible, to be avoided. The essential point, it appears to me, is to distinguish clearly the bronchial from the pulmonary changes, and still more to separate the appearances in collapse, and the secondary congestion which often follows this splenisation, from the true lobular (acinose) inflammation of the alveolar tissue of the lung. This is, I think, specially necessary in relation to the condition of 'splenisation,' whether occurring in nodular or in a diffuse form; for, although it may lead to pneumonia, it does not pathologically deserve

[1] *Lungenentzündung &c.* p. 18. [2] *Dict. Encyclopédique des Sciences Médicales.* 1870, vol. xi.

to be embraced in this category, and its inclusion within it has been, and even still remains, one of the chief sources of confusion in the study of the secondary forms of inflammation.

For the effective definition of pneumonia, it appears to be an essential condition that the vesicular structure should be filled with the products of inflammation, whether these be desquamated and multiplied epithelial cells, or their derivatives, or fibrinous or mucoid exudations. Unless this definition is adhered to, the study of most pulmonary diseases will be obscured by various fallacies. The essential criterion, in most cases of doubt, is the effect of insufflation, which rarely fails to redistend parts where the alveoli are not filled with inflammatory exudation. Where, from obstruction of the bronchi, or from long continuance of collapse, insufflation is impossible, the distinction can still commonly be made by the greater toughness of collapsed portions, as well as by their glistening appearance, and, in the majority of cases, by the smoothness of their section. The latter features are only simulated, in rare cases, by a pneumonic infiltration of the serous or gelatiniform type. The application of the test is not unimportant, even in the early condition of the mammillated islets in their red stage (see *ante*, p. 23), for many even of these are thus found to be only congested spots of collapse.

Rindfleisch has stated, as the result of his observations, that all forms of pneumonia, including the acute disease occurring in children under five years of age, are of the 'desquamative' variety, and therefore identical with the catarrhal forms. The significance of the term 'desquamative,' as inapplicable to any special class or variety of pneumonia, will be hereafter considered. I am unable, from microscopic research, to offer any opinion on Rindfleisch's statement, but some facts respecting the relation of the catarrhal to the acute pneumonia of childhood require, I think, to be specially considered. One of these is that in typical acute apex-pneumonia, at early periods of life, collapse takes place amidst and around pneumonic portions to a much greater extent than is observed in the adult, so that a large part of the apparently consolidated lung may be inflated; and I think it not improbable that in these collapsed parts, 'desquamation' of epithelium may occur, in the same manner as in the collapsed portions of lungs affected with broncho-pneumonia. Another point is that in pneumonia in the child, commencing suddenly at the apex, and ending in crisis, generalised bronchitis may occur as a complication. The bronchitis may even run its course to a fatal termination, with dilated bronchi and collapse of lung, after the primary apex-affection has resolved,—as shown both clinically and by post-mortem observation.[1] I have already attempted to show (in the section on acute primary pneumonia) that the amount of epithelial-like cells and their derivatives in the alveoli is, even in the adult, subject to many variations, and the fact that the same phenomenon is observable in the child is not therefore surprising.

Rautenberg [2] goes even farther, and asserts that fibrinous exudations or leucocytes may be found in the catarrhal pneumonia of childhood, and that, even to the naked eye, no distinction is possible between this and the 'croupous' form; while the same difficulty occurs in the clinical diagnosis. Some cases, commencing acutely, may end without crisis, and *vice versâ*. Clinically, I believe that these variations may be explained by the facts which I have just stated as coming under my own observation. Although Rautenberg is disposed to deny the value of a distinction of the catarrhal pneumonia of childhood from the acute 'lobar' form, I think that it is one which may yet be maintained

[1] See also Barthez and Rilliet, p. 480. [2] *Jahrb. der Kinderheilkunde*, N.F. 1875, viii. 105 *et seq.*

on both pathological and clinical grounds. At the same time the histological appearances cannot be made the chief support of the distinction.

Nearly the whole group of pneumonias excited artificially belong to the class of broncho-pneumonia. It was remarked by Gendrin,[1] that when an animal was made to breathe chlorine, the lungs were filled with small white nodules which were due to exudation into the alveoli, and similar results were obtained by Bretonneau from the inhalation of the fumes of hydrochloric acid.[2] The changes observed by Cruveilhier after the injection of mercury into the bronchi (by which he believed that he caused the formation of tubercles) belong also to this category; each globule of mercury was surrounded by a zone of pus.[3] Other chemical and mechanical irritants, such as hot steam,[4] excite very similar changes, but the appearances produced vary with the intensity of the inflammation excited. Thus, as Sommerbrodt remarked,[5] simple blood injected into the trachea produced only an epithelial desquamation, while perchloride of iron gave rise to fibrinous exudations with the production of leucocytes.

Similar differences have been observed by Dreschfeld[6] and Veraguth[7] in the effects of weak and strong solutions of nitrate of silver. The nodules of pneumonia thus excited, as well as those seen after section of the vagus (which are equally due to the passage of irritating matters from the mouth to the bronchi) are often apparently preceded by spots of collapse, sunken and bluish, which afterwards acquire a redder tint, and then pass into yellowish spots (like those described by Gendrin and Bretonneau), and which may eventually soften into small abscesses. Stronger irritants, such as ammonia, produce not only a membranous exudation in the trachea and bronchi, as noticed by Reitz,[8] but the lungs, as I have observed, are found studded with small solid spots, which are not prominent, are finely granular, rarely exceed the size of a pea, and break down into abscesses. When these lungs are examined microscopically, the alveoli and infundibula are found in some places filled only with granular débris, in which no cell-structures are apparent. In one specimen of this nature I found also that an intense inflammation existed around the larger and smaller bronchi, which moreover were surrounded with zones of alveolar inflammation, resembling those described by Balzer. Although there was large infiltration in the peribronchial tissue, nothing of the kind could be seen in the alveolar wall, except in places where considerable capillary extravasation of blood had occurred.

CATARRHAL PNEUMONIA IN THE ADULT.—The characteristics of pneumonia extending from the bronchi, as they have been above described, are much more commonly met with in the child than in the adult. One reason for this depends probably on the fact that acute attacks of bronchitis are not only more common in the early periods of life (partly from their general association with epidemic diseases), but also because they are more intense and more fatal, from the greater facility and extent with which collapse of the lung occurs in childhood. Wilks and Moxon have, however, recorded a series of cases where, in an epidemic of measles occurring in the crew of a ship, the lungs of those dying presented appearances identical with those seen in the same disease in childhood.[9] In diphtheria and variola the appearances seen in the child and adult are very similar, but in acute bronchial catarrh they are less common. There is indeed occasional clinical

---

[1] *Histoire Anatomique des Inflammations*, Paris, 1826, p. 302.
[2] *Des Inflammations Spéciales du Tissu Muqueux*, Paris, 1826, p. 100.
[3] *Anat. Path. Générale*, iv. 544, also *Médecine Pratique éclairée par l'Anatomie Pathologique*, 1821, p. 171, and *Bull. Soc. Anat.* Oct. 1, 1826.
[4] Heidenhain, Virchow's *Archiv*, vol. lxx.
[5] Virchow's *Archiv*, vol. lv.
[6] *Lancet*, 1876, p. 47.
[7] Virchow's *Archiv*. Bd. 82.
[8] *Sitzungsbericht K.K. Akad. Wissensch.* 1867, *Nat. Wissensch.* vol. lv.
[9] *Pathological Anat.* ed. 1875, p. 331.

evidence, in the course of acute bronchitis in middle life, that lobular extension to the pulmonary tissue has occurred. This evidence depends for the most part on the intensity of the prostration, on the severity of the fever (102° to 103°), or on the puriform character of the expectoration and the general distribution of the secretion, as shown by the abundant dissemination of fine râles. But I have only seen one such uncomplicated case prove fatal before middle life, and I have never had an opportunity of verifying the inference by post-mortem observation. In advanced life, however, bronchitis assumes more severe and dangerous forms, constituting the 'peripneumonia notha' of Sydenham. Although it frequently proves fatal, either by collapse and congestion of lung (splenisation) or by an acute inflammatory œdema (the 'pneumonia œdematosa' of Cruveilhier,[1] the 'pneumonia serosa' of Traube), genuine hepatisation, as before defined, may be wanting.

It is further to be remarked that, as has been noticed by most writers on the diseases of old age, bronchitis is a more common antecedent or complication of the pneumonia of advanced life than of middle age ; but it is probable that in a considerable proportion of these, the pneumonia differs in its essential character from the acute primary form, and cannot therefore be included in the category of broncho-pneumonia.[2] Although, however, they are less common, some of the most characteristic features of the broncho-pneumonia of childhood are occasionally met with in old age, and among these may be mentioned the dilatations of the bronchi filled with puriform secretion,[3] and also the lobular forms of inflammation. The latter, as Durand-Fardel has remarked, occur, for the most part, in the centre of portions in that state of engorgement to which the term 'splenisation' is applicable. While the greater part of the tissue may be insufflated, these islets present 'soft friable spots and greyish marblings, from which a sanious fluid escapes, which does not 'proceed from the bronchi. These isolated points, which the eye can scarcely distinguish 'in the midst of the engorged tissue, finish by uniting either into isolated nodules of the 'so-called lobular pneumonia, or into true hepatisations, which appear, as in primary 'pneumonia, smooth ("*planiforme*") or granular, red or suppurating.'[4] Even when more extended, as Durand-Fardel has remarked, this hepatisation may be distinct on insufflation, islets or tracts, where the air can still penetrate, are then seen in the midst of the consolidated tissue. This character is not unfrequently found even in the acute primary pneumonia of childhood, which is complicated by collapse to a greater extent than in the adult. In the latter this appearance may be taken as a tolerably characteristic sign that collapse and congestion have preceded the inflammation. It is thus seen that the filling of the air-vesicles with products of inflammation occurs in the adult, as a secondary consequence of bronchitis, in the same manner as in the child, but that it occurs to a still greater degree through the intervention of extensive collapse and antecedent engorgement, and the truly lobular forms are less commonly found.

A large proportion of the appearances described by the earlier writers as the broncho-

---

[1] *Anat. Path. du Corps Humain*, liv. 40, pl. iv. p. 5.
[2] The data given by Grisolle (*Traité de la Pneumonie*, p. 180) and other facts quoted by him from Laennec, Andral, and Chomel, have not their significance affected by any more recent clinical observations. Grisolle says that between the ages of 50 and 70, pneumonia is almost always preceded by either an acute or chronic bronchitis, except in the months of July, August, September, and October. Lebert also (*Klinik der Brustkrankheiten*, 1874, p. 471) says that many cases of acute pneumonia are preceded by bronchial catarrh, which, however, appears to exercise no influence on the subsequent course of the disease.

[3] Hourmann and Dechambre, *Arch. Générales*, 2 sér., xii. 274. Fauvel (*Arch. Générales*, 3 sér. x. p. 279) has also observed these cases. In one, the terminal bronchi were dilated to small cavities of the size of a pea. Another case is recorded by him (*Union Médicale*, 1847, p. 161), and another is given by Béhier (*Conférences Clinique Médicale*, p. 201). See also Durand-Fardel, *Maladies des Vieillards*, p. 473. I have likewise seen in the lungs of an adult, dying of albuminuria, the whole lower lobe collapsed, with islets of pneumonic consolidation surrounding small dilatations of the bronchi, which were filled with pus.
[4] Durand-Fardel, *Maladies des Vieillards*, p. 484.

pneumonia of old age, are, however, simply conditions of collapse. This is probably true especially of the 'planiform' variety described by Hourmann and Dechambre (whose description has been reproduced by most subsequent writers), while the form which they described as 'intervesicular,' in which the pus could be removed by pressure, was probably due to accumulations in the finer bronchi.

That in some forms of pneumonia the cut surface may be smooth instead of being granular, has been already stated in respect even of the acute disease. It depends, however, on the quality and fluidity of the exudation, and does not *per se* prove its special origin as a catarrhal affection.

The histology of the broncho-pneumonia of old age has received but little attention, and I have not had favourable opportunities for investigating it.

OTHER FORMS OF ACUTE PNEUMONIA.

The other forms of acute pneumonia still remain a subject of some obscurity, and of doubt with respect to their classification ; the obscurity is in part due to the terms employed by some writers, in part to the opinion, which has recently gained ground, that acute pneumonia is a disease of specific origin, and is to be separated, not only clinically but anatomically, from all other forms of the disease.[1] The discussion of the clinical and etiological question I must reserve for another work ; but it is desirable that the anatomical side of the subject should be considered as far as possible apart from its technical aspect. It may be here remarked that in the published cases of epidemic and pythogenic forms of the disease, which afford the strongest evidence for its specific origin, the post-mortem appearances and the changes in the lung present but little difference from the ordinary acute forms,[2] although in some the hepatisation is distinguished by softness and œdema of lung,[3] and even by a tendency to a lobular character,[4] and in some by a tendency to gangrene.[5] The other predominant features are a tendency to localisation at the apex, to a migratory character of the inflammation, to early grey hepatisation, and to multiple inflammation of the serous membranes and other parts,[6] while in those of an erysipelatous character, the fibrinous quality of the hepatisation is even denied.[7]

It is, however, needful to allude to two terms which have recently been largely applied to all forms of pneumonia not presenting the solid fibrinous coagulum typical of the acute disease, and have been employed, both etymologically and clinically, in an indefinite manner, without adequate proof of the nature of the changes which their meaning conveys. The first of these is the term 'catarrhal' applied to all forms of pneumonia in which the exudation has not the character already mentioned. This term, as is well known, was extended by the late Professor Niemeyer to most forms of phthisical consolidation, though a marked discrepancy exists between his descriptions of catarrhal pneumonia as a substantial disease, and as occurring in phthisis. Not a few writers, in following him, have

---

[1] See Jürgensen, Ziemssen's *Handbuch*, Bd. v. 'Krank. Resp. App.' ii. 145.
[2] Grimshaw & Moore, 'Pythogenic Pneumonia,' *Dublin Journal Med. Science*, May 1875.
[3] Rodman, *American Journal Med. Science*, January 1876.
[4] Ritter, *Deutsch. Archiv klin. Med.* 1880, vol. xxv.
[5] Chomel, *Dict. de Méd.* xxv. 189 ; Maclachlan, *Dis. and Infirmities of Advanced Life*, p. 180.
[6] Kühn, *Deutsch. Archiv klin. Med.* 1878, vol. xxi. and *Berliner klin. Woch.* 1879, p. 552.
[7] Strauss, *Revue Mensuelle*, 1879, iii. 695.

described as 'catarrhal pneumonia' all forms of inflammatory consolidation of the lung in which fibrinous exudation is deficient or scanty, and in which the epithelial cell-forms predominate in the air-vesicles. Although, however, this condition is largely found in some cases in which the vesicular inflammation has apparently extended from the bronchi, it does not constitute an absolute proof that all pneumonias thus characterised have had this origin (see *ante*, p. 18). Nor is the analogy perfect in other respects, for in some cases of acute pneumonia, having no other apparent origin than a chill, the predominant cell-forms in the alveoli are pyoid and of a smaller type, and *per contra*, in some cases of typical broncho-pneumonia, and notably in those resulting from section of the vagus nerve, the small cells largely preponderate over the epithelioid forms, while in some of these, actual fibrinous exudations have been demonstrated. It would therefore appear desirable to limit the use of the term catarrhal pneumonia to those cases in which the pulmonary inflammation is demonstrably the result of extension from the bronchi. To apply it to other forms is to obscure our knowledge of the etiology of pneumonia, and also to lead to erroneous aims in the study of its pathology. But it must, I think, be said that, at present, besides the character of broncho-pneumonia described in the preceding section, no special anatomical distinctive features are known, which may enable us authoritatively to assert that any case is pathologically catarrhal, apart from its clinical history and etiology. Even some forms that appear lobular to the naked eye, are not therefore certainly catarrhal, since islets of consolidation may be scattered through lungs affected with acute primary pneumonia,[1] and they are found also in certain acute diseases in which the catarrhal origin is at least doubtful, as in typhoid and erysipelas ; they also form in some cases with great rapidity after extensive burns,[2] where again their production can hardly be ascribed to a process identical with that by which they arise in the course of whooping-cough, though the pulmonary changes (with the exception of the dilatation of the bronchi) are in appearance almost identical.[3] My own conviction is that, with certain exceptions, almost all, and perhaps all, forms of the disease are due to nutritional changes in the pulmonary tissue, arising from constitutional states, and probably from changes in the blood. The exceptions are the forms of vesicular pneumonia which are demonstrably traceable to the extension of inflammation from the bronchi, and correspond to those that are produced by the direct introduction of irritants. All of these have a more or less close resemblance to the broncho-pneumonia of childhood. Apart from these exceptions this form of pneumonia is due to constitutional states. The occurrence of the inflammation may undoubtedly be favoured by local conditions, and notably by collapse and hyperæmia, but another element of causation is generally present, and is probably of the nature of a *materies morbi*. This may possibly be shown to be due to some special morbific poison, introduced from without ; although the proof of such a cause is by no means yet absolute for all the typical cases ending critically, there is a strong probability of its existence in some of the pythogenic and epidemic forms of the disease. The evidence is, however, equally strong, if not stronger, that the blood states of other acute diseases are also able to excite pulmonary inflammation. In measles, for instance, acute lobar inflammation occasionally occurs with a rapidity of consolidation equalling that of the acute primary disease ; the same is true of typhoid, of erysipelas, and

---

[1] Eppinger (*Prager Vierteljahrschrift*, vol. cxv. Post-mortem Report) divides the 'croupous' pneumonias into 356 cases of lobular, and 383 lobar = 739 cases. Of the 383 cases lobar, 255 were primary, and 128 secondary. The other forms met with in a total of 973 cases were, hypostatic, 151 ; catarrhal, 32 ; metastatic, 24 ; chronic, 27.

[2] Balzer has seen them form within twenty-four hours, *Thesis*, p. 19.

[3] See Wilks' descriptions, *Guy's Hosp. Rep.* 1860. 3rd Ser. vi. 146 *et seq.*

even of acute rheumatism. The analogy of the latter appears to render it at least quite as probable that in the diffuse forms of the disease, occurring in measles and influenza, the *materies morbi* is brought to the lung-tissue by the blood, as that it is conveyed to them simply by the air-passages, and that both the bronchitis and the pneumonia should be regarded as effects common to one morbific cause.

Another term which was introduced by the late Professor Buhl, is that of 'Desquamative Pneumonia' as applied to the forms of the disease in which the alveoli are filled with epithelial, in contradistinction to fibrinous, products. As a simple description of the histological appearances observed in some forms or phases of consolidation, the term is strictly applicable; but I think that it is incapable of being employed to define any single group of pulmonary consolidations as a basis for clinical classification—the more so as, according to Buhl's own admission, it can often only be distinguished by microscopic examination. He, as is well known, divided this variety into two classes,[1] the 'consecutive desquamative' (under which he classed all secondary pneumonias of fever, and the 'genuine,' under which he classed nearly all the consolidations of phthisis, including even, with some modification, the acute miliary tubercle. This 'genuine' form was, in his opinion, further characterised by the invasion of the alveolar wall. The latter subject will be more fully considered hereafter, under the head of phthisis. It may be sufficient to state here my own conviction that not all the diffuse pneumonias of phthisis are characterised by the large-celled desquamation of a catarrhal type, and that some are found with smaller cells, and also occasionally with fibrinous exudation. In relation to the acute and simple 'consecutive forms,' it must also be remarked that, in many of these, the pyoid cells preponderate largely over the epithelial ; and finally, as has been more recently shown by Buhl himself, an acute pneumonia, clinically indistinguishable from the typical primary disease, may be characterised histologically by the filling of the alveoli with epithelioid cells of the 'desquamative' type.[2]

By some writers, and especially by Rindfleisch,[3] the term 'desquamative' has been used as synonymous with 'catarrhal' pneumonia ; though Buhl,[4] as is well known, expressly distinguished the two forms, and even denied the existence of a catarrhal pneumonia. I have already remarked on the difficulty of maintaining this position, and would refer to the description already given of the catarrhal inflammation in support of this opinion. One variety of pneumonia appears to require, however, special mention, and of this I shall treat separately.

HYPOSTATIC, OR CONGESTIVE, PNEUMONIA.

This form of inflammation of the lung is that which holds an intermediate place between the genuine catarrhal pneumonia and most of the secondary forms of pulmonary inflammation, with the exception of those directly caused by infective emboli in pyæmia. Laennec gave to it the name of *Pneumonie des agonisans*.[5] The description by Piorry[6]

---

[1] *Lungenentzündung, Tuberculose und Schwindsucht*, 1872, p. 40 et seq.
[2] *Mittheilungen aus dem Path. Institute zu München.*
[3] *Lehrbuch*, 5th ed. 1878, pp. 353-4.
[4] *Lungenentzündung &c.* pp. 41-2.
[5] *Ausc. Méd.* 2nd ed. p. 470.
[6] *Clinique de l'Hôpital de la Pitié*, 1888. 'Mémoire sur la Pneumonie Hypostatique.'

has undergone but few subsequent material additions, and the chief point remaining for discussion respecting it is that relating to its origin and pathological position.

This form of pneumonia is figured in Plate III. It occurs in engorged and congested portions of the lung, some of which are entirely airless, while others still crepitate and float in water. The site, as Piorry remarked, is most commonly at the posterior portions, but not always at the bases, except in some rare cases in which the patient, prior to death, has been obliged to maintain the erect posture. It is generally found near the middle portions of the lung and near its root, but it is seldom strictly lobar.

The tissue in which the alveolar inflammation has occurred is non-elastic, and is usually more friable than natural, but this is common, in a greater or less degree, to all forms of engorgement except those consecutive to old-standing heart-disease, which will be described subsequently. The pneumonic process, which occurs in this engorged tissue, is marked by an increase of opacity, by a change of the deep vinous red to a grayer or whitish tint, by a greater appearance of solidity, by the fact that the part thus affected is commonly raised above the margin of the surrounding tissue, and, in the larger proportion of cases, by a more or less granular appearance of the cut surface, usually more apparent on scraping. The colour varies from a deep red, often darker than that of most forms of acute red hepatisation, to a tint as pale as that seen in the plate. The consistence is also variable. In some instances the consolidated part is exceedingly soft and friable, breaking into a pulp under slight pressure; in some, on the other hand, it is as firm as the firmest hepatisation. It tends, in the acute diseases, to pass rapidly into a soft grey hepatisation, but in the less acute affections it may apparently persist, at least during seven days, in a firm state, in which the red colour is maintained. The amount of fluid which exudes from the surface varies with these different conditions of origin, but in all it is of a more opaque and sanious appearance than is found on pressing or scraping parts which are merely the subjects of splenisation. The pneumonia always commences in islets of variable size, which tend to become confluent. It is, however, rare for them to be found isolated and diffusely scattered, as are the lobular spots of inflammation seen in catarrhal pneumonia.[1]

The *Microscopic Appearances* of hypostatic pneumonia present in many cases no essential differences from those seen in the acute and sthenic forms. The fibrinous reticulum is less marked, but the cell-forms observed are nearly identical. In large tracts the alveoli may be found filled with small pyoid cells with tripartite nuclei, like XXV. 9, *g*, *h*. Large epithelioid cells, like XXV. 9, *N*, may also be seen, and also large pigmented cells like *p* and *q*. Jürgensen has stated that most secondary pneumonias are 'catarrhal,'[2] but though tracts may here and there be found having the 'desquamative' character, I believe that, in a large proportion, the cell-types approximate more to those now described.

The mechanism of this form of pneumonia is probably complex. The chief points of interest respecting it are, firstly, its relation to catarrhal pneumonia; secondly, the mechanism by which the congestion is produced; and, lastly, the mode of origin of the inflammation.

The analogy of the splenised parts found at the termination of exhausting diseases to similar changes found in the course of acute bronchitis in children is very close, and

---

[1] Piorry, (*loc. cit.* p. 139,) described them as thus isolated, but it appears most probable that these cases may have been examples of genuine catarrhal pneumonia, inasmuch as he described the bronchi filled with pus.

[2] Ziemssen's *Handbuch*, Bd. v. '*Krankh. Resp. App.*' ii. 235. Jürgensen appears to rely in part on a statement to this effect in Rindfleisch's *Path. Gewebelehre*, p. 362. In the 5th edition of this work, p. 357, Rindfleisch appears to have modified this opinion, for he says that hypostatic secondary pneumonia may be either 'croupous' or 'catarrhal.'

led Gairdner to attribute them, when found in fever, to the same mechanism—viz. obstruction of the bronchi; and his observations clearly show that in many cases bronchitis has preceded the collapse and splenisation, as is shown by the occurrence of 'bronchial abscesses.'[1] Bronchitis, as is known, is a frequent attendant on fever, and, though collapse of lungs from this cause in the primary bronchitis of adults is rare, it is easily promoted in fever by the diminished muscular power, which prevents free expansion of the chest. This may also further explain its occurrence in the most dependent parts, for it is on these that the weight of the body presses, and thus further interferes with expansion. The frequency of the affection in the terminal stage of all exhausting diseases,[2] and in cases where no recognisable signs of bronchitis exist after death, renders it probable that congestion from defective circulation may play no small part in the production of these secondary pneumonias. In some cases, in the splenised parts, the collapse is by no means perfect, and it appears likely that in some of these it may be due to simple muscular weakness without the intervention of bronchial obstruction. The effect of position in determining the locality of congestion, and also the secondary pneumonia, is too constantly authenticated by the universal consent of all observers to permit any doubt to remain respecting the influence of this agent in their production.[3]

That mere congestion can alone be sufficient to excite this inflammation of the lung must be regarded as improbable, and hence the most adequate explanation of its origin appears to be that there is some morbid condition of the blood, which finally determines inflammatory nutritional changes in the congested and weakened parts.

While, therefore, hypostatic pneumonia has a resemblance to some phases of catarrhal pneumonia in its frequent origin in collapse, it is probable that, in a large proportion of cases, the mechanism of its production is diverse, and that it requires to be placed in a different pathological category from that variety. As in catarrhal, so also in hypostatic pneumonia, there are variations in the degree and frequency with which the pleura is affected. Both Piorry and Durand-Fardel stated that pleurisy is rarely a complication[4] of this form. The explanation appears to be that simple congestion and collapse are not attended with pleural inflammation. Such inflammation is also absent as long as the pneumonic consolidation is central; but, as far as my observation has gone, hyperæmia of the membrane, and plastic lymph upon it, are usually observed whenever the pulmonary inflammation reaches the surface of the lung.

---

[1] Gairdner, *Pathological Results of Bronchitis*, Edinburgh, 1850, p. 22 *et seq.*
[2] See Grisolle, *Traité de la Pneumonie*, p. 170 *et seq.*
[3] Grisolle (*loc. cit.* p. 178) gives a case where a patient with typhoid, obliged, by scars in the sacrum, to lie on her face, was affected with pneumonia limited to the anterior portions of both lungs; he cites numerous other instances. See also Piorry's *Memoir*; Vulpian, *Pneumonies Secondaires*; and a case from Rayer, *Malad. des Reins*, ii. 293, in which a patient obliged to maintain the sitting posture had the lower portions of both lungs affected with pneumonia. A similar case is also recorded by Jürgensen, Ziemssen's *Handbuch*, 'Krank. Resp. Apparat.' ii. 235.
[4] Piorry, *loc. cit.* p. 148; Durand-Fardel, *Malad. des Vieillards*, pp. 487, 502.

ACUTE INTERSTITIAL PNEUMONIA.

INTERLOBULAR PNEUMONIA, DISSECTING PNEUMONIA, ANGEIOLEUCITIS PULMONALIS (?),
LYMPHANGITIS PULMONALIS (?).

Plate XXIV. Figure 2.

ACUTE inflammation of the interstitial tissue of the lung is a disease that presents great rarity, though it is the common form of pleuro-pneumonia of the bovine species.[1] The illustration here given is from an unpublished drawing of Sir Robert Carswell, who has left the following manuscript description of the case:—

'*Lymphatics of the Lung containing Pus.*—A great number of lymphatics are seen 'ramifying under the pleura and running towards the glands situated at the bifurcation 'of the trachea. The larger ones follow the lobular divisions of the lung, while the largest 'traverse them indistinctly and terminate in the immediate vicinity of the bronchial glands, 'beyond which no trace of them can be seen. The pus they contained was quite fluid, and 'flowed out of them when their walls were punctured. There was no pus in the glands 'around which these lymphatics terminated; they were nearly black and very firm. 'When the lung was divided, the interlobular cellular substance' (XXIV. 2) 'was found 'to be much more conspicuous than natural, of a pale yellow colour, and infiltrated with 'pus. The lymphatics could also be seen in this substance filled with pus, and could be 'traced from it to the surface of the lung, where they were seen uniting with those lying 'under the pleura. The pulmonary substance was red, firmer than natural, and infiltrated 'with serosity. This state of the pulmonary tissue gradually diminished from the centre 'to the circumference; and in the same manner, also, those states of the lobular cellular 'tissue and lymphatics which have been described became less apparent, and ultimately 'disappeared, where the pulmonary tissue was healthy. There was no pus found anywhere 'else.

'The patient was nearly sixty years of age, and had been treated during some weeks 'for chronic inflammation of the bladder. He was a surgical patient. No affection of the 'lungs was suspected.'

The disease may apparently be due to general, or at least to unascertained, causes, or it may be attributable to local conditions in which the inflammation appears to extend along the lymphatics, either excited by some primary focus or by simple obstruction. Stokes[2] has reported a case which, admitted with 'the ordinary symptoms of pneumonia 'of three days' standing,' presented after death the following appearances : ' The substance 'of the lower lobe was completely dissected from its pleura by the suppurative inflammation 'of the subserous cellular (?) membrane. This process was also found to have invaded 'extensively the interlobular and intervesicular cellular structure, so as to cause this part 'of the lung to resemble nearly the structure of a bunch of grapes. All nearly isolated 'lobules were surrounded by puriform matter, in which they hung from the bronchial 'pedicles.' Stokes thought this case analogous to one of plastic bronchitis, quoted by him from Reynaud ; but it appears probable that it belongs to a different category, inasmuch as, except in a few cases of suppurative peribronchitis, no such appearances are commonly observed in the plastic form of the disease. It has been described by

---

[1] See Weber, of Kiel, Virchow's *Archiv*, vol. i.   [2] *Diseases of the Chest*, p. 144.

Rokitanski,[1] as met with in a single case, in terms very similar to those just quoted from Stokes. Hodgkin[2] has also seen pus in the interlobular cellular tissue in a case of œdema of the lung. The disease is also described by Buhl as an occasional complication of pyæmia in the adult, and as being most common in newly-born children who have been infected from pyæmic mothers.[3] In the latter condition the pulmonary tissue is mapped out by the interlobular septa, which are thickened, yellow, and friable. The lung itself is either airless or œdematous, or presents combinations of both these conditions. It is dense but friable, sometimes exceedingly so. The pleura is often inflamed, and is occasionally raised in vesicles over the purulent collections in the interlobular septa. Buhl described the disease as most commonly extending from the root of the lung along the bronchial vessels. Similar conditions have been seen in women dying from puerperal septicæmia.[4] It has also been observed in pneumonia, probably of a septic origin,[5] and also in broncho-pneumonia.[6] Wiedermann[7] relates a case where two children in one family suffered in this way, and questions whether they can have been infected by the milk of a cow affected with pleuro-pneumonia. Hitherto, however, there has been no proof that this disease in cattle is communicated to man.[8] Among local conditions of origin, the disease may extend from mediastinal suppuration, as I have seen in a case of retro-pharyngeal abscess. The interlobular septa of the lower lobe of one lung were thickened and yellow, and the seat of purulent infiltration. The lung-tissue between was unaffected, though several pyæmic abscesses were scattered throughout the tissue. Goodhart[9] has also described a very similar condition in a case of suppurative mediastinitis, where the lymphatics in the deeper as well as in the more superficial parts of the lung were equally affected. Spots of yellow hepatisation existed in places, but as a rule the alveolar tissue was free from change. An instance has been recorded by Virchow, where a localised dissecting pneumonia, connected with a loculate empyema, had almost separated a limited portion of the lung from the remainder, which was healthy.[10] Extension of inflammation of the pleura to the pulmonary lymphatics has been observed by Edward Wagner[11] and by Cornil and Ranvier.[12] The disease occasionally appears to be associated with previous injury to the lymphatic glands at the hilus of the lung; this, by obstructing the passage of lymph, renders the ducts from the periphery liable to inflammation from external exciting causes. This mode of origin, which was first clearly elucidated by Moxon,[13] was shown by him to exist in two cases where pleurisy was associated with extensive suppuration of the lymphatics of the lung.

Similar changes, associated with evidence of past disease of the glands, have been found

[1] Path. Anat. iii. 72.
[2] Morbid Anatomy of Serous and Mucous Membranes, ii. 129.
[3] Buhl, Lungenentzündung, Tuberculose und Schwindsucht, p. 43 et seq.; also Hecker and Buhl, Klinik des Geburtskindes, i. 202. This has now been shown to result from direct extension from the umbilical vein beneath the peritoneum to the mediastinum. See Müller, Puerperal Infection der Neugeborenen; Gerhardt's Handbuch Kinderkrankheiten, vol. ii., quoted by Silbermann, Deutsch Arch. klin. Med. xxxiv. 348.
[4] Bélier, Conférences de Clinique médicale, p. 654; also Quinquaud, Puerpérisme Infectueux, Thèse de Paris, 1872; Longuet, Annales de Gynécologie, 1874, No. 1; Heiberg, Die Puerperalen und Pyämischen Processe, Leipzig, 1873, p. 19. All cited by Troisier, Rech. sur les Lymphangites Pulmonaires, Thèse de Paris, 1874.
[5] Liouville, Bull. Soc. Anat. 1878, p. 252 (quoted by Troisier).
[6] Balzer, Art. 'Broncho-Pneumonie,' Nouv. Dict. de Méd. et Chir. Prat. 1880, xxviii. 552.
[7] Deutsch Archiv f. Klin. Med. 1880, vol. xxv.
[8] Costello (Lancet, 1881, i. 141) relates an instance where pneumonia in a regiment in Northern India became epidemic and apparently contagious, nearly 40 men being attacked out of a strength of 550, while 60 men out of another regiment died. Pleuro-pneumonia was very common at the time among the cattle in the district, but, as far as can be judged by the post-mortem reports, the disease in these troops did not present the same appearances as are observed in cattle, or as those now described. Gangrene, and also abscess of the lung, were, however, common.
[9] Path. Soc. Trans. 1877, xxviii. 87.
[10] Virchow's Gesammelte Abhandlungen, p. 469.
[11] Archiv der Heilkunde, 1870, vol. xi.
[12] Manuel d'Histol. Pathologique, 580, 2nd ed. ii. 126.
[13] Path. Soc. Trans. xxiv. 20, 28; xxvii. 46.

by other observers. They were seen by Greenhow[1] in a case of Addison's disease, and by Chevalet[2] and Darolles[3] in cases of tubercle. In the latter disease, however, the suppurative character may be indistinct, and it is more probable that the change was of a tubercular nature, similar to that earlier described by Andral.[4] Such changes have also been seen in connection with tumours invading the bronchial glands, both of the nature of lymphoma[5] and of cancer,[6] and it has also been observed by Cornil in syphilis when the bronchial glands were attacked.[7] Some cases remain still unclassified. One of this nature has been published by Damaschino, in which the affection, in a gouty person, extended throughout the lung, and beyond the hilus to the œsophagus. There was effusion of serum in the pleura, and some tubercles were present in the lungs. The condition of the bronchial glands is not stated.[8]

CHRONIC PNEUMONIA. CHRONIC INTERSTITIAL PNEUMONIA.
DILATATION OF THE BRONCHI.

This condition is one that still requires elucidation. In the opinion of some authors a large majority of cases of phthisis must be included under this category, and, according to the opinion that tubercle is a chronic lobular pneumonia, all forms of chronic ulcerative disease of the lung, other than that which arises from cancer, would be embraced under this term. I shall advance reasons to show that it is desirable that the 'tubercular' cases should be distinguished by a different terminology. and in this article I shall consider chiefly those changes in the lung which result from the non-resolution of the acute primary pneumonia or the acute catarrhal pneumonia, and also some forms of pulmonary induration the nature and origin of which are more doubtful. All these cases, when considered apart from tubercle and tubercular pneumonia, are of extreme rarity. Chomel[9] believed that only eight could be collected in the medical literature of his time. Grisolle only met with four, and there are few pathologists who have seen undoubted cases of this nature. In many cases of more recent date, in which fibroid changes in the lung have been described, there is strong reason for believing that these had a past tubercular origin, using the word 'tubercle' in the sense in which it was employed by Laennec. There is, however, both pathological and clinical evidence that acute pneumonia may fail to resolve, and that it may leave behind permanent induration, with bronchial dilatation and ulceration. Evidence of this termination exists both in the case of the acute primary (croupous) pneumonia, and also in that of the catarrhal forms.

The occurrence of this result in primary acute pneumonia was denied by Buhl,[10] but chiefly on theoretical grounds. It has, however, been demonstrated that the stage of red

[1] Greenhow, *Path. Soc. Trans.* xxviii. 231.
[2] Chevalet, *Bull. Soc. Anat.* 1873, p. 252.
[3] Darolles, *Bull. Soc. Anat.* 1875, 3rd ser. x. 35.
[4] *Clin. Méd.* iv. 28. See also Lépine, 'Sur l'Infection de Voisinage dans la Tuberculose,' *Arch. de Physiol.* 1876, p. 297.
[5] A case by Troisier and Cornil, *loc. cit.* p. 43.
[6] Raymond, *Union Méd.* 1874, Nos. 35 and 36; Troisier, Thèse, *loc. cit.* and *Archives de Physiol.* 1874, who quotes numerous other instances. See also Klein, *Anatomy of the Lymphatic Tissues,* 1875, part ii. Many of these cases are, however, illustrations of the extension of cancer rather than of inflammatory changes in the lymphatics.
[7] *Bull. Soc. Méd. Hôp.* 1874, xi. 144. Here the contents of the lymphatics were caseous rather than purulent.
[8] Damaschino, 'Angeioleucite Pulmonaire suppurée chez un Goutteux,' *Bull. Soc. Méd. Hôp.* 1879.
[9] *Dict. de Méd.* 2nd ed. 1842, xxv. 223, 225. He had himself only met with two in 20 years, and only one out of 125 cases of acute pneumonia.
[10] Buhl, *Lungenentzündung, Tuberculose und Schwindsucht,* p. 87.

hepatisation may persist for months, during which induration of tissue and a gradual thickening of the alveolar walls take place,[1] that the red colour may fade into a grey hepatisation attended by the same induration,[2] and that sometimes a yellow tint[3] may be observed, which seems to represent an intermediate stage between the red and the grey. These probably constitute the red and grey induration of Andral, and pass into the black induration described by him.[4]

This black induration is the 'fibroid induration' of some authors, the 'cirrhosis' of others. It will be shown hereafter that it most frequently results from a chronic tuberculisation. Its origin in an acute pneumonia is often uncertain, owing to the length of time during which it may persist, and in many cases it is found without any previous history. There is, however, direct pathological evidence that one of its causes may be an acute pneumonia,[5] and abundant clinical evidence that such a pneumonia may leave permanent consolidation.[6] The condition of induration is also found with a previous history of catarrhal pneumonia, and the direct continuity of the two with it may be traced in some cases.[7] A clinical history, similar to that described for the primary disease, may also be found in some cases, in which the physical signs of induration followed bronchitis, whooping cough, and measles.[8] In some of these cases, particularly in childhood, it may be questioned whether the induration has not in great measure succeeded collapse of the lung. The pneumonia of typhoid is mentioned by Jürgensen as a cause of chronic pulmonary induration, and this is supported by one of Biermer's cases of bronchiectasis;[1] but I know of no evidence, in the general literature of typhoid, proving that the association is more than occasional and rare. In addition to these there exist records of a small number of cases of non-tubercular ulceration of the lung, to which I shall subsequently allude, and these two series are the only cases to which, in strict accuracy, the term 'chronic pneumonia' can be applied. In a large number of instances, when fibroid induration has been found after death, there is no evidence of its mode of origin, and in not a few cases it has been merely an accidental post-mortem discovery. A large number are, I believe, as I have already stated, probably tubercular,[2] and a few may be traced to pleurisy.[3] The origin and nature of the remainder is a matter of inference rather than of positive proof, but I believe that in all, with the possible exception of the cases of pleurisy and collapse, an inflammatory origin is traceable—that an idiopathic fibroid induration of the lung can scarcely be held to be proved—and that, if it exists, it is an event of such extreme rarity that it can hardly be said to have a clinical existence.

The changes in the lung in the forms of chronic pneumonia which I have now described may be followed, in the descriptions of different writers, as a progressive series, to the condition of general fibroid induration. It appears desirable that they should be considered separately.

The red hepatisation differs from that of the acute stage in its progressive induration. Instead of the tissue being friable, it becomes increasingly firm and resistant, and the granular appearance may persist for a long time.[4] Even in this stage marked thickening of the interlobular septa may occur, as shown by whitish lines on the reddened ground.[5] Both the yellow and grey induration present usually a smooth section, and that of the latter is at last firm, glistening, and mottled with pigment, so as to resemble some forms of porphyry. The essential point, in which all observers[6] are agreed, is that these progressive changes depend on a thickening of the alveolar walls with a growth of round and fusiform cells, the latter predominating, which gradually encroaches on the alveolar space,[7] and may form masses projecting into the interior of the alveoli.[8] The interlobular tissue sometimes participates in this thickening, but occasionally, although the sheaths of the arteries and bronchi are thus implicated, the thickening is not general. Heschl believed that this cell-growth proceeds from the nuclei of the capillaries; but Thierfelder and Ackermann deny this, though they state that the capillaries disappear during its progress.

---

[1] Jürgensen, Ziemssen's *Handbuch*, Supplement-Band. p. 325; Biermer, Virchow's *Archiv*, vol. xix. obs. xxix. pp. 160, 274. See also Buhl, *Acute Lungenatrophie*, Virchow's *Archiv*, vol. xi. His cases appear, however, to have been chiefly a quasi-gangrenous pneumonia associated with collapse, in which dilatation of the bronchi occasionally occurred.

[2] See Reynolds's *System of Medicine*, vol. iii.

[3] Peacock, *Edinburgh Med. Journal*, 1855, p. 281; Biermer, Virchow's *Archiv*, vol. xix. obs. v. and xxvi. Dr. McDowell's case of cirrhosis was probably of the same nature (*Dublin Journal*, 1836). Barth also ascribes a pleuritic origin to some cases of bronchiectasis. Compare also two cases by Tapret reported by Regimbeau, *Pneumonie Chronique*, p. 75 *et seq*. obs. v. and vi. abridged also by Charcot, *loc. cit.* p. 789. In the latter of these the pleuritic origin is hypothetical. See likewise Steffen, *Klinik der Kinderkrankheiten*, ii. 59.

[4] See *ante*, note 1, p. 45 (Leyden and Oulmont).

[5] Corbin, *Gaz. Méd. de Paris*, 1845, p. 820, obs. vi. In this case there appears to have been an imperfect resolution, for the tissue crepitated. The history raises a suspicion of albuminuria.

[6] Lebert (*Physiol. Path.*) describes the yellow induration as caused by infiltration of the intervesicular tissue with exudation matter. Cornil and Ranvier describe a chronic catarrhal pneumonia in a child as presenting indurated nodules resembling tubercles, but their case was syphilitic (*Man. d'Histol. Path.* 2nd ed. 1882, ii. 112).

[7] Heschl, *Prager Vierteljahrsch.* 1856, vol. ii. (figure); Förster, *Path. Anat.* 1863, ii. 249, 251; Charcot, *loc. cit.*; Oulmont, *loc. cit.*; Thierfelder and Ackermann (yellow hepatisation), *Deutsch Arch. f. Klin. Med.* 1872, vol. x. (figures); Lancereaux, *Atlas Path. Anat.* pp. 95, 124, 294, 296, pl. xx. xxix. fig. 3.

[8] Thierfelder and Ackermann, *loc. cit.*

CHRONIC PNEUMONIA

In addition, recent researches have shown that part of the induration is due to an actual organisation of the exudation in the interior of the alveoli, which some observers have attributed to the organisation of the white blood-corpuscles, a fibrillar texture being formed, in which the epithelial cells are imbedded and finally disappear. This newly-formed tissue blends with that of the alveolar walls, the elastic fibres of which persist in the earlier stages.[1] That this change is not constant is apparent from the description of the authors above quoted, and also from the case which I append (*Case 32, Attwood*). In this (*see* XLII. 1) the thickening of the walls by a fibronuclear growth passing into broad-banded fibres is very distinct, and the epithelium showed no traces of organisation. In other cases of a more advanced character, when the lung has become almost wholly fibroid, the epithelium has still been found persistent, but assuming a cubical form,[2] and in some the epithelium may be found intact in the interior of the alveoli, which are much diminished in size from the thickening of their walls,[3] while in others it may be largely increased in amount, densely filling the alveoli.[4]

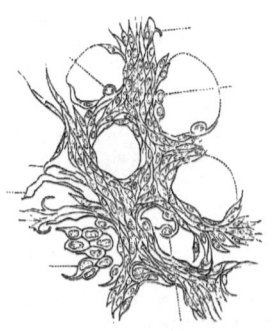

FIG. 38.— Induration of lung, thickening of wall of alveoli by cell-growth. (From Heschl, *Prager Vierteljahrschrift*, 1856, vol. ii.)

The genuine *fibroid induration*, the 'black induration' of Andral, the 'cirrhosis' of recent writers, presents a tissue resembling that of fibro-cartilage; it can be cut only with great difficulty, and creaks under the scalpel. The section is smooth and uniform, except where traversed by the bronchial tubes and vessels. It is more or less deeply pigmented, sometimes intensely so, and the surface is crossed by white bands representing the thickened interlobular septa, which are less pigmented than is the indurated pulmonary tissue. The lung is greatly diminished in size, and the pleura covering it is usually extremely thickened. The lung-tissue, thus changed, presents a structure in which the fibre element predominates in various degrees. In some parts the structure is entirely fibroid, with broad bands of anastomosing and interlacing fibres. Where this transformation is still incomplete, fusiform cells are found, and in other places round cells passing into fusiform or directly into fibre tissue.[5]

The induration of the lung which succeeds to compression by pleurisy differs in some marked features from the foregoing, and it is doubtful whether the term 'chronic pneumonia' is applicable to it, although it has been described by many as a 'chronic interstitial pneumonia.' The latter term may perhaps be applicable to some extent, inasmuch as, during the acute stage of pleurisy, the interlobular septa, extending from the inflamed membrane, are found filled with inflammatory products, and this change may sometimes

---

[1] See T. H. Green, *Pathology and Morbid Anatomy*, 3rd ed. p. 6, 4th ed. p. 356. Woronichen, *Sitz-Bericht, kk. Akad. Wiss. zu Wien*, 1868, vol. lv. ii. attributed this organisation to cells derived from the epithelium; Eppinger, *Prager Vierteljahrschrift*, 1875, vol. cxxv. (white corpuscles); Sydney Coupland, *Path. Trans.* 1880, vol. xxx. and *Lancet*, 1879 (leucocytes); Marchand, Virchow's *Archiv*, 1880, vol. xxxii. (white corpuscles).

[2] Küttner, Virchow's *Archiv*, 1876, lxvi. 21; Laveran, *Union Méd.* 1880, No. 22, supplement; Charest, *Rev. Mensuelle*, 1878, p. 784.

[3] Oulmont, *Progrès Médicale*, 1877, p. 584.

[4] Thierfelder and Ackermann, *loc. cit.* This case was of 19 months' standing. They teem in epithelial hepatisation. See also report by T. H. Green and Burdon-Sanderson on C. T. Williams's case, *Path. Trans.* 1870, vol. xvi.

[5] See Heschl's descriptions, *loc. cit.*; also the case of Attwood (Case 32).

extend for a considerable distance into the interior of the lung.[1] I have already produced evidence to show that some cases of chronic pulmonary induration may proceed from an old pleurisy, but the cases in which this mode of origin has been actually demonstrated are comparatively few.[2] Some authors have, however, placed them in a special class, under the name of 'pleurogenic pneumonias.'[3]

There is indeed strong *à priori* probability that the induration thus resulting from pleurisy would develop in this manner, but, considering the frequency of pleural effusions, it is somewhat remarkable how rarely uncomplicated cases of this nature can be met with, and in a very large proportion the lung remains simply collapsed and airless; although hard and tough, it presents no special growth of connective tissue in the alveolar walls or interlobular septa, like that resulting from acute pneumonia.[4] Some authors, and notably Lebert,[5] have ascribed a large proportion of cases of bronchial dilatation, associated with induration of the lung, to past pleurisies; but the statistics of bronchiectasis show that the theory is scarcely tenable, since a large number originate either in acute or catarrhal pneumonia or in tubercle.[6]

It is probable that collapse of the lung may lead to similar changes. Rokitanski has stated that it is attended with fibro-nuclear growth in the walls of the alveoli,[7] but the process by which induration proceeds from this has been very little studied.[8]

The term 'interstitial pneumonia' has, however, been applied in a general sense (I believe inaccurately) to a large number of all cases of fibroid thickenings of the lung (including those of tubercular origin, to which I shall refer in another section), and some authors, who use the term, expressly state that the site of this thickening is in the alveolar wall.[9] I believe that it is desirable, in a pathological sense, to regard the latter as distinct from thickening of the interlobular septa, although the two conditions may be occasionally combined. The number of cases in which thickening of the interlobular septa has been found as an independent condition, apart from the other changes, is limited to five.[10] It

---

[1] E. Wagner, 'Beiträge Path. Anat. der Pleura,' *Archiv für Heilkunde*, vol. xi.; Klein, *Anatomy of the Lymphatic System*.

[2] See ante, note 3, p. 46; also Brouardel, *Bull. Soc. Méd. Hôp.* 1872, p. 168; Parrot, *Gaz. Hebdom.* 1864 (Canstatt's *Jahrsbericht*, 1864). Ziemssen (*Pleuritis und Pneumonie im Kindesalter*, p. 93) says that from his clinical experience he believes bronchiectasis to be not uncommon, but that he has not met with pathological proof.

[3] Charcot, *Rev. Mens.* 1878; Ziegler, *Lehrb. Path. Anat.* 1889, p. 880 (figures).

[4] Goodhart (*Guy's Hosp. Rep.* 1877, p. 215) believes that fibroid change in the lung, with interlobular thickening extending along the bronchi, is almost constant in *empyema*. But in 24 post-mortems there are only three in which this change is distinctly mentioned; one of these was tubercular, in another there was bronchial dilatation. In three the lung was airless and hard; in one it was healthy; in one there were small nodules of induration (chronic tubercle?); in twelve there were either tubercles, caseous changes, abscesses, cavities, or pneumonia; and in three simple collapse. Interlobular thickening may follow induration of a pneumonic origin (see Eustace Smith, *Clinical Studies*, Obs. xxxii.) In a case by Reginbean (Obs. vi.), in which he attributes the induration to pleurisy, the apex was more solidified than the other parts of the lung.

[5] Lebert, *Brustkrankheiten*, i. 259, 280, 302, 310.

[6] Biermer, 'Bronchiectasie,' *Virchow's Handbuch spec. Path. und Therap.* vol. v. abth. i. p. 749, reckons the cases of bronchiectasis originating in acute lobar pneumonia as one-fourth of the whole number. Kaulich (*Klin. Bericht Prager Vierteljahrsch.* 1861, p. 97) found that four out of six cases of bronchiectasis resulted from a past pneumonia. M. Lebert (*loc. cit.* 622) admits that a lobar pneumonia which has become chronic may pass into bronchiectasis. With regard to the proportion of tubercle, see Grancher, *Archiv. de Phys.* 1878. There is no doubt that adhesions of the pleura are frequently found in bronchiectasis, and Biermer thinks that they aid in producing it by disturbing the respiration. He admits, however, that they may have originated in a past pneumonia, or may be secondary (see Virchow's *Archiv.* xix. 162 *et seq.*) It may be remarked that bronchiectasis occurs in an infinitely small proportion of all cases of pleural adhesions. Bollinger (*Deutsch. Archiv Klin. Med.* 1868, v. 143) found adhesions in 73 per cent. of all post-mortems, and does not mention bronchiectasis.

[7] *Path. Anat.* 1861, iii. 50.

[8] Rindfleisch (*Lehrbuch Path. Gewebelehre*, 7th ed. p. 357) deduces grey induration from collapse, but his description must refer to tubercular cases. Ziegler (*Lehrb.* 1889) refers them to thickening of the septa; his descriptions (with figures) apply chiefly to the apices (p. 853).

[9] See especially Cornil and Ranvier, *Manuel d'Hist. Path.* 2nd ed. 1882, ii. 131 *et seq.* Compare also *ib.* ii. 108, where they state that in broncho-pneumonia there is no interstitial pneumonia, because the walls of the alveoli are not affected.

[10] Greenhow (*Path. Soc. Trans.* 1877, xxviii. 231) described one in Addison's disease, but there was also disease of the bronchial glands, which, as Dr. Moxon has remarked (*Path. Soc. Trans.* vols. xxiv. and xxviii.), leads to thickening of the lymphatic tissue throughout the lung (see Interlobular Pneumonia).

is common in tuberculosis, and probably some cases described as cirrhosis belong to this category.[1] The cases in which a simple interstitial fibroid thickening has been described were all unilateral; this points to some past local conditions affecting one lung only, which, as Green has remarked, may very possibly have been a pneumonia which had undergone resolution, and has left no other traces than changes, sometimes progressive, in the interlobular septa,[2] a condition already alluded to; this opinion receives confirmation from a case by Goodhart, where the change was actually observed in progress.[3] In another, however, recorded by Wilks and Sutton, it is described as affecting both lungs, and no other circumstantial change existed to explain the appearance.[4]

Bronchial dilatation co-exists in a very large proportion of all these cases of pulmonary induration; it was present in thirty-one out of thirty-nine cases which I have analysed. Sir Dominic Corrigan, as is well known, attributed the dilatation to traction on the walls of the bronchi by the fibroid lung. This view is untenable, except in cases where the lung is firmly adherent to the pleura, since the effect of the retracting lung would be to close the tubes; even in the presence of adhesion, this mechanism appears improbable. The discussion on this point has been extensive.[5] By some the dilatation has been ascribed to retained secretion; by others, to inspiratory efforts, in consequence of which the bronchi dilate in order to compensate for the non-expansion of the lung. The explanation of the association is a matter of pure hypothesis, but the evidence seems to show that in some cases the dilatation of tubes and the induration of the lung are due to one common cause and are more or less simultaneous, as when they result from acute or broncho-pneumonia, or from broncho-pneumonia with collapse; in the latter condition, as in whooping-cough, bronchial dilatation is very common in the collapsed parts. In the whole of this group of cases, as well as in others where bronchial dilatation is found (as in the chronic indurations of phthisis), I believe that the mechanism is identical with that advocated by Sir W. Jenner[6] and Mendelssohn,[7] as effective in the production of emphysema, viz. that the dilatation results from the expiratory force of cough, acting on tissues which have lost their elasticity; this loss exists in the collapsed, consolidated, or indurated lung, just as it does in the weakened bronchial wall. The dilatation may also be increased, as Mendelssohn remarked, by the secretion in the bronchi being driven to their terminations, owing to the loss of contractile power in the lung. Charcot makes a distinction between the indurations resulting from acute lobar pneumonia and those resulting from broncho-pneumonia, on the ground that dilatations of the bronchi are present in the latter and absent in the former. It is undoubtedly true that in the broncho-pneumonia of childhood, dilatations of the bronchi are more common than in primary pneumonia, and that when the malady becomes chronic, the dilatations persist and increase in the stage of induration. It is also true that in acute pneumonia, bronchial dilatation is not a

---

[1] To this class probably belongs a case of Immermann, *Deutsch. Arch. klin. Med.* 1880, vol. v. Both lungs contained nodular masses and dense fibroid cicatricial masses. See also Reynolds's *System of Med.* iii. 700.

[2] Hilton Fagge, *Path. Soc. Trans.* vol. xx.; T. H. Green, *Path. Soc. Trans.*, vol. xxiii.; Eppinger, *Prager Vierteljahrsch.* vol. cxxv. two cases; Barlow and Sutton, *Path. Soc. Trans.* vol. xvi. Eppinger's and Barlow's cases are not cases of interstitial pneumonia, as the lung-tissue was consolidated. Eppinger thought that in his the thickening proceeded inwards from the pleura.

[3] Goodhart, *Path. Soc. Trans.* 1874, xxv. 88. A somewhat similar case, but of less certain nature, is given by Lancereaux, *Atlas*, pp. 199, 255.

[4] Sutton, *Med.-Chir. Trans.* xlviii. 809. Sections of the lungs showed that they were uniformly invaded by a tough fibre-tissue, which had destroyed their natural texture, and rendered them partially airless and very hard. There were no circumscribed masses of hard tissue, as sometimes seen, but the pulmonary tissue appeared invaded in all parts; thus the natural aspect was lost, being wrapped or interwoven with fibrous filaments. Parts of the lungs were emphysematous, the other organs being healthy. Post-mortem notes by Wilks.

[5] See Biermer, Virchow's *Handbuch*, vol. v., and *Archiv für path. Anat.* xix., also Bastian, Reynolds's *Syst. Med.* vol. iii.

[6] Sir W. Jenner, *Med.-Chir. Trans.* 1857; and Reynolds's *Syst. of Med.* vol. iii.; Mendelssohn, *Mechanismus der Respiration*, 1845, pp. 257-8.

[7] *Revue Mensuelle*, 1878, ii. 781-5.

marked feature, but evidence exists that it may be found when the pneumonia has passed into a condition of induration.¹ In another group of cases the association is probably different, and it is possible that the induration of the lung may be secondary to a primary bronchial dilatation, owing to pneumonia being set up around the enlargement. It must be remarked that bronchial dilatation, as a chronic permanent condition, is a rare affection apart from consolidative pulmonary change,² and is a much less common accompaniment of chronic bronchitis than ordinary phraseology would imply. That such secondary pneumonia does occur in cases of brochiectasis is well established. Inflammation occurs not only around the dilated tubes, but in other parts of the lung; and extension of the induration, and also of the dilatation, through the agency of the indurating pneumonia, is thus easily understood.³ Traube's observations have shown the interesting fact that putrid bronchitis, not apparently directly dependent on bronchial dilatation, may equally induce a chronic pneumonia, ending both in induration of lung and in bronchiectasis.⁴ The bronchial dilatation leads in some of these cases to ulcerated cavities, in others to gangrene, and the two are not unfrequently combined.⁵

Chronic Ulcerative Pneumonia, apart from bronchiectasis, is a disease whose origin is often uncertain. Some of the recorded cases were probably tubercular, but in others the existence of a single cavity in the lung, surrounded or not by induration, leaves a doubt as to the manner of its production.⁶ It is possible that some cases may have arisen from abscess, and others from embolism. Their most frequent cause is the passage of a foreign body into the lung,⁷ but a few cases exist in medical literature, in which none of these causes were demonstrable. Bayle's cases of 'ulceration of the lung,' as Laennec remarked, were probably instances of gangrene; but one also of these was apparently caused by a bone entering the bronchus (although the bone was not discovered), and he states that the condition may be complicated with tubercle, or with the induration of the lung which he describes as 'phthisis with melanosis' (chronic induration).⁸ That an abscess may result from acute pneumonia, and pass into a chronic state, surrounded by induration, is demonstrated by some recorded cases,⁹ though as a rule cures are not uncommon in cases of abscess having this origin.¹⁰ Traube speaks of abscess resulting from

---

¹ See *ante*, note 5, p. 54, cases by Laennec, Andral, Biermer; also Lebert, *Brustkrankheiten*, p. 558; Rapp, *Verhandlungen Würzburg. phys.-med. Gesellschaft*, p. 147, four cases.

² An analysis of Biermer's 35 cases of bronchial dilatation shows that in only 11 was pulmonary induration absent (Virchow's *Archiv*, vol. xix.)

³ Laennec's fourth case of 'Dilatation des Bronches,' *Ausc. Med.* 2nd ed. i. 229; Stokes, *Dis. Chest*, p. 158; also Biermer, *loc. cit.* obs. i. ii. xiv. xviii. xxi. xxiii. xxiv. xxix.; Ziemssen, *Pleuritis und Pneumonie im Kindersalter*, 1862, p. 260.

⁴ Traube, *Gesammelte Beiträge*, ii. 583, 590, obs. v. and vi. The converse, viz. putrid bronchitis with bronchial dilatation, arising from a chronic pneumonia, is shown in his obs. x. p. 615.

⁵ Sir B. Carswell (*Illust. Elementary Forms of Disease*, art. 'Mortification') speaks of gangrene as a result of chronic pneumonia. For cases of this nature see Andral *Clin. Med.* iii. obs. 64, p. 474; Walshe, *Med. Times and Gaz.* 1865, p. 156; Coupland, *Path. Soc. Trans.* xxx. gangrene and abscess); Greenhow, *Path. Soc. Trans.* xxiii. (ulceration); Green, *Path. Soc. Trans.* xx. (ulceration). Compare, also, Dietrich, *Lungenbrand im Folge von Bronchialerweiterung*; Rapp, *Würzburg. Verhandlungen*, vol. i.; Briquet, *Archives Générales*, 1841; Biermer, *loc. cit.*; Barth, *loc. cit.* obs. xi.

⁶ Laennec (*Ausc. Méd.* 2nd ed. p. 532) speaks of having found single cavities in the lung, but he apparently regards them as having been of tubercular origin. Another case of this nature is recorded by Louis (*Phthisie Pulmonaire*, 2nd ed. obs. iii. p. 23). The indurations of the lung reported by Portal are for the most part of tubercular nature, and especially so in his 'phthisis from inflammation'; one of these is a case of abscess of the liver. Among his cases of 'phthisis from catarrh,' is one of abscess of the lung caused by injury. Charcot's case of chronic ulcerative pneumonia (*Pneumonie Chronique*, Paris, 1860, p. 66) had tubercles in the opposite lung.

⁷ Broussais (*Hist. des Phlegmasies*, ii. 6) says that this was the only case of excavation which he ever found, except in the presence of tubercles.

⁸ Bayle, *Phthisie Pulmonaire*, obs. xxvi. p. 248. Most of Bayle's other cases were complicated by tubercles. He describes (pp. 30, 33) the walls as 'blackened, stinking, and soft.' The affection was very rare in his experience — 14 instances in 900 cases (p. 98).

⁹ Stokes (*Dis. of the Lungs*, p. 316) said that he was acquainted with several cases of chronic pulmonary abscess resulting from pneumonia. See also Andral, *Clin. Med.* iii. 474; Heyfelder, *Studien im Gebiete der Heilwissenschaft*, p. 52 (two cases quoted).

¹⁰ Graves, (*Clin. Med.* ii. 45) alludes to a number of such cases. See also Leyden, *Lungenabscesse* in Volkmann's *Sammlung klin. Vorträge*; Traube, *Ges. Beiträge*, ii. 466; and Béhier, *Conférences de Clinique Médicale*; Grisolle, *Traité de la Pneumonie*, p. 20;— for a collection of cases.

a chronic pneumonia, but some of his cases are not without a suspicion of tubercular origin, although they did not present grey granulations;[1] this remark applies also to some others to be found in medical literature.[2] Gangrene and embolism supply other instances.[3]

Apart from these conditions it remains an open question whether either acute primary or catarrhal pneumonia does, in passing into the chronic state, give rise directly to pulmonary ulceration. The remaining unexplained cases are so few (only three or four in number) that no general doctrine can be founded on them,[4] though a few cases exist where a quasi-gangrenous action appears to have occurred in disseminated spots in the course of an acute specific disease.[5] Aufrecht[6] has described an ulcerative pneumonia of which he states that he has seen seven instances. Of his four published cases, one recovered with signs of a cavity after an acute illness, which may have been pneumonia; two had tubercle; and the third (No. 1), dying within four weeks of invasion, had a grey hepatisation, breaking down in the middle lobe, a condition analogous either to abscess or gangrene.

BROWN INDURATION.

(BROWN INDURATION OF THE LUNG HASSE). INDURATION OF THE LUNG IN HEART-DISEASE.

Plate XXII. figs. 3 and 4. Plate XLIV. figs. 10 and 11.

IN the lungs of patients who are the subjects of chronic heart-disease, and particularly of mitral regurgitation or obstruction, the permanent congestion of the pulmonary tissue leads to a peculiar induration and pigmentation, which are well expressed by the term 'brown induration' introduced by Hasse. The condition has been especially described by Hasse, Virchow, and Zenker.[7] In its more advanced stages the lung is very dense and firm, but has lost some of its elasticity, and tends to pit on pressure, though it tears with great difficulty. Virchow described the lung as enlarged, and as not collapsing when the thorax is opened. The enlargement has not appeared to me to be constant unless there is also emphysema. When emphysema has preceded or attended the development

---

[1] See especially two cases by Traube, *Ges. Beiträge*, ii. 915. Each contained cavities in both lungs, and in the second case these were multiple, with numerous spots of lobular hepatisation (soft tubercle?). Traube describes these as cases of *Melanotic Phthisis*.

[2] See the second case recorded by Jürken. *Lungenabscesse*, Diss. Jena, 1874, p. 38 (cavities in both lungs, dilatation of bronchi and grey granulations). See also *ante*, notes 6, 7, 8, p. 50. Knauenberg ('Lungenabscesse' *Charité-Annalen*, 1877, iv. 224) attributes chronic abscess to a chronic pneumonia, but of his four cases the two published are probably tubercular (peribronchitis); the details of the others are not given.

[3] See, for a collection of cases, Massoine, 'Quelques Formes Rares de Cavernes Pulmonaires,' *Thèse de Paris*, 1874. One of Lebert's cases (i. 730) illustrated gangrene.

[4] The chief among these are the following:— Sir Risdon Bennett, *Path. Soc. Trans.* xii.; scarlatina 18 months before; cavity at root of lung surrounded by grey hepatisation; T. H. Green, *Path. Soc. Trans.* vol. xx.;

chronic cough, induration at base of one lung, multiple cavities in this area, moderate dilatation of bronchi; C. T. Williams, *Path. Soc. Trans.* 1870, vol. xxi.; induration and excavation of one apex; Lancereaux, *Atlas*, pl. xxix. fig. 4, pp. 199, 205; ulceration in midst of old induration at root of lung (syphilis?).

[5] Biermer, Virchow's *Archiv*, xix. 274; Buhl, *Ueber acute Lungenatrophie*, Virchow's *Archiv*, xi. 275.

[6] *Pathologische Mittheilungen*, Magdeburg, 1881, p. 80.

[7] A brown induration of the lung was described by Andral under the title of 'hypertrophy,' but he did not notice its association with heart-disease; see *Path. Anat.* ii. 516. It was also observed by Hope, *Morbid Anatomy*. Hasse (*Path. Anat. Circulation and Respiration*, Syd. Soc. ed. p. 225) appears to have been the first to associate it with heart-disease. Other descriptions are given by Virchow, in his *Archiv*, vol. i.; by Zenker, *Beiträge zur norm. u. path. Anat. der Lungen*; and by Buhl, Virchow's *Archiv*, vol. xvi.

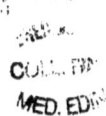

of the heart-disease, the increase of size of the lungs, and their induration, justify Andral's designation of 'hypertrophy.' In the earlier stage (XXII. 3) they show only an extreme vascularity, which often is irregularly distributed and punctiform, but at later periods they feel more uniformly solid, are of a yellowish-red or deep brown colour, and on scraping or pressure they yield a brownish-red œdematous fluid (Virchow) (XXII. 4).

The Microscopical Changes that occur in this condition are as follows. There is a great distension of the capillaries of the alveolar wall; an accumulation, to a greater or less extent, of pigmented epithelium in the interior of the alveoli, and finally a fibroid thickening of the walls of the alveoli, and also of the coats of the arteries and veins. The varicose distension of the capillaries has been insisted upon by most recent writers[1] (*see* XLIV. 10, 11), and it may exist to such an extent that the alveolar wall appears to consist entirely of distended capillaries. Orth has found not only the capillaries, but also large vessels completely obstructed by masses of pigment in the form of granules, scales, and spiculæ.[2] The epithelium-cells of the alveoli are swollen and increased in number within the alveolar cavity. They appear as cells containing hæmatoidin pigment in various stages of transformation from yellow to black, and also as larger granule-cells (Virchow). Pigment is also found largely in the alveolar walls both in a free form and also contained in cells (*see* XLIV. 10, 11). The epithelial proliferation in some cases increases until the alveoli are completely filled by these cells, and then the surface may be finely granular, sprinkled with yellow or whitish specks in the dark brown ground (XXII. 4), and in this condition the change resembles, and may even be held pathologically to be identical with, some forms of chronic pneumonia. Such portions are solid, and sink in water.[3] Friedreich has found corpora amylacea in these lungs.[4] Thickening of the alveolar walls was affirmed by Andral; it is not described by Virchow, and Zenker did not find it, but it is expressly insisted upon and figured by Rokitanski,[5] as a form of fibrous thickening. I have found it to a greater or less extent in all the specimens which I have examined, but it was not equally prevalent in all parts of the same lung. There is, in some cases, an increase in number of the nuclei of the alveolar walls, but they do not form masses or groups. In others the condensation appears to be due only to the crowding of the epithelium in the interior of the alveoli. The fibrous thickening also exists to a marked degree around the coats both of the arteries and veins, and may also be seen around the bronchi, but to a less degree. The thickening around the vessels, in some parts, is less fibrous than homogeneous, having a quasi-cartilaginous appearance, and this is especially seen around the pulmonary veins. Hypertrophy of the organic muscular fibres of the alveolar passages and alveolar walls has been described in this form of induration both by Orth and Rindfleisch.[6]

[1] Zenker, *loc. cit.*; Buhl, Virchow's *Archiv*, vol. xvi. (both with figures); also Thierfelder, *Atlas*; Rindfleisch, *Lehrbuch*.
[2] Orth, Virchow's *Archiv*, lviii. 126.
[3] They were described by Isambert and Robin under the title of 'Carnification congestiale,' *Mem. Soc. Biol.* 1855, T. 20, sec. ii. p. 3, essay.
[4] Virchow's *Archiv*, x. 206.
[5] *Path. Anat.* 1861, iii. 46. He states that in one case the condition was apparently the result of narrowing of the pulmonary artery.
[6] Orth, *loc. cit.*; Rindfleisch, *Lehrbuch*, 5th ed. p. 301 (figure). Buhl (*Lungenentzündung*, &c. p. 58) describes a muscular cirrhosis as one of the terminations of 'desquamative pneumonia.' For a further description of this hypertrophy see Eberth, Virchow's *Archiv*, 1878, lxxii. 96 *et seq.*

DISEASES CAUSED BY THE INHALATION OF DUST.

(Plate XXII. figs. 1 and 2. Plate XLIV. figs. 1–9).

THAT pulmonary disease can arise from some trades exposing the workers to the inhalation of dust of an irritating character, has been known since the writings of Morgagni. The affection thus induced resembles, in some cases, chronic pulmonary phthisis, being, like it, associated with consolidation and ulceration of the lung. In other cases these changes are absent, and the pathological consequences are those of chronic bronchitis and emphysema. The most injurious occupations are those in which mechanically irritating particles are inhaled, especially sandstone-dust and lime-dust, and next to these ranks the work in coal mines. It is probable, however, that in the latter occupation only a small proportion of the workers are affected, while in the former, as among the Sheffield knife-grinders, hardly any escape. I purpose, in this article, only to consider the phthisical changes, just mentioned, and it must be stated that even in the case of these, the amount of information respecting their precise nature is still somewhat meagre.

The direct causation of these diseases, by the irritant particles inhaled, is proved by the discovery within the lungs of the foreign bodies lodged in the tissues. This has been long recognised in the case of sand and flint, both before and since the use of the microscope,[1] and it has also been demonstrated by chemical analysis.[2] Traube[3] found charcoal in cases in which the lung-disease originated in the inhalation of dust of this nature, and iron in various forms has been found by Zenker and Merkel.[4] The penetration of dust has also been shown experimentally by Lewin, Knauff, and others.[5]

Consolidation occurs in two forms, viz. (*a*) in nodules of variable size, from a millet to a hemp-seed, scattered thickly through the lungs, and (*b*) in more extensive tracts, sometimes occupying the whole or part of a lobe, or both conditions may be found together. Their site varies, and sometimes they may be almost exclusively confined to the apices.[6] The colour of these indurations is remarkable. In a large number they are intensely black, whatever the nature of the dust inhaled,[7] but in some, where this is flinty, the nodules are whitish and are surrounded by a pigmented margin.[8] In these cases there can be but little question that the pigmentation is derived from the colouring matter of the blood—a theory of some antiquity, which has received special support from Virchow's study

---

[1] Andral (*Anat. Path.* i. 453) thought that flint particles did not penetrate, and that the phthisis in question was due to exposure. Holm (*Edin. Med. and Surg. Journ.* 1838) found, in the tubercles of a worker in certain quarries, particles of stone corresponding in character with those of the rocks.

[2] See Peacock, *Path. Soc. Trans.* vol. xii., also *Brit. For. Med. Rev.* 1860, vol. xxv., Greenhow. *Path. Soc. Trans.* vols. xvi. xvii. xx. xxi.; also Kussmaul, *Deutsch. Arch. klin. Med.* 1867; Aschen, *Bestandtheile der Lungen*; Meinel, *Erkrankung der Lungen durch Kieselstaubinhalation*, Diss. Erlangen, 1860.

[3] *Gesammelte Beiträge*, vol. ii. cases xxviii. li.; see also Manukopf, *Berliner klin. Woch.* 1864, No. 8, and Beyson, *Ed. Med. Surg. Journal*, 1864.

[4] Zenker, *Deutsch. Arch. klin. Med.* 1866, vol. ii. (see Case 4; and Pl. XLIV. 8 and 9); Merkel, *ibid.* 1871, vol. viii.

[5] Lewin, *Inhalations-Therapie*; Knauff, Virchow's *Archiv*, vol. xxxix.; Ins, *Archiv exp. Pathol.* 1876, vol. v. and Virchow's *Archiv*, 1878, vol. lxxiii. See also Rupperts, Virchow's *Archiv*, vol. lxxii. Slavjanki (Virchow's *Archiv*, vol. xlviii.) injected cinnabar and indigo into a tracheal wound.

[6] Friedreich, in stoneworkers, Virchow's *Archiv*, xxx. 403. Friedreich denied the 'tubercular' character of this affection. Hérard and Cornil (*Phthisie Pulmonaire*, p. 437), who speak of it as a chronic pneumonia, say that it is more common at the bases.

[7] Warburton Begbie, *Ed. Med. Surg. Journal*, 1857, a man working in a threshing mill; Bartholness in a miller (quoted by Oppert, 'Melanosis of Lung,' 1866); in potters where the dust is silica, see Greenhow, *Path. Soc. Trans.* vol. xvi.; (see also Pl. XXII. fig. 1); in millstone-makers, Greenhow, *ib.* vol. xvii. also in pearl-cutters, *ib.* vol. xxi.; in grinders, Fox Favel, *Trans. Proc. Med. Surg. Assoc.* 1846, vol. xiv. in sandstone-workers, Friedreich, Virchow's *Archiv*, xxx. 404; also Meinel, *loc. cit.* (several cases).

[8] See W. Thomson, *Med. Clin. Trans.* vol. xxi.; Hasse, *Path. Anat.* vol. i.; Lewin, *Inhalations-Therapie*.

of the development of pathological pigments,[1] and has been demonstrated by Nothnagel.[2] The lungs that show the most intense blackness are, however, those of miners, and this was attributed to the inhalation of coal-dust and of the smoke of the lamps by earlier writers, and especially by Sir Robert Christison and Graham.[3] This question of the source of the pigment was due to doubts whether dust could penetrate the lung.[4] This has been settled in the affirmative, not only by the experimental researches, already alluded to, but also by the demonstration, by Zenker and Merkel, that iron dust, corresponding in nature with that inhaled, can actually be found in the lung.[5] The particles are found in the epithelium lining the air-vesicles and bronchi (XLIV. 1 and 2), in the walls of the alveoli (fig. 3), in the interstitial tissue, and in the peribronchial and periarterial thickening (XLIV. 6). They are also found in adhesions to the pleura,[6] and abundantly in the bronchial glands.[7] In the interstitial tissue the black particles are sometimes found in the connective-tissue cells,[8] and sometimes free in the tissue.[9] The penetration probably occurs in two ways: first, they pass directly through the pseudostomata of the lymphatic tracts, which open between the epithelial cells of the bronchi and alveoli; in all probability the solid particles may thus directly enter the deeper tissues, ;[10] secondly, as Ins has shown, by the penetration of the particles into cells, either epithelioid or lymphoid, or derived from the white corpuscles of the blood, which pass by the same tracts into the deeper tissues, and may there be found in an enlarged form, thickening the walls of the pulmonary alveoli or the interstitial tracts.[11]

The result of this penetration is to produce the indurations described, but the process is not yet fully elucidated. There is epithelial proliferation in the interior of the alveoli,[12] and thickening of their walls and also of the interstitial tissue. The epithelial proliferation is of the nature of a pneumonic process,[13] and it has been shown that workers in irritating dust are more prone to pneumonia than those engaged in other trades,[14] and also that

---

[1] Virchow, 'Die pathologische Pigmente,' *Archiv für path. Anat.* vol. i. 'Ueber Lungenschwarz' ib. vol. xxxv. In another paper on the miner's lung *Ed. Med. & Surg. Journal*, 1858, trans. by Alexander Simpson) Virchow suggested that the blackening in these cases was due to transformed hæmatin—an opinion which he has subsequently abandoned.

[2] Nothnagel, Virchow's *Archiv*, vol. lxxi.

[3] Sir Robert Christison (*Ed. Med. Surg. Journal*, 1851) found that the black matter yielded an inflammable gas and products of distillation akin to coal naphtha. Graham (*Ed. Med. Surg. Journal*, 1834) thought the black matter akin to lampblack rather than to coal.

[4] Thus Villaret (*Cas rare d'Anthracose*, 1862) thought that the black dust entered the body by the stomach and intestines, and reached the lungs by absorption. Pigment in the intestines and mesenteric glands has also been observed in a copper worker by Lancereaux (*Atlas*, pp. 39, 297), also by Soyka in the liver and kidney (*Prag. med. Woch.* 1878).

[5] Zenker, *loc. cit.*, the peroxide of iron, see *Case 42*, and Pl. XLIV. figs. 8–9, copied from Zenker. Merkel, *loc. cit.*; this was suboxide of iron used in making ultramarine, and gave a blue colour with ferrocyanide of potassium; see also Reginbeau, *Pneumonie Chronique*, Thèse d'Agrégation, Paris, 1880, p. 104.

[6] Thomson (*Med.-Chir. Trans.* xx. 257) reports a case of a coal-miner where the adhesions of the pleura alone were pigmented, the rest of the membrane retaining its natural appearance.

[7] Knauff, *loc. cit.*; Cohnheim for Traube, *Gesammelte Beiträge*, ii. 773. See case of *Barlow, Case 58*.

[8] Greenhow, *Path. Soc. Trans.* vol. xx. pl. ii. figs. 2 and 3.

[9] Traube, *Gesammelte Beiträge*, ii. 771; charcoal.

[10] Wydozoff, 'Lymphwege der Lungen' *Wien. Med. Jahrb.* 1866, vol. xi.; Sekorski, *Centralbl. für med. Wissensch.* 1870; Klein, *Anatomy of Lymphatic System*, part ii. pp. 20, 84, and *Atlas of Histology*, 1880; Knauff, Virchow's *Archiv*, vol. xxxix.; Küttner, Virchow's *Archiv*, vol. lxvi.; Rupperts. Virchow's *Archiv*, vol. lxxii.; Buhl, *Mittheilungen aus der path. Institut zu München*, p. 191; Schottelius, Virchow's *Archiv*, vol. lxxiii.

[11] Ins, *Archiv für exp. Pathol*, vol. v. He inclines to the idea that these cells are all white corpuscles. Dr. Greenhow's plates show that some may enter the cylindrical epithelium, and Rupperts (Virchow's *Archiv*, vol. lxxii.) states that they enter the alveolar epithelium. It is therefore probable that they may also enter the proliferating epithelium of the alveoli. In his later article (Virchow's *Archiv*, vol. lxxiii.) Ins admits that the finer particles may pass direct into the pulmonary tissue, as Rupperts has stated. Ins is at variance with Rupperts as to the site of penetration. He denies that it is the floor of the alveoli, and asserts that it chiefly occurs at the angles formed by the openings of the alveoli into the infundibulum.

[12] See especially Greenhow's reports; also Virchow, *Ed. Med. Journ.* 1858.

[13] Virchow (*Edinb. Med. Journal*) described the process in the miner's lung as a chronic pneumonia with black induration.

[14] Hirt, *Krankheiten der Arbeiter*, p. 17. Pneumonia occurs in 7·4 per cent. of those exposed to dust, and only 4·6 per cent. of those not thus exposed. There are several fallacies in these data, but the result remains. Lewin (*Inhalations-Therapie*, p. 74) gives the frequency of pneumonia among stonemasons at 28 per cent.

inflammatory consolidations occur in the lungs. Part of the thickening of the alveolar walls is due to the direct accumulation of dust in them. In some cases it is attributable, as has been shown, to cell-accumulation, but whether this be entirely due to migratory cells or to a new-growth, may be open to question. In some cases certainly the pigmented cells in the septa resemble those seen in chronic pneumonia, and also in the pneumonic thickening of phthisis (see XLIV. 7). In others, however, nothing is found but a dense fibre-growth,[1] and this may extend into parts which are still pervious to air.[2]

The final result of this thickening is to produce a dense airless fibre-tissue, of great hardness and toughness, and more or less blackened. In miners it has been likened to caoutchouc,[3] but even in them some of the thickened interlobular septa may escape pigmentation, and appear as whitened bands.[4]

The nature of the nodular masses is open to more doubt. Rokitanski[5] identified them with indurated tubercles, and they have been spoken of as identical with Virchow's 'peribronchitis,' and with Rindfleisch's 'lymphangitis nodosa.'[6] Greenhow's figure shows in one case a peribronchitic thickening (see XLIV. 2); but in some cases the direct communication of these lobules with the bronchi has not been found.[7]

Meinel described tubercles in many of his cases, while Zenker denies the tubercular nature of the change and thinks it a lobular pneumonia with interstitial thickening. Merkel, however, describes the nodules in ultramarine-workers as consisting of a small-celled growth, which apparently closely resembled the structure of tubercles. My own opportunities for examining such cases have been very limited.[8] The lungs of one stonemason, sent me by my friend the late Dr. Bartlett, presented no characteristics to the naked eye, or to microscopic observation, different from those of ordinary phthisis. In the potter's lung already described, the nodules in some places presented only a dense and deeply pigmented fibre-tissue, but in others they showed a concentric arrangement of fusiform pigmented cells, which, except for the presence of pigment, bears a very striking resemblance to Schüppel's figure of indurated tubercle of the lymphatic glands.[9]

Tubercle was attributed to many of these cases in earlier periods, especially in the sandstone-workers, and even in a more recent period a large number of cases of miliary tuberculosis have been found among them.[10] I think it not improbable that the limitations which have of late been applied, as I believe too strictly, to the definition of tubercle, have, in some instances, led to its exclusion from cases in which it really existed. No explanation has yet been given why some persons suffer more than others engaged in the same mine or the same workshop,[11] and yet those who are attacked must have been more liable to disease than those who escaped.

This may indeed have been due to an inherent 'delicacy,' but there is evidence that

---

[1] Friedreich, Virchow's *Archiv*, xxx. 404; Greenhow, *loc. cit.* I have had the satisfaction, through Dr. Greenhow's kindness, of examining a large number of his preparations, and find that in most the thickening is mainly fibroid.

[2] Greenhow, *Path. Soc. Trans.* vol. xxi.

[3] Simpson, quoted by Thomson, *Med.-Chir. Trans.* xx. 253.

[4] Greenhow, *loc. cit.*

[5] Rokitanski, *Path. Anat.* iii. 87.

[6] Meinel, *Chalicosis Pulmonum*, p. 84 et seq. This is not expressly stated of these nodules either by Virchow, *Krankhaften Geschwülste*, ii. 648, or Rindfleisch, *Lehrbuch*, 1st ed. 351.

[7] See Zenker's description, quoted in a subsequent page. Case 4'.

[8] This arises in part from the objection to post-mortem examinations entertained by both miners and potters. During three years that I was physician to the North Staffordshire Infirmary, I could only obtain the lungs of two potters, and none of miners. At that period the method of hardening by chromic acid, &c. had not been introduced, and therefore microscopic research presented much greater difficulties than it does at present.

[9] Compare XLIV. fig. 6, with Schüppel's figure. *Lymphdrüsen Tuberculose*, pl. iii.

[10] Thus Burkart ('Miliar-Tuberculose.' *Deutsch. Arch. klin. Med.* 1873, xii. 276) out of 18 cases of miliary tuberculosis found 10 in workers in sand or coal.

[11] Different mines differ considerably, partly owing to the nature of the dust. Some workshops suffer more than others, though it is not long since nearly every grinder perished prematurely from his occupation.

some of these patients were actually tubercular[1] and that others belonged to tubercular families, and had either unusually delicate or tubercular children.[2] In the present aspect of the question of a specific cause for tubercle, all these may be regarded as non-essential questions; but should the tubercular nature of these diseases be hereafter more fully shown, their relation to specificity of cause will require further elucidation. It may be that both the nodules and the indurations are pneumonic, but the latter may also be akin to a diffuse tuberculisation.

Excavations constitute the most dangerous form of these diseases, though they may be absent in some cases where only indurations are found. They occur both in the larger masses of induration and also in the smaller nodules,[3] and in some cases they evidently result from the direct softening of these *en bloc*,[4] a process presenting a striking resemblance to that seen in ordinary phthisis, and differing from the ulceration of chronic pneumonia or bronchial dilatation. In some, calcareous masses are formed; their site is variable, and they are found both in the upper and lower lobes. The cavities may be simply excavated in the black induration. Their walls are usually ragged and irregular; sometimes they are traversed by bands. They may be very large, occupying the whole of a lobe or nearly the whole of a lung. Their contents are puriform and more or less pigmented. Bronchial dilatation occurs in some of the indurated masses, but the evidence that the cavities found originate in this condition is very imperfect; usually the bronchi opening into them are described as being abruptly truncated.

The bronchial glands are generally enlarged and blackened. I have found them softening (*Case 38, Barlow*); Zenker found iron dust in them. The pleura, in many cases, is intensely thickened and pigmented.[5] (*See* XLIV. 4.)

COLLAPSE OF THE LUNG.

Plates V. fig. 4; XXI. figs. 2, 3, and 4 (*Cruveilhier*); XXIII. fig. 2.

I SHALL here consider only the appearances presented in collapsed portions of lungs, and shall not discuss the theory of the origin of the condition. Collapse appears under three main conditions: (1) from congenital non-expansion; (2) from obstruction to the entry of air, combined with imperfect expanding powers of the thoracic walls; (3) from pressure, or from admission of air into the thorax. The appearances observed in the lungs differ somewhat in each of these conditions; all are characterised by an airless state, but this differs somewhat according to the amount of collapse. When this is due

---

[1] See previous note. Peacock's case had miliary tubercles in the lungs, ulcers in the larynx, and tubercular ulcers in the intestines. Traube's second case (*Ges. Beiträge*, ii. 709) had miliary tubercles in the pleura. One of Merkel's cases (*Deutsch. Arch. klin. Med.* vol. viii.) had tubercular peritonitis, as also one of Greenhow's (*Path. Soc. Trans.* xx. 44), and in Regimbeau's case (see p. 54, note 5). Nodules resembling tubercle existed in the peritoneum of one of Zenker's cases, and another was distinctly tubercular, though Zenker regarded this as accidental. See also Maurice (Schmidt's *Jahrb.* vol. cxv.) Tubercles are mentioned by many of the older writers.

[2] Thomson, *loc. cit.*; Mackellar, *Monthly Journal*, 1845, p. 650; Hamilton, *Edin. Med. Surg. Journal*, 1834, xxii. 298; 'Rep. Cornish Miners,' *Brit. and For. Med.-Chir. Rev.* 1860, ii. 60.

[3] Mackellar, *loc. cit.* Greenhow (*Path. Soc. Trans.* xvii. 36) describes the cavities as surrounded by nodules, some hard, some caseous.

[4] Mackellar describes, in a miner, a mass the size of a large apple, resembling consolidated blacking. It would appear probable that this was caseous matter, deeply pigmented; see description of bronchial glands, Barlow, *Case 38*.

[5] See Virchow's figure, *Ed. Med. Journal*, 1858, and his *Archiv*, vol. xxxv.

to pressure on the lung itself, some air may still be contained in the lung, and it may float in water, but sinks after further pressure with the fingers.

(1) *Congenital 'atelectasis,'* or imperfect expansion of the lung, may be either lobular or may extend over a considerable area. In either condition it presents certain distinctive features. The affected parts are sunk below the level of the surrounding lung. They are bluish in tint, contrasting in this respect with the redder colour of the lung into which air has penetrated. They are commonly sharply circumscribed from the surrounding tissue. When superficial, the pleura covering them retains its natural translucency (XXI. 3, 4). They are firm and resist pressure. They sink in water and do not crepitate. On section, a small amount of blood-stained fluid sometimes exudes, but this is less in quantity than in the collapse that occurs at a later period, as a result of bronchitis. The section is smooth and glistening, and retains the natural translucency of the pulmonary tissue—a characteristic by which it may be distinguished from pneumonic infiltration. The lobular arrangement is distinct, though there is no appearance of the vesicular structure. In children dying within a few days after birth the lung can be inflated, although, as West has remarked, the collapsed portions retract more rapidly than the regions which have expanded by breathing. When the child has survived for some days the power of this inflation is lost, and the tissue becomes firmer and more resistant. In some cases the colour becomes darker, but with time it gradually assumes a paler tint, and has a more distinctly lobulated appearance (XXI. 2), resembling that of a racemose gland. This condition is most common at the anterior-inferior border of the upper lobe of the left lung, and at the free margins of the lower lobe on both sides.

(2) *Collapse from obstruction of the Bronchi* may be general or partial. It is general when a main tube is obstructed, as from pressure of an aneurism or mediastinal tumour; it is partial when the bronchi of smaller calibre are occluded by mucus, and in the latter condition it may be purely lobular. This form is that most commonly found in the bronchitis of children, especially when combined with rickets. It is necessary, however, to mention that part of the collapse arising from rickets is due directly to pressure from the sinking of the ribs, and then presents the form of a vertical groove running parallel to the sternum; beyond this groove of collapse the anterior margin of the lung is found in a state of emphysema.[1]

The collapsed lobules exist in all parts of the lungs, but especially at the anterior borders and at the bases. They may, however, be found at the apices. They are distinguished by being sunk below the level of the adjacent parts, by their bluish tint, and especially by their firmness and resistance. The firmness and resistance often give the lung a mammillated aspect, and this character can also be recognised by the touch. The sunken look is not always evident when the rest of the lung collapses on removal from the thorax. When it remains distended, as in emphysema, these indurated lobules may be felt like grains of shot in the midst of pulmonary tissue, and may be mistaken for tubercles. At the bases, and especially in the groove between the diaphragm and the vertical column, the collapsed part often assumes a pyramidal form; the base of the pyramid corresponds to the pleura covering the lower part of the lung, and the apex is directed upwards. This pyramid of collapse may occupy a considerable part of the lower lobe (*see* Plate XXI. fig. 3). As in congenital collapse, so also in the acquired form, the pleura is always intact. The glistening translucency of the pulmonary tissue is also preserved, but it tends to become more gorged with blood than is usually seen in the form first described, and to pass into

[1] Sir W. Jenner, 'Lectures on Rickets,' *Med. Times and Gazette*, 1860, i. 335.

the state known as 'splenisation.' This condition also passes into pneumonia, a transition which is described in the section on 'Broncho-Pneumonia.' The regions of collapse that has originated from bronchitis often contain dilated bronchi filled with puriform fluid. During the earlier stages of this process, the lung can be inflated, and it then appears, from the large amount of blood contained in it, to be redder than the surrounding tissue, and it is also more œdematous. When pneumonia occurs, the capacity for inflation is lost. This capacity may also disappear gradually without the occurrence of inflammation, and the indurated 'pancreas-like' appearance (Sir J. Alderson) seen in the cases of congenital collapse is also found in this variety. Ultimately, the parts so affected either undergo atrophy, or possibly a calcareous change (Gairdner), or they pass into a state of fibroid induration, in the midst of which dilated bronchi are found.[1] Rokitanski showed that this induration may be due to a nuclear growth in the alveolar walls.[2]

(3) *Collapse from pressure* presents an appearance different from either of the foregoing. It is distinguished by its bloodlessness (XXIII. 2, c). When complete the tissue is airless, but when incomplete, as in some cases of pleurisy, it may still, as already stated, contain some air. The interlobular septa and the bronchial tubes and vessels may be traced in it. It is of a dull grey colour, and is tough and resistant; as in the other forms, the tissue still retains its translucency. This form of collapse undergoes fewer changes than those last described, and the power of re-expansion is long retained, as is shown by the recovery of the respiratory power even after pleural effusions of long duration.[3]

PULMONARY EMBOLISM.

THE HÆMORRHAGIC INFARCT; PULMONARY APOPLEXY; EMBOLIC PNEUMONIA; METASTATIC ABSCESSES.

Plate XXIV. fig. 1; Plate XXIII. figs. 1 and 2.

THE changes produced in the lung by obstruction of the pulmonary artery and its branches vary considerably in their appearance. They may, however, be summarised under two heads: (1) the escape of blood into the tissue—the hæmorrhagic infarct, and (2) various changes resulting from anæmia and inflammation, the latter passing sometimes into abscess and sometimes into gangrene. I purpose here simply to confine myself to a description of the appearances observed under these conditions. The mechanism of their production I hope to discuss in another work.

1. *The Hæmorrhagic Infarct* has now been traced very distinctly to obstruction of branches of the pulmonary artery, and it is capable of being produced by simple ligature of the main trunk.[4] It is possible that it may in some instances arise from other causes, such as the gravitation of blood or rupture of the lung,[5] but in the vast majority of the

---

Ziegler, *Lehrb. path. Anat.* 2 Theil, 1883, p. 853 (figure).
[2] Rokitanski, *Lehrb. path. Anat.* 1861, iii. 59 (see section on 'Chronic Pneumonia').
[3] See section on 'Chronic Pneumonia.'
[4] Küttner, Virchow's *Archiv*, lxxiii. 507. See also

Cohnheim, *Die embolische Processe*; obstructions of the artery in the tongue of the frog.
" As, for instance, traumatic rupture: see Woillez, *Maladies Aiguës des Organes Respiratoires,* obs. lxxix., p. 586. Andral in 'Phthisie,' *Clin. Méd.* iv. 158, obs. xii. Phthisis is, however, a disease in which secondary

conditions in which it occurs, as in heart-disease and in other disturbances of the peripheral circulation, it must now be considered to have merely an embolic origin.[1] Some authors, however, still hold that it may arise from rupture of the pulmonary artery in cases of atheroma of the vessel.[2] It has also been shown experimentally that the condition can be produced by obstruction of veins.[3] In its typical form the hemorrhagic infarct is wedge-shaped. It varies much in size and may occupy the whole of a lobe. It is commonly sharply circumscribed by the interlobular septa, but it may also (as Carswell remarked, in his description of 'pulmonary apoplexy') break down the lung-tissue and then assume a more diffuse character.[4] It has a tendency to be peripheral in situation, with its base at the pleura, and then this membrane usually presents petechial extravasations, and may even rupture so as to allow blood to escape into the pleural cavity.[5] It may, however, occur in the more central parts of the lung,[6] and under these circumstances the pyramidal form is often less distinct; the areas may even appear rounded in shape. They may be found in all parts of the lung, but are most common in the lower lobes,[7] and are more frequent in the right than in the left lung.[8]

A recent infarct constitutes a dense, firm, solid mass of a deep purple colour, from which all appearance of pulmonary structure has disappeared (see XXIV. 1). The surface is granular on section, owing to the coagula which fill the vesicles, and it then resembles, as stated by Wilks and Moxon, damson-cheese in aspect[9] With time, the colour becomes lighter in tint and of a brownish colour. It is probable that the effused blood may be slowly absorbed, leaving only a scar,[10] but it is doubtful whether the whiter forms of infarct, to which I shall presently allude, owe their origin to a genuine pulmonary apoplexy.[11]

The mechanism of the hæmorrhage has been the subject of much discussion. Virchow stated that its mode of production was not clear,[12] but was disposed to attribute it in part to collateral pressure, and to weakening of the capillary vessels by imperfect nutrition, which led to their subsequent rupture when the collateral circulation was re-established.[13] This view of rupture under pressure was supported by Otto Weber[14] and denied by Panum and Cohn.[15] Cohnheim[16] has laid great stress on the mechanism of venous congestion, and believes that the greater part of the hæmorrhage of the infarct is due to diapedesis through weakened vessels. He has pointed out that the wedge-shape of the infarct corresponds more with the distribution of the vein than with that of the artery, and has specially argued against an anastomosis between the pulmonary and bronchial arteries. This latter anatomical point has, however, been further elucidated by Küttner, who has shown that

embolisms are not uncommon, owing to the thromboses in the peripheral veins.

[1] Gerhardt, 'Der hämorrhagische Infarct,' Volkmann's *Sammlung klin. Vorlesungen*; Penzoldt, *Deutsch. Arch. klin. Med.* 1879, vol. xii.
[2] Traube, *Ges. Beiträge*, iii. 288; Hertz, Ziemssen's *Handbuch*,'Krank. Resp.-App.' ii. 290; Walshe, *Dis. Lungs*, 4th ed. p. 400. See also Sir James Paget, *Med.-Chir. Trans.* xxviii. 160, 186, and Dittrich, *Ueber den hämorrhagischen Lungeninfarct*; Martineau, *Comptes Rendus Soc. Biol.* 1861, pp. 166-196.
[3] Weissgerber and Perls, *Arch. exp. Pathol.* vol. vi.; see also Ponfick, Virchow's *Archiv*, vol. lx.
[4] *Illust. Elementary Forms of Disease*, 1838, art. Hemorrhage.'
[5] Carswell, *loc. cit.*; Townsend, *Cyc. Pract. Med.*, art. 'Pulmonary Apoplexy.'
[6] Penzoldt, *loc. cit.*
[7] Ogston (*Brit. & For. Med.-Chir. Rev.* 1860, vol. xxxvii.) gives the following data for 20 cases: upper lobes 10, lower lobes 27, middle lobes 6.
[8] Gerhardt, *loc. cit.*
[9] Wilks and Moxon, *Lectures on Pathological Anatomy*, 2nd ed. 1875, p. 321.
[10] Virchow, *Ges. Abhand.* pp. 364, 367.
[11] Virchow stated (*Ges. Abhandlungen*, p. 874) that in his observations the genuine pulmonary infarct did not occur from embolic closure of the pulmonary artery. Its origin from this source may, however, now be considered as proved by Cohnheim, Gerhardt, and Penzoldt.
[12] Virchow, *Handbuch spec. Path. u. Therapie*, 1854, i. 177.
[13] Virchow, *Ges. Abhandlungen*, 456. See also Rokitanski, *Path. Anat.* 1861, iii. 78.
[14] Otto Weber, Pitha and Billroth's *Handbuch der Chirurgie*, i. 97. He attributed it, however, to venous congestion—a view more fully expanded by Cohnheim.
[15] Panum, Virchow's *Archiv*, xxv. 483; Cohn, *Klinik der embolischen Gefässkrankheiten*, pp. 328, 338, 354.
[16] *Die embolische Processe*, also *Vorlesungen allgem. Pathologie*, and Cohnheim and Litten, Virchow's *Archiv*, vol. lxv.

such anastomosis does occur.[1] Litten's[2] more recent researches have led him to the conclusion that the extravasation is due to diapedesis from the distended capillaries, and to pressure through the collateral circulation, but not to venous pressure, since it occurs in parts where the veins have valves, and is increased by simultaneous ligature of the vein. He also denies the weakening of the vessels.

2. *Embolic Pneumonia.*—A considerable number of the infarcts of the lung do not present the typical appearance of the hæmorrhagic infarct just described. They have the same wedge-shape, but they have not the dark purple colour of effused blood. They are paler than those just described, have a dirty reddish-brown tint, and are surrounded by an intense zone of hyperæmia. Virchow laid special stress on the fact that these cases represent a pneumonia, that the consolidation was due to a fibrinous exudation in which were fattily degenerated cells, and that the pneumonia may be mingled with more or less hæmorrhagic extravasation.[3] Among these elements in the pneumonic process, the epithelium appears, from the concurrent testimony of most authors, to be simply desquamated, and to undergo either fatty degeneration[4] or the direct loss of vitality which has been termed by Weigert and Litten 'coagulation-necrosis.[5] There is, however, some evidence that it may also proliferate, but this process appears comparatively trifling in degree.[6] The histology of these nodules has apparently been less studied in the lung than in the kidney, but it is probable that in the lung the pale infarcts, like those in the kidney, do not depend on decoloration of hæmorrhagic extravasations, but are due to a fibrinous exudation combined with necrosis of the epithelium,[7] though even in these some proliferation may occur.[8] Varying tones of colour may, however, be imparted to them by the different proportions of blood extravasated, and it is not improbable that in the lung an hæmorrhagic zone may be produced around the central more anæmic part, from the greater pressure on the collateral circulation, in a manner similar to that which Litten has shown to occur in the kidney. It must also be stated that the inflammatory process, excited by the embolus, may extend beyond the limits of the area supplied by the affected artery, and may implicate the whole or the greater part of a lobe.[9] The differences between the two forms of infarct, the hæmorrhagic and the exudative, have not, even yet, been fully explained. Litten has clearly shown that for the production of the 'white infarct' a certain amount of circulation is still necessary. It is probable that the hæmorrhage depends on the greater amount of collateral pressure, and the reason why such infarcts are more common in the lung and spleen than elsewhere is the greater vascularity of these organs, and also the laxity of their tissue, which either permits more easy rupture of the vessels, or facilitates the escape of blood from them. Cohnheim has indeed asserted that the hæmorrhagic infarct depends on the obstruction of a terminal artery, while the inflammatory form is caused by the stoppage of a more central artery with infective material,[10] but his view of the terminal character of the pulmonary artery can now be scarcely considered to

---

[1] See Introduction, 'On the Structure of the Lung,' p. 11.
[2] Litten, *Untersuchungen über den hämorrhagischen Infarct*, Berlin, 1879; p. 29; also *Zeitschrift für klin. Med.* 1879.
[3] Virchow, *Ges. Abhand.* p. 288 et seq., also p. 673; Cohn, *Klinik der embolischen Gefässkr.* 1860, p. 354, Panum, Virchow's *Archiv.* xxv. 478 et seq. Cohnheim has also stated that these spots may go through the change of red and grey hepatisation (*Embolische Processe*, pp. 102–110).
[4] Virchow, see ante, also Cohn, *Klinik*, p. 304.
[5] Weigert, Virchow's *Archiv.* vol. lxx.; Litten, *loc. cit.*
[6] Rindfleisch, *Lehrbuch*, 5th ed. p. 387. Bälzer, *Nouveau Dict. Med. Clin. Pract.* art. 'Poumon, Embolie,' xxix. 351. Cornil and Ranvier, *Manuel d'Hist. Pathol.* 2nd ed. ii. 124.
[7] Berkmann, Virchow's *Archiv.* vol. xx; Weigert, *loc. cit.* p. 86; Litten, *loc. cit.*
[8] Litten, *loc. cit.* p. 38.
[9] Virchow's *Ges. Abhandlungen*, p. 320, 338.
[10] Cohnheim, *Die embolische Processe*, pp. 100, 102.

be tenable as supporting this explanation. There can be little doubt but the suppuration, and even the gangrene, which may be caused by the embolic processes, are due to the infecting or irritating qualities of the emboli; but it is said, on good authority, that these changes may also occur in the hæmorrhagic infarct.[1] The 'metastatic abscesses' are of very variable size, and are usually rounded in form. The process by which they arise consists more in a breaking down of tissue than in any extensive production of pus-cells, though these are also found. The transition between the softening of a part into an abscess, and true gangrene, is not a well-defined process, and the latter change (see VA, 1) may probably arise either from complete arrest of the circulation, or from special characters and conditions of the septic material.

GANGRENE OF THE LUNG.

(Plate VA, figs. 1 and 3).

I HAVE taken two illustrations of this process from the collection of Sir Robert Carswell's drawings in the museum of University College. Fig. 3 is given in his Atlas. They illustrate two of the chief forms, viz. the 'diffuse gangrene' of Laennec and the gangrene resulting from embolism. There are, however, many other varieties, differing somewhat in their appearance according to their mode of origin. I shall deal more fully with the subject of gangrene in a systematic treatise, and shall therefore limit myself here to a brief description of these variations. Gangrene was divided by Laennec into two chief forms—the 'diffuse' and the circumscribed. The former is that illustrated in fig. 3. The affected part of the lung, sometimes the whole organ, is converted into a blackened mass, which breaks down into a pulpy débris and leaves a ragged cavity. In the earlier stages, and before this breaking-down occurs, the tissue is dark, soft, pulpy, and saturated with a fetid œdema. The colour varies, being sometimes greyish, greenish, or varied shades of brown. This form of gangrene is rare. It may originate in pneumonia and also in bronchiectasis, and it has been found in workers in latrines.

Circumscribed Gangrene may have diverse appearances. It may resemble that described above, but its area is limited, and in this form it usually results from bronchial dilatation. When succeeding pneumonia, it appears as patches of dead greyish colour in the midst of consolidated tissue, which is usually in the state of grey hepatisation. There is generally no distinct line of demarcation between the hepatised and the gangrenous parts. The latter are then distinguished by their fetidity. They break down into a pulp, which is usually more or less blackened or discoloured. Although usually offensive, the broken-down tissue may, as Cruveilhier stated, occasionally be devoid of fetidity.[2] In a few cases a distinct line of demarcation, distinguished by its vascularity, separates the gangrenous parts from the surrounding tissue.[3] They have also been seen by Leyden and Jaffé of an 'intense yellow colour' in the midst of grey hepatisation.[4]

These areas tend to soften into cavities, in which sequestra of pulmonary tissue are found, and which, in a few cases, are with difficulty distinguished from abscesses. In

---

[1] *Gechwell, loc. cit.* p. 14.
[2] Cruveilhier, *Atlas.* pl. xxxii. liv. 5.
[3] Béhier, *Comp. Clin. Méd.* obs. 25, 26, pp. 246-8.
[4] *Deutsch. Arch. klin. Med.* vol. ii. obs. 5.

the majority of such cases the contents are dark in tint, sometimes chocolate-coloured, blood-stained, and fetid.

In broncho-pneumonia, the gangrenous areas may appear only as greenish striæ or as islets of a dirty brown, breaking into débris, and fetid. They tend to be superficial, and the pleura is sometimes separated from them. The gangrene that occurs in phthisis is usually found in the midst of a grey hepatisation, from which it is sometimes distinguished with difficulty. It is, however, fetid, and of a duller tint and also softer and more friable than the surrounding infiltration. In diabetic pneumonia, in which gangrene is not uncommon, the affected part may be devoid of fœtor.

The Gangrene from Infarcts caused by Embolism (VA. 1) presents a considerable variety of appearances. The most typical is that here illustrated, where the tissue changes to a dirty reddish-grey or greyish-brown, and breaks down into a ragged cavity presenting the usual fœtor. In some instances these are found in the centre of a more extended pneumonic area. In others they are circumscribed, and have the pyramidal form of a pulmonary infarct. The distinction between these spots of true necrosis and the slower changes occurring in an infarct, and also from the more rapid softening of pyæmic abscesses, is at times very difficult. In fact the border line between them is more or less arbitrary. The gangrenous process may be defined as an acute necrosis *en masse*, and is usually distinguished by a darker discolouration, and also by fetidity of the affected area. Except when surrounded by an area of pneumonic hepatisation, gangrene resulting from embolism is usually sharply circumscribed, and is sometimes separated from the surrounding tissue by a zone of dissecting pneumonia. In many of these cases the pleura is also affected with gangrene.[1] It loses its translucency, and becomes friable; perforation is not uncommon, causing in some cases fetid empyema, in others hæmorrhage into the pleura.

The condition of gangrene is essentially death of the pulmonary tissue; products of decomposition therefore abound, particularly the fatty acids, crystals of which form masses and bundles.[2] Altered blood, black pigment, fragments of lung-tissue, granular corpuscles, and triple phosphates are also present. In a large number of cases fungi have been found—Sarcina, Aspergillus, and Leptothrix mucor mucedo, and there exists evidence that the penetration of these into the lungs may prove a direct cause of ulceration or necrotic lung-disease.[3]

The further changes in the gangrenous spots consist in their sequestration or elimination. Sequestra of pulmonary tissue are not uncommon in the midst of cavities having this origin. They tend finally to soften, and there results a cavity having fetid and discoloured contents. The walls of such a cavity are usually ragged and irregular, but if the contents are evacuated by opening into a bronchial tube, the cavity may become lined by a false membrane and may finally contract and heal. The tissue around is usually indurated through an area of variable extent, by a process akin to that observed in chronic pneumonia. On the other hand, the cavity may rupture into the pleura, or may, through adhesions, open on the surface, or it may perforate the diaphragm or the œsophagus.

A peculiar form of traumatic gangrene, following a gunshot wound, has been described by Leyden.[4] The gangrene extended along the tract of the wound, which opened into

---

[1] The arrest of nutrition, as stated by Rokitanski, is shown by the absence of exudation over this area.
[2] Virchow, *Archiv für path. Anat.* 334; *Ges. Abhandlungen*, pp. 421, 728; Traube, *Ges. Beiträge*, ii. 572; and Leyden and Jaffé, *Deutsch. Arch. f. klin. Med.* vol. ii.
[3] Rothius (*Charité-Annalen*, 1877. iv. 272) found Aspergillinus niger. The case presented no fever; it began as bronchitis. Fragments of pulmonary tissue were expectorated. The patient recovered.
[4] 'Lungenbrand,' Volkmann's *Sammlung*, No. 20, p. 13.

a cavity. There was induration of the tissue around the track of the wound, and this induration extended to the sheaths of the bronchi, so as to produce a state resembling caseous peribronchitis, and, at the peripheral extremities of the bronchi, it formed nodular masses, some of which were gangrenous, while others had broken down into cavities. Caseous masses have also been found in diffuse gangrene by Banks and by Welch.[1] It is possible that these may be due to various forms of mycosis, since Buhl has observed collections of schizomycetæ in pneumonia tending to undergo this change.[2]

PHTHISIS.

The anatomical changes in pulmonary phthisis are varied and complex, and there is no tissue or structure in the lung which may not be affected by them. They consist in nodules and granulations of various size and appearance, occurring singly or collected into masses—in consolidations of a more uniform kind, affecting the pulmonary tissue, which also vary in appearance and consistence—in destruction of the tissue by ulceration or sloughing, sometimes originating in the granulations, sometimes in the more diffuse consolidation—in fibroid and cicatricial changes—and in changes in the bronchi, the vessels, the interstitial tissue, the lymphatic glands, and the pleural covering. It is necessary that these should be described singly, and also in their relation to each other. The latter subject will in part be considered separately, since the views of different authorities have varied much on many points embraced under this head.

I shall first describe the granulations, which are among the most constant appearances observed. These may be classified as (1) semitransparent granulations; (2) opaque, whitish granulations of variable size; and (3) indurated and pigmented granulations. The description of the infiltrations and other changes will follow that of the granulations. I shall describe separately the histological changes observed, and then consider the conclusions to be drawn from them.

(A) Granulations.—1. *The grey granulations*, first distinctly described by Bayle[3] as 'transparent glistening miliary granulations, sometimes marked by black lines or black shining spots; of a cartilaginous nature and consistence, varying in size from a millet-seed to a grain of wheat; never opaque and never breaking down,' has been always recognised since his definition, to which few additions have since been made. The chief of these is Laennec's statement that they might become opaque in their centres and soften. They have also been described in their early stages as somewhat soft,[4] and as occasionally red from hyperæmia (Andral).[5] The latter characteristic is, I believe, very rare, and I

---

[1] Banks, *Dublin Quart. Journ.* 1843, vol. xvii. Welch, 'Destructive Lung-disease in Soldiers,' *Alexandra Prize Essay*, 1872, p. 6.

[2] Buhl, *Lungenentzündung Tuberkulose und Schwindsucht*, Munich, 1872, p. 18 (see *Catarrhal Pneumonia*, p. 29). It may be remembered that Leyden and Jaffé found some parts of the gangrenous lung of an intense yellow colour. Virchow (*Archiv*, xx. 572) attributes this yellow colour to blood-pigment.

[3] *Phthisie Pulmonaire*, 1810, p. 26. Waldenburg's historical researches (*Die Tuberculose*, 1869, p. 32 *et seq.*) have shown that these had been already observed by Magnetus in 1700 (see later).

[4] Rokitanski, *Anat. Path.* i. 294; Förster, *Anat. Path.* 226. -Empis (*De la Granulie*, p. 39) distinctly calls attention to the softness of the earliest grey granulations in tubercular meningitis. See also Buhl, *Lungenentzündung*, etc. p. 105.

[5] Andral, *Préc. Anatom. Path.* ii. 518, and *Clinique Médicale*, iv. 6 and 27.—Thaon (*Rech. Anat. Path. de la Tuberculose*, Paris, 1873, p. 13) has made the same observation. It was even earlier noticed by Rochoux, Dalmazzone, and Mériadec Laennec, as quoted by Valleix, *Archives Générales*, 1841, x. 140. Valleix remarks that this appearance is probably due to hyperæmia preceding the granulation or surrounding it.

cannot say that I have met with the vascular appearance described by Andral. The softness in the earliest stages is also a relative term, and, though some of the smallest are undoubtedly less resisting than others apparently of older formation, distinct softness is not a common feature of the typical forms.

The essential characteristic of the typical grey granulations is their glistening translucency, and when they are thickly scattered, a section of the lung may appear as if dusted over with specks of powdered glass or white sand. They are somewhat prominent on section, but, in their most typical form, they are so only to a slight degree. When they become firmer and pigmented, the prominence is more marked. In size, they vary from almost invisible specks to granules, as stated by Bayle, of the size of a millet-seed, but they are more commonly of the dimensions of a poppy-seed. In outline they appear rounded, but they are seldom perfectly so, and they have usually an irregular margin, due, as will be stated hereafter, to the manner in which they invade the pulmonary tissue. They are often isolated, each granule appearing singly, though in close proximity to others, but they may form conglomerate groups. This is, however, less common with the typical semi-transparent granulation than with some of the more opaque forms.

They are often surrounded by a zone of hyperæmia, and where they are thickly scattered, the whole of the pulmonary tissue in which they appear is intensely vascular, and on exposure to the air becomes of a bright scarlet tinge. When, however, as is often the case, recent emphysema has supervened around them, this hyperæmia is less marked. They may also, however, be found in deeply pigmented tissue.

Whether this colour is due to pre-existing pigment in the adult, or to changes consequent on the minute extravasations in cases that have survived a certain time, is open to question, but I think that in some instances the latter is the more probable hypothesis. In number they vary considerably. In typical cases of acute tuberculosis, the lung may be densely crowded with them, so as to leave only the smallest interspaces of pulmonary tissue intervening;[1] but I would remark that when this is found the bulk of such granulations are rarely of the typical semi-transparent character, and that most of them have a whitish and more opaque appearance.

Changes in the grey granulations.—These have been the subject of dispute since the time of Bayle. On one point there has been an almost constant unanimity of opinion, viz. that with increasing age, while still retaining their translucent appearance, they may become more or less increasingly pigmented. Laennec asserted that they became opaque and were, in fact, the first stage of 'tubercle.' Andral, who denied the tubercular character of the granulations, said also that they did not undergo the change described by Laennec, though he admitted that they occasionally became opaque in their centres, or, as he expressed it, 'tubercle might appear in them.' Laennec's statement has been repeated by almost every subsequent author, but it is one difficult of proof. It is an undoubted fact that the granulations may long remain transparent, and it is equally certain that all gradations in the appearance of granulations may be found in close juxtaposition in the same lungs, from the most typical semi-transparent granulations to soft, opaque, white and yellow forms. I believe that these differences are due, in part, to the variations in the acuteness with which different granulations are produced, and also in part to variations in the amount of epithelial products which enter into their composition. I believe also that it is to this latter condition that the greater opacity is mainly due. That caseous change may and

---

[1] See cases, Christy, *Tuberculisation Aiguë à Forme Asphyxique*, Thèse de Paris, 1876. Mairet, *Tuberculisation Miliaire du Poumon*, Thèse de Paris, 1878, p. 55. Colin. *Études Clin. Méd. Mil.* p. 86, also *Arch. Gén. de Méd.* 1874; Laveran, *Rec. Mém. Méd. Militaire*, xxix. 1875.

does occur in the typical grey granulations is, I believe, histologically demonstrable, but I shall reserve the description of this until their ultimate structure is considered.

2. *Soft, opaque, white granulations* are found, of more variable size than the grey transparent form last described, sometimes even attaining the dimensions of a split pea. The smaller forms,—the 'miliary tubercles' of Bayle and Andral—are, on the whole, more common in the lung, even in cases of acute tuberculisation, than the typical grey granulations, and in some cases, when combined with the yellow granulations next to be described, they may constitute the sole granulations present in the lung in this disease. They are distinguished from the grey granulations by their whiter colour and by their greater opacity, but in both these features there is considerable variation, and it is not uncommon to find some presenting a certain degree of translucency, showing an intermediate appearance between the typical grey and a complete opacity. Like the grey, they vary in size from the smallest visible specks to a poppy-seed, or even a hemp-seed, and they tend, on the whole, to assume larger dimensions than the grey. They are also more prone to form racemose groups, which then have an irregular outline; but they may also exist in large numbers in an isolated form, scattered thickly through the lung-tissue. They are markedly softer than the typical grey form, but, except in the earliest stage, they are distinctly resisting. They are somewhat prominent, like the grey, but to a less degree. In shape, they are rounded, but their outline, even when single, is more irregular than that of the grey.

3. *Larger, opaque, white granulations*, indistinguishable in character from the foregoing, are found in all forms of phthisis, but when they are larger than hemp-seed, no translucency is observed in them, and they are then of a dead opaque white colour. They may attain the size of a pea, but in the single forms they are seldom larger than this. They are prominent and, as a rule, uniformly white, but sometimes they show a trace of yellow; they are absolutely non-vascular to the naked eye. They are generally rounded, but have a somewhat irregular and indented margin. They are homogeneous, with a finely granular section, and are easily crushed between the fingers. Some are evidently composite, and formed of groups of granulations, although this mode of origin is not always apparent, either to naked-eye or microscopic examination. Older granulations of this character, of whatever size, are sometimes surrounded by a firm and more transparent zone, which is occasionally pigmented. All forms of this granulation appear to undergo caseation, a change that will be considered hereafter.

4. *Yellow granulations*, like those last described, also occur of all sizes, from the smallest visible point to larger masses, which may attain the size of a pea, a horse-bean, or even of a hazel-nut. The smallest yellow granulations, in some cases, may be the only form present, and they may be so small and so thickly scattered throughout the lung as to merit the name of 'poussière tuberculeuse,' given them by Barthez and Rilliet.[1] In many cases, they are of about the same dimensions as the small transparent and opaque white granulations previously described, and they are generally found mingled with these. Like these, also, the yellow granulations tend to become confluent in groups of three or more, and they acquire an irregular outline, but they are also found scattered singly, round in shape, with a slightly irregular margin. They are prominent, homogeneously yellow, but finely granular; while softer than either of the forms last described, they still possess a certain degree of resistance, although they are easily crushed between the fingers. Between the smallest and the largest of these granulations, there are

[1] *Mal. des Enfants*, iii. 388 and 658.

all gradations in size. Those of medium dimensions, up to the size of a pea, are often distinctly rounded, but with a serrated margin. When larger, they are more irregular in shape and outline. Those of medium size may show no trace of composite structure; when larger, they are often visibly composed of groups of smaller granulations. These are dry, friable, and therefore soft in a certain sense, but many offer a distinct resistance to crushing. They are usually without a trace of vascularity, and are commonly finely granular on section.

5. *Indurated granulations.*—These were described by Bayle as a form of the grey granulation, and as being sometimes pigmented. Laennec paid but little attention to induration in tubercle. Andral, who denied the tubercular character of these indurated granulations, attributed their origin to a chronic pneumonia,[1] but Cruveilhier first strongly insisted on the induration as a form of cure of tubercle.[2] Rokitanski described it as 'obsolescence,'[3] while Virchow,[4] and, later, Langhans,[5] have described a 'fibrous tubercle.' Indurated granulations are found in various conditions in the lungs.

(*a*) The most typical are those in which there are small bodies identical in form and size with the grey granulation, very hard and resisting, still semi-transparent, and more or less pigmented. They exist singly or in groups. Rather larger bodies than these are sometimes found, reaching the size of a hemp-seed, still round, but often showing irregular processes of fibrous tissue extending from them. The granulations may still, in this latter stage, show a semi-transparency, or they may be so deeply pigmented that the translucency is much diminished (Plates VIII. 2, 5, and 6 ; X. 10 ; XIX. 1).

(*b*) A still larger number show a greater or less degree of opacity and caseous change in their centre, and these vary greatly in size and appearance. Some are as small as the grey granulations (X. 9 and 10), and from these, all gradations in size can be observed, to nodules equalling a pin's head or even a split pea (X. 5, 6, 10 ; XVI. 2). The proportion between the caseous centre and the indurated margin also varies considerably. In some, the former only constitutes a speck in the centre ; in others, it constitutes the greater part of the granulation or nodule, so that the fibroid pigmented periphery appears only like a capsule or cyst enclosing the central caseous part, and in different preparations the translucency of the periphery also varies. These indurated granulations, both with and without cheesy change, tend to form racemose groups which are one of the most common changes met with in chronic phthisis, and will be more fully dwelt on hereafter.

(B) INFILTRATIONS.—Infiltrations of very dense appearance are found in a variable extent of the pulmonary tissue in different cases of phthisis. They may be summarised as consisting of (*a*) red pneumonic infiltration, differing in no essential particular from ordinary red hepatisation ; (*b*) a grey hepatisation which possesses some peculiar features ; (*c*) a more gelatinous infiltration ; (*d*) caseous infiltration.

(*a*) Red hepatisation was noticed by Bayle as a complication of and cause of death in some cases of phthisis.[6] It was little insisted on by Laennec,[7] but Louis remarked that

---

[1] *Clin. Méd.* iv. 4 and 7.
[2] *Anat. Path. Gén.* iv. 560, 615, and 617. 'Tubercules de guérison, Tubercule mélanique de guérison.' See also Empis *De la Granulie*, p. 52.
[3] Rindfleisch, *Lehrb. path. Anat.* i. 298, and iii. 97, ed. 1855. In this edition he speaks of this change as being rare, and of the more common change as being caseation. In his earlier edition (1846, i. 397) he speaks of cornification (*Verhörnung*) as the only change undergone by the 'fibrinous tubercle' (the grey granulation).

[4] *Krankhaften Geschwülste*, ii. 640.
[5] Virchow's *Archiv*, vol. xlii.
[6] *Phthisie Pulmonaire*, Obs. 3 and 9, pp. 132 and 168.
[7] Laennec (*Ausc. Méd.* 2nd ed. i. 594) remarked that he had found tubercle in the midst of grey pneumonic hepatisation which had already passed into the purulent stage, but he regarded the latter as an accidental complication. Dittrich (*Prager Vierteljahrschrift*, 1848, ii. 157) found it in 11 out of 328 cases of chronic tuberculosis. He only found it lobular in one case.

he had found it in one-sixth of all his cases,[1] and that in nine of these it occupied a considerable area, while in others it appeared only as disseminated nodules. 'Engorgement,' according to him, was more frequent, but both this and the hepatisation were not more common in phthisis than in other fatal diseases. Louis' observations are probably in the main correct, and in a large number of the cases in which red hepatisations are found, they are probably a terminal stage, as believed by Bayle. It is, however, to be remarked that other observers have noticed that an acute pneumonia may appear in the course of phthisis, and may proceed to recovery, apparently uninfluenced by the tubercular disease and without accelerating the course of the latter; nevertheless, in other cases, the reverse effect is conspicuous, and even if the pneumonia be not acutely fatal, it accelerates the subsequent progress of the chronic lung-disease. It is, however, difficult to prove that such pneumonias belong clinically to the type of the acute primary disease.[2] As far as my observations have extended, this red hepatisation offers no peculiarities of naked-eye or microscopic appearance, to distinguish it from the ordinary acute disease; but in some instances it appears to pass into a chronic stage with induration, which, in general characters, resembles that found in some non-phthisical cases, when an acute pneumonia has failed to resolve. In one case of this nature the proof of the antecedent acute stage was, however, wanting (see *Case 3, Hawkins*, Plates IV. 1, XLII. 6, and XLIII. 4). I shall notice immediately a probable first stage of the condition known as grey infiltration, where a certain degree of redness and injection precedes the more uniform grey consolidation. In a few cases, where caseous change is rapidly advancing in the lung, a form of consolidation is also sometimes observed, differing but little, either in colour or in the granular appearance of the section, from the naked-eye appearance seen in ordinary red hepatisation. It is, however, firmer and more resistant on pressure, and passes insensibly at places into a consolidation which is ashy-grey in colour and presents considerable resistance. The caseous masses are scattered indifferently through both these latter forms of consolidation (*see* XII. *Case 23, Lloyd*). Whether this infiltration would, had life persisted, have passed into the more uniform grey infiltration next to be described, may be considered an open question, but I think it probable that the change would have occurred. I shall, however, under the head of caseous infiltration, have to adduce evidence that the latter change may rapidly invade portions affected with apparent red hepatisation, though I believe that the pneumonia in which it occurs is essentially different from the clinical disease 'acute pneumonia.'

(*b*) *Grey Infiltration.*—This was regarded by Laennec as a tubercular product, and styled by him the 'Infiltration tuberculeuse grise.'[3] It was also probably that described by Bayle[4] as a 'dégénérescence tuberculeuse non enkystée.' It is the most common phase of extensive pulmonary consolidation found in phthisis, though its appearance varies considerably, owing to its being mixed with caseous masses and with softening and indurated nodules, and also from ulcerations and cavities which are scattered through it. Louis,[5] who also regarded it as tubercular, noticed its occurrence in large masses and always combined with tubercles, and this statement was followed by Rokitanski.[6] Other authors have stated their opinion that it is solely inflammatory,[7] and Niemeyer identified it, as I

---

[1] Louis, *Rech. Phthisie Pulmonaire*, 3rd ed. p. 41.
[2] Andral, *Clin. Méd.* iv. 218; Huss, *Behandlung der Lungenentzündung*, pp. 23 and 182. Walshe (*Dis. Lungs*, 4th ed.) says of acute pneumonia: 'Some of the most marked examples of rapid resolution that I have met with were in phthisical persons.'
[3] *Ausc. Méd.* 2nd ed. i. 541.
[4] *Phthisie Pulmon.* p. 21; *Journ. de Chemie et Phar.* vols. ix. and x. It is not quite clear, from Bayle's description, whether he expressly includes under that head this particular form of pulmonary infiltration; but it appears to be most probable that it is to it he refers, though he describes it in more isolated nodules.
[5] *Rech. Phthisie Pulm.* pp. 4, 5.
[6] *Path. Anat.* 1861. iii. 86.
[7] Especially the late Dr. Addison (see Collected Writings, Syd. Soc. edition) and by Reinhardt, *Charité-Annalen* 1850-1.

believe erroneously, with catarrhal pneumonia, while others have regarded it as inflammation of the lung, but tubercular in character.[1] Professor Buhl has classified it among the desquamative or parenchymatous pneumonias, of which it apparently constitutes, in his opinion, the most typical form.[2] Laennec described it as existing both around excavations and also independently in other parts of the lung; it was grey, firm, indurated, smooth, glistening and homogeneous, and the characters of the pulmonary tissue were no longer recognisable. This infiltration passed into caseation, 'crude tubercle,' through the appearance in it of yellow opaque spots which coalesced. Laennec's description has remained classical to the present day, and sufficient for the recognition of this condition. The appearances of such infiltration are figured in Plates VII. 4, *a, a, a*; IX. 2, 3; X. 2; XIV. 2, *a, c*.

(*c*) *Gelatinous Infiltration.*—Laennec thought that the grey infiltration commenced with a stage to which he gave the name of 'gelatinous tubercular infiltration,' where the tissue was occupied by jelly-like material, colourless or slightly reddened, in which the outlines of the alveoli were lost, and by the latter character it was distinguished from the saturation with serum which constitutes œdema of the lung. The transformation to the grey infiltration was simply due to a gradual increase of its solidity, and its tubercular character was shown, in his opinion, by the appearance in it of yellow spots, gradually coalescing, and identical in character with those seen in the firmer variety.

There can be little doubt, in this case also, of the correctness of Laennec's description, and to it little can be added. The fluid expressed from the part thus changed is viscous and transparent or slightly turbid; it is more akin to mucus than to fibrin, but its resemblance to the former is only imperfect, and it is probably to a large extent albuminous in nature. The gelatiniform aspect can hardly be represented either by the pencil or by lithography, but it existed in parts contiguous to, and in some places passing into, the grey infiltrations here figured. In two points some addition has been made to Laennec's description of the grey infiltration, although nearly every observer has admitted the accuracy of the general description given by him. Some have asserted that the change commences with a stage of engorgement, or even of red infiltration,[3] and this appears to me to be very probable. It is certain at least that tracts are found solidified by exudation, which is firmer in consistence than the ordinary red or grey hepatisation of acute pneumonia, and has also a greater degree of translucency than those that present a more or less marked tinge of red, while the typical granular character of the latter is less marked, and indeed may be entirely absent. The tissue so changed may be identical, in general characters of firmness and translucency, with the grey infiltration, and differ from it only in the tinge of colour present (*see* X. 1, 3, 4; and XIII. 1, *a*), while in some instances the grey infiltration may be seen insensibly merging into a redder margin (XIV. 2, *c*).

In another point I believe that a slight modification of Laennec's description must be accepted. In the condition which appears to be an earlier stage of this change, the section has a certain degree of opacity and also a somewhat granular character, but it is seldom soft. Indeed the firmness and resistance described by Laennec is almost essential to its definition, though it is probable that the resistance of the tissue increases with lapse of time, and the firmness is—as remarked by Laennec—most pronounced in

---

[1] Hérard and Cornil, *Phthisie Pulmonaire*, p. 133 *et seq.*
[2] *Lungenentz. Tub. und Schwindsucht*, p. 48.
[3] Rokitanski, *Path. Anat.* ed. 1861, iii. 85.

the neighbourhood of cavities of old standing.[1] In the more opaque varieties this form of infiltration occurs in masses of variable size; sometimes large areas are thus occupied, but in other cases nodules are found of the size of a walnut or a hazel-nut, and sometimes as small as a pea. In some instances, granulations identical in character with the softer opaque granulations previously described, bear a close resemblance to these more opaque nodules, and I have seen in one case, which appeared to be commencing phthisis, such granulations standing out prominently from a grey, but firmer and more transparent, diffuse infiltration.

(*d*) *Caseous Infiltration.*—The infiltration of the lung with *crude yellow tubercle*, as described by Laennec, has been more recently termed a 'scrofulous,' or by Virchow and subsequent writers, a 'caseous' pneumonia. Laennec believed that it might originate from the transformation of the grey infiltration, whether gelatiniform or firm, but that this transformation might take place with such rapidity that the evidence of this origin was wanting. He stated that it might occur in isolated masses with irregular outlines of a dull yellow white, less prominent than ordinary yellow tubercles, and also that it occupied considerable areas where the surface is even and the shape of the lung unchanged. This infiltration has attracted much attention, though it is not comparatively so common a feature of phthisical changes as some descriptions would lead us to believe.

Of the correctness of Laennec's description of the two forms observed there can be no question. Masses are found, originating in tracts of lung solidified by a grey or reddish-grey infiltration of variable degree of firmness, and these masses are of various shades of colour, from a yellowish-white to a dull opaque yellow; are finely granular, dry, and possess a variable degree of resistance, some being distinctly firm and others more or less friable. Their size varies from a pea to a horse-bean, a hazel-nut, or a walnut, and the shape, as well as the outline of the larger forms, is irregular (*see* VII. 4; X. 4; XII. and XIV. 2). Larger areas also occur of indefinite size, shape, and outline. In all these, cavities often appear, and the areas also, by their general softening, form cavities in the midst of the firmer grey infiltration in which they may be found.

Precisely similar masses appear also in the midst of simply hyperæmic tissue, independently of the more diffuse grey or red infiltration. They are not uncommon in the acute tuberculisation of childhood (VI. 1 and 2), and also in diabetes[2] (VII. 2). In the former, they sometimes appear to originate by the confluence of smaller masses of the same nature, but this is not always the case, though in many instances an extension by this means is observable (*see* XI. 1). In these cases, however, the section is less prominent than that of the ordinary granulations previously described, even at the margins, and as Buhl has remarked, their outline is rarely sharply defined: they pass insensibly into the surrounding tissue, and in the centre the section is uniform.

In other instances, as described by Laennec, large infiltrations may occur, diffused uniformly over a considerable surface, and sometimes occupying the whole, or nearly the whole, of a lung. They are more common in childhood than in the adult, though they occur also in the latter. In childhood, Barthez and Rilliet found them in one-third of all

---

[1] Buhl (*Lungenentzündung*, p. 49) describes the 'genuine desquamative pneumonia' as slaty-grey, almost black, and finely granular, but also as markedly *soft*. The latter is not, I believe, a characteristic of this form of infiltration, and the softness appears incompatible with a cell-growth in the alveolar wall, which Buhl regards as an essential feature of the process, and also with the amount of pigment which he describes. It must be added that Buhl does not identify this with Laennec's grey infiltration, but as he describes the 'gelatinous infiltration' separately, he has left Laennec's 'grey' unidentified in his description.

[2] A good illustration of this is given by Grancher, *Archiv. de Physiologie*, 1878, 2nd ser. vol. v. pl. 1. See also Lancereaux's *Atlas*, p. 284, pl. xxviii. figs. 1 and 4.

the cases of tuberculisation, but most frequently before two years of age. They are most common in the upper lobe, but also occur in the middle and lower lobes. In ten cases one lung alone was affected, tubercle being found in the other. In one case it constituted the exclusive affection of both lungs.[1] Lancereaux has described the appearance of such lungs as if infiltrated with mastic or Rochefort cheese.[2] In some instances, where the infiltration has occurred apparently in a tissue previously emphysematous, the section may have a worm-eaten appearance (*see* VIII. 4). Here again the constituent isolated masses may remain apparent, as in a case described by Louis,[3] but occasionally the infiltration is very uniform, extending over large areas of the lung, and resembling VII. 2. This tissue is finely granular, and possesses in some cases a considerable degree of firmness. The granular character becomes more apparent on scraping or tearing the lung, which, prior to this, may appear smooth on section. The lobular character is sometimes distinctly maintained, and granulations, grey or yellow, may occasionally be observed at the margins.[4] When the change reaches the surface, it is sometimes unaccompanied by any visible inflammation in the pleura, and the yellow colour of the infiltration is then seen through the transparent membrane (XI. 2).

(C) INDURATIONS.—The other change affecting extensive tracts of tissue in pulmonary phthisis consists of a fibroid transformation by which the lung is converted into a cicatricial mass, deeply pigmented, hard, resisting, and semi-cartilaginous in texture. It occurs in various forms, the chief of which are the following:—

(*a*) Isolated granulations become, as already described, hard, semi-cartilaginous, and deeply pigmented, and these may be thickly scattered through a tissue still containing air, which may differ but little in appearance from the normal characters, or may be emphysematous, or deeply pigmented, or congested, or in some cases may present more recent grey or gelatinous infiltrations. In other cases, however, these indurated granulations, when closely examined, may be seen to present fibroid pigmented lines, proceeding from their periphery into the surrounding pulmonary tissue, like the rootlets of a plant. Sometimes a zone of thickening, some lines in breadth, is seen to surround isolated large granulations which have become entirely caseous in their centres, and from this zone also prolongations extend into the surrounding tissue (X. 10, *d*). When the indurated granulations are thickly scattered, the rootlets may join those proceeding from adjacent granulations, until a very considerable degree of pigmented but incomplete induration is produced in the pulmonary tissue, but without causing complete consolidation (X. 10). It forms, however, a step towards the next stage.

(*b*) Groups of racemose, indurated granulations, deeply pigmented, some of which are caseous in their centres, are united by tracts of fibroid induration in which no trace of granulations exist. These tracts are intensely hard and pigmented, and their section is smooth and homogeneous, showing no traces of pulmonary tissue (X. 5). An intermediate stage is, however, very common, where rootlets similar to those described as existing between isolated granulations extend between these racemose groups (XVIII. 2, 3), and it is by the extension of this process that the more uniform induration last described is apparently produced. A most extensive solidification, occupying large tracts of lung,

---

[1] Barthez and Rilliet, *Malad. des Enfants*, iii. 341-2, 661 3.
[2] Lancereaux, *Atlas*, p. 283. The whole of upper lobe was thus infiltrated. The tissue could be torn, but less easily than in ordinary grey pneumonic hepatisation. The other parts of the lung were strewn with patches of greyish-white. Herard and Cornil (*Phthisie Pulmonaire*, p. 498), who have introduced the simile of Rochefort cheese, give a case where nearly the whole of one lung was thus changed. See also Reynaud, *Archives de Méd.* xxv. 203 (quoted by Louis).
[3] *Phthisic Pulm.* obs. 40, p. 442.
[4] Barthez and Rilliet, *Malad. des Enfants*, iii. 347, 661.

may, however, be produced by the multiplication of masses of racemose granulations filling nearly the whole of the pulmonary tissue, among which caseous spots may here and there be seen (XVII. 1).

(c) Bands of interlobular thickening are not uncommon, but usually occur only in isolated patches. In them occasionally caseous masses are seen, but the presence of the latter is probably accidental, and due to the caseation of large granulations in these situations. In a few places these appear to be obstructed bronchi whose contents have become caseous [1] (X. 6, 8, 10), but in other instances the lines of thickening distinctly extend along the interlobular septa (IX. 2). It is rare to find this change to any marked extent without coincident induration of the pulmonary tissue, but I have seen it in a few cases as a very distinct feature, though associated with indurations and caseous changes in other parts. Such bands may traverse the lungs in all directions, marking out the larger lobules and dividing the tissue like the septa of an orange.[2]

(d) Large areas of indurated tissue are produced by the combination of the two last-named processes. They sometimes present an irregular fibroid structure, quasi-reticulate, with a certain uniformity in the branching of the fibres, which extend over large areas, sometimes interspersed with isolated caseous granulations, as in XIV. 1, XV. 1, and XVIII. 3. In other instances the tissue becomes almost entirely homogeneous, as in XVII. 2 c, 3 a. In many of these cases, however, racemose masses of indurated granulations are seen at the margins of these indurated parts.

(e) Extensive indurations, generally more or less homogeneous, but sometimes showing caseous nodules within their area, are probably produced by a gradual fibroid change in the indurated 'grey infiltration' of Laennec. The proof of this mode of origin is partly inductive, partly histological; it may be seen, in some cases, proceeding at the margins of parts thus infiltrated, and in other cases it occupies considerable areas of a lung in which, elsewhere, the predominant change consists of this infiltration (see XIII. 1, 3).

This induration, as Laennec remarked, proceeds to a very large extent around cavities, and here also it takes origin chiefly in the 'uniform' infiltration by which they are surrounded, though the process may be combined with that of induration by means of racemose granulations.

(f) The final result of these changes, singly or combined, is in some cases to produce a fibroid change of the whole, or nearly the whole of one lung, attended with great retraction and diminution of its bulk, as in cases observed by Portal[3] and Quain.[4] Cavities may occupy more or less of this area, and a few dilated bronchi may traverse it, but the preponderant condition is fibroid contraction. The pleura covering such lungs, or parts of lungs, is greatly thickened—to the extent, it may be, of a quarter or even half an inch (see XIX. 2); the thickened pleura blends with the fibroid lung; and though it may be actually distinguished from the latter by its whiter, more fleshy, and more vascular appearance, it sometimes sends thickened prolongations deeply into the interlobular septa.

(g) Dilated bronchi are common in these tracts of general induration (see XIII. 3, XVIII. 1). Sometimes, however, they are entirely absent. I am disposed to believe

---

[1] See Carswell's *Illustrations of the Elementary Forms of Disease*, art. 'Tubercle,' pl. iv. fig. 4.
[2] See a case by Reynaud, *Mém. Acad. Méd.* 1845, p. 160; also Andral's description, *Clin. Méd.* iv. 375. I have seen two cases presenting these features.
[3] Portal (*Obs. Phthisie Pulmonaire*, ii. 365) says that the lungs may be reduced to a quarter of their natural size, and may be of such density as to be 'coriaceous' and 'like burned leather.' He quotes also older observers.
[4] Quain. *Lancet*, 1852, and *Trans. Path. Soc.* 1851, vol. ii. The left lung, indurated and contracted, displaced only 9 ounces of water; the right displaced 23 ounces.

that they tend to occur most commonly in the indurations that proceed from pneumonic infiltrations, and that when the induration arises from the fusion of groups of racemose granulations, they are very commonly absent; even in these, however, they may be occasionally traced (XIV. 1, XVIII. 3, 4).

(D) CAVITIES.—The most important feature in pulmonary phthisis consists in the destruction of the lung-tissue and the formation of cavities. This condition has attracted attention from the earliest times, and ulceration of the lung has been throughout regarded as the characteristic feature of pulmonary consumption, although, as is well known, other diseases had been included under this category prior to the writings of Laennec. It is at this point that much of the confusion in pulmonary nomenclature commences.

Without here entering into the history of the views of different authors respecting this process, it may be sufficient to enumerate the chief sources of destruction of lung-tissue other than those associated with the changes already described. These are cancer, gangrene, syphilis, bronchial dilatation, abscess of the lung occurring in acute pneumonia, and some cases of ulceration occurring among workers in dusty trades—knife-grinders, miners, &c. All these are, comparatively speaking, individually rare. They present certain characteristic features, and they do not present the changes common to pulmonary phthisis. In phthisis, on the other hand, excavation originates from the changes in the lung already described, and from some hereafter to be mentioned as occurring in the bronchi.

The characters and appearances of cavities vary in some degree with their modes of origin. They may commence in any of the forms of granulations, single or conglomerate, which have been already described, with the exception probably of the hard pigmented granulation of Bayle. A common mode of origin is also in caseous masses, either existing singly or occurring in the midst of grey or yellow infiltration. Bayle and Laennec limited their descriptions of the origin of cavities principally to the softening of 'tubercles,' with some attempt at classification of these into encysted and non-encysted varieties. Very important additions to the history of the formation of cavities have been made by Louis, Cruveilhier, Barthez and Rilliet, and by Hérard and Cornil.

The fact that isolated small cavities may occur from the direct softening of single granulations is well illustrated in many cases of acute tuberculisation in the child. It is not improbable that, though Bayle's definition of the grey granulations included the statement that they do not break down (*ne fondent pas*), these bodies, when originating acutely, may occasionally do so in the lung, in the same manner as Virchow has shown that they may ulcerate in the larynx without antecedent caseation.[1] This event is, however, rare. In the majority of cases of this nature a certain degree of caseation precedes the softening and excavation, which as Villemin has shown, may occasionally attack the grey granulations during their formation and lead to their acute liquefaction.[2]

The softening of the yellow granulations in an isolated form has been well illustrated by Louis, who showed that this process might lead to pneumothorax.[3] They were observed by Fournet to form small excavations no larger than the head of a pin,[4] and in some cases of acute tuberculisation in children, small, isolated cavities of this nature, which usually have a caseous margin, may be found thickly scattered through the pulmonary tissue.[5]

---

[1] Virchow, *Krankhaften Geschwülste*, ii. 644; Rindfleisch, (Ziemssen's *Handbuch*, Krank. Resp.-App. ii. 180) has made the same statement with regard to tubercle of the mucous membrane, and I can confirm it in respect of the bronchi.
[2] *Etudes sur la Tuberculose*, p. 103.
[3] Louis, *Phthisie Pulmonaire*, p. 3.
[4] Fournet, *Phthisie Pulmonaire*, 1839, p. 701.
[5] Moxon, *Path. Soc. Trans.* 1872, xxiii. 300.

The more common and extensive cavities are, however, associated with the softening of the larger single granulations, or of the racemose groups of granulations, which are either caseous, or may be partially caseous with an indurated margin.

Softening of isolated caseous masses is the common type of acute phthisis (*see* VII. 1, 3 ; XIII. 1 ; VI. 5). Here again, as in those last described, the centre is often found softened while the cheesy periphery extends more or less irregularly into the lung-tissue. Excavation of caseous matter, surrounded by a margin of induration, is not common unless some more diffuse pneumonic infiltration has occurred around these bodies, and it will be described under this head. Caseous matter thus encapsuled is, however, very common, and has been already referred to under the head of induration.

The most common form in which excavation occurs is from the softening of caseous matter surrounded by a grey or red infiltration. Here the masses which soften may be of very variable size, from a pea to a hazel-nut—at least cavities of these sizes may be found excavated in the firmer infiltration surrounding them. In a few places they appear as if sharply cut out with a punch from the surrounding infiltration,[1] but in the very large majority of cases a margin of softening caseous matter intervenes between them and the infiltrated tissue. It appears probable that in some cases the excavation increases in size by the further extension of this caseous matter ; but in others it is not improbable that the cavities presenting this appearance are those seen in process of formation (*see* VII. 4 : X. 1, 3, 4 ; XI. 1 ; XII. ; and XIV. 1 and 2). These excavations rapidly become very irregular in shape and size, as is seen in the figures.

The nature of the association of cavities with indurated *masses* is more difficult to trace. It appears to me to be often due to a secondary process of softening occurring in parts in which there has been a previous attempt at repair, and to be very frequently due to an inflammatory process taking place around them, and probably also to a deterioration of vitality due to fever and to fresh extensions in other parts. Such ulcerations are, however, very common in patients dying of an acute exacerbation after a long history of chronic phthisis. The softening occurs in scattered spots, in the midst of the indurations, probably by the extension of the caseous matters remaining in such tracts as are figured in X. 5. In other cases, which are on the whole more common, the process appears to be due to fresh caseation occurring in islets of pulmonary tissue which had previously been unaffected by the phthisical processes (XVII. 2, *a*, *b*) ; having once commenced in these, it extends to the indurated portions (*ib.* fig. 3).

Prior to evacuation, the softened caseous matter assumes a more or less fluid form ; it resembles in some instances a thick pus, or, as remarked by Laennec, it has the aspect of a milky fluid in which float fragments of caseous material. These softened areas constitute potential cavities, and when their contents are evacuated, the wall is usually found lined with a softening material akin to that of the contents. They may be more or less circumscribed by a zone of homogeneous transparent infiltration, but this is less apparent in the acute forms.

In some cases, instead of a gradual softening, necrosis *en bloc* occurs in the caseous matter, which may be separated from the surrounding tissue by a process of sequestration and suppuration, and may hang, as a mass, by a few filaments to the containing walls. This process, which was first described by Louis,[2] was regarded by Cruveilhier[3] as a species of gangrene, but without the characteristic odour. When the softening and ulceration have

---

[1] These were termed 'Géodes' by Cruveilhier. *Anat. Path. Générale,* iv. 574.

[2] *Phthisie Pulm.* p. 18.
[3] *Anat. Path. Gén.* iv. 578, 591.

reached the nearest permeable bronchus, the matter is evacuated; this evacuation may take place suddenly, and when in large quantities may cause death by asphyxia.[1] The occasional delay in this evacuation is due to the fact that the bronchus leading to the mass of induration is closed, both by growth in its walls extending to the interior, and also by its own inspissated contents. It is only when the softening and ulceration extend beyond the point of obstruction, that the free communication with the open part of the tube is established. The bronchus opening into a cavity is thus abruptly truncated, and its mucous membrane at once ceases. In a few cases the softened material opens laterally into a bronchus, in which the cavity may form a diverticulum, but this event, as Laennec remarked, is rare.[2] The smaller softened isolated 'tubercles' are also found occasionally as closed cavities, filled with puriform fluid, but as their communication with the bronchi is comparatively more direct, their contents more easily escape.

After the evacuation of their contents, cavities undergo various changes. In the simple form they are lined by a soft whitish material, which may be smooth and homogeneous, or may contain masses of caseous matter; these masses are often round, and present the characters of softening granulations. They may be more or less deeply imbedded in the wall, and may even extend into the subjacent tissue. This material presents the character of a very soft false membrane, but may also have that of a quasi-diphtheritic exudation extending even into the adjacent bronchi. Beneath it is an intensely vascular stratum of a semi-transparent substance, homogeneous and somewhat firm, resisting pressure, but tearing out with a fibrous structure. In its outer portions, where the vascularity is less marked, it passes into the 'grey infiltration' of Laennec, the 'melanosis' of Andral, the 'iron grey induration' of Addison. In this tissue, tubercular granulations are often to be found by the microscope.[3] It may be interrupted by caseous nodules, or by nodules of induration of older standing, projecting into the interior of the cavity; but these are accidental, and in a typical case the cavity presents the characteristic now described. In some cases the cavities are lined by a highly vascular 'granulation tissue,' which may pass into an almost fungoid growth, and give to the whole interior a villous appearance. Such cavities probably represent a stage of 'cure' to which allusion will be made hereafter.

Composite and sinuous cavities are much more commonly found *post mortem* than the foregoing simple forms. They result from the coalescence of numerous foci of softening; hence they assume very irregular forms, and often attain a large size. They occupy, in some cases, a great portion of a lobe, and burrow deeply in all directions, so that their connections are only traceable by dissection. Early stages of this process may be seen in VII. 1, 4; IX. 1; X. 1. 3, 4; XI. 1; XII. and XIV. The larger sinuous cavities can hardly be represented in a drawing, but a partial illustration is afforded in XI. 1; XII.; and XIV. 2. This peculiarity is due to tracts of induration, or of inflammatory infiltration intervening between the softening portions, so that the latter only communicate with one another at the points at which they are in contact. Many bronchi may open into these irregular excavations; their truncated ends being apparent when the cavities are cut open. The tissue intervening between them consists in great part of the indurated portions of lung-tissue, but as this gradually becomes involved in the destructive process, only the thickened interlobular septa remain, and these constitute the bands or septa by which such composite cavities are traversed. Such septa contain

---

[1] Andral. *Clin. Méd.* iv. 123 4. obs. vi. and vii.
[2] *Ausc. Méd.* 2nd ed. i. 547.
[3] Cornil and Ranvier, *Manuel Histol. Path.* 2nd ed. 1882, ii. 176.

branches of the pulmonary arteries and veins, and also occluded bronchi. The vessels are also occluded, in the vast majority of instances, by fibro-plastic growth, and hence Laennec asserted that they were not present in these bands. In some cases, however, they remain patent, and may have aneurismal dilatations in their course; these may be the source of fatal hæmorrhage.[1] The septa tend generally to break down, and may remain only as cord-like prominences in the walls, or their ends may be apparent as wart-like projections. In other respects the lining of the cavity presents appearances resembling those described in the simple forms.

When a cavity has arrived at this stage, it is commonly impossible to state with any certainty in which of the various processes above enumerated it has originated. Many of the most extensive excavations are found in lungs which are largely indurated by fibroid growth, or occupied by masses of indurated or pigmented granulations (see XIX.), but the clinical history and analogy would lead us to conclude that the process of excavation has for the most part commenced and proceeded by acute softening, and that the conditions last-named, with which, *post mortem*, the cavities are found to co-exist, are solely the result of the lapse of the phthisis into a more chronic state.

By some writers the formation of cavities has been largely attributed to changes in the bronchi. I believe that changes in these tubes only rarely constitute the first or most prominent feature in excavation, which is accomplished mainly at the expense of the lung-tissue. That they are necessarily invaded by processes of ulceration is self-evident. The manner in which this proceeds in them, and also the cases in which ulceration commences in them, will be considered hereafter.

Encapsuling and Cicatrisation of Cavities.—This process was described at great length by Laennec, who based upon the processes thus observed the doctrine of the curability of pulmonary phthisis.

It has been admitted by all writers that 'tubercle' (including granulations and caseous matter) *may* be entirely eliminated by the process of excavation, and that a cure would be thus more commonly effected, were it not for the tendency of fresh granulations to appear in other parts of the lung; these, as Laennec remarked, frequently radiate around the cavity.[2]

Laennec's description of the gradual formation and thickening, around the cavity, of induration-matter more or less pigmented, which he described as semi-cartilaginous and

---

[1] The first instance recorded of this with which I am acquainted is by Stark (*Works*, edited by J. Carmichael-Smyth, 1788, p. 31). Another is given by the late Mr. Fearn of Derby (*Lancet*, 1841; see *Path. Soc. Trans.* vol. xxii. p. 42). Others are given by Dittrich (*Prager Vierteljahrsch.* 1846, xii. 160, and 1848, ii. 151), and by the late Dr. Peacock (*Edinb. Med. Surg. Journ.* 1843). Collected cases of this nature are given by Rasmussen (*Hospitals-Tidende*, 1868, translated into *Edinb. Monthly Journal*, 1868, vol. xiv.), by Fränzel (*Charité-Annalen*, 1875, vol. ii.), by Samuel West (*Med.-Chir. Trans.* 1875, vol. lxviii.), and by Douglas Powell (*Trans. Path. Soc.* vol. xxii.). Numerous isolated cases exist in the *Path. Soc. Trans.*; see index to these. Hilton Fagge (*ib.* vol. xxviii.) records one case in a child aged 2½ years. Rasmussen found one in a child aged 3½. In one case, by John Williams (*ib.* vol. xvii.), several varicose dilatations were found on two branches of the pulmonary artery in a single cavity. Rasmussen also gives examples of multiple aneurisms in a single cavity; in one case two existed, and in another four. Douglas Powell has given an instance where, although an aneurism was present, rupture of the artery took place at a different spot. His explanation of their origin is the most probable, viz. that they are due to inflammatory softening of the coats. Rasmussen says that laminated coagula are rarely found in their interior. Rokitanski, however, states that even after their rupture, the opening may be closed by coagula, and Damaschino (*Bull. Soc. Méd.* 1879) has found laminated coagula in their interior. He has not only found them multiple in cavities, but existing in both lungs. For other references see Cotton (*Med. Times and Gaz.* 1866); Peacock (*St. Thomas Hosp. Rep.* 1870); Reginald Thompson (*Pulmonary Hæmorrhage*, p. 115). An erosion of the pulmonary artery by an ulcerating bronchus is figured by Sir R. Carswell, *Illust. Elementary Forms Disease*, art. 'Hæmorrhage,' pl. ii. fig. 5.

[2] Laennec, *loc. cit.* Barthez and Rilliet (*Mal. de Enfants*, iii. 667) met with eight cases of cicatrised cavities in children; four died of other diseases, four of relapse of 'tuberculisation.' Boudet (*Comptes Rendus de l'Académie des Sciences*, 1848, vol. xvi.) reports ten instances of such cicatrised cavities without recent tubercles, and eight more in the presence of recent tubercles.

sometimes more or less vascular, has remained one of the most perfect yet afforded. The result, as he stated, is to contract the cavity to a condition which he likened to an almost innocuous fistula. The cases which he described do not afford illustrations of complete closure, though this is sometimes effected by the occlusion of the bronchus and cretification of the contents of the excavation, such as were described by Roger.[1] The proof that these matters had an origin in a cavity which had ever opened into a patent bronchus is, however, wanting, and in many cases these cretaceous matters have probably proceeded from non-evacuated, caseous material. Andral, however, has given several conclusive instances of the contraction and almost complete obliteration of bronchi penetrating the fibroid tissue surrounding old cavities.[2]

The absolute closure of a cavity of any considerable size to a linear cicatrix, not including cretaceous matter, is a rare event, and its occurrence has been doubted by competent observers. It nevertheless appears occasionally to occur, and an excellent illustration of the process has been given by the late Dr. Hughes Bennett.[3] Most of the puckered cicatricial masses of the apex are, however, probably the result of indurated conglomerate granulations, or of indurated grey infiltrations, which have not proceeded to excavation.

An old inert cavity with thickened walls is usually attended with a marked cicatricial contraction and puckering of the surface of the lung. There also the pleura is usually thickened and adherent, and sometimes contains many vessels of new formation, which give rise to anastomoses between the intercostal and the bronchial arteries—a fact that was pointed out by Schröder van der Kolk and Guillot.[4] An instance is shown in XVI. 1 and 2. On cutting through such a cicatrix the cavity is found to be surrounded by a variable thickness of deeply pigmented induration-matter, which is usually hard, dense, semi-cartilaginous, and almost black in colour, but is sometimes very vascular. This radiates in deep puckerings in all directions around the cavity and the fibrous bands of the enclosing masses of old caseous and cretaceous matter, and it may be mingled with groups of granulations. These puckerings pass into crepitant pulmonary tissue, which is frequently highly emphysematous.

The lining membrane of the cavity tends, with time, to become smooth and to lose its vascularity. The soft false membrane, with the highly injected tissue beneath, also tends to disappear, and the smooth lining blends insensibly with the cartilaginous wall. The junction of the cavity with the bronchus becomes less defined than in a recent excavation, and its lining assimilates more to the appearance of the bronchial mucous membrane. The fusion is possibly rendered more complete by the previous ulceration of the latter where it joins the cavity. In some cases, as before stated, the bronchi leading to these cavities are contracted, and some are obliterated.

The cavity continues to secrete pus, but in varying degrees ; in addition, old or more recent clots may be found in them,[5] and sometimes confervoid growths.[6] Cavities, sometimes of large, sometimes of smaller size, are also found in the midst of dense, indurated tissue. Their lining membrane is either smooth or vascular, according to the activity of the processes proceeding in them (see XIII. 1 (below c) ; XIV. 1 ; and XIX. 1 and 2).

Instead of the limitation of the cavity by fibroid thickening, the lung may be per-

---

[1] Roger (Essai, 'Curabilité de la Phthisie Pulmonaire,' Arch. Gén. 3rd sér. 1839, vol. v.
[2] Clin. Med. iv. 308 et seq.
[3] Pulmonary Tuberculosis, 1853, pp. 88, 89. Two illustrations of a 'cicatrix of dense white fibrous tissue, varying in breadth from one-fourth to three-fourths of an inch and measuring about three inches in length.' A similar linear cicatrix was described by Andral (Clin. Méd. iv. 372). Barthez and Billiet (loc. cit. iii. 669) give eight instances of the cure of cavities. Lebert (Brustkrankheiten, ii. 191) says he has met with a series of cases.
[4] Schröder van der Kolk, Obs. Anat. Path. p. 67 ; Guillot, L'Expérience. i. 545.
[5] Louis. Rech. sur la Phthisie, p. 22.
[6] Bristowe, Trans. Path. Soc. 1858, v. 88.

forated during the softening and excavation of caseous masses. This usually occurs in the acutest stage, during the softening of caseous matter, and it may arise from very small isolated granulations, but also from the larger masses. Ulcerative excavation may also extend through pleural adhesions, and may perforate the aorta [1] or the pulmonary artery ; [2] it may penetrate the spinal canal [3] and cause paralysis, or it may pass into or through the thoracic walls, and sometimes extend even to the neck. [4] In some of these latter cases the penetration of the thoracic wall is incomplete, and the skin becomes distended with air when the patient coughs ; the subcutaneous emphysema thus produced may even be fatal. [5]

Cretification.—Instead of softening and excavation, the caseous material may cretify, and form the origin of the calcareous masses which are found in the apices and other parts of the lungs in chronic phthisis. Such masses may, in some cases, be expectorated. This change induced Bayle and Portal to erect this class into a separate variety, under the title of ' Phthisie Calculeuse' ; the latter of these authors has given instances where these masses were expectorated in large quantities, and he distinguished them from gouty concretions. They had been recognised by Morgagni, who associated them with asthma. [6] Laennec also pointed out that they occurred in people who had no other pulmonary symptoms, and he attributed them, in many instances, to the ' cure' of a past phthisis. [7]

They are found in the lungs in two forms : in the one as a putty-like mass, surrounded by a dense, pigmented capsule of fibroid tissue of varied extent, from which radiating lines frequently extend ; in this case the mass is usually rounded, and the contents homogeneous. They occur also as calcareous bodies of stony hardness, frequently very irregular in shape, and surrounded, like the first form, by a fibroid capsule. They may, however, be found surrounded by lung-tissue that is apparently but little altered.

Virchow has stated that he knows of no evidence proving the cretification of tubercle, and that the majority of these concretions result from the retention of pus in small cavities, or, still more frequently, in dilated bronchi. [8] Considering the frequency with which they are found, [9] to refer them to dilated bronchi is to ascribe to such dilatations a larger share in the pathology of phthisis than they appear to possess ; and, on the other hand, the frequency of the formation of such concretions in bronchial dilatations is not borne out by the evidence respecting the latter in man, though they often occur in the bovine species. [10] That the softened contents of a potential cavity, which have not been evacuated through a bronchus, may easily undergo this cretaceous or calcareous change, is in the highest degree probable, and it is to this origin that Gairdner [11] attributes most

---

[1] Dittrich, *Prager Vierteljahrsch.* 1848, ii. 151.
[2] Carswell, *Illust. Elementary Forms of Disease,* art. 'Hæmorrhage,' pl. iii. fig. i.
[3] Cruveilhier, *Anat. Path. Gén.* iv. 580.
[4] I have seen a case of this nature. See also Cruveilhier, *loc. cit.,* and Buhl, *Sec. Anat.* 1856, vol. xxxi. 2nd ser. i. 33; also *Atlas,* liv. xxxii. For other references see Rayer, *Archives de Méd. Comparée,* 1843, i. 207 ; Williams, *Dis. Chest,* p. 102 ; Schmidt's *Jahresbericht,* 1856, vol. xci.; Bonchut, ' Des Fistules Pulmonaires Cutanées,' *Gaz. des Hôp.* 1854, No. 54 (twenty-three cases) ; Biermer, *Schweiz. Zeitschr. für Heilkunde,* ii. 139 (several references) ; Stokes, *Dubl. Hosp. Gaz.* p. 185 (penetrated glenoid cavity) ; Lebert, *Klinik der Brustkrankheiten,* ii. 207 ; Flammarion, *Des Fistules Thoraciques,* Thèse de Strasbourg, 1869 (several cases).
[5] Cruveilhier, *Bull. Soc. Anat.* Paris 1856, and *Gaz. Hebdom.* 1856 ; Cleland, *Glasgow Med. Journ.* 1878.
[6] *De Sedibus et Causis Morborum,* Epist. xv. 15.
[7] *Ausc. Médiate,* 2nd ed. ii. 24.

[8] ' Ueber das Verhalten abgestorbener Theile im Inneren des menschlichen Körpers,' *Verhandl. Berliner med. Gesellsch.* 1865, pp. 257, 267.
[9] Roger (' Essai sur la Curabilité de la Phthisie Pulmonaire,' *Arch. Gén. de Méd.* 1839, 3rd ser. vol. v.) found in the bodies of ten old people, fifty-one instances of calcareous concretions in the lungs. In the apex alone there were 39 ; scattered through all parts of the lung, 6 ; in other parts than the apex, 6 ; in both lungs simultaneously, 24 ; in the right alone, 17 ; left alone, 10. They often co-existed with tubercles. They were either surrounded by induration, or by healthy lung. The bronchial glands sometimes contained concretions when the lungs did not. See also Boudet, ' Rech. sur les Transformations des Tubercles Pulmonaires,' *Comptes Rendus Acad. des Sciences,* 1843, vol. xvi.
[10] See later, Bronchial Dilatations in Phthisis.
[11] *Path. Anat. of Bronchitis.* See also Rindfleisch. Ziemssen's *Handb.* bd. v.

of these concretions. The fact that occluded and contracted bronchi are often found leading to them, points rather to this mode of origin than to the origin in bronchial dilatations. Similar concretions, as is well known, are frequently found in the kidney when the disease is attributable to tubercle rather than to any mere dilatation of the pelvis by occlusion of the ureter; the same is true of the Fallopian tube. The best proof of the origin of these calcareous masses from caseous degeneration of pre-existing tissue ('tubercle') is, however, that afforded by the lymphatic glands, in which there is no question of the retention of products of viriated secretion or of mere suppuration. Seeing how closely the changes in the glands are allied to those in the lungs, it is easy at least to comprehend that the caseous masses in the latter may undergo the same metamorphosis. It is further worthy of remark that cretification, even of acute miliary tuberculosis, has been described as a cure of this process by Burkart, the lungs in such cases having the feeling of sand-paper;[1] and it has been seen in miliary tubercle of the liver by the late Professor Ed. Wagner.[2] Sir Robert Carswell believed that the calcareous nodules proceeded from cretified bronchial glands, perforating the bronchi,[3] and a case of this nature is recorded by Rühle.[4]

The calcareous masses yield a large quantity of lime-salts, mingled with cholesterin. Virchow has stated that when the former are dissolved out, traces of cell-structure are still apparent, but no other element of tissue. The fact is, however, that when complete caseation and softening has occurred (a change probably preliminary to most forms of cretification), the structural elements of the lung have almost entirely disappeared. Reynaud,[5] however, stated that he found elements of pulmonary tissue among them, and the fact is easily credible.

Gangrene must be reckoned among the occasional destructive changes of the lung in phthisis. It is, however, comparatively rare, a fact which is remarkable, considering the occasional intensity of the processes and the extent to which the circulation is arrested. It sometimes occurs in the sloughing walls of cavities, but it is more common in the grey infiltration or in the softer pneumonic processes. It seldom passes into the black variety, or breaks into cavities, but is usually found in the form of a grey softening of a dirty appearance, passing into a fetid and ichorous pulp I have met with it in six out of a hundred cases of phthisis, and always in the acute pneumonic forms of the disease.[6] In one case it appeared to be due to the contraction of a branch of the pulmonary vein by induration-matter, and here it had broken down into a blackened pulp.[7] Lebert also states that in his experience it is rare. The sequestra of caseous material occasionally found free in cavities can hardly be included in this category.

Changes in the Bronchi.—Extension of cavities further takes place by the implication of the bronchi.

By some recent writers, and notably both by Virchow[8] and Rindfleisch,[9] pulmonary tuberculisation is held to be in a large measure a bronchial affection. Buhl also, under the title of 'purulent peribronchitis,' for which he claims the place of a substantive disease, has advanced the theory that much of the destruction of the lung is due to this

---

[1] Burkart, *Deutsch. Archiv klin. Med.* 1873, vol. xii.
[2] *Archiv der Heilkunde,* 1861, ii. 37.
[3] *Illust. Elementary Forms of Disease,* art. 'Tubercle.'
[4] Ziemssen's *Handb.* bd. v. abth. ii. p. 48.
[5] 'Oblit. des Bronches,' *Mém. Acad. Méd.* 1855, p. 148.
[6] Three of these were in the midst of pneumonic infiltration, three in cavities.
[7] *Klinik der Brustkrankheiten,* ii. 100.
[8] *Verhandl. Berliner med. Gesellsch.* 1865.
[9] *Path. Gewebelehre,* ed. 1878, and Ziemssen's *Handbuch,* vol. v.

cause.¹ I shall have hereafter to allude to these views, and will here simply remark that no theory or statement of facts not directly applicable to the pulmonary (alveolar) tissue appears capable of covering the most important changes which lead to its destruction. I must confess that I have never seen this purulent or caseating peribronchitis apart from other phthisical processes affecting the substance of the lung, although in various degrees it may be found connected with them; and participating in the changes which they produce.

I shall here discuss the chief changes visible to the naked eye which affect the bronchi in phthisis.

Tubercle of the terminal bronchi can, for the most part, only be recognised by the microscope, and will be described later. It is not commonly found very extensively diffused in the mucous membrane of the larger bronchi, except in the immediate neighbourhood of cavities,² and in these cases the tubercular ulceration only contributes to the extension of the cavity by the erosion of the bronchus, *pari passu* with that of the lung-tissue surrounding it. It may then be seen as isolated grey granulations, becoming cheesy, and passing into spots of ulceration which tend to become confluent, and it may resemble very closely the more superficial erosions of the laryngeal mucous membrane. In other cases, apart from cavities, the mucous membrane is swollen and thickened, and largely infiltrated with the growth, passing into caseous change and generally into ulceration.³ This process may be bilateral, and may extend to the bifurcation and thence to the trachea; there are confluent granulations, passing into caseous masses of a diameter of one-eighth to one-quarter of an inch, and in some places leading to deep ulcerations between the cartilages (XX. 1).

In other instances, however, there is a manifest peribronchitic thickening passing into cheesy change, which apparently leads to more extensive ulceration, as in VII. 1, *c*, *b*; X. 3, *a*; XII.⁴; XIV. 2, *d*; XVIII. 4, *f*.⁵ In many of these cases it is, however, difficult to define strictly the change in the bronchial wall from that of the adjacent pulmonary tissue, as the one often passes insensibly into the other (*see* VI. 3). It must also be added that, though some thickening of the bronchial wall takes place in all parts adjacent to cavities, a distinct peribronchial growth is with difficulty recognised by the naked eye before the occurrence of this caseation, although it is observable with the microscope.⁶

In some cases, however, there is a manifest thickening of the wall, and in one instance of sloughing quasi-gangrenous pneumonia, occurring in a case of old phthisis, I found soft granulations scattered through the infiltrated tissue, and the bronchi were surrounded by a soft material, similar in character to the granulations, which was invading the walls and passing into ulceration.

The mucous membrane of the bronchi is reddened, swollen, and thickened. This change tends to be general in all cases of acute phthisis. In the more chronic forms it is chiefly noticeable in the neighbourhood of cavities. The swelling of the membrane may coincide in some places with thickening of the outer coats, so that a noticeable diminution of the calibre of the tube may ensue.

---

¹ *Lungenentzündung, Tuberculose u. Schwindsucht,* pp. 89, 92 *et seq.*
² Cruveilhier has described submucous tubercle in the bronchial mucous membrane of the cow. *Anat. Path. Gén.* iv. 597.
³ Cf. Rokitanski, *Path. Anat.* iii. 28.
⁴ In the left-hand upper corner of the figure.
⁵ Cf. also Hérard and Cornil's coloured plates in *Phthisie Pulmonaire.*

⁶ Goodhart (*Brit. Med. Journ.* 1879, i. 542) has recorded a case where peribronchitis was found in the midst of hepatised tissue, no other change being present than caseation of the mediastinal glands. He thinks the pneumonia was due to a caseous change extending along the bronchi. It appears to me probable that this was excited by the surrounding pneumonia. The case has some analogy with those of interlobular lymphangitis associated with obstruction of the glands; see later.

Ulceration of the mucous membrane is not uncommon, and it often assumes a serpiginous form, with islets of deeply injected and swollen mucous membrane intervening between the ulcers. These ulcerations commonly extend from cavities, but may, in rare cases, occur in other parts.[1]

The bronchi may be either dilated or contracted. Dilatations are common, and occur in two distinct phases of phthisis.

(a) They are met with as part of the phenomena of acute tuberculisation of childhood,[2] where they probably occur under the same conditions of origin as prevail in acute broncho-pneumonia (see ante, p. 24). The dilatation sometimes coincides with thickening of the wall, which is usually tubercular in character,[3] the 'peribronchitis tuberculosa' of Virchow, and the tube is then rigid and its diameter much enlarged. But dilatation may exist without this thickening; the walls are then thin, and the tube dilated. Buhl attributed to 'purulent peribronchitis' a large share in the production of bronchial dilatation.

(b) Dilatations are still more common in tracts of fibroid induration, though in these, as will be noticed presently, contraction is also not uncommon. The dilatations in these parts may be either fusiform or globular. The former occur also in parts not thus indurated, but both varieties are most marked in the fibroid portions (see XIII. 3; XIV. 1; XVIII. 1; and XIX. 2). The fibroid induration belongs to the class before described; as a general rule the walls of the bronchi are fused with it, and are indistinguishable from it.

The mucous membrane in both these forms of dilatation is commonly inflamed and swollen, and ulceration is occasionally present, but to a variable degree. It may sometimes proceed to a considerable degree, but this is rare.[4] Reinhardt[5] attributed a large share of the excavations found in phthisical lungs to bronchial dilatation, and in this he has been followed by Ruhle and by Niemeyer,[6] but I believe that this view is untenable.

The distinction of a cavity formed by a dilated bronchus from one originating in the destruction of the pulmonary tissue and communicating with a bronchial tube, is at times a task of great difficulty, as was recognised by Laennec.[7] The difficulty exists in three directions. The first is in rare cases where all the bronchi of a lobe present sacculiform dilatations separated only by thin septa, which septa are perforated by communications between the dilatations, giving rise to the appearance of multilocular cavities. This event is, however, singularly rare in the upper lobes.[8] In a second class a difficulty exists, as pointed out by Gairdner, when a single cavity connecting with a bronchus is lined by a smooth membrane. The third is when a dilated bronchus has undergone secondary ulceration.

---

[1] Barthez and Rilliet (*Malad. des Enfants*, iii. 709) say that the ulcerations may occur when miliary tubercles alone are disseminated through the lungs. Louis found them in 22 out of 49 cases: in 5 out of 19 females, and 17 out of 30 males. He thought that there was a greater tendency to secondary ulcerations of the mucous membrane of the upper air-passages in the male than in the female sex. He remarked that bronchi leading to solid masses of 'tubercle' were seldom inflamed.

[2] This was noticed in an adult by Fournet, *Rech. Cliniques*, ii. 707.

[3] Förster, *Path. Anat.* 1863, ii. 228.

[4] Barth ('Rech. Dil. des Bronches,' *Mém. Soc. Méd. Obs.* 1856, vol. iii.) found ulcerations of the bronchi rare in the general disease, having only met with three instances in 48 cases. Biermer, however (Virchow's *Archiv*, vol. xix.), found such ulcerations common in tubercular lungs.

[5] *Charité-Annalen*, 1850, i. 273-4.

[6] Ruhle, 'Untersuchungen über die Höhlenbildung in tuberculösen Lungen,' *Habilitations-Schrift*, Breslau,
1853; Niemeyer, *Klin. Vorträge*, p. 67. Gairdner (*Path. Anat. of Bronchitis*, Edinb. 1850, p. 76) took precisely the opposite view, and attributed 'almost all' so-called sacculated dilatations of the bronchi to enlargement of the lungs, which he says may be lined by a smooth membrane, and an imperfect reproduction of epithelium.

[7] *Ausc. Méd*, 2nd ed. i. 208. Laennec, who in this article gave the first detailed description of bronchial dilatation, announced his intention of describing, in the chapter on phthisis, the distinction between these dilatations and cavities, an intention which he did not fulfil. The first accurate definition was given by Virchow (*Verhandlungen Würzburg. phys.-med. Gesellschaft*, ii. 24 *et seq.*), and to this paper I am mainly indebted for the data here given. The distinction given by Stokes (*Dis. Chest*, p. 171) applies only to simpler cases. See also Walshe, *Dis. Lungs*, pp. 235-6, and Barthez and Rilliet, *Malad. des Enfants*, iii. 665.

[8] See a case by Barth (*loc. cit.* p. 480) where the tube leading to these dilatations was almost closed.

In most ordinary cases the continuity of the mucous membrane in dilated bronchi, and its abrupt cessation when the bronchus opens into a pulmonary excavation, is a sufficient criterion. In other cases, when through excessive dilatation of the tube the mucous membrane has been almost effaced by stretching, the distinction may be made by the continuity of the vessels, which are abruptly truncated in the case of a cavity. Further, as Virchow has pointed out, the elastic membrane of the bronchus is still continued in the walls of the dilatation. It must, however, be admitted that a smooth-walled cavity, continuous with a bronchus and surrounded by indurated tissue, may at times be very difficult to distinguish from bronchial dilatation, even under careful microscopic observation.

The distinction of a dilated bronchus, the subject of secondary ulceration which has completely destroyed its walls, from a cavity originating in the lung, can only be a matter of inference from the state of the surrounding pulmonary tissue. In the vast majority of cases of phthisis, evidence exists of the disease of the lung, while in simple bronchial dilatation the surrounding tissue is either simply inflamed and possibly gangrenous, or is indurated. A practical difficulty of this kind is therefore comparatively rare. If any traces of mucous membrane are still discoverable within the cavity, they would be conclusive evidence of its origin in bronchial dilatation.[1] Even in genuinely phthisical cases the bronchial dilatation may be unilateral, and limited to a single portion of the lung. It is, however, in these conditions much more common in the upper than in the lower lobes. The mechanism by which these dilatations are produced in phthisis is probably the same as that by which they originate in other conditions of chronic induration. The wall is weakened and loses its elasticity by inflammatory change, and possibly by tubercular infiltration ; it then yields to the expansile influence of chronic cough.

Contents of the Bronchial Tubes.—In most cases of phthisis ending fatally, the tubes contain everywhere a large amount of mucus, which is often blood-stained. In some acute cases this is only of the ordinary type of a thickened mucoid secretion ; in others it is to a variable degree fluid or puriform. The tubes traversing the portions of lung affected with pneumonic consolidation, whether this be grey or caseous, are often obstructed with a solid and more or less fibrinous material, which may occasionally be found in various stages of softening,[2] but in other cases of this nature they are only filled with a puriform mucus. Plastic exudation into the interior of the tubes, resembling diphtheritic false membrane, is not uncommon near large cavities in which a similar membrane is found. It sometimes extends considerably beyond the neighbourhood of such cavities, and may be found independently.[3] Raynaud[4] has described a case where a plastic exudation obstructed nearly the whole of the tubes.

A point which has received much attention during recent periods has been the question of the retention and caseation of the secretions in the interior of the bronchial tubes, and the opinion that these retained secretions have been widely mistaken for tubercles of the lung. This view was first put forward by the late Dr. Addison,[5] who, however, combined it with a statement that the walls of the tubes were themselves so thickened as to resemble ' a boiled pipe of maccaroni.' It was represented in very similar terms by Reinhardt[6] and Rühle,[7] and has received the support of Virchow, who added that most of the ' encysted

---

[1] Rokitanski, *Path. Anat.* iii. 91.
[2] Hérard and Cornil, *Phthisie Pulmonaire*, pp. 137, 140.
[3] Louis, *loc. cit.* p. 27 ; Lebert (*Klinik der Brustkrankheiten*, ii. 36) met with it four times, twice in chronic, and twice in acute cases.
[4] *Mém. Acad. Méd.* 1865, p. 160.
[5] *Collected Writings*, Syd. Soc. ed. pp. 54, 61, 62.
[6] *Charité-Annalen*, 1850, i. 371–4.
[7] Rühle, *Untersuchungen Höhlenbildungen in tuberculöse Lungen*. Diss. Inaug. Breslau, 1858.

tubercles' of Bayle and Laennec were only bronchi with retained contents,[1] and he cited, in favour of this view, Carswell's celebrated figure.[2] In reference to these opinions I venture to make the following observations. Carswell, as is well known, held tubercle to be a secretion on the free surfaces of mucous membranes. The appearance illustrated by him in Fig. 1 is so rare that I have not met with one resembling it. It has, however, been figured by the late Professor Colberg,[3] but I think it is more than open to question whether these are truly bronchi laid open, or only racemose caseous masses. Carswell's Fig. 2 corresponds very closely with Addison's figures of supposed thickening of the bronchial tubes simulating tubercles. Carswell, however, held that this apparent thickening with a central opening was due to a 'gradual secretion' from the wall into the interior, and on this subject I would make the following remarks. It has been stated by Virchow that a large proportion of tubercles, miliary and other, are entirely of bronchial or peribronchial origin, and that when this growth occurs in their walls, their contents are retained and contribute to the caseous or 'scrofulous' mass found in their interior, in this respect resembling the ureter and Fallopian tubes.[4] This view has been very fully adopted by Rindfleisch, and if true it removes the discussion to another basis, viz., not whether these conditions are purely fallacious appearances, resembling tubercle, but whether they are due to tubercle in special situations. In this sense also Addison's view may be held to be capable of reconciliation with that of Virchow and Rindfleisch. The question as to the seat of tubercle in the pulmonary tissue and bronchi is in a great measure histological, and as such these views will be considered hereafter. I may, however, state that, apart from the appearance of granulations softening in the centre, I have hitherto found it impossible to trace any bronchial tubes ending in dilated extremities filled with thickened pus, such as have been described by Addison, Reinhardt, and Ruhle. One other point insisted on by Addison also requires allusion. He lays great stress on the proof that these bodies are thickened tubes, afforded by the fact that a bristle can be pushed through their centre into other bronchial ramifications. That this can be done, does not, however, prove that they are solely changed tubes, because it can be effected also in any softened 'tubercle' when the connection with the bronchus is free. Moreover this apparent central passage may exist in 'tubercles' in the serous membranes where no such fallacy is present.[5] I shall hereafter have to show that bodies such as are figured in X. 6, 7, 9, 10, which very closely resemble cut sections of bronchi filled with inspissated pus, are really in large measure changes in the structure of the lung-tissue, and that the implication of the bronchi, when this occurs in such formations, is only a part of this change, involved of necessity by the relation of the tubes to the alveolar structures.

The contents of dilated bronchi are sometimes inspissated and caseous, but very frequently they are semi-fluid and purulent, and do not differ from those found in bronchial dilatations under other conditions. The opinion that these may calcify, and form the chief origin of the calcareous concretions found in the apices of the lungs in cases of healed phthisis, has been already alluded to. This opinion receives, however, but little support from the general history of bronchial dilatation in other diseases than phthisis, and though it appears to be not uncommon in the bovine species, it is rare in man.[6]

---

[1] *Krankhaften Geschwülste*, ii. 648-9.
[2] *Illustrations, &c.* art. 'Tubercle,' pl. i. figs. 1, 2.
[3] *Deutsch. Arch. klin. Med.* 1868, ii. pl. vii. fig. 7.
[4] *Krankhaften Geschwülste, loc. cit.* 1863; and *Verhandlungen Berliner med. Gesellschaft*, 1865, i. 263.
[5] Aufrecht, *Centralbl. für med. Wiss.* 1869, p. 433.

This description refers to the omental forms of tubercle in the artificial disease in the rabbit. Lebert (*Klinik der Brustkrankheiten*, ii. 81) considers that in the lung a central opening demonstrates a peribronchial formation.
[6] See above, p. 77.

Contraction and obliteration of the bronchi was shown by Andral (see ante, p. 76) to take place in the neighbourhood of most of the masses of induration, and the tubes traversing these are for the most part no longer recognisable. Marked atresia of the bronchi in other parts of the lungs is, however, a rare event, and is seldom the result of direct changes in the wall, except at places where the lung-tissue is especially affected by phthisical changes. In some cases, however, it is produced by the contraction of cicatricial tissue around a bronchus,[1] and a similar effect may result from the pressure of enlarged bronchial glands. Closure of the bronchus by tubercular growth into its interior will be again alluded to.

Histology of the Granulations.

In commencing the histology of phthisis I have to remark that, although I have described separately the different naked-eye appearances of granulations found in the lung, it is by no means easy to give a corresponding histological classification. One reason for this is that in the typical disease acute tuberculosis, as occurring in childhood, very great variations are observable in the histological characteristics of granulations which are, to the naked eye, very similar, and that these differences are found in apparently similar granulations in the same lung. Another reason is that a very large proportion of the granulations, in some cases of acute generalised tuberculosis, have not the typical glistening characters of the grey granulation, but are more or less opaque and soft, while some, still maintaining the form and size of the smaller granulations, are distinctly caseous. This is true, not only in childhood, but also in cases of acute tuberculisation in the adult, and is a point on which considerable stress will be laid hereafter in considering the unity of nature and origin of these states. Similar differences to those which I shall have to notice, but in a more pronounced form, have been observed by Klein in the acute tuberculisation of the lungs of children. It is probably these differences that have occasioned the great variety of description, classification, and interpretation, which has of late prevailed in the literature of tubercle.

I have hitherto avoided, as far as possible, using the word tubercle in reference to these granulations, but in the admitted disease—acute tuberculosis—it can hardly be avoided without inconvenience. I shall attempt to show hereafter that all changes occurring in this disease are also met with in the lungs in phthisis, whether this is acute or chronic.

Granulations in the Lung in Acute Tuberculosis. (a) *Grey Granulations.*— The classical tubercle of Virchow,[2] the typical granulation,—composed of a small-celled growth, dense, becoming caseous in the centre, and gradually extending in a more scattered form at the periphery,—may be regarded as having formed the basis of most of the discussions on the nature of phthisis during the past twenty years. It is, however, as compared with other forms of granulation, by no means common in the lung. In fact it is more characteristic of tuberculisation of the serous membranes, although here also it is not the sole form present; diffuse infiltrations, of the same nature as regards structure and change, occur also in them. Granulations of

---

[1] A case of this character is given by Williams, *Pulmonary Consumption,* case 47, p. 200. The pulmonary artery was also contracted.   [2] *Cellular-Pathologie,* 1858, p. 442.

this nature are, however, met with in the lung (see XXX. 1). They sometimes appear to arise in the interlobular septa, but they also occur in the alveolar tissue, and may be seen filling the alveoli, where they become fused with the alveolar walls (see XXXIX. 7). Nodules like these are composed of a dense small-celled growth, separated by a reticulum with which the walls of the cells are often so blended that only the nuclei, which nearly fill the cells, are visible. The cells vary in size from the $\frac{1}{4000}$ to the $\frac{1}{2800}$ of an inch in diameter. When the nucleus can be distinguished from the cell-wall, it measures from $\frac{1}{5000}$ to $\frac{1}{3000}$ of an inch. Both cells and nuclei may, however, be smaller than the foregoing measurements. Some cells may have only a transverse diameter of $\frac{1}{4000}$ inch, and the nuclei may be as small as $\frac{1}{5000}$, $\frac{1}{6000}$, or even $\frac{1}{7000}$ of an inch. The mean of measurements are, however, generally, for the cells, between $\frac{1}{3500}$ and $\frac{1}{3300}$ inch, for the nuclei from $\frac{1}{4000}$ to $\frac{1}{3000}$.[1]

Extravasation of blood is sometimes found both in the firmer granulations and also in the softer forms presently to be described, and is probably the source of the pigmentation to be observed in them.

The reticular structure, with cells imbedded, may occupy considerable areas, as in XXX. 2, 9, without being present in the whole of a granulation; and, as in fig. 2, it may invade the whole of the wall of the alveolus, but without the intermixture of other cell-forms; the alveolus, as in this instance, maintaining its cup-shaped form.[2] This appearance, however, is rare, since in the vast majority of instances the cavity of the alveolus is more or less filled, either by a small-celled growth, or by epithelioid or small round cells, the nature of which will be more fully considered hereafter.

The reticular appearance here described has been the subject of considerable dispute. In some of my drawings and particularly in XXX. 1, 2, 5, the fibrillated appearance is somewhat exaggerated.[3] By some authors, however, 'tubercle' is described as a mass of small round cells or nuclei without any intervening material, the latter being attributed solely to the effect of hardening agents employed in the investigation.[4]

I would, however, venture to remark that the use of these reagents cannot *make* this material, but can only bring it into prominence. In some nuclear accumulations of rapid growth, and where epithelioid cells are rapidly produced, it is not apparent, and some authors have even divided tubercle into the reticulated and non-reticulated forms.[5] This intervening material tends to increase in amount with time, and finally becomes fibrillated,

---

[1] The foregoing are given from my own measurements. The numbers of authors who have given detailed measurements of the cells of tubercle is comparatively small. Lebert (*Malad. Scrof. et Tub.* p. 7) gives the size of the tubercle-corpuscle as having a mean of $\frac{1}{2000}$. Rokitansky (*Path. Anat.* 3rd ed. i. 294) describes tubercle as composed of *nuclei* varying in size from $\frac{1}{2500}$ to $\frac{1}{6000}$, mingled with some larger cells. Hérard and Cornil (*Phthisie Pulmonaire*) describe the cells as varying from $\frac{1}{3000}$ to $\frac{1}{2170}$ and the nuclei as $\frac{1}{6000}$ to $\frac{1}{5000}$. Cornil and Ranvier (*Manuel*, 2nd ed. 1881, vol. i.) give the size of the *cells* as from $\frac{1}{5000}$ to $\frac{1}{10000}$. Wagner (*Handb. allg. Path.* 1876) describes the *nuclei* as from $\frac{1}{3000}$ to $\frac{1}{7500}$, and the cells as about the size of white blood-corpuscles. Grancher (*Arch. de Physiol.* 1878, v. 23) gives the cells as varying from $\frac{1}{2000}$ to $\frac{1}{3500}$ inch. Delafield (*Studies Path. Anat.*) has given his drawings of the natural size, and the following measurements are taken from his pl. 44, 50, 67, 69: cells, $\frac{1}{1500}$ $\frac{1}{2500}$ $\frac{1}{3700}$ $\frac{1}{2100}$ $\frac{1}{2500}$ $\frac{1}{2000}$ $\frac{1}{7500}$; nuclei, $\frac{1}{5000}$ $\frac{1}{7000}$ $\frac{1}{7500}$ $\frac{1}{8000}$ $\frac{1}{7500}$ $\frac{1}{7000}$. Burdon-Sanderson (*10th Rep. Med. Off. Privy Council*) has given the following measurements: spherical corpuscles, granulations, lungs, $\frac{1}{4000}$ to $\frac{1}{300}$; nuclei of interalveolar thickening $\frac{1}{4000}$: liver, nuclei of adenoid growth $\frac{1}{2500}$ to $\frac{1}{5000}$; nuclei in spleen $\frac{1}{4000}$ to $\frac{1}{6000}$; nuclei of perivascular growth in peritoneum $\frac{1}{2500}$ to $\frac{1}{4000}$.

[2] I found it difficult, with such limited artistic powers as I possess, to represent the hollow of the alveolus, but in the original the whole depth of the cavity could be traced in a very marked form by altering the focus of the microscope.

[3] It has, however, been figured with quite as strongly a marked fibrillated structure by Delafield in his drawings made with the camera lucida. See *Studies in Pathological Anatomy*, pl. 44, 48, and 49. Baumgarten (*Zeitschr. klin. Med.* 1885, ix. 126) says it may be found in frozen specimens.

[4] This has been most distinctly asserted by Cornil. *Leçons Anat. Path.* and *Sur les Signes fournis par l'Auscultation dans les Maladies du Poumon*, Paris, 1874, p. 57. A reticulum has also been denied by Thoma (*Bech. Anat. Path. Tubercle*, 1879, p. 16) and by Friedländer ('Ueber locale Tuberculose' *Volkmann's Sammlung klin. Vorträge*, No. 64, p. 2).

[5] Hering (*Studien über Tuberculose*, pp. 84, 108) divides 'miliary tubercle' into two forms: the 'endothe-

as seen in XXX. 9 ; XXXI.; XLII. 2 ; and XLIII. 1, 2 ; and, except by the authors above quoted, its existence is generally admitted in a large number of tubercular formations.[1] The discussion has turned in part on the question whether the presence of this reticulum constitutes any analogy between tubercle and lymphatic formations, and by some who deny this analogy, the existence of this structure is nevertheless admitted.[2] In most cases it originates, I believe, as a species of ' formed material ' (Beale), or intercellular substance between the cells of new formation, and in this sense it was first described by Lebert, as a solid material intervening between the cells of tubercle.[3] In some places, however, as in XXX. 10, it appears to be in part formed out of the empty capillaries,[4] which blend with the fibroid substance ; in others it may be formed, as Klein believes, from the alveolar connective tissue.[5] It plays an important part in the fibroid transformations of tubercle hereafter to be considered.[6]

Where this small-celled growth is proceeding rapidly, the reticular structure is often less apparent. In some places it is limited to the alveolar wall, and may resemble a purulent inspissation. In others, the granulations appear to consist of a mass of small cells, filling the alveoli, and resembling the appearance in some forms of pneumonia. From both these conditions it may be distinguished by the comparative uniformity and smaller size of the cells, and in the vast majority of instances, when such appearances as those now described are met with, transitional forms occur between them and the firmer reticulate granulations, such as are seen in XXXVIII. 7, XXXV. 6, and XLI. 6. I shall have hereafter to describe, in connection with the acute caseation-processes of the lung, how closely some phases of the production of this small-celled growth are allied to those of inflammation. The granulation-form, however, when distinct, is peculiar and characteristic. When these granulations thus invade the lung-tissue, all traces of pulmonary structure disappear, but the elastic fibres may, as Grancher[7] has shown, be again demonstrated by the use of liq. sodæ.

A large proportion of the granulations in the lung in the acute tuberculisation of childhood are, however, differently constituted from those last described (A), and may be thus classified—(B) Granulations containing giant-cells. (C) Granulations containing a variable amount of epithelioid elements. (D) Granulations almost amorphous or entirely caseous. (E) Granulations presenting more or less induration.

(B) *Granulations containing giant-cells.*—It will save repetition if the subject of the granulations containing giant-cells is here considered *in toto* in their relation to phthisis.

Cells with multiple nuclei were described, as occurring in tubercle, by Rokitanski, under the title of ' mother ' cells.'[8] It is not very clear from his figure whether these are the genuine ' giant cells ' which, though previously recognised by Lebert[9] as forming a

---

lial ' and the ' reticulated.' He, however, states that the ' reticulated ' tubercle may change into a ' cellular ' tubercle, and *vice versa*.

[1] See Wagner, *Das tuberkelähnliche Lymphadenom*; also Schüppel, *Untersuch. über Lymphdrüsen-Tuberculose*; Talma, *Untersuch. über Lungenschwindsucht*; Rindfleisch, *Lehrb. path. Gewebelehre*, and Ziemssen's *Handbuch*, 'Krank. Resp.-App.'; also Delafield, *loc. cit.*

[2] Grancher, *Arch. de Physiol.* iv. 625, and v. 25.

[3] Müller's *Archiv für Anat. u. Phys.* 1844, p. 194.

[4] This has been asserted by Schüppel, *Lymphdrüsen-Tuberculose*, p. 93.

[5] *Anat. Lymphatic System*, part ii. p. 66.

[6] This has been much insisted on by Talma.

[7] *Archives de Physiol.* 1872, iv. 626.

[4] Rokitanski, *Lehrbuch path. Anat.* 1855, i. 90, 205. They had previously been described as ' mother-cells ' by Johannes Müller, *Ueber den feineren Bau der Geschwülste*, Berlin, 1838, p. 6. The literature of this subject has become so extensive that I will only refer to the following authors who have given the most complete historical *résumé*: Malassez and Monod, *Archiv. de Physiologie Normale et Pathologique*, 2nd ser. 1878, vol. v., to which I am under special obligations for many of the references in the text; Schüppel, *Ueber Lymphdrüsen-Tuberculose*, p. 87 ; Wagner, *Das tuberkelähnliche Lymphadenom*, 1871 ; Langhans, Virchow's *Archiv*, vol. xlii. ; Brodowski, *ib.* vol. lxiii. ; Lubimow, *ib.* vol. lxxv. ; Klein, *Anatomy of the Lymphatic Tissues*: see also *Lancet*, 1879, i. 414.

[9] *Physiologie Pathologique*, 1842, ii. 125.

constituent of certain sarcomata, and by Robin[1] as occurring in the development of bone.[2] were first described by Virchow[3] as occurring occasionally in tubercle in bovine tuberculosis, and also in lymphatic glands and tubercular peritonitis in man. To Virchow the name of 'giant cells' is due. They were soon afterwards recognised by Wagner[4] in tubercles of the liver, and a few years later by Busch in those of the choroid.[5] They were brought, however, into special prominence by Langhans, who asserted that they were an almost constant element of tubercle in all parts of the body, and they have been minutely described not only by him but by Schüppel, Wagner, Hering, Ziegler, Klein, and other authors.[6] They have been regarded by some authors, and especially by Köster, Charcot, and Hamilton, as one of the best criteria for the histological definition of tubercle, an opinion which is now scarcely tenable, since they have been proved to occur in other diseases.

Description of giant-cells.—The description first furnished by Virchow has received but few essential additions. In size, when fully developed, they may vary from $\frac{1}{1200}$ to $\frac{1}{105}$ of an inch, and Köster has described them as being as large as $\frac{1}{30}$ of an inch in diameter. They are, however, very irregular in shape; the larger ones are usually elongated, and the long diameter may considerably exceed the transverse (*see* measurements in descriptions of Plates XXXI. XXXII. and XXXIII.).

In the earlier stages they are highly diaphanous, and are best brought into view by Müller's fluid or chromic acid; the contents, even under these reagents, are, in addition to the nuclei, only an almost amorphous or occasionally very finely granular basis-substance. In those which are probably older, the apparent solidity and density of their basis-substance becomes more marked, and in some a line of fat-drops appears in the circumference, between the nuclei and the outer layer (Langhans). In some there is a granular interior layer, and a clear centre (Köster). Pigment is very abundantly deposited in some of old standing[7] (*see* XXXII. 7), and the tubercle-bacilli have been observed in them by Koch.[8]

With time there forms around some of these bodies a thick capsule ('mantle' Langhans) as originally described and figured by Virchow. It is glistening, transparent, homogeneous, and apparently structureless. It may attain a thickness of from $\frac{1}{2000}$ to $\frac{1}{100}$ of an inch (Langhans—*see* his figure of a ruptured cell), and in those of old standing it undergoes various transformations, by which it becomes blended with the surrounding tissue, and more or less fibrillated (*see* XXXIII. 6, 10. 11). The cells in their earlier stages are often, but not constantly, rounded (XXXI. 1, *b*, *d*; 3, *k*, *l*); many, however, soon acquire a serrated margin (XXXI. 1, *f*; 4, *c*), and from this margin pass off processes which blend in various ways with the surrounding tissue. In some places it would appear as if the processes were only fibroid prolongations of the capsule, but in others it is apparent that they are part of the cell, and contain nuclei (XXXI. 4, *b*; 5, 6).

The nuclei and their arrangement within these cells form one of the most important and

---

[1] Robin, *Compt. Rend. Soc. Biol.* 1849, p. 119.
[2] Robin termed them 'myeloplaxes.'
[3] *Würzburg. Verhandlungen*, 1857, vii. 143 and 228; and *Archiv für path. Anatomie*, 1858, xiv. 50 (figures).
[4] *Archiv der Heilkunde*, 1861, vol. ii.
[5] Virchow's *Archiv*, 1866, vol. xxxvi.
[6] Schüppel, *Lymphdrüsen-Tuberculose*; Wagner, *Das tuberkelähnliche Lymphadenom*; Hering, *Histol. u. exp. Studien über die Tuberculose*, Berlin, 1873; Ziegler, *Exp. Untersuch. über die Herkunft des Tuberkel-Elements*, Würzburg, 1873; Klein, *Anat. Lymph. Syst.*; Köster, *Die fungöse Gelenkentzündung*, Virchow's *Archiv*, 1869, vol. xlviii.; Lubimow, Virchow's *Archiv*, 1879, vol. lxxv.; Schüller, *Scrofulöse und tuberculöse Gelenkleiden*, Stuttgardt, 1880.
[7] Observed by Klein, *Anat. Lymph. Syst.* p. 64; also by Cornil, *Gaz. Méd.* 1880, p. 580. Langhans also pointed out that they take up pigment in the choroid.
[8] *Berliner klin. Woch.* 1882, No. 15.

characteristic features of the structure of these bodies. They appear either round or ovoid, and the latter shape is so constant that I am disposed to believe that the round forms are merely transverse sections of the ovoid, or the latter looked at end-ways. They are exceedingly numerous; there may often be from 200 to 300 in the larger cells. They may contain one or more highly developed nucleoli (Köster). Their outline is well defined against the ground-substance of the cell.

The elongated nuclei measure from $\frac{1}{1500}$ inch to $\frac{1}{3000}$ inch in length, and $\frac{1}{5000}$ inch to $\frac{1}{7200}$ inch in breadth. The majority are about $\frac{1}{2000}$ inch in length and $\frac{1}{6000}$ inch in breadth, and the breadth of most of those that appear round is from $\frac{1}{5000}$ to $\frac{1}{7000}$ inch. Some that are slightly ovoid measure $\frac{1}{4000} \times \frac{1}{6000}$. Indications of the multiplication of the nuclei by fissiparous division may occasionally be observed, although I have not found it easy to satisfy myself on this point. It has, however, been seen both by Langhans and by Klein.

The most remarkable feature of the nuclei is the manner in which they are grouped at the periphery of the cell. They tend to form a circle within this, with their long diameter pointed towards the centre (see XXXI. 1, 2, 4; XXXIII. 11). In some of the larger cells, viewed from the surface, they form a group, also at the periphery but less regularly arranged (XXXI. 2, a), and sometimes they are apparently central (XXXI. 3, h; XXXII. 9). In others, while still maintaining this character of grouping, they accumulate predominantly at one part only of the periphery of the cell (XXXI. 1, b; XXXII. 1), and in many specimens portions of the periphery are left free. In some cells of earlier formation only a few of the nuclei are visible (XXXI. 3, l, k), while in others, also apparently in course of development, the whole cell appears to be densely crowded with them (XXXI. 1, g, 2 e). When the prolongations pass from the cells into the surrounding tissue, these elongated nuclei may extend abundantly with them, until both the nuclei and the prolongations blend with the fibrillated tissue of the surrounding growth, in which similar nuclei exist (XXXI. 1, g, 4, b, 6); but in many places the prolongations exist without the nuclei. It is also not at all uncommon to find less definite forms, in which the cell-outlines are indistinct, but which are characterised by a similar grouping of nuclei in a quasi-protoplasmic material, passing insensibly into the surrounding fibro-nucleated growth (XXXI. 1, ll, 4, d).

The origin of these cells has been attributed to nearly every structure among which they are found.

(a) Virchow[1] originally ascribed their formation to the enlargement of the cells of the connective tissue, and he believed that he had traced their progressive stages from these and also from fat-cells. Wagner also observed their development from the cells of the reticulum in tubercular growths.[2]

The other supposed sources of these bodies may be thus classified:—

(b) Sections of blood-vessels or development from the interior of vessels.[3]

---

[1] *Archiv*, xiv. 51. For the history of these views see Malassez and Monod's article; also Lubimow, Virchow's *Archiv*, vol. lxxv.; Wagner, *Handbuch der allg. Pathol.* 9th edit. p. 492; Arnold, Virchow's *Archiv*, vol. lxxxviii.; Marchand, Virchow's *Archiv*, vol. xciii.

[2] *Das Tuberkelähnliche Lymphadenom*, p. 31. Billroth, finding them in granulations, attributed their origin to branching cells (*Ueber die Entwickelung der Blutgefässe*, Berlin 1856). Ziegler has also deduced them from fat-cells (*Tuberculöse u. Schwindsucht*, Volkmann's *Sammlung*, No. 151, p. 10).

[3] Schüppel (*Arch. der Heilk.* xiii. 80) from protoplasmic masses in the interior of vessels. In *Untersuch. über Lymphdrüsen-Tuberculose*, p. 93, he still believed in this origin, but admitted that they might equally arise within lymphatics. Cornil (*Comptes Rendus Soc. Biol.* 1878, p. 100) regarded them as sections of vessels. Rindfleisch (Ziemssen's *Handbuch*, 'Krankh. Resp.-App.' ii. 165) has figured them in the interior of capillaries. See also Thaon, *Rech. Anat. Path. Tuberculose*, p. 16, and Thin, 'On Pathology of Lupus,' *Med.-Chir. Trans.* vol. xlii.; Kiener, *Arch. de Phys.* 1880, vii. 825, 866; also discussion on scrofula, *Bull. Soc. Méd. Hôp.* 1881.

(c) Sections of lymphatics or developments from their endothelium.[1]

(d) Enlarged epithelial cells of the pulmonary alveoli, or a fusion of these, or from the epithelioid cells of tubercle in other parts.[2]

(e) From confluence of other cells,[3] as granulation-cells[4] or the endothelium of the iris.[5]

(f) From the white corpuscles of the blood.[6]

(g) It has been held that they represent modifications of the process of formation of blood-vessels ('angeioplastic').[7]

(h) From masses of protoplasm.[8]

(i) Lastly must be named a classification which accepts various modes of origin, which has been adopted in part by Langhans, and specially by Grancher, Lubimow, and Arnold.[9]

Some of these views are opposed to what is seen of the formation of the cells in tubercle of the lung. Thus the opinion that they merely represent sections of blood-vessels is scarcely applicable to a process in which one of the primary changes is a destruction of the vessels. Rindfleisch's drawing [10] has indeed a parallel in one instance, which I have figured, of what appears to be an early stage of these formations (see XXXI. 3, k), but the majority of the forms seen can scarcely be attributed to this origin.

The theory of development from lymphatic endothelium, except in so far as that may

---

[1] The latter opinion was first proposed by Klebs, Virchow's *Archiv*, xliv. 289. It was also supported by Köster, Virchow's *Archiv*, xlviii. 115, and by Aufrecht, *Die chronische Bronchopneumonie*, Magdeburg, 1873, p. 45. Rustizky has also seen them produced from the endothelium of the lymph-sac of the frog (Virchow's *Archiv*, lix. 218). These, however, may possibly have been due to the same origin as those found by Senftleben, see note 6. Schüppel, however, pointed out that these cells originate in the centres of lymphatic glands where no lymphatic vessels proper exist; and Langhans had shown that they are found in portions of the omentum free from lymphatic capillaries. Hering regarded them as sections of lymphatics (*Studien über Tuberculose*, 1878, p. 105), Treves (*Scrofula and Gland Disease*, pp. 147, 154) considered that they arose from lymph-coagula including a greater or less number of cellular elements.

[2] This opinion has been strongly supported by Klein for the lung, though he admits that giant-cells in other parts may have a different origin, *Anatomy of the Lymphatic Tissues*, part ii. pp. 64, 77; by Hering, *loc. cit.* p. 20; by Friedländer in desquamative pneumonia, Virchow's *Archiv*, lxxvi. 348; by Grancher, *Archives de Phys. Norm. et Path.* 1878, who attributes more than one origin to these cells; by Gombault, *Comptes Rendus Soc. Biol.* 1878, xxx. 281; and lastly in a recent article by Arnold (Virchow's *Archiv*, lxxvii. 140, and lxxxviii. 426). Arnold points out their derivation from the epithelial cells of the testicle by Gaule (Virchow's *Archiv*, vol. lxix.), Lubimow, and Waldstein—from those of the liver and kidney by himself—from epithelium in chalazion by Vincenti, and from corneal epithelium by Zielonko (*Centralblatt med. Wissensch.* 1873, No. 56). See also Talma (*Studien über Tuberculose*, p. 49). It must be remembered that these epithelioid cells may be derivatives from the connective tissue, and in this sense Marchand (Virchow's *Archiv*, vol. xciii.) refers the origin of giant-cells to them as well as to endothelium and possibly to epithelium.

[3] Langhans, *loc. cit.*

[4] Weiss, Virchow's *Archiv*, vol. lxviii. He finds them formed around hairs introduced into the subcutaneous tissue. Martin (*Arch. de Phys.* 1881, viii. 57) found, in the interior of giant-cells in tubercle of the peritoneum, pieces of thread which had been injected with the infective material.

[5] Ewetzki, quoted by Lubimow, Virchow's *Archiv*, vol. lxxv.

[6] Ziegler, *Ueber die Herkunft der Tuberkelelemente*, Würzburg, 1875. He watched the development of white corpuscles placed between plates of glass into cells resembling giant-cells. Similar results have been obtained by Senftleben (Virchow's *Archiv*, vol. lxxvii.) and by Tillmanns (*ibid.* vol. lxxviii.) by introducing pieces of tissue hardened in alcohol into the abdomen of living animals. Also by Martin, *Arch. de Phys.* 1881, viii. 51 *et seq.*

[7] Wegener (Virchow's *Archiv*, vol. lvi.) has ascribed this origin to the 'osteoclasts' of Külliker (*Die Normal-Resorption des Knochengewebes*. Leipzig, 1873), who, however (*Würzb. Verhand.* 1872), still holds to his original opinion that they are the derivatives of the original osteoblasts or bone-cells. Brodowski (Virchow's *Archiv*, vol. lxiii.) deduces them from protoplasmic formations from the capillaries, similar to those by which the new formation of blood-vessels proceeds, and he proposes the name of 'angioblasts.' This view has been adopted by Malassez and Monod; also in part by Grancher, *Archives Physiol.* 1878, p. 30, and more fully by Creighton, who has found them in the placenta, *Jour. of Anat. and Phys.* 1878, xiii. 9. See also Virchow (*Archiv*, iii. 450, and xiv. 51), who refers to this growth as analogous to giant-cells. Ziegler (*loc. cit.* p. 70) has also in part adopted this view.

[8] Rindfleisch (*Lehrb. path. Gewebelehre*, ed. 1878, p. 88) considers them merely masses of protoplasm which, under the influence of defective oxygenation and excess of carbonic acid, have not divided into cells.

[9] Thus Brissaud (*Arch. Gén.* 1880, ii. 147) thinks some are formed from vessels, some by fusion of ordinary cells of tubercle, and some from endothelium of vessels. Baumgarten (Virchow's *Archiv*, 1881, lxxxvi. 208) thinks they may arise from the endothelium of either blood-capillaries or lymphatics. Arnold (Virchow's *Archiv*, lxxxii. 389–391) has observed them in tubercle of the liver formed in the biliary passages.

[10] See note 3, p. 87.

be regarded as part of the connective tissue series, has also not been supported by conclusive figures of the progressive stages of these cells.

Ziegler's, Senftleben's, and Rustitzky's observations on the changes of the white corpuscles into cells resembling giant-cells must be accepted at present as deserving of further inquiry. I may, however, remark that with the exception of one figure by Zeigler,[1] neither his, nor Senftleben's, nor Tillmanns' figures have shown the reproduction of forms of cells identical with the giant-cells that ordinarily exist in tubercle. In the absence of any very positive proof of the first stage of the process, the possibility of this origin must, however, be admitted. One difficulty in accepting it is due to the occurrence of such forms as some of those in XXXI. Where a single giant-cell appears in each alveolus,[2] it would be necessary to assume that of the multitude of white corpuscles which are supposed to have emigrated, one only has enlarged in each alveolus.

Their origin from the fusion of epithelioid cells of the pulmonary alveoli has received the important support of Klein, and has its analogy in the observations of Gaule on the testicle. In the lung a very large number of preparations may easily be found to support this view, which I was at one time strongly disposed to entertain. It is easy to find abundant instances in which such apparent fusion occurs side by side with fully formed giant-cells (see XXXII. 2, 3, 4, 5, 11; and XXXIII. 3). In some of these finally the whole floor of the alveolus is occupied by the apparently single, large cell, while in others, adjacent to these, the process of apparent fusion may be observed (XXXII. 8, 10; XXXIII. 3). Moreover, as Klein has remarked, indications of their having been originally formed out of multiple elements may sometimes be observed between them, and in some, larger cells occasionally appear to be imbedded (XXXIII. 3, d). Klein believes that in the lung they are a secondary formation, and are often preceded by an amorphous exudation into the vesicles. In many cases, moreover, they have appeared to me to be coincident with a general cell-multiplication in the floor of the alveoli, of which they form a part, although a peculiar one. Further observation has, however, made me feel several difficulties in accepting this hypothesis.[3] I find it exceedingly difficult to believe that such forms as are seen in XXXI. 2, 3, 4, 5, 6, are developed out of cells which have simply formed from the fusion of pre-existing epithelial cells. In this general difficulty I include the peculiar arrangement of the nuclei, differing so remarkably from that which would be expected out of a mere agglomeration, and further, the fact that they have materially altered in shape. They appear to me to suggest an abortive and misshapen attempt at a lymphatic growth from some of the reticulate cells of the wall of the alveolus, and in this sense they would find their parallel in the theory which, in other tissues, seeks their origin in abortive processes of the formation of blood-vessels,[4] but which, for the reasons already stated, is not, I believe, applicable to tubercle. Klein has objected to the theory that they can in any case be sections of lymphatics; but some round forms, which appear to be early stages of the formations of these cells, strongly suggest this origin (see XXXI. 3, l, k; XXXII. 1 and 1A). In some cases also an origin from reticulate cells is clearly suggested (see XXXII. 11, a[5]; XXXIII. 2, a).

---

[1] Loc. cit. Taf. v. fig 3, and p. 42.

[2] See also Klein's fig. 26, Anat. Lymphatic System, part ii.

[3] I may mention that I once held this opinion so strongly that some of the figures in Plates XXXII. and XXXIII. were selected in part to illustrate the process.

[4] See especially a figure by Billroth, Uber die Entwickelung der Blutgefässe, Berlin, 1856, p. 32 and pl. ii.

[5] In this case the contrast between the enlarging reticulate cell, and the non-fusion of the multitude of epithelioid cells, is very distinct.

I must confess that, although the enlargement of single fully-formed epithelial cells of the alveolar wall, and the multiplication of the nuclei, must be admitted as a possibility, yet the fusion of these, after they have attained maturity, appears to present many difficulties. Frequently, in acute tuberculosis, this fusion of the multiplied epithelial cells can be seen to occur without the production of giant-cells. That younger protoplasmic masses, from which these epithelial cells are regenerated, may thus blend by fusion is very possible, but even this is not proven as regards such a complex structure as a fully-formed giant-cell. The matrix or source whence the epithelial cells of the pulmonary alveoli are regenerated has not yet been identified, though one must be admitted if they are replaced after desquamation, as is most probably the case, e.g. in recovery after catarrhal and also after acute pneumonia. It is probable that this regeneration may take place from the connective tissue of the alveolar wall, although the analogy of the pulmonary epithelium with an endothelium is now generally held to be untenable. Apart, however, from this speculation, it appears to me that the chief origin of the giant-cells may well be from the connective-tissue cells of the alveolar wall, since these, both lymphoid and reticular, are the elements most concerned in the characteristic changes of the granulations found in phthisis. This view stands also in direct relation to the origin of similar cells in bone and in the sarcomata, as well as in other formations and tumours. The variety of situations in which they are found, and the multiplicity of pathological conditions in which they occur, exclude any single origin—such as that from the pulmonary epithelium—and equally involve of necessity that they should either have one common origin, such as the connective tissue, or result from the fusion of protoplasmic masses, or of the white blood-corpuscles. Of these theories the weight of evidence appears to be at present in favour of the connective tissue.

Pseudo-giant Cells.—There are some appearances in the lung which may properly bear this name. The chief of these are when groups of large cells accumulate in the bronchioles, as in XXXII. 6, or when the latter are filled with nuclei imbedded in the products of inflammation hardened by the reagents employed (XXXIII. 9). These, however, do not present the arrangement of the nuclei characteristic of the true giant-cell.[1]

Site of the Giant-Cells.—In a very large proportion of cases they are found in the central portion of the alveoli, and in some of the most typical forms a giant-cell is seen in the centre of each alveolus of the group by which a tubercular granulation is constituted (see XXXI. 1; also Klein's 'Anatomy of the Lymphatic System,' Part II. pl. vi. fig. 26). In many, however, they are less regularly arranged, though it is rare to find more than one giant-cell in each alveolus (XXXI. 2, 3). In almost all cases they have an alveolar rather than an interstitial origin.[2] Langhans, whose statement has been repeated by Grancher[3] and by Charcot,[4] described them as occupying the space between the caseous centre of a granulation and the surrounding zone of small-celled growth, and this arrangement undoubtedly occasionally occurs, particularly in some forms of chronic phthisis (see XXXII. 7), but is by no means constant. In tubercles of other

---

[1] Jacobson (Virchow's *Archiv*, vol. lxv.) classifies as varieties of 'pseudo-giant cells'—(1) sections of lymphatics, (2) thrombi in blood-vessels, (3) sections of capillaries filled with white corpuscles, (4) conglomerates of detritus containing nuclei, (5) masses of micrococci, (6) sections of hypertrophied muscular fibres, (7) sections of gland-tubules and other epithelioid structures, (8) sections of nerves.

[2] Delafield (*Studies Path. Anat.* p. 77) states that they have no special site and may be entirely absent.
[3] *Archives de Physiologie*, 1878, vol. v.
[4] *Revue Mensuelle*, 1877, p. 876 et seq. Charcot states that in most cases the giant-cells form at the centres of the alveoli, and that traces of them may also be found in the caseous centres.

parts, as in the lymphatics, and in granulations found in scrofulous joints, they are generally central,[1] but in many cases of acute tuberculosis, when the granulations are of alveolar origin, they are not absolutely central, but may occur in one or more alveoli irregularly situated in the nodule.

The structure of the granulations, in which the giant-cells are found, differs in but few particulars from others in which they are not present. From this, however, I except some of the softer forms of granulation hereafter to be described, which consist largely of epithelioid cells, and in which a reticular structure is less apparent. The remainder of the granulation consists of small cells and nuclei imbedded in a reticulum, and among which epithelioid cells are mingled (XXXI. 2, *e, m*). In some, the reticulum is very distinctly fibrillated (*see* XXXI. 1), and the nuclei in many parts are fusiform rather than round (XXXI. 4, 5). The branching processes of the giant-cell, when these exist, pass into the reticulum intervening between the small cells and the epithelioid cells surrounding the giant-cell, and become insensibly blended with these. In a great many instances, a space may be seen around the giant-cell, but this is, I believe, in most cases artificial. Charcot regards the 'mantle' as the equivalent of a lymph-sinus, but I am disposed to believe, with Langhans, that its evolution can be gradually traced from the thickening of the wall, and that it is to be regarded only as part of the cell. It may be recalled that Wagner and Schüppel have described lymph-sinuses as existing around some tubercular granulations as a whole.[2]

Changes in the Giant Cell.—Caseation and calcification were both noticed by Virchow; the latter appears to be confined to the bovine species. Fatty degeneration is common,[3] but in some cases the change is more of the nature of a fine molecular transformation, to which the names of 'vitreous' or 'hyaline' have been given; in this much of the firmness of the original tissue is preserved[4] (*see* XXXI. 3, *a*).

There can, however, be no doubt that in some cases these cells have a remarkable persistence, especially in the fibroid forms of tubercle. In these they remain visible in some degree, while the rest of the tubercle has undergone a more or less complete fibroid transformation, which may be blended with caseation.[5] In some the nuclei disappear and the cell remains, either pigmented, or sometimes distinguished only by its outline as a glistening amorphous-looking body in the midst of the gradually increasing fibroid structures, among which nuclei imbedded in a reticulum may here and there be seen (*see* XXXII. 7). In other cases the nuclei shrivel and wither, but continue apparent, retaining their peculiarity of form and of arrangement in the midst of cells that have undergone great apparent thickening (*see* XXXIII. 6, 11, 12). In others, again, a very peculiar form is retained, of which I have seen several instances, when a more or less globular 'cell,' showing a similar disposition of nuclei, but crowded in the centre, gives off one elongated process, which may be traced for a considerable distance into the surrounding fibroid tissue, with which it insensibly blends (*see* XXXIII. 10). In other instances the giant-cell itself participates in the fibroid changes which affect the rest of the granulation. At first this appears to advance from the periphery; the nuclei remain crowded in the centre, or in some cases may disappear; but the process by which the cell has blended with the reticulum, and also the whole reticulum of the remainder of the granulation, become converted into broad bands between which nuclei and epithelioid cells may not

---

[1] Schüppel, *loc. cit.*; Köster, *loc. cit.*
[2] Schüppel, *Lymphdrüsen-Tuberculose*, p. 42.
[3] Langhans, *loc. cit.*; Köster, *loc. cit.*
[4] Arnold (Virchow's *Archiv*, lxxxviii. 426).
[5] Baumgarten (Volkmann's *Sammlung klin. Vorträge*, No. 218) has asserted that they may be found in old fibroid indurations.

persist. In the latter case their absence is marked by spaces in the reticulum (see XXXII. 8, 9; XXXIII. 7, 10). The nuclei of the cell itself appear to blend with the reticulum and form clear outlined spaces, while the reticulum advances gradually towards the centre. Probably in these instances the whole finally blends in the more or less homogeneous indurated mass of fibroid change which will be described later.

Relation of Giant-Cells to Tubercle.—It has been held that these bodies are an essential part of its structure;[1] they have even been strongly insisted upon as an element in its anatomical diagnosis, but this position is no longer tenable. In the first place they are not, as a rule, discoverable in tubercular granulations of the pia mater,[2] and as these are among the most typical of the forms of tubercle, their absence in a large number of the granulations of the lung is not *per se* sufficient to make us place such granulations in a separate category, and to class them as pneumonic, as distinguished from tubercular. It is further to be observed that cells of this nature have been observed in simple broncho-pneumonia, artificially excited by occlusion of the bronchi,[3] and also in ordinary inflammations of the serous membranes.[4] They have further been found in other acute and chronic inflammations of very diverse characters,[5] including some distinctly specific,[6] and others to which this character may be more or less attached.[7] They are found also in various processes akin to inflammation,[8] in simple granulation-tissues,[9] and also to a large extent in the group of tumours classified as sarcomata.[10] They are found also in other seats of rapid tissue-formation, as in the placenta,[11] and they appear occasionally during the process of formation of blood-vessels,[12] and even in some degenerative processes,[13] as well as in lupus and elephantiasis, of which the pathological position in relation to tubercle must be considered more doubtful.[14] It is evident, therefore, that neither their presence nor absence can be in any sense relied on for a definition of

---

[1] Köster, Virchow's *Archiv*, xlviii. 111, who, however, remarked that they are not peculiar to tubercle; Hamilton, *Path. Anat. of Bronchitis*.

[2] Baumgarten (Virchow's *Archiv*, lxxxvi. 208) states that they are commonly absent in the tubercles found in the adventitia of the vessels, but that they may be found in those existing in the meshes of the pia mater. Cornil and Ranvier (*Manuel Histol. Path.* 1882, ii. 152) say that they may sometimes be found in the perivascular granulations of the lung.

[3] Friedländer, Virchow's *Archiv*, 1876, lxvii. 342. See also Lichtheim, *Arch. exp. Pathol.* x. 66—broncho-pneumonia from division of recurrent nerves. This observation is open to the objection that it was made on a rabbit—an animal which easily becomes tubercular after operations. In the numerous observations of this class on dogs, giant-cells have not been described, so far as I am aware. See Frey, *Lungenveränderungen nach Lähmung der Nervi Vagi*.

[4] Cornil and Ranvier, *Manuel Histol. Path.* 2nd ed. 1884, i. 505; also Kundrat, quoted by Friedländer, *Berlin. klin. Woch.* 1874, No. 37.

[5] Stucker and Heizmann, inflammation of sclerotic and bones; quoted by Friedländer, *Berliner klin. Woch.* 1874. Ziegler (*Herkunft Tuberkelelemente*, p. 88) says that any inflammation may, under certain circumstances, produce giant-cells.

[6] Weigert, in rete Malpighii of small-pox pustules, *Anat. Beiträge Lehre von Pocken*, Breslau, 1874 (quoted by Friedländer, *loc. cit.*); Klein, Anatomy of Scarlatina, *Path. Soc. Trans.* vol. xxviii. in the lymphatic glands (see figures by him); in syphilis, Köster, *Centralbl. med. Wiss.* 1873, p. 914.

[7] Around concretions in a gouty joint. Kiener. *Arch. de Phys.* 1880, vii. 919.

[8] Abscess of mamma; ulceration of os uteri, Friedländer, Volkmann's *Sammlung*, No. 64, p. 4. Köster, *Centralblatt*, 1878; in the walls of an echinococcus-cyst, Weiss, Virchow's *Archiv*, vol. lxviii.

[9] Förster, *Handb. path. Anat.* 8te Auflage (this edition has been inaccessible to me); Baumgarten (*Centralbl.* 1876, No. 45) after ligature of vessels; *ib.* 1878, p. 228, ' any foreign body placed under the skin will excite their formation'; Heidenhain, around foreign bodies introduced into peritoneum; Langhans, in capsule forming around blood introduced under skin, quoted by Friedländer, *Berliner klin. Woch.* 1874.

[10] See Virchow, *loc. cit.*; Malassez and Monod, *Arch. de Phys.* 1878, vol. v. In fibro-sarcoma of uterus by Baumgarten, Virchow's *Archiv*, vol. lxxv.

[11] Virchow, *Archiv*, iii. 450, and *Gesam. Abhandl.* p. 213; Friedländer, *Anat. u. phys. Untersuch. über d. Uterus*, 1870; Creighton, *Journ. Anat. and Phys.* vol. xiii. 1878.

[12] See Billroth, note 2, p. 87; also Malassez and Monod, *loc. cit.*; Ranvier, *Arch. Physiol.* 1874; Leboucq, *Rech. Dév. des Vaisseaux*, Gand, 1876.

[13] Friedländer (*Berliner klin. Woch.* 1874) observed them during the rapid atrophy of fatty tissue. Arnold (Virchow's *Archiv*, lxxxvii. 146) considers that they are the results not of a formative but of a degenerative process; he regards them as resulting from cell-fusion.

[14] The bibliography of lupus is very extensive. See Grancher, art. ' Scrofulose,' *Nouv. Dict. Enc. des Sciences Méd.* ' Elephantiasis,' Köster, *Centralblatt*, 1878.

tubercle,[1] and though they are common events in some forms of this disease, they are by no means invariable, and they appear in many cases to be associated in greater degree with the chronic than with the acute forms of the disease.

Charcot[2] has indeed stated that the giant-cells of tubercle may be distinguished from others by the fact that they are multipolar, presenting numerous prolongations which pass into the surrounding tissue, while the varieties found in other conditions than tubercle, except lupus, do not present this character. It may be sufficient to remark that these prolongations are figured by Billroth in granulation-tissue, and also by Malassez and Monod in the myeloplaxes of epulis and cancer, and Baumgarten has asserted that all variations in the appearance of these, as well as in those observed in simple granulations, may be also found in tubercle.[3]

(c) *Granulations containing epithelioid elements.*—In the acute tuberculosis of children, in many cases the granulations do not present either of the forms last described. They consist of more or less circumscribed masses composed of two elements, viz. epithelioid cells, and a growth, in variable proportions, of small round cells imbedded in a reticulum, such as those described under (A) and (B). A typical example of this is seen in XXX. 3. The centre, already becoming caseous and granular, is composed mainly of shrivelled nuclei, nebulous masses in which no nuclei are discernible (measuring $\frac{1}{4000}$th to $\frac{1}{6000}$th inch), and a few remains of epithelioid cells, while here and there remnants of the walls of the alveoli may also be seen. Beyond this is a dense mass of small-celled growth, such as was described under (A), imbedded in a solid reticulum of intercellular substance; among these small cells are a few epithelioid cells, e. In the outer zone are remains of alveoli e e, where epithelioid cells, measuring from $\frac{1}{2500}$th to $\frac{1}{2000}$th inch, are more abundant, and it would appear probable that the epithelioid cells remaining in the more central parts are of the same nature, and have been gradually enclosed by the small-celled growth, which elsewhere is seen encroaching on the alveoli and has grown in their wall.

Thaon[4] has described the return of the epithelium of the alveoli to the cuboid form of embryonic life, as one of the first stages of this process, and his statement has been endorsed by Charcot.[5] I have only seen very imperfect and rudimentary forms of this transformation within the alveoli, but it may occasionally be well seen in the alveolar passages and bronchioles (*see* XXXVIII. 6, from acute phthisis). I think that the origin of these epithelioid cells may be attributed to the epithelium lining the alveoli; but it must be remembered that they are found in tubercle of other parts, as in the lymphatics and peritoneum,[6] and that they are, therefore, deducible from the connective tissue,

---

[1] Baumgarten (*Centralblatt*, 1878, p. 228 *et seq.*) appears to consider that giant-cells, other than tubercular, do not caseate. But some of those found in tubercle do not undergo this process, but present a fibroid change.

[2] Quoted by Malassez and Monod, *Arch. de Phys.* 1878, v. 308.

[3] *Centralblatt med. Wiss.* 1878; and Virchow's *Archiv*, vol. lxxxii.

[4] *Anat. Path. Tuberculose*, 1878, p. 78. See also Ziegler, *Ueber die Herkunft der Tuberkelelemente*, 1875, p. 32.

[5] *Revue Mensuelle*, 1877, p. 886. See also Grancher, *Archives de Physiol.* 2nd ser. vol. v. pl. vi. fig. 5. Friedländer (Virchow's *Archiv*, 1876, lxviii. 359) has termed this a 'typical epithelium.' It is not peculiar to tubercle, for he has seen it around a sarcomatous tumour of the lung. Küttner (Virchow's *Archiv*, 1876, lxvi. 21) has also described it in cirrhosis, and as resulting from a new formation of epithelium in confined spaces.

[6] Lebert (*Phys. Path.* i. 402) described some cells in tubercle as measuring from $\frac{1}{500}$ to $\frac{1}{1000}$ inch. See also Virchow, *Krankhaften Geschwülste*, ii. 618; Schüppel, *Lymphdrüsen-Tuberculose*, p. 86; Arnold, Virchow's *Archiv*, lxxxvii. 135; Langhans, *ib.* vol. xlii.; Köster, *ib.* vol. lviii.; Klebs, *ib.* vol. xliv.; Villemin, *Etudes sur la Tuberculose*, p. 103. See also Rindfleisch, Virchow's *Archiv*, vol. xxiv. and *Lehrbuch path. Gewebelehre*, for large cells in tubercles of pia mater. In his article in Ziemssen's *Handbuch*, 'Krankh. Resp.-Apparat.' ii. 162, Rindfleisch appears to regard these large cells as the germinal tissue (Keimgewebe) and the histological acute of tubercle. See also Virchow's *Archiv*, 1881, lxxxv. 76. In the lung, certainly, they disappear with the gradual invasion of the alveolar wall by the small-celled growth. Thaon (*Clinique Climatologique des Malad. Chron.* p. 11) has similarly described large cells in laryngeal tubercle, and Lebert (*Brustkrankheiten*, xi. 27) in the pleura.

or the endothelium of the lymphatics,[1] or even from emigrated white blood-corpuscles.[2] The proportion of these cells also varies, and in some recent granulations, nearly the whole of the formation may consist of large epithelioid cells[3] much swollen and granular and sometimes containing multiple nuclei[4] (see XXX. 5, 6, 8), while in others the granulations are almost entirely occupied by small free cells or leucocytes (XXX. 10). Under both these circumstances, however, a gradual invasion of the wall by a small-celled growth may be seen to be progressing, which tends to the obliteration of the alveolar cavity.

In some of these granulations, sections of the alveolar ducts may be found, filled either with granular débris or with small or large epithelioid cells (XXX. 4. d, and 7, a a).

(D) *Soft amorphous or caseous granulations*.—These, as has been already stated, sometimes constitute a considerable proportion of the granulations found in acute tuberculosis. They may be mingled with both the forms last described, or may be almost the sole change observed.

Their general microscopic characters are seen in XXVIII. 6, 8, and in XXXVIII. 3. In these advanced stages, they consist of little but a granular yet purely fibrillated material, in which, however, markings of the alveolar structure still exist. In other instances the same granular fibrillated material is seen filling the alveoli, the walls of which are still apparent. In this stage, no traces of cell-structure are discoverable, but intermediate processes may be observed such as are seen in XXVIII. 7, where a small-celled growth is forming in the alveolar wall, mingled with an epithelial desquamation in the interior of the alveoli. It is probable that it is to the acuteness of the latter process that the rapid caseation is due. I shall return to this subject later.

(E) *Indurated Granulations*.—The granulations in acute tubercle sometimes assume a more fibroid character. I shall, however, discuss this change later in considering the transformations of the granulations.

GRANULATIONS IN ORDINARY PHTHISIS.—A very large proportion of the granulations found in ordinary phthisis differ in no essential particulars from those met with in acute tuberculosis. Some varieties, however, are occasionally found, which require special description. They relate chiefly to the size of the granulations, and to processes of softening and of induration, found in composite granulations and in masses apparently originating from the fusion of several granulations. Single granulations, identical with the typical grey granulation (XXX. 1) are found in all forms of phthisis, but especially in the acute varieties and where much pneumonic infiltration exists (see XXXVIII. 7, from *Case 24, Hall*, Col. Pl. XIV. 2). They are also found in the more chronic forms. See XXXV. 6 (*Smith*) and XXXIX. 6 (*Overall*).

Caseous granulations, similar to those found in acute tuberculosis, are also met with in all varieties, even in the indurating forms. See XLIII. 5 (*Case 26, Heath*, also X. 5, 6).

The main variations in the naked-eye appearance are in the large granulations, sometimes softening in the centre, which are found either singly or associated with

---

[1] I do not include under this the epithelial lining of the lung. Buhl (*Lungenentzündung*), as is known, regarded this as the analogue of an endothelium, and this opinion has been repeated by Thaon and also by Martin. It must now be abandoned. See Klein, *Anatomy of the Lymphatic System*, and Küttner, Virchow's *Archiv*, vol. lxvi.

[2] Talma (*Studien über Lungenschwindsucht*, p. 42), in the more diffuse growth, considers these to be cells of lymphoid origin, which have become epithelioid.

[3] Green, *Pathology of Consumption*, p. 8; Arnold Virchow's *Archiv*, lxxxviii. 423, 437; Delafield, *Studies in Path. Anat.* p. 77.

[4] Green(loc. cit.) believes that this granular appearance is due to a mucoid transformation of the contents of the epithelioid cells.

pneumonic processes. The majority of these correspond in type with those shown in X. 1, 2, 3, 4, and with XI. XII. XIII. 1, and XIV. 2. Their histological characteristics are seen in XXXVI. XXXVII. XXXVIII. XXXIX. Viewed with a low power they present the appearances seen in XXXVI. 1, 3, and XXXVII. 4. They may either form distinctly circumscribed masses, softening in the centre, where remains of alveolar structure are still apparent (XXXVI. 1), or appear as less defined areas with several spots of caseation scattered through them, as in XXXVI. 3, *a*, and XXXVII. 4, or as nodules which have passed into absolute caseous débris, as in XXXVI. 5, or XXXVIII. 9.

The origin of these spots is of considerable interest. It is desirable here to state that the pneumonic infiltration, in the midst of which they occur, resembles in its histological characters that seen in XXVI. 7, XXXVII. 6, XXXVIII. 1, 2, 4, 5, XXXIX. 1, 2. The alveoli are filled with varied forms of epithelial proliferation and exudation, and their walls are more or less infiltrated with a small-celled growth. Destructive changes are also present, which will be described hereafter.

The circumference of the caseating nodule shown in XXXVI. 1, is seen, in fig. 2 of the same plate, to be composed of a small-celled growth imbedded in a reticulum of fibroid type, and within this is a débris of nuclei, similar to that which characterises the soft granulation of acute tuberculosis, as seen in XXX. 3, 4. As in that instance also, the remains of the alveolar structure of the lung are seen in the softening centre. A similar small-celled infiltration extends indefinitely into the surrounding pulmonary tissue, gradually becoming less dense, until it meets the margins of similar nodules of caseation in its neighbourhood (XXXVI. 1, *d*, *e*). The line of demarcation of some of the larger nodules appears to be the interlobular septa, and the softening proceeds until these are reached. The septa are themselves invaded by the same growth, and it extends beyond them into the alveolar tissue. Other and smaller granulations in this lung present the characters of XXXVII. 5, where an epithelial proliferation is mingled with a small-celled growth, again almost identical in appearance with the soft granulation last noticed. Giant-cells were found in some instances in the tissue surrounding these masses.

In many of these granulations the process is identical with that occurring in the more diffuse pneumonic infiltrations that pass into detritus, from which the granulations are only distinguished by their more circumscribed character. The essential characteristic is the small-celled growth in the alveolar walls, and this is combined, in varying proportions, with an epithelioid proliferation in the interior of the alveoli. In some, the growth causes the granulations to assume the character of dense masses, like that seen in XL. 1, 2 (*Heath*); but most of the granulations characteristic of this lung are those seen in XXXVII. 5, together with some in which the acute destructive changes next to be described are observed.

The process by which the granulations form and perish is illustrated in XXXVII. 1, 2, 3: a fine nuclear growth takes place in the floor of the alveoli, either arising from the natural reticular texture or from the nuclei of the capillaries; the latter also disappear (as is seen in XL. 6, a process likewise reproduced in this specimen, and in many others), and the growth appears to pass early into caseation. In some of these masses there is no appearance of epithelial proliferation, while in other and adjacent alveoli the latter may be observed (*see* XXXVII. 1). In the former case it is probable that the epithelium has perished at the commencement of the nuclear proliferation; at any rate no demonstrable traces of it remain.

Those granulations, therefore, formed of a small-celled growth, tend to perish more or less rapidly, and the amount of the growth observed is in inverse ratio with the acuteness of the process. The destruction in these early stages is, I believe, in no small measure due to the implication of the capillaries.[1] The nodules shown in VII. 1 (*Price, Case 12*) resemble those last described, but many are of the same nature as those of VI. 1, 2 (*Polley, Case 6*). A very large number are, however, caseous and finely fibrillated, like XXXVIII. 3. The early stages of these latter are seen in XXXIX. 4. Here, as in the soft nodules last described, a small-celled growth has entirely filled the alveoli, growing from the floor, and this passes into caseation, commencing from the centre of each alveolus. A fibronuclear growth, sometimes with fusiform nuclei, surrounds this dense mass, and the alveolar wall is occupied by masses of dense, small-celled growth. These nodules may attain variable sizes, the larger ones being formed by confluence of smaller, until the process is circumscribed by an interlobular septum. This form of nodule, composed almost entirely of a small-celled growth filling the alveoli, like XXXV. 6 and XXXIX. 6, 7, is very common in all forms of phthisis, both acute and chronic, and it alternates and is intermingled with others in the same lung, in which epithelial proliferation, like XXXVII. 5 and XXXVIII. 7, is more or less mingled with this growth.

INDURATED GRANULATIONS.—I shall under this head describe the more indurated grey granulations of acute tuberculosis, the conglomerate masses of indurated, pigmented granulations met with in chronic phthisis, and the larger nodules of indurations, sometimes caseous in their centre, which are found both in acute and chronic phthisis.

The induration of the grey granulation consists in a gradual thickening of the reticulum into broad bands; these advance for the most part from the periphery to the circumference by a process which, in some cases, presents a striking resemblance to that seen in the process of ossification from the periosteum (*see* XLII. 2, from a child). The interlobular tissue also thickens, and encloses the granulation in a species of capsule; such granulations may become caseous in their centres, or may apparently persist long in the condition shown in this figure.

In other cases nearly the whole of the granulations, as seen in XXXI. 8 (*Beale, Case 11*), may have their reticulum thickened into broad-banded fibres, which, in some cases, enclose nuclei in their meshes, while in others the nuclei may disappear. Perilobular thickening of the same nature accompanies this process, and the granulations, densely crowded in the lung, may apparently undergo no other change (*see* XLIII. 2).

In other instances, specimens may be found where a similar induration to that last described occurs in combination with an amorphous and granular centre, as in XLIII. 1. Soft or caseous granulations may coexist with these in the same lung. I think it probable that induration of the same nature may occur in granulations associated with a certain degree of epithelial proliferation, but it is difficult to trace this, inasmuch as the large epithelioid cells disappear during the formation of the small-celled reticular growth, in which this process of induration proceeds. It can, however, be traced in some forms of chronic phthisis (*see* XL. 10).

The induration-nodules in chronic phthisis present several variations, but all may be included within the types last described.

(A) A common form, which is also one of the most simple, is that seen in XLI. 5, where, without caseation, there only remains in the centre of the nodule a pigmented

---

[1] An excellent illustration of this process is given by Lionel Beale, *The Microscope in Medicine*, pl. xlvi. p. 330. I have figured it also in the *Rodentia*, 'Lecture on the Artificial Production of Tubercle,' pl. ii. p. 5.

fibroid reticulum, without traces of cell-structure, while around this is a dense small-celled growth, much pigmented, and passing, from the centre to the periphery, into the same fibroid change. It appears probable that the nuclear growth has perished in the centre by a granular disintegration, analogous to that seen in XXXVIII. 3 (*Case 35, Roberts*, Coloured Pl. XVIII. 1, 2), but that the fibroid basis has remained more distinct.

(B) Another and a common type is that seen in XLI. 2, 3. Fig. 2 so closely resembles the process of induration as described in acute tuberculosis, that it requires no further description. In other places, however, the centre of these nodules becomes an almost uniformly indurated, fibroid, glistening mass, like the section of fibro-cartilage, while lines of fibrillation connect it with the periphery, which is composed of an alveolar structure concealed by a small-celled growth imbedded in reticular fibres. Much pigment also occurs in these. The agglomeration of these masses produce tracts of tissue like XLI. 1, where considerable areas are occupied by glistening, broad-banded fibres—some homogeneous, some fibrillated, enclosing lacunæ in which nuclei may or may not be found—and also by remains of alveoli still marked by epithelial proliferation. Some of these granulations are caseous in their centres. In all these nodules, an alveolar origin is apparent, and whether they indurate or caseate, indications of this persist. Giant-cells exist in many of these nodules, and pass through processes of induration such as are figured in XXXII. 7, 8, 9, and XXXIII. 7, 8, 10.

(C) Another variety, closely akin to the foregoing, is seen in XLI. 7, where the whole nodule of induration consists of a small-celled growth, among which fibres are extending, but not in the broad-banded reticular type of that last described.

(D) In the same specimen (XLI. 7), and also in many other preparations, are seen nodules almost entirely fibroid and deeply pigmented, like XLIII. 1. The fibrillation is very fine, and not in broad bands, and it is arranged consecutively—distinctly showing that it has developed out of a series of alveoli ; masses of pigment are abundant, and retain in parts the form of nuclei and cells, which, however, have almost entirely disappeared as independent structures. (*Case 33, Coppin*, Coloured Pl. XVII. 2, 4.)

(E) A large number of indurated granulations, in all specimens, present a combination of a caseous centre with a densely indurated margin, consisting of a small-celled growth, invaded by fibres and mingled with pigment. Adjoining granulations may consist entirely of small-celled growth, among which fibres are extending ; and this small-celled growth may or may not be caseous in the centre. *See* XXXIX. 5, 7 (*Cases 25, Overall,* and *10, Unwin*), and XLI. 6, (*Case 34, Cox,* and Coloured Pl. XVIII. 3, 4). In the earlier stages of some granulations of this nature, the cell-growth may be seen to be proceeding from a reticular structure in the floor of the alveoli, apparently arising from the nuclei of capillaries ; even where it is more dense, it still shows traces of this origin (*see* XL. 7, 8, 9).

(F) The large indurated nodules, with or without caseous centres, are a subject of some interest, as they have frequently been described as peribronchial thickenings ; to the naked eye, and even with low powers of the microscope, they strongly suggest this origin. A careful examination of the majority of such formations as are figured in X. 5 to 10, shows, however, that they have an alveolar origin, and are formed out of a thickening of the pulmonary tissue by processes which are practically identical with those last described. I may also add that a large number of nodules found in the lungs in cases of acute and chronic phthisis arise in the manner which I have now to describe.

In the lungs of *Heath* (*Case 26* and Coloured Pl. X. 5, 6) the appearances seen are of three kinds : tracts of fibroid induration like XL. 2 ; nodules of caseation of various kinds which will be described later ; and finally granulations of the structure seen in XL. 1, 3, and 6. These granulations are seen to consist, like others before described, of a great thickening of the alveolar walls with a small-celled growth, which, as in XL. 6, may be observed to form the floor of the vesicles, sometimes with fusiform and sometimes with round nuclei, entirely obliterating the capillary structure. Much pigment is seen in them. Giant-cells exist in places among this growth, but large tracts, and sometimes whole nodules, appear within these structures. The alveoli in the central parts of these nodules show but little trace of epithelioid cells ; these probably disappear before the small-celled growth. In the peripheral parts, the alveoli still show an abundance of epithelial cells. These nodules attain a considerable size, and appear only to be bounded by the larger interlobular septa. The whole nodule may present the characters here described, but in some, as seen in XL. 3, caseation commences in the centre, and may gradually extend until the thickened interlobular septum is reached. In the earlier stages of this caseation, and even in some cases where it is considerably advanced, the alveolar origin may be observed, as in this figure. In some of the large nodules of caseation thus bounded, a very remarkable appearance of dilated alveolar ducts may be occasionally seen ; these are filled with a dim nebulous matter, or with traces of cells and nuclei, faintly defined and disintegrating, but sufficient also to mark the lobular rather than the bronchial origin of these caseous masses (see XL. 4).

The conglomeration of these masses, especially when they assume the forms of rows and lines, presents a very singular resemblance to bronchi ; and the same resemblance may be produced by the agglomeration of nodules such as that seen in XXXV. 4. This may be the case even with the caseation of soft granulations in acute phthisis in a pneumonic area, as in X. 1, 2, and XXXVI. 1 ; but here, as already stated, the examination with a high power reveals the remains of alveolar walls. When, however, these rows of nodules, caseous in their centre, are surrounded by much fibroid induration, and the interlobular septa on which they rest are much thickened, the resemblance is still more deceptive, for they may even appear to branch and bifurcate, and longitudinal and cross sections can hardly be distinguished from bronchi except by the higher powers of the microscope. When thus examined they are found, as in XLIII. 3, to show remains of the alveolar structure, and even when this has almost disappeared in the caseation, bands of fibres may be seen extending into the area in a manner which shows its true origin.

After a prolonged and repeated investigation of this subject, I believe that the very large majority of these caseous and soft masses with thickened periphery ('encysted tubercles' of Bayle) are not sections of bronchi, as was held by Addison, or accumulations of caseous matter in the interior of dilated bronchi, as has been frequently stated, but that they are formed in the manner which I have now described. They are due to the invasion of the pulmonary tissue by a small-celled growth, which may pass into a more or less extensive caseation in the centre of the nodule thus formed, or may indurate in a variable proportion of the area. It may further be remarked that, even in these lungs, entirely caseous nodules, surrounded by a dense margin of thickening (interlobular septum), and showing the most undoubted proofs of their alveolar origin (XLIII. 5), exist side by side with the formations just described and with others, and from these they are, to the naked eye, indistinguishable.[1]

[1] Delafield (*Studies Path. Anat.* 1882, p. 93) has stated that nodules with a caseous centre, and undergoing fibroid induration at their periphery, must not be mistaken for sections of bronchi. Barthez and Rilliet (*Malad. des Enfants*, iii. 344) had already distinctly given this warning.

Some of these nodules, such as are shown in X. 8, 9, 10, are also formed out of the softening of large areas of small-celled growth, invading the pulmonary tissue and bounded by the thickened interlobular septa, as seen in XXXIX. 5.

It must, however, be added that in cases where extensive peribronchial infiltration has occurred, and has passed into caseation, the contents of the bronchi are inspissated and form a continuous mass with the wall. When this softens, ulcerations occur, spreading into the adjacent tissue. These ulcerations have usually a caseous margin (X. 3, 4), which has resulted from the extension of the small-celled growth beyond the peribronchial sheath into the alveolar tissue. In the early stages of these changes, and before ulceration has occurred, such bronchi present caseous nodules identical in appearance with the large caseous granulations before described, and are indistinguishable from them except by microscopic examination—the crucial distinction being, as already stated, the discovery in the latter of the remains of pulmonary tissue. Indeed, in some lungs it is not uncommon to find both forms of granulations side by side in the midst of a grey pneumonic infiltration.

Many also of the indurated granulations which have been described as 'indurating peribronchitis,' are seen to have an alveolar origin by the fact that the fibroid change extends entirely to their centre, which could not be the case were they merely tubes (*see* XLI. 2, 3, 5).

Seat and origin of the Granulations.—By the older authors, two distinct opinions were held regarding the site of the granulations of the lung. These may be briefly stated as being, whether tubercle was vesicular or extra-vesicular. The leading authorities were about equally divided between these views, and the discussion, even with the aid of the microscope, has continued to the present day, but with some modifications. The statements now made respecting the granulations are that they are alveolar, perialveolar, or interalveolar, or may occupy the same position with respect to the infundibula, or that they are interstitial, perivascular, or peribronchial.

The opinion which has received most support is that tubercle in the lung is for the most part a peribronchial growth. It was first stated by Virchow that in a large proportion of miliary tubercles, the growth begins in the submucous tissue of the bronchi,[1] and this view has been extended by Rindfleisch,[2] who makes it the invariable character of all the tubercular formations of ordinary phthisis, only excepting acute tuberculosis (in which he regards the granulations as being interstitial) and some other forms which he describes as being of lymphatic origin. Rindfleisch (whose views have been adopted by Charcot)[3] asserts that tubercle, in all ordinary forms of phthisis, commences at the angle where the peribronchial tube breaks up into the alveolar passages, *i.e.* at the point where there is an enlargement of the tube, and where secretions, which, in his opinion, are the source of the infective origin of tubercle, are the most easily retained; it is to this mode of growth that the lobular or trefoil form of tubercle is due.

Of all the authors who have written on tubercle, none have given, as far as I am aware, any distinct drawing of tubercle having this origin, though a diagrammatic repre-

---

[1] *Verhand. Berliner med. Gesellschaft*, 1865, p. 268 *et seq.* See also *Krankhaften Geschwülste*, ii. 649. Virchow, as far as I am aware, has made no general statement respecting the site of tubercle under all circumstances in the lung.
[2] *Lehrbuch path. Gewebelehre*, 5th edition; and Ziemssen's *Handb.* 'Krank. Resp.-App.'
[3] *Revue Mensuelle*, 1879, p. 900. Charcot admits an interstitial, a perivascular, and an alveolar variety, the two former chiefly in acute tubercle. See *ib.* 1877. Martin also asserts that the majority of the granulations found in the lung have a bronchial origin; *Rech. Anat. Path. Tubercule*, 1879, p. 46.

sentation of it has been furnished by Rindfleisch.[1] I venture to remark that such a circumscription of a growth which must, under these circumstances, be infinitesimally small, would necessarily be extremely rare, and I confess that I have not seen it. The site of most granulations in the lung is alveolar, and so is their essential growth, but some are undoubtedly peri- and interbronchial, some are perivascular, and some exist in the interstitial tissue. It may be better, however, for the sake of perspicacity, to consider the site of the granulations which occur elsewhere than in the alveolar tissue, and then to discuss the relations of the latter to the former.

Bronchial Tubercle.—This occurs in two situations, viz. the submucous tissue of the smaller bronchi, and the peribronchial sheath. Those in the former were described by Virchow, and later by Rindfleisch, as consisting of very small granulations in the submucous tissue,[2] which begin as white spots, and may be traced as far as bronchi of $\frac{1}{8}$th of an inch in diameter.[3] They are also described by Cornil and Ranvier as projecting into the interior of the bronchus and covered by ciliated epithelium.[4] Histologically the growth of tubercle in the submucous tissue of the bronchi is seldom unassociated with a similar growth in the wall,[5] and the two together present appearances such as are seen in XXXIV. 5, XLII. 5, XLIII. 6. There is a proliferation of the epithelium in the interior of the bronchus, which in the smaller ones may lead to their complete obstruction, and in addition a small-celled reticular growth takes place in the wall, which, as seen in XLIII. 6, may also grow irregularly in the form of granulations into its interior —a condition which has been described by Martin as 'obliterating bronchitis.'[6] Thaon has also described an extensive caseous infiltration of the submucous tissue of the bronchi, the epithelium at first remaining intact, but subsequently disappearing in the process of ulceration, while in the larger bronchi the same change is observed, but suppurative rather than caseating.[7] These thickenings of the bronchial wall, with growth into their interior, take place in all forms of phthisis, and in the indurating varieties they pass into sclerotic, almost homogeneous, glistening, fibroid tissue, as will be considered hereafter.

I have already described the caseous masses which these peribronchial growths form, and the manner in which they may be distinguished from similar masses arising from the pulmonary tissue. They are, as I have already stated, less common than the latter, but when present they may contribute largely to the breaking down of the lung, especially when surrounded by a grey pneumonic infiltration. The infiltration of the peribronchial sheath with a small-celled reticular texture, which is one of the common forms of change in the artificial tuberculosis of the rodentia, occurs also in acute tuberculosis, with the formation of nodules of adenoid tissue. These were observed by Schröder van der Kolk, and likened to glands.[8] They have been minutely described by Burdon-Sanderson,[9] and

---

[1] Ziemssen's *Handbuch*, 'Krankh. Resp.-App.,' ii. 171. Rindfleisch's description of his method of preparation is given in the *Berlin. klin. Wochenschrift*, 1873, p. 81. I venture to remark that two drawings given by Grancher (*Arch. de Physiol.* 2nd ser. vol. v, pl. v, fig. 3, pl. vi. fig. 1) do not appear conclusive as regards the bronchial origin of the granulations. The former would represent almost any granulation in the lung which had become caseous in the centre, and the latter, filled almost entirely with epithelium-cells and the remains of a retiedum, appears to me to represent an alveolus. Ziegler (*Herkunft der Tuberkelelemente*, p. 30) states that the smallest miliary tubercles commence in the alveolar passages.

[2] Klein (*Anat. of Lymph. Tissues*, part ii. p. 230) describes masses of lymphatic tissue, akin to the lymphatic follicles of other mucous membranes, as existing normally in the submucous tissue of non-cartilaginous bronchi.

[3] It must be remembered that the terminal bronchi are seldom more than $\frac{1}{50}$ inch in diameter.

[4] *Manuel Path. Histol.* 1882, ii. 153.

[5] An illustration of this is given by Hérard and Cornil, *Phthisie Pulmonaire*, p. 111.

[6] Martin, *Rech. Anat. Path. Tubercule*, 1879, p. 51.

[7] Thaon, *Rech. Anat. Path. Tuberculose*, 1873, p. 68 *et seq*.

[8] *Obs. Anat. Path.* 1826, pp. 71–2.

[9] *Rep. Med. Off. Privy Council*, 1867, 1868.

by Klein.[1] They are met with in the child, but to a much less extent, as far as my observations have extended; and it is only comparatively rarely that they are distinctly found in an isolated form in the phthisis of the adult. This is probably due to the fact that the lungs in the latter are commonly examined in more advanced stages, when the lymphatic masses which normally exist in this situation, have become blended with, and indistinguishable from, the changes in the adjacent pulmonary tissue. I have already described the invasion of the peribronchial wall and the process by which this occurs.[2] Cornil and Ranvier have described this peribronchial growth as surrounded by dilated lymphatic vessels.[3] Klein has stated his belief that in the rodentia, caseation rarely occurs in the peribronchial growths, nor does he appear to consider that the process often extends from them to the lung, but he rather believes that they are secondary in point of time to the alveolar and perivascular changes.

The *pericascular growth of tubercle*, first observed by Dr. William Addison of Brighton,[4] and attributed by him to the exit of white corpuscles, was shown by Virchow to be the common form in the meningeal variety,[5] and was again asserted by Heschl, Deichler, and Otto Weber, to be one of its modes of origin in the lung. This statement was confirmed by Colberg, who, however, asserted that it began in the capillaries, and thence extended to the adventitia of the arteries.[6] It was also asserted by Schüppel for the larger vessels[7] and Klein[8] regards it as one of the earliest appearances in artificial tuberculosis of the rodentia, and as the source of much of the implication of the pulmonary tissue. The latter describes it as finally forming a dense reticular small-celled growth in the peri-arterial sheath, which may develop in places into solid nodules. The wall of the artery is similarly invaded, and at the same time a proliferation of the endothelium occurs in the interior, greatly narrowing the calibre of the vessel.[9] Similar changes, but to a less extent, were observed by Klein in the veins. Mugge, however, has found the latter more frequently affected,[10] and the granulations in them may exist as small round tumours. In the rodentia, Klein regards the periarterial changes as the starting-point of most of those which occur in the alveoli, to which they extend, apparently by continuity, but

[1] *Anat. of Lymph. Tissues*, part. ii. pp. 28, 78.
[2] Cf. Rokitanski, *Path. Anat.* iii. 28.
[3] *Manuel Histol. Path.* 2nd ed. 1882, ii. 155.
[4] Addison, *Healthy and Diseased Structure*, 1849, pl. iii. fig. 9. It is open to question whether this was not observed by Schröder van der Kolk, *Obs. Anat. Path.* 1826, pp. 71–2.
[5] Virchow, *Wien. med. Woch.* 1856, p. 3, and *Gesamm. Abhand.* 1856, p. 217; also Buhl, *Zeitsch. Rat. Med.* 1857, viii. 58. See also Rindfleisch, Virchow's *Archiv*, vol. xxiv., and Bastian, *Edinburgh Med. Journ.* 1867.
[6] Heschl, *Prager Vierteljahrschrift*, 1856, iii. 17. Deichler, *Beiträge Hist. des Lungengewebes*, Göttingen, 1861. The original of this has been inaccessible to me, and I know it only from quotations. Deichler appears to have recognised the origin in the adventitia. Colberg (*Deutsch. Arch. klin. Med.* ii. 471) says that the growth begins in the capillaries, and thence extends to the adventitia. See also Otto Weber, 'Ueber die Betheiligung der Gefässe in den Neubildungen,' Virchow's *Archiv*, vol. xxix. In the brain it was also observed by Cruveilhier, *Atlas*, liv. vi. pl. ii. figs. 3 and 4. See also Hérard and Cornil, *Phthisie Pulmonaire*, p. 39 *et seq.*; and Wagner, *Tuberkulöhutisches Lymphadenom*, p. 11.
[7] *Lymphdrüsen-Tuberculose*, p. 80.
[8] *Anat. Lymphatic Tissues*, part ii. pp. 55, 59, 78.
[9] Thaon (*Rech. Anat. Path. Tuberculose*, 1873, p. 28) has described in tubercular pneumonia an 'endartérite végétante' which closes the vessels. Friedländer (Virchow's *Archiv*, 1876, lxviii. 357) has described this as an 'arteritis obliterans.' See also Orth, Virchow's *Archiv*, lxxvi. 229. Martin (*Rech. Anat. Path. sur le Tubercule*, 1879) has adopted Friedländer's terms. See also Kiener, *Arch. de Phys.* 1880, vii. 718, 'Tubercule vasco-formatif.' Pauli (Virchow's *Archiv*, lxxvii. 60) has found the arteries in cavities closed by a small-celled growth containing giant-cells. Weigert (Virchow's *Archiv*, lxxvii.) has also found tubercle in the wall of an aneurism of the pulmonary artery (for the structure of these, see Cornil and Ranvier, *Manuel Histol. Path.* 1882, ii. 178). Similar changes exist in syphilis; see Wagner, *Archiv der Heilk.* vol. vii.; Heubner, *Die luetische Erkrankungen der Hirnarterien*, Leipzig 1874. Ref. also to Baumgarten, Virchow's *Archiv*, vols. lxxiii. and lxxxvi. Peculiar thickenings occur in the arteries in other conditions. See Kussmaul and Maier, *Deutsch. Arch. klin. Med.* 1866, i. and Meyer, 'Periarteritis Nodosa,' Virchow's *Archiv*, lxxiv. 1878.

[10] Mugge (Virchow's *Archiv*, lxxvi.) thinks the intima is affected by the tubercular poison passing through the coats of the vessel. Weigert had made earlier observations on this subject; see *Deutsche med. Woch.* 1881, No. 24. In Virchow's *Archiv* (lxxviii.) he has given two instances, and thinks this may be a source of general infection. See Huguenin, Ziemssen's *Handbuch*, quoted by Frerichs (*Beiträge Lehre Tuberculose*, 1882, p. 61), who has found similar instances. Cohn (*Klinik der embolischen ticfiiss*, 1860, p. 230) observed perforation of the pulmonary vein by tubercle.

though they were also found by him in the acute tuberculosis of children, he does not describe them as having a similar connection. Martin describes a gradual thickening of the coats of the vessels until they are 'complely occluded,' as is shown in the accompanying woodcut by him.[1] The small-celled growth in the arterial wall is seen in XLII. 3, 4. This perivascular thickening, like the peribronchial, is common to all forms of phthisis ; but in none of these, including the acute tuberculisation of childhood, have I been able to observe that it forms a predominant element, or appears to be the primary change, or that the bulk of the granulations in the lung are in any way connected with the growth in the wall.

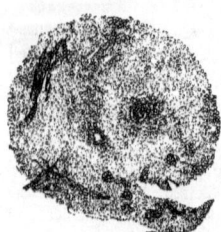

FIG. 39.—Growth surrounding and obliterating vessel of lung. 'The inflammation develops simultaneously in the whole circumference of the artery, and soon surrounds it with a considerable zone of embryonal tissue, in the midst of which the wall proper has entirely disappeared. The vasa vasorum and the alveolar capillaries are attacked in their turn, so that a section shows the vessel in the centre of a mass of sarcomatous tissue. . . . The figure shows this alteration. The vessels are injected with Prussian blue' (Martin, loc. cit. p. 57).

Alveolar Granulations—Exclusive of the peribronchial and periarterial growths, the vast majority of all the granulations found in the lung, whether these be small-celled or whether they contain epithelioid cells or giant-cells, are alveolar or infundibular. There is no proof that they have any other origin, and their structure shows, I believe very conclusively, that they commence in the pulmonary vesicles.

In this growth the bronchi and alveolar passages are doubtless occasionally surrounded, and when these are not occluded by cell-proliferation, they have the appearance of round openings, as in XXVIII. 3 and 4, which suggest that the growth may have had a peribronchial origin, though, as in fig. 3, solid granulations of purely alveolar structure are seen side by side with the others.[2]

At the periphery of the lung in acute tuberculosis, both in the epithelioid and giant-cell variety, granulations may be found conical in shape and almost purely infundibular,[3] without any evidence of extension either from the bronchioles or from the vessels (see XXVIII. 1 and 2, XXXIV. 1), and these infundibular infiltrations, consisting of a small-celled growth in the walls of the alveoli[4] and alveolar passages, mingled with more or less epithelial proliferation in their interior, may be found side by side with lobulettes or acini which are yet unaffected. Moreover, in some cases a purely alveolar origin may be traced in granulations not exceeding $\frac{1}{120}$ of an inch in diameter.[5]

Sections at all depths through an apparently single granulation show that it is made up of groups of alveoli, the walls of which are invaded by a small-celled growth with more or less epithelial proliferation in their interior ; the latter disappears, as has been already described, before the advancing neoplasm (see XXXIX. 1 to 5). Traces of alveolar passages and bronchioles may be seen in the sections, but these are involved only *pari passu* with the alveolar walls. The composite granulation must of necessity assume a *racemose* or *trefoil* shape from implication of adjacent alveoli, infundibula, and acini, and for the production of this shape it is not necessary to assume that the new

---

[1] Martin, *Rech. Anat. Path. Tubercule*, 1878, p. 58. Similar changes are figured by Grancher, *Arch. de Phys.* 1878, vol. v. pl. iii. fig. 1 ; pl. vi. fig. 2.

[2] Aufrecht (*Centralblatt*, 1866, p. 433) has described a similar central opening in tubercles of the omentum, which he regards as a section of a lymphatic vessel.

[3] Described by Cornil, *Leçons*, p. 59.

[4] This alveolar growth has been figured by Moxon, *Path. Soc. Trans.* 1872, xxiii. 300.

[5] Ziegler (*Herkunft der Tuberkelelemente*, p. 8) has also stated that the smallest miliary tubercles commence in the septa of the alveoli, where they form *circles* of induration.

growth has commenced in the bronchioles. I would here remark also that, although in all gland-structures inflammation may extend from the duct to the acini, the latter are not unfrequently primarily affected; and under nearly all other conditions, while the affection of the duct often remains superficial, that of the gland-tissue tends to become parenchymatous.[1] I have reinvestigated (1881) every specimen which I possess, in order to find appearances bearing out the statement of Rindfleisch and Charcot as to the primary seat of tubercle in the lung, and I must confess that none have shown any traces of an origin at the passage of the bronchial tube into the infundibula. I cannot therefore but believe that this mode of origin must be exceptional and rare. Tubercles tend to form at the periphery of the lung, under the pleura, and also along the interlobular septa (*see* XXVIII. 5). In this respect also all the extra-lobular bronchi, and even some of the intralobular, stand to the infundibula in the relation of bases on which the latter rest, and hence bronchi, and even arteries, may occasionally be seen surrounded by groups of granulations which are not of bronchial but of alveolar origin.[2]

The growth of the alveolar granulations has been very minutely described by Klein,[3] and more recently by Arnold.[4] Klein, in the artificial tubercle of the rodentia, found that the granulations commenced by an exudation into the interior of the alveoli, followed by epithelial proliferation, while in the walls there formed a series of trabeculae, filled with lymphoid cells, out of which a solid reticular or cytogenic tissue developed. The trabeculae have their anatomical origin in the lymphatics of the interalveolar tissue; the reticulum is formed, in part at least, from their endothelium; and many of the lymphoid cells are probably, in Klein's opinion, emigrated white blood-corpuscles. He found a similar structure in most cases of acute tuberculosis of children, and he gives to some of these granulations the name of a 'catarrhal pneumonia.' I think this term is best avoided for reasons already stated (*see* 'Catarrhal Pneumonia'), and especially because the implication of the alveolar wall with a solid growth is not the ordinary feature of a genuine catarrhal pneumonia, but involves a superadded process which entirely changes its character. In some cases of acute tuberculosis, the nodules may be apparently entirely pneumonic: I say 'apparently' because they are also at once destructive, and I shall have hereafter to consider the nature of this destructive change.

I have already described the epithelial proliferation, though I confess I am disposed to lay less stress on it than Klein has done, as a constant element in this process. In some of the smallest microscopic granulations, involving only two or three alveoli, and which therefore may be presumed to represent an early stage, their growth may be seen to take place almost *ab initio*, without enlarged or desquamated epithelial cells forming any essential part of the process.

Klein has most perfectly elucidated the origin of the greater part of the small-celled growth. Part of this, however, in the floor of the alveoli, has appeared to me to arise from the nuclei of branching cells in this position, and another part is preceded by a growth of fusiform cells which are gradually replaced by the small round cells (*see* XXX. 7 and 10; XXXI. 1, 2, 3, and 4). Another part arises from the proliferation of the nuclei of the capillaries, which Klein has confirmed (*see* XXX. 6 and 10; XL. 6, 7, and 8).

From the alveoli, the small-celled infiltration extends to the alveolar passages and

---

[1] This is, I believe, the interpretation of Hérard and Cornil's figures. *Phthisie Pulmonaire*, p. 110.
[2] Granchér (*Arch. de Phys.* 1st ser. 1872, iv. 629) says that, although analogy might lead us to expect that the seat of tubercle in the lung might be peribronchial or perivascular, the vast majority of tubercles of any appreciable size in this organ are alveolar.
[3] *Anat. Lymphatic Tissue*, part ii. pp. 44–64.
[4] Virchow's *Archiv*, vol. lxxxviii.

bronchioles, thickening their walls. The interior of these is occupied by epithelial proliferation; the cells are large, and tend to pass into amorphous débris, and conjointly with the rest to form part of the general mass of solidification.

Interstitial Granulations.—The occurrence of these has been asserted by many writers,[1] but apart from those existing in the peribronchial and perivascular sheaths, it is difficult to prove their independent existence, since the alveolar tissue becomes implicated at an early period. The interstitial tissue between the ultimate lobules is difficult to trace in the normal lung, and also in cases where any extended change has taken place in the alveolar structures. I am disposed to believe, however, that granulations may form in the interlobular septa, though these generally participate in the small-celled growth in a more extended form, akin to an infiltration.

HISTOLOGY OF INFILTRATIONS AND CASEATION.

The histology of the infiltrations of phthisis necessarily includes those that are caseous, but I shall first describe infiltrations that have not assumed this character. The subject of caseation will be considered both as affecting all the forms of granulations previously described, and also as occurring in a diffuse form.

The minute structure of these infiltrations will be considered in the same order as was adopted in the description of their naked-eye appearances.

(*a*) *Red Hepatisation.*—The ordinary red hepatisation met with in phthisis differs apparently but little from that which occurs as an independent disease, but its special histological characters have not received much attention.[2] In some cases, however, a red hepatisation (XII. *Case 23, Lloyd*), which passes into caseation, corresponds in its main characters with those of the grey hepatisation, and will be subsequently described. In other instances, while still maintaining the red appearance, it may pass into extensive tracts of fibroid induration (IV. 1, *Case 3, Hawkins*), which also will be considered later. Frerichs has also given an account of the red pneumonic infiltration that attends acute tuberculisation, as presenting epithelioid cells similar to those hereafter to be described in tubercle, and also large cells practically indistinguishable from giant-cells.[3]

(*b*) *The Gelatinous Infiltration* of Laennec has been described by Niemeyer as a 'chronic catarrhal pneumonia,'[4] by Buhl as one of the varieties of the condition which

---

[1] Grancher (*Arch. de Physiol.* 2nd ser. v. 569) has asserted this especially for acute tuberculosis, which he considers to follow the course of the lymphatic tracts. See also Arnold, Virchow's *Archiv*, vol. lxxxviii.

[2] Hérard and Cornil (*Phthisie Pulmonaire*) describe it as differing in no respect from the exudation of ordinary acute pneumonia. Cornil and Ranvier (*Manuel Histol. Pathologique*, 1882, 2nd ed. xi. 166, 169) describe a fibrinous pneumonia in phthisis, which they state to be as frequent as the 'catarrhal' form. Green (*Pathology of Consumption*, p. 36) describes the pneumonia of phthisis as presenting a fibrillated coagulum within the alveoli, precisely similar to that seen in acute croupons pneumonia, although the fibrillation is less abundant and less distinct. Small and large cells are mingled in this exudation, but in some cases there may be but little epithelial proliferation. Delafield (*Studies in Pathological Anatomy*, p. 90) describes, in acute phthisis, a red pneumonia presenting a fibrinous exudation.

[3] Frerichs, *Beiträge Lehre Tuberculosis*, Marburg, 1882, p. 37.

[4] Niemeyer, *Vorträge uber die Lungenschwindsucht*, pp. 15, 16, and *Spec. Path. u. Therapie*, ed. 1868,

pp. 235, 245. Niemeyer left Laennec's 'grey infiltration' almost undescribed. I shall allude to this subject hereafter, and attempt to show that the application of the term 'catarrhal' to this form of infiltration is essentially incorrect. The term 'catarrhal' has been used in different senses by various writers on phthisis, as applied to the consolidations found. Thus Hérard and Cornil use it in reference to the soft granulations, and apply it also to the gelatinous infiltration and to Laennec's grey infiltration. They term these, however, 'tuberculous pneumonia,' because they define the catarrhal form as chiefly characterised by epithelial proliferation; *loc. cit.* pp. 129, 134; also Hérard, *Bull. Congrès Internat. de Paris* 1867. Buhle (Ziemssen's *Handbuch*, v. § ii. 10 and 26) rejects catarrh as a cause of phthisis. I believe that it will best serve the interests of science if we apply the term 'catarrhal pneumonia,' to that which originates in catarrhal causes. Its application to phthisis is purely hypothetical, and something more is needed to convert a catarrhal pneumonia into phthisis, although it is true, as Cornil and Ranvier have remarked, that the bronchial catarrh common in phthisis may easily cause catarrha pneumonia (*Manuel Histol. Path.* 2nd ed. 1882, xi. 166).

he termed 'genuine desquamative pneumonia,'[1] and by Rindfleisch[2] as a desquamative pneumonia associated with œdema.

It is mainly characterised by the filling of the alveoli by an amorphous, finely granular exudation, in which only a few swollen epithelial cells are found (*see* XXXVIII. 2, 4). These cells may be very large, measuring from $\frac{1}{2500}$ to $\frac{1}{1000}$ of an inch, and may contain a single nucleus or sometimes two or three nuclei. They may also swell to transparent bodies, apparently undergoing the mucoid transformation. A few blood-corpuscles and pyoid non-nucleated cells may be mingled with these larger cells. The exudation in the interior of the alveoli is probably albuminoid in character; at least no appearances of a fibrinous network are seen in it. In some specimens, when the alveoli are thus occupied, it would appear as if the amorphous matter resulted from the breaking down of the epithelial-like cells, but in the majority of instances the material filling the alveoli is probably exudation of the albuminoid or possibly mucoid class.[3] The walls of the alveoli are rarely thickened in the typical form, and in some instances the capillary network is still preserved. In others, however (*see* XXXVIII. 4), a nuclear growth may be observed to be commencing in them, and probably marks a stage of transformation to the grey infiltration.

This gelatinous infiltration is commonly diffuse, but in some cases of acute tuberculosis it may be found in a lobular form[4] and it appears to pass subsequently into the inflammatory type of granulation, in which epithelial proliferation blends with a small-celled growth. When specimens of different phthisical lungs are examined with the microscope, this amorphous filling of the alveoli is found to be not uncommon. It exists in both the acute and chronic forms of the disease, but appears to be more common in the former, and it is also found in acute tuberculosis.

The conditions to which it is due are uncertain. It is believed by Rindfleisch to arise from capillary obstruction, but it is not unlikely that its peculiar characters are due to defective blood-states, since it occurs, as was remarked by Rokitansky, most extensively during the terminal stages of phthisis. He, however, appears to regard a colloid change as sometimes resulting from epithelial degeneration.[5] Talma[6] believes that the origin of the change is an infiltration of the spaces of the peribronchial and interlobular tissue with granular exudation and lymphoid cells, some of which attain the size of epithelioid cells, while the alveoli are simultaneously filled with a gelatinous exudation. I have not seen this as clearly as has been described by him, but it would appear probable that the implication of the interstitial tissue is the origin of this gelatinous exudation.

---

[1] Buhl. *Lungenentzündung*, p. 71, and *Mittheil. aus der Path. Inst. zu München*, 1878, see also *ante*, p. 80. The name 'desquamative pneumonia,' chosen by Buhl, has the disadvantage of imperfectly expressing his meaning. He defined it as 'parenchymatous,' meaning that the walls of the air-vesicles are implicated, and that this distinguishes it from the 'croupous' variety. (He denies the existence of a 'catarrhal' pneumonia.) The epithelial changes are, in his opinion, only secondary to those in the wall, although so far characteristic that they continued throughout the whole process, and pus-corpuscles were absent—points of distinction from the croupous variety. Caseation and induration occurred in consequence of this parenchymatous change, and miliary tubercle was only a variety of the disease. I have endeavoured to show that the epithelial changes are not special to this form. (See *ante*, Acute and Catarrhal Pneumonia.) Friedländer (Virchow's *Archiv*, lxviii. 341, 345) appears to define 'desquamative pneumonia' as the filling of the alveoli with large cells, and 'catarrhal pneumonia' as a similar filling with small cells. He also applies the latter term to the inoculation-disease in the rabbit, to which he denies a tubercular character, because giant-cells are not found in it. It must be added that, in many places, little or no epithelial desquamation is to be found in the gelatinous infiltration.

[2] Rindfleisch, Ziemssen's *Handb. Krank. Resp. App.* ii. 201. He describes the gelatinous infiltration as lobular and the œdema as due to capillary obstruction.

[3] Virchow (*Würzb. Verhand.* i. 8 4) found in it much albumen, and material akin to casein.

[4] Klein (*Anat. Lymphatic Syst'm*, ii. 72) has described some of the early stages of acute tuberculosis as presenting nodules filled with a *fibrinous* exudation. This differs from the amorphous material which I have observed.

[5] *Path, Anat.* 1861, p. 86.

[6] *Studien über Lungenschwindsucht*, Utrecht, 1879, p. 80.

Caseous spots, as Laennec pointed out, are found in the midst of this infiltration. Their nature and origin will be considered hereafter.

(c) The *Grey Infiltration*, as stated by Laennec, exists in two forms, the diffuse and the lobular, and both (also as described by him) pass into caseation. It is characterised by three chief conditions, viz. (1) by filling of the alveoli with epithelial cells, leucocytes, and their derivatives, mingled with exudation matter; (2) by the thickening of the walls of the alveoli with a small-celled growth; and (3) in some places by a destructive change, akin to suppuration, which may take place over considerable areas.

(1) *Distension of the alveoli.*—The exudation into the interior of the alveoli seems to be frequently of a mucoid or albuminous character; at least it does not always fibrillate. Fibrinous exudation has, however, been observed in it by Hérard and Cornil.[1]

The *epithelial cells*, within the alveoli, are often very large, measuring $\frac{1}{1500}$, $\frac{1}{1200}$, and even $\frac{1}{1000}$ of an inch, and containing one or more well-defined nuclei. They may also enlarge to 'physalides,' or into large, clear, mucoid bodies. Large tracts may be found thus occupied, in which but little change can be found in the alveolar walls, and in which the capillaries are still pervious (*see* XXVI. 7, *Case 17, Ellsom*). In some cases these cells appear to undergo a granular disintegration, but it seems also not improbable that they may persist for some time unchanged, and no sign of caseous degeneration occurs in parts thus infiltrated unless other processes have supervened. In other parts of the same lung, alveoli may be found filled with smaller cells, varying in size from $\frac{1}{3000}$ to $\frac{1}{2500}$ of an inch, generally with a single nucleus and resembling those common in acute pneumonia. These alveoli may also have their walls apparently unchanged. The cells are imbedded in an amorphous exudation-matter. Such parts tend to pass into changes akin to suppuration. The majority of the purely pneumonic changes in phthisis present, however, large rather than small epithelioid cells.

The *diffuse thickening of the alveolar walls* by a small-celled growth was figured by Rokitanski,[2] in 1861, described by Förster,[3] in 1863, by Meyer,[4] in 1864, and re-asserted by Villemin, in 1867.[5] It appears to me to be one of the most important and characteristic features in phthisical pneumonia, and to be the main condition which induces subsequent caseation or induration; and I cannot but believe that the neglect of this change has been the cause of much of the confusion which has existed during the last twenty years on the subject of the nature of phthisis.[6] In spite of Villemin's statements, it only received full recognition in Germany when Buhl called attention to

---

[1] *Phthisie Pulmonaire*, p. 135. It has also been described as occasionally fibrinous by Thaon, *loc. cit.* p. 64. It is described by Grancher as fibrinoid, *i.e.* as not possessing the firmness of the exudation of acute primary pneumonia; *Archives de Physiol.* 1878, v. 36. Cornil and Ranvier (*Manuel Histol. Path.* 2nd ed. 1882, xi. 171) appear to refer the grey infiltration to an acute red fibrinous pneumonia which has become chronic, a proposition which I think doubtful.

[2] Rokitanski, *Path. Anat.* 2nd ed. 1861, cxi. 86.

[3] Förster, *Path. Anat.* 1863, ii. 226-9.

[4] Ludwig Meyer, Virchow's *Archiv*, xxx. 46. He speaks distinctly of this as a tubercular infiltration.

[5] *Etudes sur la Tuberculose*, 1867, p. 146. It is more distinctly stated by him in *Bull. Congrès Intern. Méd. de Paris*, 1867, p. 61. See also his figures of tubercle in the kidney and testicle; *Du Tubercule*. Paris, 1861, pl. ii. figs. 3 and 4.

[6] The reason why this condition has been so much overlooked has been the tendency to attribute the majority of the caseations in the lung to epithelial changes, and the denial by Virchow that an 'infiltration' of tubercle occurred in the lung, though he admitted it, by confluence of granulations, for other tissues. See his *Krankhafte Geschwülste*, ii. 600, 601, 644. Hérard and Cornil described an infiltration of the alveolar walls around grey granulations, but did not describe it as an element of these tuberculous pneumonias (*loc. cit.* pp. 112-14). Niemeyer (*Spec. Path. u. Therapie*, 1868, i. 265) admitted an occasional implication of the alveolar wall, but only as a rare event. In his sense the destruction of the lung was mainly due to intra-alveolar changes. In 1868 the growth was described in the rodentia by Burdon-Sanderson (*Rep. Med. Off. of Privy Council*) and by myself (*Artificial Production of Tubercle*). See also Klein, *Lymphatic Tissues*. In

HISTOLOGY OF INFILTRATIONS

it under the name of 'desquamative pneumonia.' This change is found in all forms of phthisis, and is not uncommon in the diffuse caseous infiltrations of acute tuberculosis (see XXVIII. 7). It occurs, as has long been known, around all forms of tubercular granulations[1] (see XXXVIII. 4, XXXI. 1, m, and XXXIV. 1). Cornil and Ranvier have stated that it is limited to the neighbourhood of the peribronchial and perivascular growths,[2] but I believe that it exists in tracts where such growths cannot be seen in an isolated form, and it is to this condition that I shall now specially refer.[3]

In these infiltrations in acute tuberculosis, the change is found as a small-celled growth, thickening the alveolar walls and narrowing their cavities. In the earlier stages it is associated with cell-proliferation into the interior of the alveoli, both of large epithelioid cells and also of leucocytes (see XXX. 5 and 6). The small round cells of the growth are imbedded in a reticulum,[4] sometimes transparent, sometimes more or less fibrillated; but they may, in places, be so densely crowded that no reticulum can be seen. The alveoli are greatly narrowed by the growth, and this, where it is of considerable duration, tends to become fibrillated and granular, and to occupy nearly the whole structure of the lung, while the cells often disappear from the interior of the vesicles (XXVIII. 9 and 10). The elastic fibres are first separated by the growth,[5] but later they disappear from view, although they may be made again apparent by the use of dilute solution of soda.[6]

Similar changes in the alveolar wall are found in the grey infiltration of all forms of phthisis, acute and chronic, as well as in acute tuberculosis.[7] In the former, as well as in the latter, the same extreme thickening of the walls, and gradual closure of the lumen of the alveoli by the growth, may be observed[8] (see XXXVIII. 1). It surrounds also the bronchioles and alveolar passages, and in these the cubical change of the epithelium, described by Thaon,[9] can be seen.[10] (XXXVIII. 6). In earlier stages the growth may be observed to commence with a gradual thickening of this nature, even in the

---

[1] I stated it to be one of the most important conditions of phthisis (Reynolds's *Syst. Med.* iii. art. 'Chronic Pneumonia,' 754). Wagner (*Das Lymphadenom*, 1871, pp. 29-42) described a diffused growth in the lung, which he asserted to be identical with miliary tubercle. In 1872, Grancher (*Archives de Physiol.*) made a similar statement which he has subsequently expanded more fully. (See *Unité de la Phthisie*, Thèse de Paris 1873, and *Archives de Physiol.* 1878, vol. v.) It was observed by Aufrecht, but attributed by him to inflammation (*Chronische Bronchopneumonie*, 1873). The identity of the 'infiltration' with the granulation has also been asserted by Thaon, *Rech. Anat. Path. de la Tuberculose*, 1878. In an earlier paper he had described the grey infiltration of Laennec as consisting of a mass of miliary granulations, but the latter as filling the interior of the alveoli, the walls of which remained entire (see *Comp. Rend. Soc. Biol.* 1872). The same opinion has been approved by Charcot (*Rev. Mens.* 1877, pp. 42-5) and by T. H. Green (*Path. of Consump.* 1878, pp. 42-5). Buhl's views have been more or less fully adopted by Friedländer (Virchow's *Archiv.* lxviii.) and by Rindfleisch (Ziemssen's *Handbuch*, v. 195), who asserts that it is the most important feature of the infiltration; by Arnold (Virchow's *Archiv*, vol. lxxxviii.) and by Baumgarten ('Latente Tuberculose.' Volkmann's *Samm-lung klin. Vorträge*, No. 218, 1882), who has, partly on this ground, accepted the doctrine of the unity of phthisis. The thickening of the alveolar walls has also been described by Talma, under the name of a 'Granulation-Pneumonie' (*Studien über Lungenschwindsucht*, 1879).

See also Dollinger, *Arch. exp. Pathol.* 1878, i. 376, and Martin, *Rech. Anat. Path. sur le Tubercule*, 1879.

[1] Figured by Hérard and Cornil, *Phthisie Pulmonaire*, pp. 112, 113; Thaon, *Anat. Path. de la Tuberculose*, pl. ii. fig. 1; Martin, *Rech. Anat. Path. sur le Tubercule*, 1879, figs. 1 and 2; Shepherd, *Pulmonary Consumption*, Gulstonian Lectures, pl. i. and iii.; Green, *Pathology of Consumption*, 1878, p. 16. See also Charcot, *Revue Mensuelle*, 1877, p. 880.

[2] *Manuel Histol. Path.* 1882, ii. 171.

[3] This subject will be considered later.

[4] See Wagner, *Tuberkelähnliches Lymphadenom*, 1871, p. 30; Talma, *Studien über Lungenschwindsucht*, p. 37.

[5] Ludwig Meyer, Virchow's *Archiv*, vol. xxx.

[6] Grancher, *Archives de Physiol.* 1872.

[7] Wagner (*Das Lymphadenom*, p. 42) described the 'non-miliary diffuse lymphadenoma' as especially characteristic of chronic phthisis, but I believe that it occurs equally in all forms.

[8] A similar appearance is figured by Martin in an artificially-excited pneumonia; *Archives de Physiol.* 1880, vol. vii. pl. i. fig. 1.

[9] Thaon describes this change as occurring within the alveoli, and he is confirmed by Martin, *Rech. Anat. Path. Tubercule*, p. 78; see also Arnold, Virchow's *Archiv*, Bd. 83, p. 428.

[10] Rindfleisch (*Lehrb. path. Gewebelehre*, 5th ed. 350) says that this thickening of the alveolar septa may occur in extensive tracts of the caseous pneumonia of children, without desquamation of the epithelium.

presence of infiltration (XXXVIII. 2 and 4), when the first stage appears to be the growth of fusiform cells in the alveolar wall, which gradually passes into a round-celled structure (XXXVIII. 5). In a similar manner it can be seen extending indefinitely around nodules both of induration and caseation (XXXVI. 3 and 4; and XL. 1 and 3), while in others it occupies the tissue intervening between the small-celled nodules of miliary granulations (XXXIX. 4 and 7). In all these situations giant-cells are found, as described by Wagner, often pigmented. They are mingled with the growth, but their number is variable, and sometimes they may be entirely absent through considerable areas. The growth also tends to assume, at times, a very diffuse form, in which only traces of the alveolar structure are apparent, since the vesicles become almost entirely filled with the small-celled formation (XXXVIII. 8, XL. 2). In some of these instances (as in the figures last referred to) the epithelial cells and the leucocytes filling the alveoli remain long unchanged, and occasionally the granulations may grow, in a more or less pedunculated form, into the cavity of the air-vesicles, as described by Charcot and Martin.[1] (See XXXVII. 7.) In some cases of this nature the growth may be nodular, and may occupy only one side of the alveolar wall. In other parts and instances, a rapid caseation takes place in the interior of the alveoli, and, in some places, appears to occur in the small-celled growth that fills them (XXXVII. 6); in others it is seen in the exudation of epithelial products (XXXIX. 2).

It remains to be stated that in some places, and especially in acute pneumonic phthisis, this thickening of the alveolar walls, instead of being firm and reticulated, presents an appearance more resembling suppuration; the cells are rather large and more irregular than those of the small-celled growth, and they are nucleated, the nucleus nearly filling the cell. All stages of transition between such appearances and a reticulated growth may, however, be observed in the same specimen.

Origin and nature of the growth.—By a certain number of writers this growth is styled 'interstitial,'[2] a term which is, I think, inaccurate. The growth essentially affects the alveolar wall; little, if any, interstitial tissue, in the ordinary sense in which the term is employed, can be traced between the individual alveoli of each acinus. Such tissue is only recognisable as perilobular. There can be little question but that this perilobular tissue is also invaded, but the main effect on the pulmonary tissue is produced by means of the implication of the alveoli. The growth doubtless extends to the alveolar passages and bronchioles,[3] and involves the coats of the vessels[4] in these situations. It leads to the occlusion of the capillaries and smaller arteries, while, in some of the larger vessels,

---

[1] Charcot, *Revue Mensuelle*, 1877, p. 880; Martin, *Rech. Anat. Path. Tubercule*, p. 82. Martin speaks of this growth as a vascular granulation which may involve several alveoli. I have not seen vessels in them. A growth of this nature is figured by Cornil and Ranvier, *Manuel Histol. Path.* 1882, ii. 150. Delafield, *Studies in Path. Anat.* p. 95, has also described polypoid growths extending from the walls into the interior of the air-vesicles.

[2] Hérard and Cornil, *Phthisie Pulmonaire*, p. 123. 'Cloisons interlobulaires'; Cornil and Ranvier, *Manuel Histol. Path.* 2nd ed. 1882, ii. 179; Friedländer (*Untersuchungen chronische Pneumonie*, Virchow's *Archiv*, 1876, lxviii. pp. 342, 355) speaks of the growth as being in the interstitial tissue (walls of bronchi and vessels), but also (p. 341) he speaks of it as occupying the alveolar walls. Thaon retains the term 'interstitial,' although he applies it to all connective-tissue growth, whether affecting the bronchioles, the vessels, or the alveolar walls. *Rech. Anat. Path. Tubercule*, p. 72. Talma (*Studien über Lungenschwindsucht*, 1879, p. 41) says that it begins in the interstitial tissue, and thence extends to the alveolar walls. This sequence appears difficult of proof as a general proposition, although undoubtedly peribronchial and periarterial growth may have this extension.

[3] See Wagner, *Das Tuberkelähnliche Lymphadenom*. I have already expressed my opinion that, as a general rule, this thickening does not necessarily commence with the bronchioles in the granulation-form, and I believe that this statement equally applies to the diffuse forms of small-celled growth affecting the pulmonary tissue.

[4] Wagner; Friedländer; Buhl; Martin; Talma; Charcot. Martin has laid special stress on this implication of the vessels.

thrombi are occasionally found.¹ It is to the arrest of the circulation thus produced that the exsanguine appearance of the tissue, as well as its liability to subsequent caseation, are mainly due.

The origin of the growth has been a matter of considerable discussion. Wagner, though tracing it in all the tissues already mentioned, professed himself unable to pronounce positively upon this point. Martin lays great stress on the 'endo-arteritis,' but in some parts the vessels and capillaries remain apparently more or less permeable until the growth has somewhat advanced. Talma ascribes its origin to lymphoid cells, around which a reticulum subsequently forms, while some of these cells undergo a change to epithelial structures—an opinion closely resembling that expressed by Addison,² and repeated by Von Waldenburg,³ that tubercle consists of emigrated white corpuscles. This view has also been in part supported by Rindfleisch, as respects the development of the large cells.⁴ It cannot be denied that, in the present aspect of the pathology of inflammation, such an origin is possibly attributable to some of these cells. It must be remarked, however, that an extensive proliferation of the nuclear elements of the alveolar wall occurs in these growths, as shown by the early production of fusiform cells, and that the nuclei of the capillaries also participate. Klein has described⁵ it in the rodentia as consisting of an excessive development of the interalveolar tissue into an almost uniform reticulum of nucleated cells, with very numerous and finely-branching, anastomosing processes—a structure closely resembling an early lymphatic growth, and I am disposed to believe that it is from the connective tissue of the alveolar wall, as representing a lymphatic element, that the growth mainly proceeds.⁶ In this sense it may represent an 'endothelial lymphatic growth,' as has been said by Talma, and this was originally stated by Klebs⁷ to be the origin of the grey granulation.

DESTRUCTIVE CHANGES.—I have postponed the consideration of the destructive changes in the granulations previously described until now, because it has appeared to me that they would be best considered in relation to those which occur in the more diffuse infiltrations, and because great differences of opinion have existed, during the last twenty years, in respect to their nature in both situations.

They occur in two main forms—as caseation and as an acute softening which is akin to suppuration; the former is by far the most common.

Caseation.—I shall have hereafter to discuss certain of the opinions expressed with regard to this change. Some of them have become widely known, and they may be stated briefly to have originated with Virchow's observation that other morbid products than tubercle may undergo the caseous change.⁸ Almost simultaneously, Reinhardt⁹ stated that *all* the processes of phthisis were inflammatory, including the grey granulation, and that most of what had been termed crude or yellow tubercle was pus inspissated in the terminal bronchi. Virchow, recognising the difficulty of distinguishing tubercle from other caseous matters, proposed to confine the term to the grey granulation, and regarded

---

¹ Hérard and Cornil, *Phthisie Pulmonaire*, p. 138.
² Addison, *Healthy and Diseased Structure*, p. 100.
³ Waldenburg, *Die Tuberculose*, p. 414, see also Aufrecht, *Bronchopneumonic, Tuberculose und Schwindsucht*, 1878; Martin, *Études sur la Tuberculose*, pp. 15, 16.
⁴ Ziemssen's *Handbuch*, 'Krankh. Resp. App.' ii. 193, also *Die Tuberculose*, Virchow's *Archiv*, 1881, lxxxv. 76.
⁵ *Anatomy of the Lymphatic System*, part ii. p. 66.
⁶ Many French writers, and especially Grancher and Charcot, give this tissue the term 'conjunctive embryonique.' Thaen and Martin style it 'sarcomatous' or 'caseo-sarcomatous.'
⁷ Virchow's *Archiv*, Bd. 44.
⁸ *Würzburg. Verhandlungen*, ii. 72, iii. 99, and 'Die Entwickelungsgeschichte des Krebses.' Virchow's *Archiv*, vol. l. Caseous change had gradually come to be regarded as almost synonymous with tubercle, and Virchow showed that the two were not necessarily identical. The term 'caseous' appears to date from Bonetus, 'Sepulchretum,' 1700, quoted by Peski, *Études Historiques Tuberculose Pulmonaire*, 1880, p. 19.
⁹ *Charité-Annalen*, 1850, vol. i.

most of the other caseous substances in the lung, especially all infiltrations, as the result of a caseous pneumonia either miliary or diffuse,¹ while the indurated nodules were in many instances not tubercular but due to a peribronchitis.² Virchow insisted on the caseation of the granulation, but stated that after this change its origin was incapable of recognition, and the nature of some changes could only be determined from the co-existence of other recent tubercular granulations in their neighbourhood.³ Virchow, as is well known, placed the seat of tubercle in the interstitial or connective tissue, and also in the bronchial and arterial walls. He denied its alveolar situation, and, refusing to regard tubercle as an infiltration, he does not appear to have recognised a growth in the alveolar wall.⁴

Nature of the caseous change.—Engel and Reinhardt attributed it chiefly to the inspissation of inflammatory products with loss of water;⁵ Virchow, to the fatty degeneration of such products, with shrivelling of the cells and necrosis of the tissue, due to arrest of the circulation.⁶ The necrosis has been, until recently, too much left out of sight in the consideration of this process,⁷ and an almost undue prominence has been given to the fatty degeneration, since, as Engel remarked, the yellow matter consists in greater part of protein material akin to casein (Preuss), and contains only a small proportion of fat.⁸ In many cases no distinct fat-drops can be seen, and only a fine molecular disintegration is observable (see XXXI. 3. 7).

Recent observations have shown that the degenerative change thus undergone by tubercle is of a more complex nature, and has analogies with various forms of degeneration occurring under other pathological conditions, which have been termed by different observers ' hyaline,'⁹ ' vitreous,'¹⁰ or ' waxy.'¹¹ Grancher describes it as chiefly affecting the epithelial cells, which present enlargement of their nuclei, acquire a glistening aspect and become brittle, as shown by fissures. In some cases the wax-like substance forms globules, which stain with osmic acid but not with carmine, and which therefore Grancher believes to be of a fatty nature, though differing from the ordinary appearances of fat-drops. It has been described in similar terms by Gombault, as affecting the giant-cells of tubercle.¹²

---

¹ *Wien. med. Wochenschr.*; 'Cellular-Pathologie' ed. 1858, pp. 162, 419 *et seq.*; *Krankhafte Geschwülste*, ii. 600; 'miliare käsige Pneumonie ' *ib.* p. 601. He terms these a scrofulous broncho-pneumonia, and says they may be associated with tubercles.
² *Krankhafte Geschwülste*, ii. 634.
³ *Ib.* ii. 610. This refers especially to the fibrous tubercle.
⁴ See *Verhand. Berliner med. Gesellsch.* 1865, i. 207. He says that the only condition in which this can occur is in a lung thickened by previous chronic pneumonia, and with this exception there is no form which can rightly be called a tubercular infiltration, in which truly demonstrable tubercle is deposited in the alveolar tissue of the lung.
⁵ Engel, *Zeitsch. der Gesellsch. der Aerzte zu Wien*, 1844, vol. i.; Reinhardt, *Charité-Annalen*, 1850, i. 368-9.
⁶ Virchow, *Verhand. phys.-med. Gesellschaft zu Würzburg*, 1850, i. 85; 1852, ii. 73.
⁷ Thus Waldenburg (*Die Tuberculose*, 1869, p. 164) wrote of this thickened caseous matter as ' thickened pus.'
⁸ *Loc. cit.* p. 557. In a later work he speaks of fatty degeneration and tuberculisation, ' Fettmetamorphose oder Tuberculösewerden' (*Prager Vierteljahrsch.* 1855, xlv. 27).
⁹ This change is probably the same as that figured by Rokitanski as a ' colloid ' or ' amyloid ' transformation in the interior of the alveoli. (*Path. Anat.* 1862, iii. 86.) It was mentioned by Villemin (*Cong. Méd. Internat. de Paris*, 1877) who describes the cells as becoming glistening, and at the same time shrivelled as if dried, and he attributes to Kuss a similar observation under the title of 'mummification.' The latter author is inaccessible to me. Two papers by him are quoted by Hérard and Cornil from the *Gazette Médicale de Strasbourg*, 1847 and 1855. It is mentioned by Ranvier in the bones. He describes the tissue before caseation as becoming translucent, and the cells shrivel and fuse together; *Arch. Physiol. Normale et Path.* 1868, i. 95. An historical account of it is given by Vallat (Virchow's *Archiv*, 1882, vol. lxxxix.) and he ascribes to Schüppel (*Lymphdrüsen-Tuberculose*, 1871, pp. 46, 77) an early observation of the same character. Rindfleisch (*Berlin. med. Wochenschrift*, 1878, p. 68) describes the cells as transparent and glassy. Buhl (*Lungenentzündung*, p. 59) described a waxy change in the tissue and its vessels. See also *Handbuch path. Gewebelehre*, ed. 1878, p. 348. The term 'hyaline' is employed by Hering (*Studien über Tuberculose*, Berlin, 1878, p. 83), and it was brought into more common use by Recklinghausen in 1879 (*Tageblatt 52ste Versammlung Deutsch. Naturforscher u. Aerzte, Baden-Baden*), and it has since been adopted by Arnold and Vallat.
¹⁰ The term vitreous, as far as I can discover, first appears in a paper by Charcot ; he calls it ' mortification vitreuse ' (*Rev. Mensuelle*, 1877, pp. 877, 886.) A fuller account of the change is given by Grancher (*Archives de Physiol.* 1878, pp. 19, 33.) He claims priority for its employment in the *Comptes Rendus Soc. Biol.* 1877, and Vallat attributes it to him in the *Comptes Rendus Soc. Biol.* 1872, but I cannot find a description of this appearance in either of the papers by Grancher in those volumes.
¹¹ Grancher, *Arch. de Phys.* 1878, v. 33.
¹² *Comptes Rendus Soc. Biol.* 1878, p. 281.

Arnold has also observed it, both in the giant-cells and in the epithelioid cells of tubercle of the lung.[1]

As regards the frequency of this hyaline or vitreous change, there is some discrepancy of statement. Grancher regards it as almost a necessary condition of all caseations of the tubercular or scrofulous nature, though less apparent in the smaller granulations.[2] Vallat found it only occasionally in granulations in the lung, but with greater frequency in other organs, in some of which, but especially in the spleen, it may appear in the so-called caseous pneumonia, independently of the presence of granulations.[3] On the other hand, Arnold found it most frequently in the disseminated nodules. The origin of the change has been ascribed by Rindfleisch to an escape of the protoplasm of the cells. Grancher describes it as a direct result of cell-transformation ; a conclusion which is doubted by Vallat, though it appears to be confirmed by Gombault and Arnold. The tendency is to commence in the centre of the granulations (Vallat), although, as it speedily passes into caseous degeneration, this latter condition is often found centrally, surrounded by a zone of hyaline material.[4] In some places, as in the brain, it affects chiefly the reticulum, but it invades all other cell-forms of tubercle, and also those which thicken the alveolar wall (Vallat).

Vallat, following Langhans, regards this material as fibrinous and as being probably an exudation from the vessels, which undergo a similar degeneration. It bears a close resemblance, as was noted by Schüppel, to the reticulum of diphtheria, and also to the waxy degeneration of muscles,[5] and to the amyloid and lardaceous change, from which latter it is distinguished, however, by not colouring so intensely with iodine.[6]

It is evident, from numerous observations, that this material subsequently undergoes the granular caseous degeneration, but there remains strong ground for doubt whether it is a necessary antecedent of this degeneration, inasmuch as it is not observed in the ulcerative forms of phthisis (Vallat), and extensive pulmonary caseation has been observed by Leyden without its appearance.[7]

The whole group of caseations has been classified by Weigert under the term, introduced by Cohnheim,[8] of 'coagulations-necrosis,' a process that Weigert and Cohnheim regard as having, in tubercle, a specific origin.[9] The tendency of recent research is to show that the whole of this group of degenerative processes requires further investigation ; although some features are common to all, yet further differences, both in the chemical processes and in the nature of the changes undergone by the tissues, will probably be hereafter ascertained. It is evident that the classification together of such processes as smallpox, diphtheria,[10] simple fibrinous exudations, the degeneration of muscles in fever, infarcta,

---

[1] Virchow's *Archiv*, vol. lxxxviii.
[2] *Dict. Encycl. des Sciences Médicales*, art. 'Scrofule,' 3rd ser. viii. 308. Rindfleisch, *loc. cit.*, also appears to speak of it as constant.
[3] Thus Vallat found it in one-half of his cases of splenic tubercle. In other organs he found it in the following proportions:—serous membranes, twice in ten cases ; liver, five times in twenty cases ; kidney, twice in twenty cases, and never in the latter in connexion with miliary tubercles, but only with diffuse caseation. In twenty-five cases of the lungs he only found it with difficulty in isolated spots, 'hie und da.' He cites Arnold (Virchow's *Archiv*, vol. lxxxviii.) as having found it in thirty-eight out of ninety cases of tubercle of the lymphatic glands. It may be noted that Vallat found it in two out of three cases of gummata.
[4] Rindfleisch, *Lehrbuch*, ed. 1878, p. 348.
[5] Rindfleisch, *loc. cit.*
[6] Rindfleisch. *loc. cit.* Vallat, *loc. cit.*, p. 213. He states that, in some cases of sago-spleen, tubercle undergoing this change may be found side by side with nodules of amyloid degeneration. Schüppel. however (*Lymphdrüsen-Tuberculose*, p. 19), describes the giant-cells as staining deeply with iodine, but not coloured by the subsequent addition of sulphuric acid. It may be recalled that Dickinson described the lardaceous degeneration as a de-alkalised fibrin. (*Med.-Chir. Trans.* 1867. l. 53.)
[7] Leyden, *Zeitsch. klin. Med.* 1882, iv. 208 *et seq.*
[8] *Vorlesungen allg. Pathologie*, pp. 452, 458, 471, 616.
[9] Weigert, Virchow's *Archiv*, 1879, lxxvii. 272. Cohnheim, *loc. cit.* 616.
[10] It may be remembered that Buhl wrote of caseating (or 'tuberculising') pneumonia as akin to, if not identical with, diphtheria. (Henle and Pfeuffer's *Zeitschr.* 3rd ser. 1857, viii. 57. See also *Lungenentzündung*, p. 74.)

and the caseation of tubercle, can only be provisional; they must be due to different conditions of arrest of vitality, differences which are fully recognised by the talented workers who have commenced these observations, though the detailed discussion of the variations observed would be unsuitable to this place.[1]

As regards the changes in tubercle, one feature stands out prominently from recent observations, viz.: that its caseation is due largely, if not entirely, to arrest of the circulation, which, though noticed by Schröder van der Kolk,[2] has only of late received the attention which it deserved.[3] The caseation is not due, as was believed by Niemeyer and others, to the simple accumulation of inflammatory products.[4] In a few cases it may possibly be caused by the pressure of these products on the capillaries,[5] but in the majority it is owing either, as was formerly believed, to coagula within the pulmonary vessels [6] or more commonly to cell-growth closing their cavity (which has received the name of 'endarteritis' [7]) and possibly also to simple degeneration of their walls of the so-called 'hyaline' type.[8]

It has been shown conclusively by Litten's experiments that a partial or temporary arrest of the circulation can give rise to a fibrinous coagulable exudation into the cell-elements of the tissue, followed by a necrobiosis in which the nuclei disappear or become incapable of receiving certain colouring matters, and through which the whole tissue acquires a hyaline or vitreous aspect, later changing to an opaque and caseous appearance. He has also shown that parts in which the circulation has been entirely cut off die, but

---

[1] See especially Weigert's papers, Virchow's *Archiv*, vols. lxx. lxxii. lxxvii: also Cohnheim, *loc. cit.*; Vallat, *loc. cit.*; Neumann, *Archiv für mik. Anat.* vol. xviii. It may be remarked that a 'hyaline' degeneration was observed in cancroid by Köster (Virchow's *Archiv*, 1867, xl. 480). See also Weigert, *Hyaline Entartung der Lymphdrüsen*, Virchow's *Archiv*, 1870, vol. lxxviii. He regards this change as not peculiar to any one disease, but as common to many conditions of dyscrasia.

[2] Schröder van der Kolk, *Obs. Anat. Path.* 1826, pp. 66, 77.

[3] Some of the authors who referred the formation of tubercle to the walls of the capillaries, did not speak of this as the cause of caseation. Ref. Charcot, *Rev. Mensuelle*, 1870, p. 907.

[4] Many authors have spoken of caseation as due solely to the mutual pressure of the cells. Cf. Niemeyer *Klin. Vorträge*, pp. 15–17, who, however, admits that in some cases it may be due to invasion by cell-growth of the alveolar walls, *ib.* p. 18. Caseation by cell-pressure was asserted by Ruhle, Ziemssen's *Handbuch*, vol. v. *abth.* ii. p. 13; also in part by Schröder van der Kolk, *Niederland Lancet*, 1852 (Canstatt's *Jahresbericht*, and *Brit. and For. Med.-Chir. Rev.* 1853). Rindfleisch, in the first edition of his *Lehrbuch*, attributed it to mutual cell-pressure; see pages 381–87. In his later writings he attributes it, in part, to peculiar products of scrofula, in part to pressure on the vessels (*Lehrbuch*, 1878, pp. 85 6, 358; also Ziemssen's *Handbuch*, v. 153 195). Though he recognises the influence of this invasion in the production of haemorrhage, he speaks of it only doubtfully as a cause of caseation; *ib.* pp. 200, 203; see also *Berliner klin. Woch.* 1878. Mutual cell-pressure is recognised by Cornil and Ranvier as a cause, but combined with the obliteration of vessels, *Manuel Hist. Path.* 1882, ii. 149; *ib.* i. 136.

[5] Virchow, *Cellular Pathologie*, 1858, p. 423, and by Friedländer, Virchow's *Archiv*, lxxiii. 351.

[6] The direct causation of tubercle by obstruction of the vessels, owing to coagula or cell-accumulation in the interior and aided by an abnormally small size of the pulmonary capillaries, was asserted by Campbell in 1841 (*Observations on Tubercular Consumption*, p. 156), and by Henle (*Rationelle Pathologie*, 1847, ii. 701–5).

Coagula were found in the pulmonary arteries by Hérard and Cornil (*Phthisie Pulmon.* 1867), but they do not ascribe caseation to this cause. Cornil (*Arch. de Phys.* 1868, i. 102) has recognised it in numerous situations. Cf. also Cornil and Ranvier, previous note.

[7] Cf. Schröder van der Kolk, previous note. Förster (*Path. Anat.* 1863, ii. p. 227) distinctly ascribed caseation to invasion of the vascular wall by the tubercular growth. Bastian (*Edinb. Med. Journ.* 1867) ascribed the central softening of the brain in tubercular meningitis to the tubercular growth in the walls of the meningeal arteries. In the lungs and other parts, this was recognised as a cause of caseation by Villemin (see *Cong. Internat. Méd. de Paris*, 1867, and *Etudes sur la Tuberculose*, 1868, pp. 141, 150, 161). Colberg (*Deutsch. Anat. klin. Med.* 1867, vol. ii.) attributed it to the invasion of the capillaries, although in the diffuse form he ascribed it to cell-pressure, see pp. 470, 474–5. Tubercular growth in the walls of the vessels was regarded as the cause of caseation in bones by Ranvier. *Arch. de Phys.* 1868, i. 94, and also by Cornil, *ib.* p. 102, also *Cong. Internat. de Paris*, 1867, p. 100. Cf. also Buhl, *Lungenentzündung* p. 72; Thaon, *Rech. sur le Tubercule*, p. 42; Fox, *Trans. Path. Soc.* 1873, vol. xxii.; Martin, *Rech. sur le Tubercule*, 1879, pp. 50, 67, 84, 89; also *Mém. Laboratoire d'Histologie de France*, 1880, p. 195. The latter also states (*ib.* p. 191) that caseation from this cause is the link between all varieties of tubercle and that the caseation is due to endarteritis. Ref. also to Levy, *Arch. der Heilkunde*, 1877, vol. xviii. (diffuse form); Talma, *Studien über Lungenschwindsucht*, Utrecht, 1879, pp. 43–5. Orth, Virchow's *Archiv*, 1879, lxxvi. 229 (diffuse form); Cohnheim, *Vorlesungen*, ii. 616; Leyden, *Zeitsch. klin. Med.* 1882, iv. 298 *et seq* (diffuse form). Delafield (*Studies in Path. Anat.* pp. 109 10) regards 'coagulations-necrosis,' affecting large areas, as due to obstruction of the pulmonary artery, but as differing from the cheesy change in tubercle.

[8] Vallat, *loc. cit.*; Buhl, *Lungenentzündung*, p. 59. In the testicle, see Wahlstein, Virchow's *Archiv*, lxxv. 408. Radcliffe Hall, Birt. and Fox (*Med.-Chir. Rev.* 1855, vol. xvi.) described fatty degeneration of the pulmonary arteries as the cause of haemoptysis.

retain their nuclei.[1] It would appear not improbable that both these forms of change may go on at different rates and at different times in tubercular formations, and that the variations in aspect may thus be accounted for — especially the fact that in many tracts of caseation there is no hyaline appearance and the nuclei persist, though in a shrivelled form and with a loss of their power of imbibing colouring matter.[2]

The main fact which requires recognition is that this change is a true necrosis, and affects the intercellular substance as well as the cells and nuclei,[3] and fatty degeneration is only one of its phases, and is not its most essential feature. These conditions are more prominent in tubercle than in any other pathological product, and the caseous process is common to the whole series of phthisical changes, and is that by which the destruction of the lung-tissue is most frequently induced.[4]

I shall now consider the anatomical conditions in which it most frequently occurs.

(A) *In acute tuberculosis.*—(a) *The typical grey granulation* undergoes a molecular disintegration, commencing in the centre, exactly as was described by Virchow (*see* Plates XXX. 1; XLI. 6). The change affects both the cells and the intercellular substance, and the result is an almost amorphous product, yellow to the naked eye and granular under the microscope, in which no further traces of structure are discernible. I must, however, repeat here that many of these granulations become fibrous rather than caseous, though the two conditions may be combined, and the granular disintegration may be seen extending into the thickened reticulum (XXXI. 2, 8). In some granulations also, though the cells have perished, traces of the reticulum still remain (*see* XXXII. 7, *a*; XXXV. 4). It must further be remarked that in the larynx, as described by Virchow, the grey granulation may possibly break-down without undergoing caseation.[5]

(b) In *granulations containing giant-cells* the caseous change may appear in these structures, as stated by Langhans, in the form of fat-drops, but as Schüppel observed, the giant-cells may long resist the caseous change,[6] and those at the margins of a caseous mass often show little but atrophy and pigmentation (*see* XXXII. 7). In some, however, there are indications that it commences in them (XXXI. 2), and Gombault, moreover, as already stated, has seen them becoming 'vitreous.' In other respects the later stages of caseation in these granulations resemble those described in granulations in which giant-cells are absent.

(c) *The soft epithelioid granulations* (XXX. 3, 4; XXXVII. 5; XXXVIII. 7) which contain a variable amount of small-celled growth in the alveolar wall (*see* XXVII. 2, 7; XL. 1), and which also sometimes contain giant-cells, caseate from their centre to the periphery. The change does not apparently commence in the epithelial cells alone, though these fuse into an amorphous débris; it appears rather to commence in the smaller cells (*see* XXX. 3). The final result of the caseation of most nodules of this description is to form a fibrillated granular nodule like XXVIII. 8; XXXVIII. 3;

---

[1] Litten, *Untersuch. über den hämorrhagischen Infarct,* Berlin, 1879. He has found that such parts of the kidney are also specially given to take up lime-salts. Weigert has shown that if a fresh portion of tissue be inserted into the abdomen of another animal, its cells and nuclei are preserved, but if it be first killed by immersion in alcohol, the cells and nuclei disappear—a result which Weigert attributes to the action on them of fibrin. See Virchow's *Archiv,* lxx. 488, and lxxix. 99.

[2] See Baumgarten, Virchow's *Archiv,* lxxxvii. 47 *et seq.*; Vallot (*ibid,* lxxxix. 224, 225) has noticed this abundance of nuclei in caseous masses. As they are not visible in the hyaline change, he doubts whence they come when the latter is transformed into the former. See also Virchow, 'Der Untergang des Zellenkerns,' *Archiv,* vol. lxxxv.

[3] Baumgarten, *loc. cit.* The origin of the change in the intercellular substance was noticed by Lebert, Müller's *Archiv,* 1884, pp. 194, 488. Ref. also to Virchow, *Würzb. Verhandlungen, loc. cit.,* and to Buhl. *Lungenentzündung,* &c. pp. 77-8.

[4] *Krankhafte Geschwülste,* ii. 644.

[5] The direct influence of bacilli in the production of caseation will be considered later.

[6] *Lymphdrüsen-Tuberculose,* p. 99.

XLIII. 5. Caseous nodules of this description may be distinctly traced to a small-celled growth invading the capillaries and reticular cells in the floor of the alveoli, as are seen in XL. 6, 7; XXXVII. 1, 2, and the caseation extends to the reticulum as in XXXIX. 1.

(d) *The small yellow granulations*, sometimes conglomerate but more often occurring singly, produced in acute tuberculosis (*see* VI. and XXVIII. 6), are those concerning which the greatest difference of opinion has existed. They present, in the more advanced portions, an almost uniform granular débris, in which but few traces of structure can be seen ; in other and less degenerated parts, they show the alveoli filled with an amorphous granular substance ; the walls, as Green has remarked, exhibiting but little small-celled infiltration. In the outer zone, on the other hand, the alveoli are filled with large epithelial cells, more or less fattily degenerated and sometimes deeply pigmented. The first inference would be that the caseation results directly from the breaking down and fusion of these cells, but I believe that this is not the fact. It is true that the cells do thus break down, and their débris, mingled with the exudation contained within the alveoli, contributes to the caseous mass ; but this is, it seems to me, preceded by another change, which, however, is not easy to trace in all specimens. The destruction and complete caseation of the epithelium does not appear to occur until a small-celled growth has taken place in the floor and walls of the alveoli, affecting, as in the granulations last described, the capillaries and the reticular cells of the floor. This is seen in XXX. 7, 8, and 9, where the small-celled growth is mingling with the epithelioid cells, while in fig. 7 are some alveolar passages filled with amorphous débris.[1] Changes like XXX. 5 are also seen in parts where the alveoli, containing large epithelial cells, are surrounded by walls thickened by a small-celled growth, but this is not common. The more usual features are those represented in XXVIII. 6, and at the margins of these are alveoli resembling XXXIX. 2, interspersed with, or passing into, those like XXX. 8, 9, but sometimes attended with a more distinct small-celled growth, as in XXVIII. 7. The small-celled growth is usually scanty and not reticulated. The cells are often distinctly nucleated, and the growth is mingled with fusiform cells which appear to spring from the nuclei of the capillaries ; the latter in many parts distinctly participate in the change. The growth can also be traced through stages like XXXVII. 1, *a c b*, and 2 ; and also like XL. 6.

The peculiarity of the process is the acuteness with which it occurs ; general necrosis appears to ensue before any considerable amount of small-celled proliferation has taken place, and sometimes apparently during the earliest stages of this, so that it is only in some places that it can be traced. I believe, however, that this change in the alveolar wall, to which I shall have hereafter to recur, is the antecedent of the caseation and is its true cause, owing to the arrest of the circulation produced by the implication of the capillaries, coupled, in all probability, with a more acute inflammatory process than attends the formation of the grey granulation.[2] In many parts of the lungs in which this acute production of yellow miliary nodules is proceeding, a lobular pneumonia may

---

[1] These figures are drawn from parts where a more diffused caseation existed, but the change was equally seen around nodules like XXVIII. 6.
[2] The acuteness of formation of the yellow granulation was urged by Green as the cause of the early necrosis, *Med. Times and Gaz.* 1872, ii. 457. Green recognised also the scanty small-celled growth, but did not attribute to it the influence which I am disposed to ascribe to it. Rindfleisch, in the fourth and fifth editions of his *Lehrbuch der path. Gewerbelehre*, 1875 and 1878, p. 353 (the third edition is inaccessible to me) has described this caseation as arising in a similar manner from a small-celled growth, to which he applies Buhl's term of 'desquamative pneumonia,' and he styles it a 'tubercular broncho-pneumonia.' In his first edition (1869, p. 341) he called it a 'pseudo-tubercular bronchopneumonia,' and attributed the caseation solely to the accumulation of epithelial products. *See* p. 399.

be found, differing in no essential particular from that seen in the typical broncho-pneumonia of childhood ; the infundibula are filled with large desquamated epithelioid cells, mingled with more or less exudation-matter, and the process assumes a pyramidal form, with the base on the pleura or on the interlobular septa. In some of these, a small-celled growth of the nature of that now described may be found, proceeding in the walls of the alveoli and of the alveolar ducts ; coincidently with this, caseation may be observed in various stages of progress (*see* XXVIII. 2). Lobules or acini thus affected may be found side by side, in absolute juxtaposition, with others where the only apparent contents of the alveoli are epithelial, and where no signs of caseation are apparent. The conclusion appears to be justified, that many of these granulations commence with a process akin to that seen in broncho-pneumonia, but owe their caseation to the small-celled growth. The proportions between the epithelial and small-celled growth vary, however, considerably in different specimens. It has been repeatedly stated that many of these granulations are purely epithelial in character, but as far as my observation has extended, it is not common to find granulations of this nature, in any form of tuberculosis or phthisis, entirely unattended by small-celled growth, except in their initial stages, although such granulations undoubtedly do exist. In some cases, indeed, the small-celled growth may be seen commencing in the alveolar walls, while the epithelium in the floor is still flat, and shows no signs of proliferation ; in others a small central nodule of this growth may be observed passing into caseation, while the surrounding alveoli exhibit epithelial proliferation. Giant-cells are not seen to precede this process of acute caseation. They appear to require a certain time for their production, which is not allowed in the rapidity of the destructive process.

The perivascular and peribronchial growths in acute tubercle do not show as great a tendency to caseation as is observed in the granulations of alveolar origin. Klein[1] believes that in the artificial tuberculosis of the rodentia, caseation does not occur, or only at advanced stages, but I have observed it in the perivascular growth in childhood, though apparently extending from the adjacent alveolar infiltration. The peribronchial growths in ordinary phthisis tend to caseate, and the cavity of the tube may then be found obstructed by caseous material.

(B) *The caseation of the granulations in ordinary phthisis* proceeds apparently by processes identical with those now described as occurring in acute tuberculosis. In some cases where absolute identity of apparent origin does not exist, there is, however, an essential unity in the character of the process, viz. that it takes place subsequently to, or coincidently with, a similar small-celled growth and obstruction of the capillaries. Thus caseous nodules like XXXVIII. 3, and XLIII. 5, may be traced to earlier conditions like XXXVII. 5, XXX. 3, XXXVIII. 7, and XL. 1, and in some places to stages like XXXIX. 1, and XXXIX. 4. They can also be traced to processes where the invasion of the capillaries can be distinctly seen, as in XL. 6. In many instances, both in acute and chronic phthisis, the caseation of nodules consisting almost entirely of small-celled growth can be seen, interspersed among the other forms of this change (*see* XXXIX. 7 ; XLI. 6). It remains to notice the process of caseation in some of the larger conglomerate nodules, the large soft granulations, and the combinations of caseation with fibroid degeneration.

(*a*) The process in some of the *conglomerate nodules*, like XXXII. 7. XXXV. 4, begins with changes like XL. 1 and 2, combined with those seen in XL. 6, which

[1] *Anatomy of the Lymphatic System*, part ii. p. 52.

have been already described. Other conglomerate caseous masses proceed direct from the caseation of the soft, epithelioid nodules, like XXX. 1 and 3, XXXIV. 1, XXXVII. 5, and XXXVIII. 7.

(*b*) The *large yellow granulations* (IX. 1 ; X, 1, 2, and 4) may also originate, like those last described, by the fusion and caseation of the softer epithelioid granulations, but in many instances they arise from larger areas of infiltration, embracing lobules of various sizes, formed of the whole of the terminal acini of individual bronchioles. The types of these may be seen in XXXVI. 1, 2, and 3, and XXXVII, 4. They consist essentially of epithelial desquamation in the interior of the alveoli, mingled with small-celled growth in the wall, and the latter apparently causes the caseation of the masses by the obstruction of the vessels. The process of the formation of these masses has been already described. See pp. 93 and 102.

A somewhat peculiar form of soft caseous nodules, generally also of large size, and bounded by thickened interlobular septa, but sometimes without any distinct limits, is seen in XL. 4. It is met with both in acute and chronic phthisis. (*Heath, Case 26*, and *Gardiner, Case 22.*) There is a greater persistence of the alveoli and alveolar passages than is usual, and also of the terminal bronchioles, and the latter appear to be dilated within these masses, though this change is not observable in the adjacent portions of pulmonary tissue. They can be distinctly seen to proceed out of masses like XL. 1, 2, and 3. There is but little epithelial proliferation, and the lobule caseates directly on the appearance of the small-celled growth, the invasion of which can be distinctly traced in some specimens, though the caseation takes place before the growth has proceeded to the extensive thickening seen in XL. 5.

(*c*) *Indurated nodules* are found combined with various amounts of caseous change, which is generally limited to their central parts, but may occur also in spots within the nodule, the remainder of which is fibrillated or pigmented. This caseation is seen to affect both the cell-elements and the reticulum. It occurs in the indurating nodules of acute tuberculosis (*see* XXXI. 7 and 8). It is, however, more commonly found where a certain amount of epithelial proliferation has preceded the small-celled growth, as in XXXIX. 5 ; XL. 9, and nodules of caseation of this origin may be distinctly traced to amorphous or caseous masses like XXXII. 7 ; XXXV. 4. It is also observed when the small-celled growth has proceeded to a dense reticulate fibroid formation, as in XLI. 2, 3, and 5, and some of these nodules, partly caseous, are also intensely pigmented, as in XL. 10. Nodules of small-celled growth, like XLI. 6 (*Case 34, Cox*), also occur in the midst of fibroid reticulate growth, like XLI. 7 (*Case 33, Coppin*).

All the forms of caseation described, both in acute and chronic phthisis, may be surrounded by a zone of fibroid thickening containing giant-cells, as in XXXI. 7 (*see* also XXXVI. 1, XL. 3 and 4, and XXXIX. 5 and 7). This fibroid thickening for the most part corresponds to the interlobular septa, and the giant-cells are in the adjacent alveoli. These latter are not always so regularly disposed as in XXXI. 7, but may be found scattered in varying numbers irregularly in the adjacent tissue.

In other parts, the nodules of caseation are not thus abruptly circumscribed, and show at their margins either alveoli filled simply with epithelioid cells, or alveoli in the walls and floors of which small-celled growth is proceeding (*see* XXXVI. 3 ; XLIII. 5). In many places the alveoli adjacent to the caseous nodules are found presenting changes like XL. 6, and XLI. 6 ; while some indurating nodules are bounded by a dense small-celled growth, like XLI. 5.

The Diffuse Caseations of Phthisis, which are still occasionally termed 'caseous pneumonia,' originate in various ways, but essentially, in all their characteristics, they reproduce the processes described as conducing to similar changes in the granulations. They may arise from the confluence of granulations, of either the small-celled or of the epithelioid types, in all the forms which I have described, and this confluence may be observed with more or less trace, in their periphery, of the fibroid zone containing giant-cells, as described by Charcot.

(*a*) Forms of caseation, identical in character and appearance with those described as arising from the caseation of granulations, may often be observed in a diffuse form extending over considerable areas, without any definite circumscription, and not only without any evidence that they have originated in the confluence of granulations, but, on the other hand, with distinct evidence at their margins that they are proceeding indefinitely and irregularly through altered pulmonary tissue. The greater part of these may be seen in tracts of grey pneumonic infiltration (*see* VII. 4; X. 4; XIV. 2), while others may be seen in a redder pneumonic infiltration (XII.); others again may extend in more or less irregular masses into highly injected pulmonary tissue (VII. 2; XI. 1), and others again may occupy considerable tracts of tissue having a more or less worm-eaten look, or like Rochefort cheese[1] (VIII. 3). These undefined areas may be irregularly intermingled with nodules evidently proceeding from the confluence of granulations, and the distinction between the two forms is not always easy, even with the microscope. I have, however, no hesitation in again expressing my opinion that diffuse caseations arise, in these pneumonic tissues, through processes in which the grey granulation proper forms no necessary part, but which are due to a small-celled growth, having characters similar to those of the granulations, but infiltrating the alveolar wall, destroying the circulation, and arresting the vitality of the part.

Thus the type of caseation seen in XXVIII. 8; XXXVIII. 3; XLIII. 5—where a more or less fibrillated structure remains among the amorphous débris—may be traced to changes, occurring in a diffuse form, similar to those which have been described in the shape of nodules, in which the same characteristics may be observed. It may thus be seen to proceed from indefinite areas having the appearances of XXVIII. 7; XXXVII. 1 and 2; XL. 6. It may also arise out of areas of diffuse small-celled growth, more or less mingled with epithelium, like XXXV. 6, and XL. 2, and also from changes like XL. 1, but occurring in extended and non-circumscribed areas. In some places similar tracts may be seen proceeding in parts where the alveolar wall is becoming thickened through undefined areas, by processes resembling XXXVII. 6 and XXXIX. 2.

(*b*) Large areas of caseous pneumonia, like VI. 2; VII. 2;[2] VIII. 3, proceed by thickening of the alveolar walls with a small-celled growth in a diffuse form, and having the character of XXVIII. 9 and 10; XXX. 5 and 6; XXXVIII. 1. They are also seen like XXXVI. 4, a condition that arises from infiltrations like XXXVII. 6 and 7; XXXIX. 2 and 3. In some of these, as in XXXVI. 4, a dense homogeneous small-celled growth invades portions of the tissue, filling the alveoli and leading to a uniform caseous mass. Such infiltrations, in their earlier stages, result from changes like XXXVIII. 8, and XL. 2, and they may also be traced back to diffuse changes like XL. 1, or to changes like XXXVIII. 7, occurring in indefinite areas, while in some

[1] *See* p. 70, note 2.
[2] This figure is one of a diabetic lung (*Case 14*). In it all the caseating processes were traceable to one or other of the two forms here described.

cases, large areas of a similar character may be seen arising from infiltrations of mingled epithelial and small-celled growths, like XXVIII. 2 and 7.

In this and also in the foregoing process (*see* ante, *a*) masses of small-celled growth may be seen, in some specimens, to be filling the alveoli and participating in the caseation, without, however, forming distinct granulations, except from their position within the alveoli.

(*c*) Areas like XL. 4 may also be seen in a diffuse form, owing their apparent origin to processes similar to those in which the same appearances arise in a nodular form (*see* p. 116).

(*d*) Caseation without apparent thickening of the walls, like XXXVI. 5, and XXXVIII. 9, occurs also in extensive areas, and then resembles XXVIII. 6. This form has been especially attributed to the caseation of epithelium accumulated in the interior of the alveoli, and this opinion has been one of the chief reasons for the use of the term 'caseous pneumonia' in its application to the whole of the diffused caseous processes. Similar conditions in the nodular form have been already described (*see* p. 114), and I believe that, in all cases, identical changes can be traced in those of a similar character that occur diffusely. The epithelium, though occasionally becoming granular, does not, I believe, *per se* undergo the caseous change until conditions different from those found in ordinary pneumonia have arisen in the floor and walls of the alveoli, and I think it very doubtful whether the epithelium as such constitutes, except in rare instances, any large proportion of the caseous mass. Indeed I believe that caseation in the pneumonia of phthisis, in whatever variety it may appear, does not ensue, except as due either to granulations or to the changes that have been already described, or those to which I have now to direct attention, and in which all the tissues of the lung are destroyed except the elastic fibres. These areas proceed from the implication of the floor and walls of the alveoli with a small-celled growth, mingled with fusiform cells, which also invades the capillaries, as is seen in XXXVII. 1, 2, and XL. 6. Large areas, caseating like XXXVIII. 9 (where remains of small-celled growth may still be seen), may also be traced to infiltrations resembling XL. 9. In some cases, epithelioid cells may be seen mingled with this growth, as in XXVII. 7; XXX. 7, 8, 9. The amount of small-celled growth is not large, though some alveoli may be seen more densely filled and resembling XXXVII. 6, *a a b*, and it may be traced, passing at once into débris with shrivelled cells and nuclei, as in XXXVII. 3. In all these instances there is but little evidence of epithelium in the interior of the alveoli. In fact the epithelium appears to perish in proportion as the growth of the small-celled structure advances (*see* XXXVII. 6).

In some places, before this stage is reached, a degeneration of the nuclei and reticulum may be seen (XXXIX. 1, and XLI. 6), and the nuclei finally disappear, leaving a reticulum like XXXV. 5. This process is less acute than that seen in XXXVI. 5, but the naked-eye appearances of the two are indistinguishable, and the final histological results are almost identical; in fact, all stages of variations between these two changes may often be found in the same specimen.

Acute softening.—In many parts, processes like those last described present a striking resemblance to suppuration. This apparent suppuration differs, however, from a true pus-formation in two important particulars. It does not give rise to any accumulation of pus-cells, like genuine abscess, but it passes at once into a destructive change of the caseous kind, like that last described. Further, in some places, and in immediate juxtaposition with the latter, it forms solid nodules of reticulate small-celled growth, which are indistinguishable from the miliary granulations of tubercle. Such nodules, in some cases, are seen to fill the alveoli, and in considerable areas they resemble a small-celled pneumonia, while in other parts they are seated in the walls of the air-vesicles, and in those of the bronchioles and of the alveolar ducts. The caseation of this destructive kind cannot, therefore, in any way be referred to the inspissation of accumulated pus, for no such accumulation occurs, and when the cells constitute solid masses, they differ markedly from purulent deposits, and in many cases a reticulate structure can be traced between them. The caseation is due to a rapid degeneration of cells of new formation, arising in the walls and floor of the alveoli in a manner identical with that in which the dense small-celled growth originates. The apparent resemblance to suppuration depends also, I believe, on the greater rapidity of production of these cells. In consequence of this, in the first place, they appear rather more rounded and more distinctly nucleated than the ordinary cells of the reticular growth; and, in the second place, they perish before a reticulum has time to form between them, and to constitute a solid texture. This apparent suppuration is not, however, very common, except in some cases of very acute phthisis (*Griffin, Case 19; Gardiner, Case 22;* and *J. Thomas, Case 20*). It is sometimes found in a diffuse interstitial form, but it may be observed also in the acute pneumonic infiltrations of ordinary phthisis, and also in the granulations of acute miliary tuberculisation of childhood, when all gradations may be noticed between the acute destructive processes now described and the solid granulations composed almost entirely of small-celled growth, or of this growth mingled with epithelial products. Similar gradations to an acute softening can also be traced in the epithelial granulations of ordinary phthisis, such as XXXVII. 5, and XL. 1; and in some instances there may be transitions to such changes as that seen in XL. 6. Cells may in some cases be seen to grow into a solid mass of small-celled growth (grey granulation) or they may at once break down before this has time to form.

The histological boundary line between these processes and suppuration is, however, undefined, and I think it not improbable that in the rapid extension of cavities, especially of the peribronchial class (*see* X. 3, 4), a genuine suppuration may ensue, though most of the appearances which I have observed would point, even in these instances, to the rapid caseation and liquefaction of a diffuse tubercular growth, rather than to the formation of pus in the ordinary manner. In fact, the suppuration, if it occurs, would be aptly termed 'tubercular' in its origin and progress.

Genuine suppurative changes do, however, occur in some forms of infiltrating pneumonia of phthisis, but the process differs from those which have now been described, and the tissue liquefies at once (*see* XIII. 4, *Case 18, Brodrick*). The softening is apparently lobular, though the grey infiltration is diffuse; it seems to extend upwards to the bronchioles and bronchi, and the walls of the latter participate in the process. It is seen with the microscope (XXXV. 1) rapidly to break down large tracts of lung by a process of liquefaction, but even here, in some parts (fig. 1 *a, a,* and figs. 2 and 3), there is an attempt at reticular formation, passing, however, immediately into granular disintegration.[1]

Apparent suppuration leads also to destruction of the lung in some cases where diffuse pneumonic infiltration occurs without visible granulations. I have only seen two instances of this. One of them is depicted in V. 5 (*Case 5, S. Brown*) and the micro-

---

[1] This case presented well-marked instances of genuine tubercular formations, both recent and indurating, in other parts of the lung; and also large tracts of fibroid induration, the result of an earlier attack. See Plate XIII. fig. 3.

scopic appearances are seen in XXXV. 7. Here again the lung-tissue appears to break down at once into suppuration, though in other parts of the lung small-celled infiltrations may be found, both diffuse and nodular, resembling those already described as constituting the chief characteristic of phthisical change.

I have found, though comparatively rarely, suppurative areas like these, in other cases of grey, and also of red, pneumonic infiltration in phthisis. The tendency to reticular formation distinguishes them, as far as my observation has extended, from any similar changes of a destructive character either in acute pneumonia[1] or in broncho-pneumonia. This suppuration, when present, breaks down the lung at once by an acute liquefactive process, which differs entirely in appearance from the softening of caseous masses.

The softening of caseous matter has received various interpretations, which may be fairly summarised as represented by two main theories :—

(*a*) That the caseous material itself softens. This is the opinion of Laennec, Rokitansky, and Virchow.[2]

(*b*) That it is due to a liquefaction by pus secreted by the adjacent tissues,[3] an opinion expressed by Andral, Cruveilhier, Hasse, and still more recently, without qualification, by Hérard and Cornil.

I confess that I am strongly disposed to adhere to the view, expressed especially by Virchow, that the softening is a chemical process occurring in the caseous matter. Its almost constant occurrence in the centre of the granulations renders the theory that it is due to liquefaction by pus, extemely improbable ; and though this argument may be met by the statement that these tubercles are peribronchial, and that the softening proceeds from pus secreted in their interior—a view of their structure which I have already combated—it must be remembered that this change equally occurs in the interior of lymphatic glands, where such a source of liquefaction is impossible. It is true that tubercular granulations are less given to softening in some regions than in others, and notably less in the serous membranes, though even there they may undergo acute caseation and ulceration.[4] But it must also be remembered that softening may occur in the brain,[5] kidney,[6] testicle[7]

---

[1] I have not had opportunities of observing any genuine cases of abscess of the lung in acute pneumonia which I could submit to microscopic observation.

[2] Laennec, *Traité d'Auscultation médiate*, 2nd ed. i. 584, 589, 544 ; Lobstein, *Anat. Path.* i. 388, 472; Rokitanski, *Path. Anat.* 1855, i. 208. Rokitanski believed that the products of this softening might mingle with the surrounding exudation. Virchow, *Handbuch der spec. Pathol. und Therapie*, pp. 282, 285, 302 ; *Cellular Pathologie*, pp. 164, 286 ; *Die krankhaften Geschwülste*, ii. 596, 598, 644, 649. The main point dwelt upon by Virchow, in his account of softening from caseation, is that the caseation is a fatty metamorphosis in a finely granular form, which subsequently liquefies by a chemical process. He terms it an 'anæmic necrosis' or 'necrobiosis,' due to the arrest of the circulation —an opinion asserted by Schröder van der Kolk, *Obs. Anat. Path.* 1826, p. 67, though this author believed that the liquefaction was assisted by purulent secretion from the non-obstructed vessels. Virchow specially insists that this softened matter is not pus. Ref. also to his observations on the softening of thrombi (*Cellular Pathologie*, p. 179,) and on the softening of atheroma, (*ib.* 321, 327) and also of embolism (*Gesammelte Abhandlungen*). Similar opinions have been expressed by Förster, *Path. Anat.* 1863, ii. 229; Lebert, *Traité Malad. Scrofuleuses et Tuberculeuses*, p. 16; Wagner, *Handb. allg. Pathol.* 7th ed. p. 610. See also Louis, *Rech. sur la Phthisie*, 2nd ed. p. 9, and Waldenburg, *Die Tuberculose*, p. 156. Many other authorities might be cited in support of this view.

[3] Andral, *Préc. Anat. Path.* i. 415. He quotes Lombard, *Essai sur les Tubercules*, 1826, as the first who expressed this theory. Cruveilhier, *Anat. Path. Générale*, iv. 535 *et seq.*; Hasse, *Diseases of the Circulation and Respiration*, Syd. Soc. Trans. p. 530; Cornil and Ranvier, *Manuel Histol. Path.* 1882, ii. 168, 169, 174. These authors appear to consider softening almost entirely a suppurative process, and state that an islet of caseous matter cannot suppurate (p. 169.) Part of the liquefaction is, in their opinion, attributable to secretion from the bronchi, an opinion akin to that of Carswell, who, regarding tubercle as seated in the interior of the bronchi and air-vesicles, considered its liquefaction as due to further secretion from those parts; see *Illustrations Elementary Forms of Disease*, art. 'Tubercle.'

[4] Virchow (*Krankhafte Geschwülste*, ii. p. 652) for the pleura and peritoneum, and not for the meninges, Dohrlich, *Studies in Pathological Anatomy*, p. 77 ; Lebert, *Brustkrankheiten*, ii. 133.

[5] *Krankhafte Geschwülste*, ii. 665; Meyer, Virchow's *Archiv*, xxx. 29.

[6] *Ib.*; also Frerichs, *Beiträge zur Lehre von der Tuberculose*, Marburg, 1882, p. 52. This was found in a case of acute tuberculosis.

[7] Virchow, *loc. cit.* 685 ; Gaule, Virchow's *Archiv*, 1877, vol. lxix.; Reclus, *Tubercule du Testicule*, 1876, pp. 57, 59.

spleen,[1] and liver,[2] and in these latter situations it may form cavities, actual or potential. In some situations, indeed, and notably in the larynx [3] and trachea, tubercle may apparently soften without antecedent caseation. On the other hand, it must be admitted that caseous matter, once formed, may persist long unchanged, and may pass, as already stated, into various degrees of inspissation and calcification.

The tendency to softening may, I believe, in a large number of cases, be attributed to the acuteness of the process in which the tubercles originate,[4] and in many instances it may be due to pneumonia arising around them, which destroys the remaining vitality. At least, softening of granulations, evidently of some standing, may be constantly observed in the midst of pneumonic infiltrations of apparently more recent date. In many cases in acute tuberculosis, however, the caseation found is only a stage in the rapid softening of the granulations, and those varieties which have been described as passing directly into caseation break down very acutely.

It is highly probable that when these areas have thus softened, further liquefaction and extension may occur through processes which are indistinguishable from suppuration, but even in many of these, this suppuration appears to present rather the tubercular character (see p. 119) than the ordinary inflammatory type.

Diffuse Induration.—The large areas of almost cartilaginous firmness, deeply pigmented, smooth on section, sometimes enclosing caseous masses, sometimes small cavities, or which are traversed by dilated bronchi, chiefly characterise the chronic forms of phthisis. They may, however, be found occasionally in large tracts, in cases running apparently a more acute course, and in some of these they may be distinctly traced to an antecedent attack of a phthisical nature (see *Cases S. Brown* (5), *Broadrick* (18), *and Smith* (28), V. and XIII.).

These areas may, in the majority of cases, be traced to one of two processes, which, however, are variously intermingled.

(*a*) They may arise from the confluence of indurating granulations before described, as seen in X. 5; XIV. 1; XVI. 2; XVII. 1 and 3; XVIII. 4; and XIX.; but in some of these (as in XIX. 2) the origin in granulations may be no longer discernible.

(*b*) In other parts they arise, conjointly with the foregoing, from diffuse infiltration of the alveolar walls with a small-celled growth, identical in characters with that described as passing into areas of caseous pneumonia. In fact, in some places in the same lung, changes like those figured in XLI. 7, and XLIII. 2, may be seen in extensive areas, passing in one part into fibroid induration, and in another into diffuse caseation or even into acute softening, and these again may be traced, in their earlier stages, to a diffuse small-celled growth identical in appearance with XXXVIII. 8, and XL. 2.

(*c*) Large areas of fibroid change may be seen, as in XLII. 1, to proceed from a small-celled infiltration in the walls of the alveoli, similar to those observed in XXX. 6 and 7; XXXVII. 6 and 7; and XXXIX. 2 and 3. In some parts of the pneumonic infiltration, where the contents of the alveoli may be either epithelioid or pyoid cells, little

[1] Paget, *Surgical Pathology*, ed. 1863, p. 818.

[2] Frerichs, *loc. cit.* p. 104. Lebert (*Brustkrankheiten*, ii. 147) says that softened masses of tubercle are common in the livers of monkeys. Cf. also Rayer, *Arch. Méd. Comp.* vol. i. 1843, pp. 210-11.

[3] Virchow, *Krankhafte Geschwülste*, ii. 640. Rindfleisch (Ziemssen's *Handbuch.* Bd. v. 'Krankh. Resp. App.' ii. 189) has expressed similar opinions for other mucous membranes. The tubercle-cells in these softenings play the part of pus, but are not true pus.

[4] Burdon-Sanderson has communicated to me the result of an interesting experiment performed by himself and Klein (see *Path. Soc. Trans.* vol. xxiii.). A guinea-pig, rendered tuberculous by the ordinary process, was subsequently injected with the poison of acute pyæmia; the result was a rapid softening of the tubercles. See also Villemin, *Études sur la Tuberculose*, p. 105.

can be seen of the small-celled growth here described, and only a fibroid change can be observed, proceeding directly from fusiform cells (see XLII. 6). In all such instances, however, that have come under my notice, in which granulations and other evidence of phthisical change were present in other parts of the same lung, these purely fibroid changes were only very local; in other and adjacent portions, small-celled growth coexisted, either diffuse, or forming granulations, and passing into indurative changes, and furnishing evidence of the nature of these fibroid processes. Such combinations of tubercular and purely fibroid induration, arising in pneumonia, are also seen in XLI. 1, and very similar conditions were observed in the tracts of fibroid induration seen in XV. Like the granulations before described, these fibroid areas may arise from a small-celled reticular growth, which may undergo one of two changes. It may pass at once into caseation, or it may form a dense fibroid structure by the thickening of the reticulum and the gradual disappearance of the cells. This structure, in some places, shows considerable vascularity, as remarked by Moxon and by Greenfield. The vascularity, however, is usually on a large scale; the vessels, as these authors have observed, appear dilated, and I have seen but little evidence of fine capillary vascularity. This vascular appearance is not, moreover, either constant or very common.

In some of these tracts, great thickening of the bronchi and of the coats of the vessels may be observed, and it may even appear as if radiating lines of induration extended from them (see XLII. 7).

This induration has been termed 'interstitial,' but, except in such cases as that last mentioned, I believe that it is essentially alveolar. The thickening, whether diffuse or in firm conglomerate granulations, primarily affects the alveolar tissue. Although the interlobular, the peribronchial, and periarterial connective tissue takes part in and contributes to the general thickening, it does not constitute either the starting-point, or even the principal or most essential portion, of this change.

SYPHILITIC DISEASES OF THE LUNG.

SYPHILITIC affections of the lung have in recent years been brought prominently under the attention of the profession, although some allusion was made to them by earlier writers. Much doubt still exists whether all the changes in the lung, lately described as having this origin, are truly specific in their nature, or have any special relation to syphilis. I shall, however, enumerate the chief of these, and discuss the grounds on which they have been included in this category.

Gummata of the lung constitute the only evidence of syphilis recognisable with certainty, but they are, comparatively speaking, rare. They have been fully described by Wilks,[1] Wagner,[2] Virchow, and other more recent writers. Illustrations of them are given in Plates IV. 2, 3, XXVI. 8, and XXVII. They are found in two stages, the period of formation and the period of caseous change. In the earlier stages they form masses of a grey, reddish-grey, or brownish-red tint, and are pigmented in parts. The section is smooth and semi-transparent. They are markedly firm, and yield but little fluid either on scraping or on pressure. At still earlier periods, they have an almost gelatinous

---

[1] Wilks, *Guy's Hosp. Rep.* 1863, and *Trans. Path. Soc.* vol. ix. [2] E. Wagner, *Archiv der Heilkunde*, vols. iv. v. vii.

aspect,[1] and commence as 'specks and streaks of glutinous material, thickly studding limited districts of the pulmonary parenchyma.[2]

They sometimes send irregular prolongations into the surrounding tissue.[3] In the earlier stages they are not encapsuled,[4] but later become sharply defined,[5] and a distinct capsule sometimes surrounds them when the caseous stage is attained. Caseation usually commences in spots and streaks in the midst of the grey, firm ground of the gumma, but sometimes it begins in the centre.[6] When the caseous change is completed, the gummata form 'circumscribed nodules of a firm, yellowish, dry substance, totally unlike any 'ordinary inflammation or scrofulous deposit;' they correspond in all particulars to the gummata found in the liver, 'only less firm,'[7] and within them, all traces of pulmonary tissue have disappeared. They tend to soften, sometimes into caseous matter resembling that which results from ordinary pneumonia,[8] sometimes so as to resemble masses of firm, white, pottery clay, and they may contain crystals of cholesterine.[9] In some instances, they form cretaceous masses;[10] in other cases they produce puriform masses, which have led to doubt whether they were not circumscribed pyæmic formations, but from these they may be usually distinguished by the firmness of the wall surrounding them.[11] They may also soften into cavities, and of this process numerous instances exist in medical literature.[12]

In size, these masses vary. The most typical and characteristic are single, and attain dimensions from a bean to a small orange.[13] In many instances they are described as smaller;[14] Fournet[15] indeed states that they vary in size from a hemp-seed to a hazel nut, and are seldom larger than this. In some cases, when small, they are multiple, and have even been so numerous as to make the lung feel like a bag of peas, the individual gummata not exceeding the size of a lentil.[16] With regard to site, they seem to have no special predilection. The larger masses are commonly single, and when of medium size they seldom exceed two or three in number and then may be limited to one lung or may affect both, but large and small may coexist in considerable numbers.[17]

When the smaller bodies are numerous, the distinction between them and indurated tubercles becomes more difficult, and indeed in some cases it may be doubted whether some nodules thus described as syphilitic ought not to be classed as tubercle, inasmuch as they correspond more closely with these formations than with typical gummata. Virchow,[18] as is well known, is disposed to classify as syphilitic various nodular forms of indurative 'peribronchitis' and also multiple caseous nodules; but he admits the difficulty of distinguishing these from tubercle, and this difficulty has not yet been overcome.

---

[1] Meschede, Virchow's *Archiv*, 1866, xxxvii. 567; Lacnge, *Essai Phthisie Syphilitique*, Thèse de Paris, 1870, p. 78.
[2] Welch, *On Destructive Lung Disease among Soldiers, &c.* Alexander Prize Essay, 1872, p. 66.
[3] Schnitzler, *Lungensyphilis*, p. 31; Mahomed, *Path. Soc. Trans.* 1877, xxviii. 339.
[4] T. H. Green, *Path. Soc. Trans.* xxviii. 331.
[5] E. Wagner, *Arch. der Heilkunde*, iv. 331.
[6] Fournet, 'Leçons Phthisie Syphilitique,' *Gaz. Hebdom.* 1875, p. 760.
[7] Wilks, *Guy's Hosp. Rep.* 1863, and *Path. Soc. Trans.* vol. ix. (figures).
[8] Goodhart, *Path. Soc. Trans.* xxv. 32.
[9] Moxon, *Guy's Hosp. Rep.* 1867, p. 344.
[10] Lancereaux, *Gaz. Hebdom.* 1867, p. 644.
[11] Depaul, *Bull. Soc. Anat.* 1857; *Gaz. Méd.* 1851; *Mém. Acad. Imp. de Méd.* 1853; also Ricord, *Clin. Iconograph.* pl. 28.
[12] Schröder van der Kolk, *Obs. Anat. Path.* p. 130.

Fournet, *loc. cit.* p. 760, says that these cavities may be anfractuous, when several gummata have coalesced. See also Wilks, *Path. Soc. Trans.* vol. ix. (figure). Von Cube (Virchow's *Archiv*, 1880, lxxxi.) describes a case in which the breaking down of a gumma (characteristic fragments of which appeared in the expectoration) led to the signs of a cavity.

[13] Wilks (*loc. cit.*) compared the size to that of a 'marble.' Masses the size of an orange have been described by Gowers and by Green (*Path. Soc. Trans.* vol. xxviii.), and one the size of a hen's egg by Fleischl and Klob (*Wien. med. Woch.* 1860, quoted by E. Wagner).
[14] That of a pea, Sidney Coupland, *Path. Soc. Trans.* vol. xxvii.
[15] *Gaz. Hebdom.* 1875, p. 760.
[16] Lancereaux, *Bull. Acad. de Méd.* Oct. 1877.
[17] Heuop, *Deutsch. Arch. f. klin. Med.* 1879, xxiv. 250 (figure). One was the size of a goose's egg.
[18] *Krankhafte Geschwülste*, ii. 467.

Indeed, if all nodules of this nature occurring in syphilitic patients are to be regarded as specific, the range of syphilitic pulmonary disease must be vastly extended, and I venture to adhere to the opinion that in the majority of these, the disease is essentially tubercular in nature, and not syphilitic. The indurated nodules sometimes form conglomerate racemose masses, which, judging from the descriptions given, must very closely resemble those found in ordinary chronic phthisis, and their nature will be discussed hereafter. Virchow indeed admits that no marked distinctions exist between them and the masses found in 'grinder's phthisis.'[1] Rindfleisch[2] has even described as syphilitic a tuberculisation which he admits is indistinguishable from miliary tubercle. The real questions as regards these forms are—whether they are instances of ordinary tubercle in syphilitic subjects; whether they are bodies, not tubercle but resembling it, produced by syphilis; or whether they are tubercles modified by the syphilitic diathesis. Baumgarten has recently stated that there is evidence of the occurrence of genuine miliary syphilomata in the lung.[3] That miliary nodules may be of a syphilitic nature (demonstrated by their association with gummata), is evidenced by Gowers' woodcut (see later). When these have been described in other organs, there is, in many instances, some doubt whether the cases may not have been of tubercular nature.[4] In other cases the evidence is stronger in favour of syphilis,[5] and Virchow is disposed to regard some nodular thickenings of the pleura as being of this nature.[6] Cornil and Ranvier have described gummata of the liver as being surrounded by smaller nodules.[7] The difficulty of diagnosis is increased by the fact, as shown by Baumgarten, that the smaller supposed syphilomata have a structure identical with that of miliary tubercle, and undergo the same changes.[8]

Among the variations that have been described in the appearances of supposed gummata, must be mentioned those in which a certain resemblance exists between these bodies and pulmonary infarcts. The most remarkable of these is by Henop,[9] who describes a wedge-shaped mass, the size of a goose's egg, situated in the upper lobe, with its base at the pleura and the apex at the periphery of the lung. It was yellow, firm, dry, and surrounded by a hyperæmic zone of healthy tissue, but its syphilitic character may be regarded as proved by the co-existence of other gummata in the lungs. Smaller nodules, which caused Cornil to doubt whether they were not of embolic origin, are described by Martineau;[10] the opinion stated by them was that they were syphilitic rested on the freedom of the pulmonary artery and on microscopic examination.

Syphilitic Pneumonia.—Various forms of inflammatory consolidation of the lung have been attributed to syphilis. The most characteristic is that which was described by

---

[1] See Sacharjin, *Berl. klin. Woch.* 1878, p. 35. Recent pneumonia at the bases; bronchiectasis at the apex of the right lung; much induration throughout both lungs in the form of small nodules, the size of pins' heads, collected into groups and connected by bands of fibroid tissue. Vogt and Papinoff (Virchow's *Archiv*, vol. lxxv.) describe conglomerations of the dimensions of a hazel-nut, consisting of small bodies, the size of pins' heads, sometimes showing thickenings, in which the lamina of bronchi appear, passing into diffuse thickening. See also Ramdohr, *Arch. der Heilk.* 1877, vol. ix., most of whose cases appear to me tubercular. (See my Plates X. figs. 5, 6, 7, and XVII. XVIII. XIX. for the same appearances in chronic phthisis).
[2] Rindfleisch, Ziemssen's *Handbuch*, vol. v. 'Krank. Resp.-Apparates,' ii. 223 (figured).
[3] Virchow's *Archiv*, 1881, lxxxvi. 197–8; see also Von Bärensprung, *Deutsche Klinik*, 1858, No. 17.
[4] Thus Wagner (*Arch. der Heilk.* iv. 441) speaks of some miliary nodules in the liver, associated with supposed syphilomata of larger size, as being miliary tubercles. Tubercles existed in this case in other parts, but he calls other nodules 'syphilitic' on account of their structure (*ib.* v. 139). See also *ib.* obs. 32, vol. iv. 437, where there was no direct evidence of syphilis; likewise vol. v. 124, (liver syphilitic, lungs miliary tubercles), and v. 133, (diabetes, lungs tubercular, liver syphilitic). Ref. also to Ramdohr, note 1.
[5] Virchow, *Krankhafte Geschwülste*, ii. 425, (liver). For other references see Baumgarten, Virchow's *Archiv*, 1879, lxxvi. 487.
[6] Virchow, *Krankhafte Geschwülste*, ii. 468.
[7] *Manuel d'Histol. Path.* 2nd ed. i. 228. Baumgarten *loc. cit.*) denies that this is common.
[8] Virchow, *Archiv*, lxxvi. 488, lxxxvi. 198.
[9] Deutsch. *Arch. kl. Med.* 1879, vol. xxiv. (figure).
[10] Martineau, *Bull. Soc. Anat.* 1862.

Virchow[1] and Weber[2] as 'white hepatisation,' and as affecting the lungs of children in intra-uterine life. An appearance apparently identical was described still earlier by Cruveilhier[3] as a form of pneumonia occurring in syphilitic children, and its association with syphilis was later asserted by Hecker,[4] by Lorain, and by Robin[5] (who named it 'epithelioma of the lung,' and traced its connection with syphilitic pemphigus), and also by Howitz[6] and Wagner.[7] It has also been found in the lungs of the adult by Moxon,[8] and recently by Vierling.[9] Lungs in this state are distended so as to fill the cavity of the thorax, and bear the impress of the ribs. The pleura is sometimes found unaffected, but there may be recent inflammation of this membrane.[10] They occasionally admit of partial insufflation, but this is not constant. They are dense, and usually so firm as to resist pressure, although in some cases described by Weber, the finger may be pressed into them as into a fatty liver. They may be four or five times heavier than natural. Their colour is whitish with a shade of yellow. The cut surface is smooth and shining, and allows but little fluid or débris to be removed by pressure or scraping. The lobular texture is still apparent, and the interlobular tissue is sometimes slightly reddish. The bronchi contain a tough mucus. The bronchial glands are enlarged, greyish, homogeneous, and in parts present a cheesy aspect. The extent of infiltration varies; sometimes the whole of both lungs are affected,[11] sometimes only one,[12] and sometimes only portions. When the affection is partial, isolated spots may be found of the same nature in different parts, varying in size from a pea to a pigeon's egg;[13] in adjacent parts, more recent pneumonia may also be found.[14] There is evidence that this form of pneumonia may soften into cavities and even become gangrenous (Moxon's case, see p. 127). Looking, however, to the comparative frequency with which cases are reported in which physical signs of pneumonia have disappeared under an anti-syphilitic treatment, it may be questioned whether the condition last described (and which, as will presently be mentioned, presents certain histological peculiarities) is not to be regarded as an advanced stage of a simpler form of consolidation of the nature of chronic grey hepatisation, which may advance either to the firm white hepatisation, or else to excavation by the softening of caseous nodules of gummata scattered through the tissue. Some illustrations of these are found in Pancritius' observations, where all these latter combinations were met with, and where, also, still earlier stages of red hepatisation were occasionally found. But no distinctive criteria of the syphilitic nature of either of these forms have yet been established, and it is possible that, in these earlier stages, the specific nature of the disease may be incapable of absolute demonstration.[15]

Welch has described a grey infiltration, closely resembling that found in some tubercular lungs.[16] The excavations may be extensive and numerous, surrounded either by caseous or white nodules, or by hæmorrhagic extravasations. Pancritius lays great stress on the origin of these consolidations and excavations in the central portions of the lungs.

---

[1] In his *Archiv*, i. 146, and also *ib.* vol. xv. and *Krankhafte Geschwülste*.
[2] *Path. Anat. der Neugeborenen und Säuglinge*, ii. 47.
[3] *Anat. Path. du Corps Humain*, liv. xv. pl. ii. and text. Lungs of a child, born syphilitic and dying immediately; the lungs could not be insufflated; they were greyish-white, and indurated throughout. There was a small, cartilaginous nodule in the middle of one lung. The two lungs weighed 3 ounces; normal weight 2 ounces.
[4] *Verhand. der Berliner geburtshülfliche Gesellsch.* 1854, viii. 130.
[5] *Gaz. Med. de Paris*, 1855.
[6] *Behrends, Syphilologie*, 1862, iii. 611.
[7] *Archiv der Heilkunde*, 1868, vol. iv.
[8] *Guy's Hosp. Rep.* 1867, case 12, p. 368.
[9] *Deutsch. Arch. klin. Med.* 1878, xxi. 325.
[10] Greenfield, *Path. Soc. Trans.* vol. xxvii. See Plate XXVII. figs. 6, 7, and description.
[11] Wagner found both lungs affected in four out of six cases.
[12] Greenfield's case.
[13] Köstlin, *Arch. der Heilk.* vol. xvii.
[14] Moxon's case, *loc. cit.*
[15] Pancritius, *Ueber Lungensyphilis*, Berlin, 1887, obs. C. 1, p. 254. C. 6, p. 265.
[16] Alexander Prize Essay 1872, p. 61.

Grandidier[1] also has made the remarkable observation that in twenty-seven out of thirty cases he found the middle lobe of the right lung attacked, but the recorded cases of other observers, either with or without post-mortem examinations, shows no such preponderant frequency of affection in this part, and numerous apical and basic affections are recorded.[2]

Another form of pneumonia met with in adult syphilitic patients has been described by Virchow,[3] as resembling the 'brown induration' of heart-disease. The lungs are firm and the alveoli are filled with pigmented epithelium. Virchow, in his large experience, had only met with it twice, and it has not been commonly found by others. Pancritius has, however, met with two cases in which the lung was indurated, with the character of 'dried liver.'[4]

The relation of this condition to syphilitic processes has yet to be elucidated. I have met with a somewhat similar condition in a case of chronic pulmonary induration in a syphilitic patient, but here there was evidence of chronic tuberculisation (?), and the peculiar pigmentation described by Virchow was absent (see *Case 3, Hawkins*, Plates IV. 1, and XLII. 6, and description of latter).

Lobular Pneumonia or *Broncho-pneumonia*, in both the indurative and suppurative forms, has of late been brought increasingly into prominence as a manifestation of pulmonary syphilis. It must be remembered that most of the changes in phthisical lungs (in which no question of syphilis exists) have been described of late in terms practically identical with those applied to the supposed syphilitic processes, and this in the period from 1860 to 1875, at least among German and among many French writers. The question, as regards these broncho-pneumonic forms, is whether they owe any of their individuality to syphilis—whether or not they originate in it—and if so, whether, under these circumstances, they present any characteristics by which they may be distinguished. I confess that as yet I have found nothing, in the descriptions hitherto given of their changes, to show that any such criteria have been established. Until this is accomplished, the question must be regarded as still *sub judice* whether they are, or not, merely ordinary phthisical (or as I believe, tubercular) changes occurring in syphilitic persons.

The indurated masses, which these processes form, have been already described. Förster[5] observed that these lobular, or broncho-pneumonias, are very common in the lungs of children who are the victims of hereditary syphilis and die soon after birth, but that, in the majority of cases, they are identical with the ordinary forms of broncho-pneumonia in childhood. In some of these cases suppuration occurred,[6] in others induration with thickening of the interstitial tissue, but in the latter again no special distinction is drawn from chronic tuberculisation. Virchow, however, remarks that in his experience tubercle is not found in fœtal lungs,[7] though changes such as Förster has described (and which are ordinarily considered to be of tubercular nature) may commence in the lungs of children dying of atrophy.[8]

---

[1] *Berlin. klin. Woch.* 1875, No. 15. A case of this nature, in which the upper lobe of the left lung was attacked, is given by Beger, *Deutsch. Arch. f. klin. Med.* 1879, xxiii. 619.

[2] *Krankhafte Geschwülste*, ii. 470.

[3] See a synopsis of 76 cases by Carlier, *Etude de Syphilis Pulmonaire*, Paris, 1882. Pancritius indeed also gives clinical evidence, apart from post-mortem observation, of a frequent commencement of physical signs in the central portions of the lung, and several of his cases presented cavities in the central parts, though others showed both apex and basic affections.

[4] *Loc. cit.* obs. A, 4, p. 80, C. 10, p. 282.

[5] *Würzburg. med. Zeitsch.* iv. 4.

[6] A suppurative lobular pneumonia had been earlier described by Cruveilhier as occurring in the lungs of syphilitic children, and as holding an intermediate place between tubercle and inflammation. (*Atlas Anat. Path.* liv. xx. pl. ij).

[7] *Krankhafte Geschwülste*, ii. 460.

[8] Virchow, 'Constitutionell. syph. Affectionen,' *Archiv*, xv. 3-12. How doubtful this point remains, is shown by the fact that Wagner claimed as syphilitic a case that Virchow had described as tubercular, and which Virchow later still maintained to have been of the latter nature. (See *Krankhafte Geschwülste*, ii. 465.)

Welch has described syphilitic pneumonia in different terms from those employed by most other writers on this subject, and from his large opportunities of observation, his descriptions deserve careful consideration from pathologists. He does not appear to have met with white hepatisation, but regards the syphilitic pneumonias as lobular, although tending to confluence, and distinguished by the following features: 'the marked limi-'tation of the diseased strand, the variation in degree of the affected parts, and the 'absence of all marked congestive œdema or swelling in the surrounding tissue. 'The tissue is not diminished in firmness, and the colour varies from a pale liver to 'almost waxy white, the latter interspersed among the former, with portions inter-'mediate in hue. The pale portions average about one-third of an inch in diameter, 'and are often arranged in a serpiginous manner among the less advanced disease or 'even ramify among crepitant normal parenchyma. It is evident that the lesion is 'lobular, very variable in dispersion, of different stages, and approaching chronic in 'character; there is but little if any undue vascularity in connection with it. Looking 'at these lobules with a hand-lens, some of the component vesicles will be observed to 'project above the cut surface; others are uniform with it; others are depressed below 'the general level; the intervesicular textures are very prominent; there is a firm, glis-'tening aspect pervading all. The microscope shows vesicles swollen out with cell-con-'tents, other sparsely occupied, others empty, the fibrous framework decidedly in excess.'

Welch adds that this is not the only form of pneumonia observed in syphilis. 'It is, 'however, far from uncommon, seems to accompany the evolution of the virus, and is 'regarded as dependent on it. It is the form with which this variety (the caseous) of 'pulmonary consumption is linked as a sequel.'

From Welch's description, as here quoted, and also as given in subsequent passages, it would appear that he regards a caseating pneumonia from which gummata are absent as a specifically syphilitic lesion. I shall endeavour to show hereafter that these caseating pneumonias must be for the most part regarded as being of tubercular nature, and again I venture to raise the question whether such conditions, when found in syphilis, are not accidental concomitants, representing ordinary phthisis in a syphilitic subject, rather than anything specially due, as Welch believes, to the virus. I have, it is true, met with analogous conditions in syphilitic persons (see *Case 23, Lloyd*, XII. and XXXIX. 1). Three other cases of acute pneumonic phthisis illustrated in the Atlas had also suffered at earlier periods from venereal sores, and one from a sore-throat (viz. *Case 22, Gardiner*, XI. and XXXIX. 3). These, however, as will be seen hereafter, presented typical tubercular characters, and differed in no respect from two other cases of acute caseous pneumonia where there was no suspicion of syphilis (*Case 19, Griffin*, X. 1, 2, 3, 4; XXXVI. XXXVII., and *Case 24, Hall*, XIV. 2, and XXXVIII. 8). Two other cases of destructive pneumonia had also a syphilitic history (*Case 15, Scarrow*, VII. 3, and *Case 18, Brodrick*, XIII. 3, 4). The latter will be made the subject of special discussion, but the former differed in no respect from other forms of yellow tubercle. As yet no one has shown that 'caseous pneumonia' can be regarded as specially or exclusively syphilitic, or that, when occurring in syphilitic subjects, it presents any peculiar features. Until this is accomplished, I believe that its special association with the syphilitic poison must be regarded as doubtful. Moxon regards gangrene as an occasional result of syphilitic pneumonia.[1]

---

[1] *Guy's Hosp. Rep.* 1867, p. 372. A case of gangrene of the lung in a syphilitic subject is described by the late Dr. Budd (*Dis. Liver.* p. 410). It is probable that in this instance the gangrene had a pyæmic origin.

Syphilitic Indurations.—Cicatricial contractions of the lung from thickening of the interlobular tissue, limited to the lower lobe, and producing changes and appearances closely resembling those found in syphilitic contractions of the liver, were first noticed by Dittrich.[1] A remarkable case of an analogous character was shortly afterwards published by Vidal de Casis,[2] where thickening extended inwards around the bronchial tubes of the lower lobes, forming an indurated mass resembling a periostitis. Since this period many fibroid indurations of the lung have been ascribed to syphilis. They may, according to the descriptions given, be classified in four chief groups. (*a*) Thickening extending from the hilus around the bronchi and vessels. (*b*) Isolated masses of fibroid tissue found in different portions of the lung. (*c*) Diffuse changes, occupying the whole or the greater part of one lung. (*d*) Peculiar puckerings and thickenings around cavities.

(*a*) The most typical and characteristic forms are those of the first class. In some instances, as in Vidal's case, the extension is decidedly peribronchial,[3] and occasionally proceeds from the trachea through the mediastinum;[4] in others it has been traced down the bronchial sheath into the pulmonary tissue.[5] It has also been traced along the blood-vessels,[6] or along these and the bronchi simultaneously;[7] while in others it has extended inwards from the root of the lung, causing extensive induration, and has then been associated with much thickening and puckering of the pleura.[8] The tissue forming this induration is described, in some cases, as being remarkably vascular (Greenfield and Goodhart). The vascularity of the growth in early stages has been noticed by other observers in the more diffuse forms.[9]

(*b*) The appearance of isolated nodules of fibroid tissue, found in different portions of the lung, is open to more fallacy and is less certainly of syphilitic origin, since such nodules may be only the remains of various antecedent processes, particularly of obsolescent tubercle. Allusion has already been made to the indurated masses, which, as Virchow remarked, are scarcely if at all distinguishable from these, or from the chronic indurations produced by the inhalation of dust, as in the 'grinder's phthisis.' When, however, such nodules occur, without other evidence of phthisical change, in the middle or lower parts of the lung, there would appear to be strong reason to regard them as specific in origin.[10] In some of the recorded instances, caseous spots may be found, and in others a tendency to secondary ulceration—conditions which again raise doubts as to their nature, but which are doubtless compatible with a syphilitic origin. It is probable that in some of these instances the masses found in a later stage to be fibroid, may have commenced as gummata or in some form of chronic pneumonia. A support to this latter view is afforded by a case of Beer's,[11] where the change was actually found to be progressing. It would appear to me not improbable that the illustration given, in Plates XV. and XX. 3, and XLII. 7 (*Case 29, Brown*), of fibroid change extending from the hilus, may have belonged to the same category. In some cases also

---

[1] *Prager Vierteljahrschr.* 1850, xxvi. 42. See also Wilks, *loc. cit.* Another case is given by Wagner, *Arch. der Heilkunde,* vol. iv.
[2] *Malad. Vénériennes,* 1855, quoted by Lancereaux, *Traité de la Syphilis,* p. 490.
[3] Welch, *loc. cit.* p. 65, relates a remarkable case in which indurated syphilitic ulceration extended down the interior of the bronchial tubes, and was associated with caseous masses in the lung.
[4] Moxon, *Guy's Hosp. Rep.* 1867, p. 338.
[5] Pye-Smith, *Path. Soc. Trans.* xxviii. 354. Colomiati, *Wien. med. Woch.* 1878, No. 28.

[6] Payne, *Path. Soc. Trans.* vol. xxv.
[7] Greenfield, *Path. Soc. Trans.* xxviii. 258 *et seq.*; Tiffany, *Amer. Journ. Med. Science,* July, 1877.
[8] Mahomed, *Path. Soc. Trans.* xxviii. 340.
[9] Andreu, *Lungenaffectionen syphilitischer Kinder,* Diss. Würzburg, 1878, p. 31.
[10] See Virchow, *Krankhafte Geschwülste,* ii. 465, also Schutz, in Klebs' *Beiträge Path. Anat.* 1878. Hft. i. 58; Goodhart, *Path. Soc. Trans.* 1874. xxv. 31. and *ibid.* xxviii. case 2. (induration of both bases); Beer, *Die Eingeweide Syphilis,* pp. 75, 149.
[11] Beer, *loc. cit,* p. 150.

fibroid thickenings have been found extending into the lung from the nodular masses in the pleura.[1]

(c) More general fibroid change has been found in the lungs of syphilitic children,[2] and by such cases a presumption is afforded that the lesion may have this specific origin in other instances. In these cases it begins in the interlobular tissue, and thence extends to the alveolar walls.[3] Induration of the whole of one lung, with bronchial dilatation, has been attributed to this cause both in syphilitic children[4] and in adults.[5] At the same time, it must be remembered that the large proportion of all cases of fibroid induration of the lung are due either to chronic tuberculosis or to chronic pneumonia.

(d) A peculiar puckering around a cavity has been described by T. H. Green,[6] as significant of syphilis, but in the case in question no other evidence of the condition existed than the shape of the incisor teeth. Goodhart[7] is disposed to believe that fibroid changes found in the lungs of syphilitic patients, are, to a great extent, due to the constitutional disease. In 189 cases of visceral syphilis, he found prominent fibroid changes in the lung in twenty-six, of which, however, six contained tubercles. Even when the latter are deducted, a doubt must remain whether some of the remaining twenty may not have had a tubercular rather than a syphilitic origin, and this doubt must specially be felt with regard to such changes situated in the apices. Goodhart lays special stress on the bilateral symmetry of this lesion. It must, however, be remarked that this presents a marked contrast to the ordinary history of gummata and of other syphilitic affections. Lanceraux, indeed, has stated the precise converse, viz. that a unilateral phthisical affection affords grounds for suspicion of syphilis. A bilateral character would suggest rather a tubercular than a specific origin of such induration, although, *per contra*, unilateral phthisical affections, when the disease is chronic, are not altogether uncommon. Finally it must be remembered that Rindfleisch ascribes to syphilis an influence in producing fibroid induration in tubercles. This theory appears, however, to require a proof which it would be difficult to render positive.[8]

Changes in the lymphatics of the lung were first described by Hermann Weber[9] as among the occasional phenomena of syphilis. They presented on section the appearance of pale yellow spots which were found to be masses of coagulated lymph, partly caseous, containing enlarged lymph-cells and granular corpuscles. The bronchial glands were enlarged to the size of a pigeon's egg or hazel-nut. Some of those of larger size were softened and creamy; others, which were less enlarged, had a marbled appearance, due to lardaceous-like tissue interspersed with very vascular tracts. A very similar condition has been described by Cornil,[10] where also there was chronic inflammation both of the bronchial and lymphatic glands. In both these cases it is probable that the changes in the lymphatics were secondary to those in the glands (*see* Interstitial Pneumonia). Rindfleisch, in describing a form of miliary tuberculosis as syphilitic (*see* ante, p. 124), regarded these spots as of lymphatic origin, but only apparently so far as he attributes a similar origin to other forms of miliary tuberculosis.

---

[1] Beer, *ib.* case 7, p. 62.
[2] Andral, case 1, p. 10 (figured).
[3] Fournier, *Gaz. Hebdom.* 1875, p. 760.
[4] Andral, *loc. cit.* case i. p. 19.
[5] Lanceraux, *Traité de la Syphilis*, pp. 326-30. Pye-Smith, *Path. Soc. Trans.* 1877, xxviii. 394. A case of unilateral induration of one lung in a syphilitic patient is given by Williams, *Consumption*, case 85, p. 288.
[6] *Path. Soc. Trans.* 1873, xxiv. 31.
[7] *Ibid.* 1877, vol. xxviii.
[8] Rindfleisch, Ziemssen's *Handbuch*, v. 161.
[9] *Path. Soc. Trans.* 1866, xvii. 153; two plates of appearances in lungs, bronchial glands, and liver.
[10] *Bull. Soc. Méd. des Hôp.* 1874, xi. 144.

SYPHILITIC DISEASES OF THE LUNG

MICROSCOPIC APPEARANCES: (A) *Gummata*. These consist, in the earlier stages, of a swelling of the alveolar walls, which passes into a fibroid tissue mingled with fusiform cells, and sometimes with small, round cells. Von Cube[1] regards the latter as characteristic, and among them he has found also giant-cells.

Green[2] thinks that this growth of small cells proceeds mainly around the interlobular blood-vessels, thus distinguishing it from tubercular formation, but there is evidence that syphilitic new-formation also takes place in the bronchial wall, where it may even form prominences under the submucous tissue, and in some cases, as shown by Gowers, the extension may be chiefly along the course of the bronchioles.

The growth in some places, as seen by the woodcut (Fig. 40), tends to form isolated masses of small-celled formation. The epithelium of the alveoli presents some proliferation, but only to a moderate degree. Evidence of inflammatory change is, however, seldom wanting (see XXVII. 2, *a*). From this small-celled growth, fibroid change proceeds, as seen in XXVII. 1 and 5 (which are drawn from sections of a gumma kindly lent me by Dr. Goodhart). The small-celled growth forms, in places, dense masses, as at *b*, fig. 2.

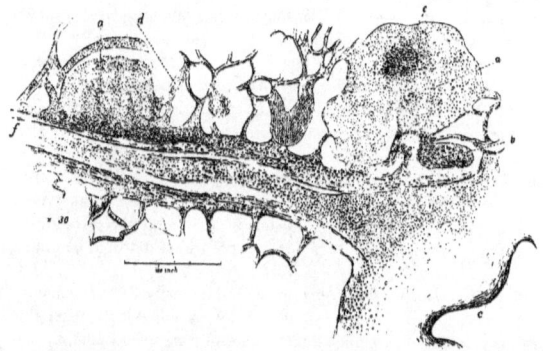

FIG. 40.— Syphilitic growth in the lung. *a a*, small-celled syphilitic growth; *b*, mixed growth and pneumonic products in centre of the air-cells; *c*, commencing cascation of new-growth; *d*, infiltration of alveolar walls; *e*, interior of large bronchus with thickened walls, the inner portion of which is plicated; *f*, a thickened smaller bronchus along which the growth is extending.—Gowers, 'Syphilitic Diseases of the Lung,' *Path. Soc. Trans.*, xxviii. 330.

Between these, a reticulum of fibres gradually forms (as at *a*, fig. 1), and this reticulum thickens (*b b*, fig. 1; *c*, fig. 2), enclosing within its meshes groups of cells (*c, d*, fig. 1) which may remain a single or double nucleus in the interstices of the reticulum (*f, g*, fig. 1), and finally only as oval nuclei imbedded in broad-banded fibres (*k*, fig. 1). In some places, the cells are seen to assume a stellate form (*h h h*, fig. 1, *f f*, fig. 2), with branching fibres, probably the commencement of a lymph-canalicular system, which is seen more highly developed in figs. 3, 4, and 5 (XXVII.). The reticulum gradually thickens into broad-banded fibres, highly refracting, from the interstices of which the cell-growth gradually disappears (*d*, fig. 2; *b*, fig. 1), or only remains as elongated processes in the centre of the spaces. The final development is to an almost homogeneous structure (such as is seen in figs. 3 and 5) of broad-banded fibres, between which stellate cells form a lymph-

---

[1] Virchow's *Archiv*, 1880, vol. lxxxii. See also a case by Sydney Coupland, *Path. Soc. Trans.* 1876, vol. xxvii., in which these small round cells predominated.   [2] Green, *Path. Soc. Trans*, xxviii. 388.

canalicular system. In its later stages, this thickening presents the characters seen in XXVI. 8 (drawn from another specimen of gumma from the same lung as that described by Dr. Gowers). Here the same arrangement of broad-banded interlacing fibres is seen, and this in many places has proceeded to the complete obliteration of the whole alveolar structure. In other parts the alveoli can still be seen greatly narrowed ; in some (a, a) destitute of epithelium, in others, (b, b) still crowded with epithelial-like cells, while in other parts again (c, c) the invasion of the alveoli and their gradual obliteration by the broad-banded fibro-nucleated growth can be traced. Thickening of the blood-vessels can also be seen (d). Among the small-celled growth, giant-cells have been seen by Von Cube,[1] and also by Mahomed.[2]

It is probable that these cases, in which the fibroid change is thus distinctly marked, are such as have a tendency to pass into cicatricial tissue rather than into caseation. Gowers found some tendency to caseation in parts of the specimen which he examined (fig. 40, c). In the more marked case of this change figured in Pl. IV. fig. 2 the specimen was lost, and no full account has yet been furnished of the metamorphosis, but it is easily intelligible that necrosis, instead of fibre-growth, should occur in a tissue so entirely non-vascular, and that this necrosis should present the caseous transformation, and subsequently pass into softening.

(B) The *Syphilitic Pneumonias*, or diffuse syphilomata, have been already described, except in the case of the white hepatisation of the lungs of childhood. The characteristic change in this condition is very closely akin to that observed in gummata. The essential feature is the thickening of the alveolar walls and interlobular tissue by a growth, consisting of small cells mingled with fusiform cells, and in some cases highly vascular ;[3] it may form prominences in the interior of the alveoli. Fibre-tissue is not always formed from this growth,[4] but in some cases it is very conspicuous, and may resemble the bands existing in the gummata ; this is well seen in the drawing given by Greenfield (*see* XXVII. 6 and 7), and it is also shown in drawings by Von Bärensprung[5] and by Thierfelder.[6]

The changes undergone by the epithelium of the alveoli are variously described. Probably they differ according to the stage of the disease. Virchow and Weber[7] observed its proliferation, while Wagner remarked that nothing could be removed by brushing the surface of a section of the lung. Lorain and Robin,[8] on the other hand, found such an extensive multiplication of the epithelium that they described the change as an epithelioma. This process is also illustrated in Greenfield's drawing (XXVII. 7), though in this case it does not prevail to a considerable extent.

The subcutaneous tissue of the bronchi has been found by Wagner, infiltrated with a small-celled growth similar to that seen in the gummata. In a form of pneumonia, which Colomiatti regards as syphilitic, but which does not appear precisely to correspond with this white hepatisation, he has found giant-cells both in the interstitial tissue and also in the interior of the alveoli.[9]

The *fibroid form* presents the least marked characteristics. It has been found, however, by Goodhart and Mahomed proceeding by a small-celled growth in the walls of the

---

[1] *Loc. cit.*
[2] *Path. Soc. Trans.* 1877, xxviii. 339. Ref. also Baumgarten, Virchow's *Archiv*, lxxvi. 487.
[3] Andrea, *Lungenaffectionen syphilitischer Kindern*, obs. A., obs. N ; also an illustration by Cornil and Ranvier, *Manuel d'Histol. Pathologique*, 2nd ed. 1881, ii. 221.
[4] Wagner, *Archiv der Heilkunde*, 1868, iv. 359.
[5] Von Bärensprung, *Die Hered. Syph.* Taf. vii.
[6] *Atlas Path. Histol.* 1872, Lief. i. Taf v. fig. 3.
[7] Virchow's *Archiv.* i. 146.
[8] *Gaz. Méd. de Paris.* 1855.
[9] *Wien. med. Presse.* 1878, No. 28. The original of this has been inaccessible to me.

alveoli, which are thickened by it and sometimes show epithelial proliferation of their contents.[1] Mahomed has also seen this growth forming nodular masses, in which giant-cells were found,[2] and whence the fibroid change extended. The vascularity of this fibroid growth has been already noticed. In their later stages, the fibroid growths, attributed to syphilis, have not been described as offering any special peculiarities, and the recognition of their syphilitic origin (which is still doubtful in many instances) must depend rather on their distribution than on their histological characters.

Syphilitic Phthisis.—It may here be perhaps desirable to append a few remarks on the so-called 'syphilitic phthisis.' Apart from the phthisical symptoms caused by a purulent bronchitis, with pyrexia, in the syphilitic patient, which may occasionally progress to a chronic condition of pulmonary consolidation, and has not yet been elucidated by post-mortem examination [3]), the anatomical changes implied by this term must be among those which have now been enumerated. I have already ventured to express the opinion that, in a large number of the cases—both of small nodular masses described as broncho-pneumonia, of peribronchitis, and of fibroid induration—the disease found was of a tubercular rather than of a syphilitic origin. That, on the other hand, a phthisical affection may originate from the effects of the syphilitic virus on the lung, is established in two directions. First, by the evidences of the cure, through an anti-syphilitic treatment, of consolidation associated with phthisical symptoms in infected subjects,—evidence which is abundant in medical literature. Secondly, by the formation of cavities without any association with tubercle, to which allusion has already been made; these may have originated either in gummata, or in more diffuse forms of pneumonia.[4] These are, however, the only indubitable forms, and their distinction rests rather on the naked-eye appearances than on the histological structure. In the latter the resemblance between tubercular and syphilitic formations is very striking, and is so close that positive criteria cannot yet be established between them. Thus Gowers' figure of a gumma (see Fig. 40, p. 130) presents a very close analogy to the formation of the series of grey granulations (compare XXVIII. 4 and 5), while Greenfield's figure of syphilitic pneumonia (XXVII. 7) and Goodhart's of progressive fibroid induration,[5] very closely resemble some forms of tubercular pneumonia (see XXXVIII. 8, and XXXVII. 7). The fibroid structure of gummata (see XXVII.) resembles not only the characters of typical indurating tubercular granulations (compare XLII. 2), but the more extensive invasion of the alveoli (in XXVI. 8) has its analogy also in chronic phthisis (see *Case 30, Carr*; XLI. 1), while the mode of extension of the fibroid growth, as described by Mahomed, has a remarkable analogy, even to the presence of giant-cells, with some forms of tubercular growth. Scarcely any writer who has treated on this subject has failed to notice the close correspondence of the histological characters of the two diseases; Cornil and Ranvier even remark that in most cases described as pulmonary syphilis they have been unable to find any characters conclusively distinguishing the lesion from tubercle.[6]

In the discussion on syphilis at the Pathological Society, Greenfield [7] pointed out the following features as distinctive:—that the syphilitic growths are more vascular, and that the cells are larger, less crowded, and more mingled with fusiform cells than in

---

[1] Goodhart, *Path. Soc. Trans.* 1877, xxviii. 313, and pl. xvii.
[2] Mahomed, *Path. Soc. Trans.* 1877 xxviii. 339.
[3] Walshe. *Dis. Lungs*, 1871, pp. 231-2.
[4] It appears to me not improbable that a remarkable series of cases of ulcerative pneumonia described by Aufrecht (*Path. Mittheilungen*, Magdeburg, 1881) may have had this origin. Two of them were, however, tubercular. They all showed cavity-formation in the middle of the lungs.
[5] *Path. Soc. Trans.* vol. xxviii. pl. xvii.
[6] Cornil and Ranvier, *Manuel d'Histol. Path.*, ed. 1881, i. 232.
[7] *Path. Soc. Trans.* xxviii 277.

tubercle. This, however, is only a question of degree, and in both syphilitic new-formations and tubercular growths, considerable variations are met with in each of these particulars. Pye-Smith, in the same discussion, admits that the only ground for the pathological diagnosis of the nature of the fibroid change is that afforded by the history of syphilis, the presence of similar changes in other organs, and the absence of tubercle. But this latter distinction will scarcely apply when bodies are found in numbers in the lungs which are otherwise indistinguishable from tubercular granulations. Goodhart[1] has published drawings of 'indubitable tubercle,' spreading from caseous masses which he regards as gummata, but which histologically were also indistinguishable from tubercular formations. His figures show also a close identity with appearances which are very commonly found in ordinary phthisis, and if his conclusions are correct, we must admit one of three things—either that syphilis can actually produce tubercle (a proposition which has been before affirmed,[2] but which I must regard as doubtful) ; or that it can produce changes both to the naked eye and to the microscope indistinguishable from tubercle, a view which has no parallel in any other organ than the lung, and from which I also venture to differ ; or, finally, that these appearances are only cases of ordinary tubercular change occurring in a syphilitic subject. The last opinion appears to me the most probable.[3]

CANCER OF THE LUNG.

Plates XXII. figs. 5 and 6 ; XXIII. fig. 2[1] ; XXIV. figs. 3 and 4, XLV.

THE lungs may be the subject of nearly every known form of morbid growth, but in most instances these are secondary to similar affections in other organs. Many are comparatively of great rarity, and I shall here only describe the recognised forms of genuine cancer. I shall not describe mediastinal tumours as a class in this place.

Cancer of the lungs occurs, in its more marked characteristics, in two chief forms, viz. as nodules and as infiltration. Histologically it assumes two chief types : cancer in the ordinary sense of the word, and epithelioma. I use these words in their common significance, fully aware that the definitions of both are as yet a matter of discussion. The differences of opinion respecting them are, however, of only secondary importance in pulmonary pathology. In fact, primary cancer of the lung-tissue is rare, and clinically, except in a few infrequent instances of such disease, the chief importance of malignant intrathoracic growths depends on those occurring in the mediastina. These are for the most part sarcomata of glandular origin or lymphadenomata, and their direct effects are chiefly produced by pressure, sometimes indeed on the lungs, but with nearly equal frequency on other parts. All forms of cancer have been occasionally found in the lung,

---

[1] See *Path. Soc. Trans.* 1879, xxx. 232 et seq. (two plates), and *Lancet*, 1878, ii. 809, for discussion on these appearances.

[2] Von Bärensprung (*Deutsche Klinik*, 1858, p. 170), who refers probably to the caseous change. See also Jonathan Hutchinson, *Trans. Path. Soc.* 1876, xxvii. 354, on the absolute non-identity of syphilis on the one hand and tubercle and scrofula on the other.

[3] A similar view has been expressed by Hilton Fagge, *Trans. Path. Soc.* 1876, xxvii. 382. Pye-Smith (*ibid.* 1877, xxviii. 334) has stated that in his opinion most of the cases of so-called syphilitic phthisis are instances of 'true tubercular phthisis in a syphilitic subject, which runs its course uninfluenced by the latter disease.'

[1] This figure should be properly classified as a small-celled sarcoma, probably of mediastinal origin ; a class which I shall not attempt here minutely to describe.

but colloid and melanotic cancers have hitherto only been met with as secondary growths, except in one case, quoted by Walshe, where primary colloid and encephaloid coexisted.[1]

Colloid Cancer is generally described as resembling the same disease in other parts, a semi-transparent, soft, gelatinous tissue, though the traces of the lobules may be still preserved. In some instances this condition merges into one of a more opaque and whiter appearance. The sub-pleural lymphatics, and also those of the lung, may be filled with a similar material, and the external surface of the lung may be rendered nodular by the growth.[2] Melanotic tumours resemble for the most part a deeply pigmented encephaloid, but the pigmentation varies much in amount and may be slight. They may, however, become confluent and form a deeply pigmented and almost black tissue, breaking down into cavities.[3]

Scirrhus Cancer may also form in the lungs, as hard masses, striated from their centre, like those seen in the mamma and stomach. In other cases it contracts the lung into a series of uneven masses, resembling a 'hobnailed liver.' In some cases the growth appears to follow principally the interlobular septa, but it may also extend into the lung in masses and nodules, yielding on pressure a creamy juice. Combinations of encephaloid and scirrhus are not uncommon.[4]

The majority of the cancerous growths in the lung come either under the general term of *encephaloid* or of '*mixed*' growths, while to some of the 'infiltrations' only the general term of 'cancer' can be applied. In the form of tumours, cancer appears in nodules of variable size, from an orange or larger, to miliary growths which are with difficulty distinguished from tubercles, but have no special tendency to appear at the apex. In a certain number of cases the nodules are mainly subpleural, and these were termed *plaques cireuses* by Cruveilhier, from their resemblance to drops of wax.[5] When these extend more deeply into the lung they may even have a mushroom-like appearance.[6]

Infiltrating cancer of the lung-tissue (see XXII. 6) may either preserve the lobular form, or be almost homogeneous and with difficulty distinguished from ordinary inflammatory consolidation. In fact it has in some cases been called a 'cancerous pneumonia.'[7] In other cases it presents the manifest characters of colloid, scirrhus, or encephaloid. The latter is more or less vascular, and is traversed by large vessels, or mottled with extravasion of blood, the 'fungus haematodes ;' but in many cases the colour is uniformly greyish, although more vascular than the ordinary grey pneumonic infiltration. It is also softer, easily broken down, though with a somewhat crisp fracture, and yields a creamy juice both on section and on scraping. The infiltration may not be general, but may be limited to particular portions of the lung-structure. Thus it may affect the lymphatics alone, without implicating the pulmonary tissue.[8] It then forms a white network in the

---

[1] Walshe, *Dis. Lungs*, p. 516.
[2] Warren, *Med.-Chir. Trans.* vol. xxvii.; Hasse, *Path. Anat.*; Wilks and Moxon, *Path. Anat.* p. 532; Bristowe, *Path. Soc. Trans.* xvii. 136, xix. 230; Virchow's *Archiv*, iv. 200; and *Atlas path. Anat.* pl. 44, Text, t. 321, 666.
[3] Carswell, *Illus. Elementary Forms of Disease*, art. 'Carcinoma'; Lebert, *Atlas path. Anat.* pl. xcii. (horse); Sir George Burrows, *Med.-Chir. Trans.* vol. xxvii.; Kohler, *Krebs der Lunge*, Diss. Inaug. Tübingen, 1847, a case by Roger; Sieveking, *Path. Soc. Trans.* vol. i.; Bryant, *ib.* vol. xiv.; Pemberton, *Midland Quarterly Journal*, 1857, quoted by Beigel, art. 'Cancer,' Reynolds's *System Med.* vol. iii.
[4] Albers, *Erläuterungen*, quoted by Kohler; Mayne,

Dubl. Hospital Gazette, 1857; Gordon, *Dublin Quart. Journ.* 1861, xxxvi. 210. Sir Risdon Bennett, *Intrathoracic Growths*, p. 55 (figure); Bristowe, *Path. Soc. Trans.* vol. xi.
[5] Cruveilhier, *Atlas*, livr. xxii. xxviii. xxxi.; Lebert, *Atlas*, pl. lxxxv. and text, i. 731.
[6] *Atlas*, pl. xxiv. fig. 2. See also Lebert, *Atlas*, livr. xxiii. pl. 5; Carswell, *Illust. Element. Forms Dis.* art 'Carcinoma,' pl. iii. fig. 6; Walshe, '*Cancer*,' p. 341; Bristowe, *Path. Soc. Trans.* vol. xi.
[7] Skrzeczka, Virchow's *Archiv*, vol. xi.; Rokitanski, *Path. Anat.* iii. 83; Schnyder, Canstatt's *Jahresbericht*, 1864, vol. iii. p. 254.
[8] Fränzel, *Charité-Annalen*, 1876; secondary to cancer of stomach.

pleural surface, interspersed with nodular masses. The same network may be traced in the interior of the lung, and the nodular masses may be found to be chiefly situated within the lymphatics, though the growth may extend from them into the pulmonary tissue.[1] These lymphatics may sometimes contain cancerous cells, at other times caseous matter (Bristowe), or their contents may present the characteristics of epithelioma, when a tumour of this nature has been present in other parts and has affected the lung[2] (see XXIV. 4).

In other cases the infiltration extends through the alveolar septa,[3] involving principally the walls of the bronchi and the vessels. In the bronchi it commences apparently in the adventitia, and thence extends to the submucous tissue, but Langhans has shown that the submucous glands may be the origin of the growth.[4] Schottelius is of opinion that it extends in the lymphatic sheaths of the bronchi.[5] This extension of 'malignant' growths along the bronchi has been noticed in other forms of tumours, as in lymphadenomata and in sarcomata.[6]

The vessels may be invaded in a similar manner, and the cancerous growth may be limited principally to their sheaths (see XXII. 5, and Case 45, Parsons, also XLV. 1, 2, 3), though the bronchial sheaths are also commonly involved.

The invasion of the lung-tissue may take place in one of two ways, either by a growth within the cavities of the alveoli or by a gradual thickening of their walls; combinations of both processes also occur.[7]

The filling of the alveoli, in some cases of ordinary carcinoma, takes place by a process akin to pneumonia. There is a proliferation of cells in their interior, and they gradually assume the form of cancer-cells, a process described by Rokitanski and Skrzeczka, as a cancerous pneumonia. A stroma is, however, described by Rokitanski in these cases, though Skrzeczka found none, and some alveoli were filled only with detritus and fat-drops. Rokitanski also figures pedunculated masses growing from the walls, and extending into the interior, of the alveoli.[8] That the growth occurs in the alveolar walls, and produces a uniform infiltration of the lung-tissue, is seen in XLV. 4, 5, 6, 7. It has also been figured by Thierfelder as extending into them from the bronchi.[9]

Epitheliomata of the lung reproduce both the ordinary forms of epithelial growth, the squamous and the cylindrical. Both are most commonly secondary, but instances of each are recorded as having their primary seat in the lung. The naked-eye characteristics of these epitheliomata vary. The most minute description of the squamous form is that by Sir James Paget;[10] he describes the nodules as opaque, white, marbled with pale yellow and pink, intersected by lines of grey and black, and marked with blood-vessels. They were brittle, crumbled under pressure and yielded no creamy juice, and they permeated the bronchi and also the pulmonary artery. Arnott describes them as of a pinkish-white colour, having a granular appearance. The friability was remarked by Perls, but Virchow speaks of them as being firm, though softening in the centre. Columnar epitheliomata are described by Malassez as closely resembling encephaloid, soft and of a pinkish-white, passing into a yellow tinge, and yielding a milky juice. Finlay and Parker found them of a yellowish-white colour, stained with extravasated blood, and of soft consistence. Greenfield found them vascular, soft, and pinkish. In my case they were remarkably firm and resembled scirrhus, umbilicated where they reached the pleural surface, but softening into cheesy masses in the centres.

Primary squamous epithelioma has hitherto only been recorded in one case by Perls,[1] and here there were secondary deposits in the pleura, the sphenoid bone, the choroid, and the liver. In some cases of its secondary occurrence in the lung, it may possibly have

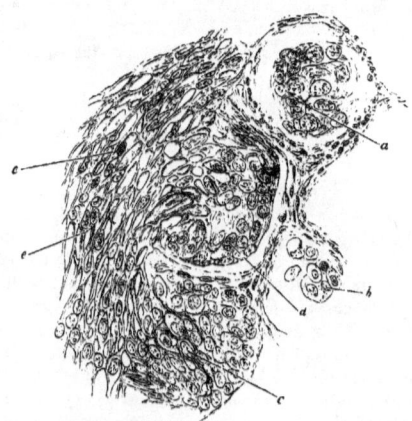

FIG. 41.—Cancer of lung. *a a*, large squamous cells within the alveoli; some, as *b*, very large and presenting two nuclei; *c*, cells with appearance of intervening stroma; *e e*, similar growth extending into adjacent tissue.

been due to direct transplantation of cancer-cells, gravitating into the air-passages from the œsophagus, or during operations for cancer of the tongue,[2] but in other instances, as those recorded by Virchow,[3] and one by Arnott[4] (where the lung-affection was secondary to epithelioma of the clitoris), the infection must have arisen by means of the blood or lymphatics. In most of the cases hitherto recorded, the lung-affection appears to arise from the interior of the pulmonary alveoli by a proliferation of cells which gradually assume the character of squamous epithelium.[5] The late Prof. Otto Weber, however, believed that the new-growth originated from the connective tissue, and not from the epithelium of the alveoli.[6]

[1] Virchow's *Archiv*, 1872, vol. lvi.
[2] Moxon, *Path. Soc. Trans.* vol. xx. (secondary to œsophageal epithelioma); Wilks and Moxon, *Pathol. Anat.* p. 852 (secondary to laryngeal cancer); Gollee, *Path. Soc. Trans.* vol. xxxii. secondary to operation on tongue. Here a large mass of epithelial cancer existed in the mediastinum.
[3] *Gazette Hebdomadaire*, 1855; case communicated to Velpeau, obs. i. This case showed multiple epitheliomata secondary to a tumour of the tongue.
[4] Arnott, *Trans. Path. Soc.* vol. xxii. (figure). Arnott does not describe the mode of growth of this tumour in the lung. He cites instances of other secondary epitheliomata in the supra-renal capsules.
[5] See figure by Perls, *loc. cit.*
[6] Virchow's *Archiv*, xxix. 179 (figures).

Through the kindness of Mr. Godlee I have been allowed to take a drawing from one of his preparations, and, as is seen in the accompanying woodcut (Fig. 42), the growth begins by an epithelial proliferation, in which the alveoli are crowded with large squamous cells. Similar cells appear gradually in the alveolar walls, and finally the growth extends to the surrounding tissue in a manner which leaves it doubtful whether this extensive infiltration consists of a stroma with cells and nuclei imbedded, or whether the appearance of the stroma is not simulated by cells which have assumed an epidermic character, and lie flattened against one another. Perls noticed the absence of stroma in the growths in the lung, though it was present in those of the liver. In the alveoli some cells show broad spaces or vacuoles. There was, in this instance, as remarked by Godlee, only an imperfect formation of nests, but these have been noticed by Virchow, Perls, and Arnott.

Columnar or cylindrical epithelioma has hitherto been usually found to be secondary, though some cases are recorded of its primary appearance.[1] Secondary columnar epitheliomata of the lung have invariably reproduced the character of similar formations in other parts, and particularly in the liver, stomach, and ovaries.[2] In the case which I have illustrated (XXIV. 4; XLV. 8, 9, 10, 11, 12), the lung-affection was secondary to that of the liver. Both were so firm, and the surface of the tumours in the lung so markedly umbilicated, that I took them for scirrhus, and the liver was unfortunately not preserved for microscopic examination. In the lung, in this instance, the growth appears to commence with an epithelial proliferation, which fills the alveoli and bronchioles (XLV. 10). The cells in some alveoli are at first round, then, as described by Malassez, cubical or club-shaped. Flat cells, as observed by him, were not seen in this specimen, but I find them in the preparation kindly lent me by Mr. Godlee, which I shall describe subsequently. The cells gradually acquire a cylindrical shape, and the growth then assumes one of two characters, either bulbous (figs. 8, 9, 11), or else tubular or gland-like (fig. 8, *c*).[3]

Although the alveoli, for the most part, constitute closed spaces filled with these masses of growth, as described by Malassez, yet a gradual invasion of the pulmonary tissue also takes place (*see* fig. 12) ; the alveoli also fuse into one another by a growth of cells in the interlobular tissue, which sometimes constitutes a uniform structure (*see* next woodcut) and sometimes assumes the form of tubercles.[4] Tubular growths also occur in the interlobular spaces, probably arising from the lymphatics[5] (*see* XLV. 8, *e*), and these may afterwards assume the villous character. Extensions around the bronchi, similar to those described in the other forms of cancer, have been found by Finlay. In a primary case, Norman Moore believed that the growth commenced in the tubular glands of the bronchi. The bronchial glands in several other cases, as well as in my own, presented alveolar spaces filled with a similar growth, so that sections of these were indistinguishable from those of the lung. In a case where an epithelioma of the bladder showed nests

---

[1] Finlay and Parker (*Med.-Chir. Trans.* 1877, vol. lx.) record a case where the two organs affected were the lungs and liver; the former in a preponderant degree. They quote also Ettore Marchiafava, *Rivista Clinica di Bologna*, 1874 (primary cylindrical epithelioma of lung, secondary deposits in brain and frontal bone) and also Lataste and Malassez's case, *Bull. Soc. Anat. de Paris*, 1875, and *Archiv. de Physiol. Norm. et Path.* 1876 (lungs, mediastinal lymphatics, and pleura alone affected). See also a case by Norman Moore, *Path. Soc. Trans.* xxxii. 32.

[2] Virchow's third case, *loc. cit.*, appears to have been of this nature; he describes some of the cells as elongated, and the structure of the growths as 'acinous.' Here the ovaries and vagina were the first affected. Cf. also, Greenfield, *Path. Soc. Trans.* vol. xxv, when the lung-affection was secondary to a columnar epithelioma of the liver; also one by Finlay, *Path. Soc. Trans.* 1883, xxxiv. 102 : multiple cylindrical epitheliomata, secondary to growth in the stomach and remarkable as associated with a similar growth in multiple subcutaneous tumours.

[3] These tubular forms are figured by Greenfield, *Path. Soc. Trans.* vol. xxv.

[4] Greenfield has described tubules growing in the alveolar walls.

[5] Virchow (*Gaz. Hebdom.* 1855, case iii.) has described these. Malassez has figured the mode of extension in pleural adhesions.

of horny epithelium, observed by Godlee, the growths in the lung assumed the villous type, mingled with flat epithelium, and from this combination 'nests' of imbricated epithelial cells were found, as shown in the accompanying woodcut, drawn from one of his specimens.

Cancer of the lung occasionally softens into cavities which are distinguished by their ragged and irregular walls.[1] They may in some cases be multiple, in others solitary. The mode of their formation has not been minutely studied, but Perls has noticed a peculiar gelatiniform degeneration in his case of squamous epithelioma. Virchow and Sir James Paget have found this form breaking down into cavities.[2]

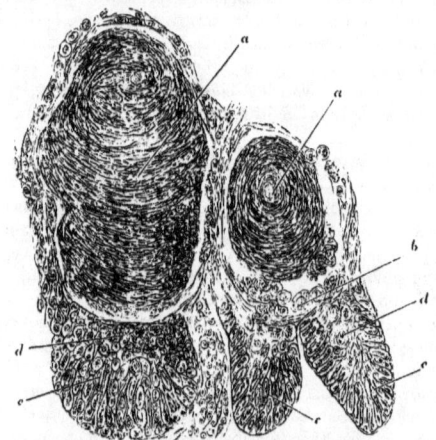

FIG. 12.—Growth in lung secondary to epithelioma of the bladder. *a a*, nests of imbricated epithelium cells; *b*, flat epithelium cells seen laterally; *c c*, portion of growth assuming villous type; *d d*, epithelial proliferation of rounder cells.

The changes resulting from the pressure of mediastinal tumours on the root of the lung are usually the consequence of occlusion of the bronchi and of pressure in the vessels. The former give rise to bronchial dilatations which are filled with retained secretions, and set up secondary pneumonia and gangrene.

[1] Bayle, *Phthisie Pulmonaire*, obs. xxxvi. p. 399; Maclachlan, *Lond. Med. Gaz.* 1843; Lebert, *Klinik der Brustkrankheiten*, ii. 658; and *Atlas*, text, p. 665, 745; Sir Andrew Clark, *Trans. Path. Soc.* vii. 76; Stokes, *Dublin Quart. Journ*, 1842, p. 234; Cailliot quoted by Cockle, *Intrathoracic Cancer*, p. 42; Lobstein quoted by Köhler, *Thèse*, p. 20.
[2] Virchow, *loc. cit.*; Paget, *Surgical Path.* ed. 1863, p. 706.

ON THE ARTIFICIAL PRODUCTION OF TUBERCLE.

It may not be without value to append a summary of the chief anatomical changes observed in the experimental production of tubercle in the lower animals. I shall not, however, attempt to present an exhaustive history of the literature of this subject, which is very voluminous, particularly as this has been already done by Spina, Johne, Klein, and Watson Cheyne.[1] Further, I do not propose to enter into a discussion of the question whether tubercle can be produced by the inoculation of other substances than tubercle. As I have formerly expressed the opinion that this is possible,[2] I wish now distinctly to state that I regard the more recent experiments on this subject by Cohnheim and Fränkel, by Koch, Baumgarten, Aufrecht, and Watson Cheyne, as conclusively proving the negative and thus supporting Villemin's original position,[3] and I have to add that Dawson Williams' experiments, which I had the opportunity of watching throughout, have convinced me that there was some fallacy in my own on this subject, due probably either to imperfect disinfection of my instruments or to imperfect isolation of the animals.[4]

All the more recent researches tend to show that tubercle can only be produced by the introduction into the system of tubercular products, or of the blood or some other fluid of tubercular animals,[5] either directly by the transference of these from one animal to another, or indirectly through fluids in which tubercular material has undergone culture and in which micro-organisms are for the most part demonstrable. The introduction may be effected either by wounds penetrating the integuments, the serous cavities, the veins, the eye, the joints or other parts,[6] by deglutition and entrance into the intestinal canal, or by inhalation or direct injection into the air-passages or lungs; in all these methods, efficiently cultivated fluids are practically as effectual for the production of the disease as is tubercle taken direct from the human body. The effect of such introduction, except that directly into the blood, is to produce, in the first instance, a local[7] and subsequently, in most instances,

---

[1] Spina, *Studien über Tuberculose*, Wien, 1883; Johne, *Geschichte der Tuberculose*, Leipzig, 1883; Klein, *Practitioner*, 1881, vol. ii.; Watson Cheyne, *Practitioner*, 1883, vol. i. Most of the writers on this subject have given a history; cf. also Schmitt, *Tuberculose Expérimentale*. Concours d'agrégation, Paris, 1883, with bibliography; Hering, *Experimentelle Studien über Tuberculose*. In Burdon-Sanderson's papers (*Rep. Med. Off. Privy Council*) will also be found a summary of the results obtained by the earlier observers.

[2] *On the Artificial Production of Tubercle*, Lecture Royal College Physicians, 1868, published in the *Lancet* and *Brit. Med. Journ.* 1868, and also separately with plates.

[3] Villemin (*Études sur la Tuberculose*) made numerous experiments of this kind with a negative result. Cf. also *Gaz. Hebdom.* 1865, and *Bull. Acad. Méd.* 1865, 1866, vols. xxxi. xxxii. and *Bull. Cong. Internat. Méd. de Paris*, 1867. Cf. also Cohnheim, *Vorlesungen allg. Path.* ii. 609; Koch, *Berliner klin. Woch.* 1882, and *Mitth. k.k. Gesundheitsamt.* Berlin, vol. ii. 1881; Baumgarten, *Berliner klin. Woch.* 1880, and Volkmann's *Sammlung klin. Vorträge*, 1882; Aufrecht, 'Pathologische Mittheilungen.' *Deutsche med. Woch.* 1882, viii. 206; and Watson Cheyne, *Practitioner*, 1883. For instances of fallacies in inoculation resulting from purely accidental contamination, see Klein, *Rep. Med. Off. Privy Council to the Local Government Board*, 1883-4, xiii. 148.

[4] Dawson Williams repeated a series of experiments on guinea-pigs with most of the non-tubercular substances with which I had previously produced tubercle in these animals in 1868, but with an entirely negative result. The animals thus inoculated were, however, carefully kept distinct from those inoculated with tubercle, in a set of hutches made new for the purpose, in a part of the building not previously employed for this object, and a series of fresh trocars was used. Cf. *Lancet* and *Brit. Med. Journ.* Dec. 1883, and *Trans. Path. Soc.* 1884, vol. xxxv.

[5] Villemin, *Études sur la Tuberculose*, p. 567; Baumgarten, *Centralblatt med. Wissensch.* vol. xxxii. Micro-organisms have been found in the blood of tuberculous patients by Weigert, Weichselbaum, and Meisels (*Fortschritte der Medicin*, 1880-3, and *Wien. med. Woch.* 1884); cf. also Pench, *Mém. Acad. Sciences*, 1880; Damsch, *Deutsch. Arch. klin. Med.* 1882 (Spina). For references on the infectiveness of milk, see Cornil and Babes, *Les Bactéries*.

[6] Langhans employed the conjunctiva; *Uebertragbarkeit der Tuberculose auf Kaninchen*, Habilitationsschrift, Marburg, 1867. The employment of the anterior chamber of the eye, which has led to such valuable results, is due to Cohnheim and Salomonsen, *Sitzungsbericht der Schlesisch. Gesellsch. für vaterländische Cultur*, 1877 (Baumgarten); 1878 (Spina), or *Wiener med. Blätter*, 1879 (Klein).

[7] Stricker (*Path. Infections-Krankheiten*) has shown that the introduction into the eye of tuberculous material may occasionally only produce a local effect, and this also was observed by Schottelius, of tuberculous material in

a generalised outbreak of granulations in different organs, and of other changes, identical in their essential features, both anatomical and vital, with those found in generalised tuberculosis in man. The disease thus produced is again capable of being reproduced in other animals, either by direct inoculation with the diseased parts, or by means of fluids cultivated from these, and finally the observations of Schüller have shown that when these substances are introduced into the system a special localisation of their effects may be produced by injury. It is true that non-tubercular substances, when introduced into the serous membranes and other parts, will give rise to local granulations, which, in their chief anatomical structure, closely resemble the earliest forms of some miliary tubercles. They do not, however, produce the generalised disease, and the granulations caused by them are incapable of reproducing the same disease when reinoculated.[1] I believe that all experiments tending to show that they possess either of these properties have been fallacious. Further, they rarely undergo caseation, although this is sometimes observed.[2]

It may therefore be affirmed that the artificial reproduction of generalised tubercle by inoculation, conducted under proper precautions, is a fair and, practically, a conclusive test of the tubercular nature of any pathological product.[3] On this point it is of importance to remark that this property is found to reside in nearly all the morbid products variously classed as tubercular or scrofulous, and concerning whose nature much dispute has prevailed during the past twenty years. It is found in caseous pneumonias, caseous glands, the white swellings of joints, caseous osteomyelitis, the pus of scrofulous abscesses, the caseous (tubercular) testicle, and the large tubercular tumours of the brain.[4] The position of lupus is more doubtful. Cohnheim denied that these effects could be produced by it,[5] but Koch has observed them by direct introduction of lupus-tissue.[6]

The identity of bovine with human tuberculosis has long been and still remains a subject of dispute. Virchow originally believed the two to be different diseases, and has even recently appeared to regard the question as open to discussion.[7] Others also have maintained their diversity,[8] and

---

haled (*Centralblatt med. Wiss.* 1878), and also by Tappeiner under similar conditions (Virchow's *Archiv*, 1878, vol. lxxiv.

[1] A great number of the statements on this subject are based on granulations containing giant-cells, but these bodies, as I have attempted to show (p. 92) cannot be regarded as a test of tubercle. Cf. Martin, *Archives de Phys.* 1881, viii. 58 *et seq.* and *Revue de Méd.* 1882, ii. 280, 908; also Baumgarten, *Zeitschr. f. klin. Med.* 1885, vol. ix. figs. 1, 2. In one of Martin's cases, where irritant non-tubercular matters were injected into the peritoneum, granulations resembling tubercle were formed in the mucous membrane of the intestine. Martin also (*Rev. de Méd.* 1882) found that animals, inoculated with tubercle rendered sterile by exposure to a high temperature, died marasmic but not tubercular. There was probably here some form of septicæmia.

[2] Baumgarten (*Latente Tuberculose*; Volkmann's *Sammlung klin. Vorträge*, No. 218, 1882) says that they never caseate; Martin (*Archiv.de Phys.* 1881) and Stricker (*Infections-Krankheiten*, p. 148) both state that they do.

[3] This test was first proposed by Marcet (*Med.-Chir. Trans.* 1808, vol. vi.) as a mode of distinguishing phthisis by the sputa.

[4] Cohnheim, *Die Tuberculose von Standpunkt der Infections-Lehre*; Koch, *Mitth. k.k. Gesundheitsamt*, vol. ii. and *Congress Med. Wiesbaden*, 1882, p. 61. (Koch did not find bacilli in all cases of fungoid joints, and in the cases in which they were absent, tubercle was not reproduced by inoculation. *Berliner klin. Woch.* 1882, p. 226.) Cf. also Baumgarten, *Latente Tuberculose* Volkmann's *Sammlung klin. Vorträge*, p. 81; Schüller, *Exp. Untersuchungen üb. Gelenkleiden*; Stuttgart, 1880.

[5] Cohnheim, *loc. cit.* p. 16.

[6] Koch, *Mitth. k.k. Gesundheitsamt*, ii. 38. Vidal, on the other hand, failed to inoculate lupus (*Bull. Soc. Méd. Hôp.* 1881, p. 87); see also Kiener, *ib.* p. 64. Baumgarten (Virchow's *Archiv*, lxxxii. 422) denies the tubercular character of lupus, on histological grounds. Koch (*loc. cit.*) and Schüller (*loc. cit.* pp. 62 and 74), however, reproduced tubercle by inoculation with culti-

vated fluids from lupus. Klein (*Micro-organisms and Disease*) considers the bacilli of lupus different from those of tubercle. For other references to lupus, see Cornil and Babes, *Les Bactéries*.

[7] Cf. Virchow, *Die Krankhaften Geschwülste*, vol. ii.; also *Archiv für wissensch. und prakt. Thierheilkunde*, 1880, vol. vi., and *Berliner klin. Woch.* 1880.

[8] The most important of these is Semmer (Virchow's *Archiv*, vol. lxxxii.), who states that the injection of bovine tubercle into pigs reproduced the appearances found in the cow, *whereas ordinarily the tubercle of the pig resembles that of man*, but the disease produced in the sheep by the *same* process resembled human tubercle. The data as regards the natural tubercle of the pig and sheep, and also respecting the effects of inoculation in these animals, appear to be contradictory and uncertain. Förster (*Handbuch path. Anat.* ii. 287) says that there is very little information respecting tubercle in these animals. Rayer (*Archives Méd. Comp.* 1848, i. 194) states that pigs are liable to a form of chronic pneumonia which is a kind of bovine tubercle, an observation confirmed by Koch (*Mitth. k.k. Gesundheitsamt*, ii. 41), who, however, found bacilli in this pneumonia. (Koch does not state the resemblance to the bovine disease.) Virchow (*Berliner klin. Woch.* 1880 and *Archiv Thierheilkunde*, 1880, vol. vi.) states that pigs are liable to enlargement of the cervical, sub-maxillary, mesenteric, and bronchial glands, which is practically identical with scrofula, and that they are also subject to growths in the liver and kidneys resembling tubercle, but whose nature it is difficult to determine. Lydtin and Fleming (*Propagation of Tuberculosis*, p. 49) give similar descriptions, and add that pigs are liable to tubercle of the lungs and intestines, where it assumes the form of nodosities or of caseous degeneration. They quote Baumgärtel (*Sächs. Bericht*, 1881) as having met with a pig whose lungs contained tubercular nodules, but on whose pleura there were growths as large as a pea, resembling those seen in bovine tubercle. The evidence respecting the natural disease in sheep and goats is still more imperfect. Villemin, *Études sur la Tuberculose*, doubted whether

Creighton believes that bovine tuberculosis is a specific disease which is communicable to man, and in the human subject assumes characteristics similar to those found in the cow, so that man is liable not only to human tubercle but also to the disease of cattle. Creighton has not given direct evidence of this mode of communication, but bases his opinion on certain peculiarities of changes ordinarily classed as tubercular, and found in some cases in man which he has examined. The appearances that he describes as characteristic may be occasionally found in post-mortem examinations of tubercular cases, and would, I believe, serve equally as arguments to show the similarity of the two conditions.[1] One point on which Creighton lays especial stress is the presence of giant-cells in bovine tuberculosis, and Baumgarten has also stated that in the inoculation experiments, these are more common in the changes produced with bovine than in those obtained with human tubercle.[2] Giant cells are, however, so common in cases of chronic phthisis in man, that they must be regarded rather as evidence of chronicity than of specificity, and their occurrence in so many and diverse pathological processes necessarily deprives them of any claim to the latter character.[3] It will be seen in the accounts of different organs, particularly of the peritoneum and of the lungs, that giant-cells occur among the results of inoculation with human as well as with bovine tubercle.

Koch has maintained the identity of the bacilli in the two diseases, but Klein has pointed out that they vary in size, and somewhat also in their distribution in the affected parts, and particularly in the fact that bovine bacilli are only found in the interior of the cells of the affected parts, while the bacilli of human tubercle are found in the interstices of these.[4] There can be very little doubt but that (apart from the greater predominance of giant-cells), the results of inoculation and feeding with bovine tubercle are, in nearly all animals, practically identical with those produced by inoculation with human tubercle, and that in the rabbit and guinea-pig they correspond very closely with the original disease in man, and have very little resemblance to that in the cow,[5] and

sheep were liable to tubercle. Lydton and Fleming give some evidence which tends to show that in goats the disease has a tendency to assume the character of bovine tubercle. Bollinger (*Arch. exp. Pathol.* i. 371) says that he has seen spontaneous miliary tubercle in the sheep. Koch (*loc. cit.*) describes tubercular nodules in the sheep's lung and also calcified bronchial glands. In the goat he found cavities. If, owing to peculiarities of the natural tissues in certain animals, spontaneous tubercle assumes in them certain characters, the inoculated disease would probably show the same tendencies.

There are, however, as already stated, but few experiments on the inoculation of human tubercle in the pig and sheep. As regards bovine tubercle, Gerlach (Virchow's *Archiv*, vol. xli.) found in pigs and lambs, fed with the milk of a tubercular cow, changes analogous to those of bovine tuberculosis, including a tendency to calcification in the lamb. Bollinger (*Archiv exp. Pathol.* i. 366-8), from an analysis of cases by different authors, found similar changes in these animals, including sheep and goats; but in some cases of pigs the appearances of gland-affection resembling scrofula were found as described by Virchow. In one the pig had been fed with artificial tubercle from the sheep; in another, miliary tubercle existed. Virchow (*Berliner klin. Woch.* 1880) found in some pigs fed with milk from a tubercular cow only enlarged glands, in others *tubercle*. (Virchow's definition of tubercle must be accepted as excluding other conditions.) In one pig, however, not thus fed, but killed for the sake of comparison, *appearances resembling bovine tubercle* were found. Toussaint (*Comptes Rendus Acad. des Sciences*, 1880 and 1881), in a series of experiments on pigs by feeding, and also by inoculation with bovine tuberculosis, found, in some, extensive gland-enlargement, in one instance with calcification, in others miliary tubercles. The former infected rabbits with ordinary tubercle. Wagner (*Handb. allg. Pathol.* 1876, vol. lxv.) quotes from Zürn that feeding and inoculation with bovine tubercle affects pigs, sheep, and rabbits with miliary tubercle. Bollinger (*Archiv exp. Pathol.* vol. i.) injected bovine tubercle into the peritoneum of two goats and produced miliary tubercle. In another, into

which he injected a human scrofulous gland, he produced appearances more resembling those of the bovine class. Vemguth (*Archiv exp. Pathol.* 1883, xvii. 267-8), in two goats inhaling human phthisical sputa, found larger masses than ordinary, and also calcification in the lungs and omentum, and in one, smooth-walled cavities with much connective tissue. Villemin (*Études*, p. 536) inoculated a sheep with bovine tubercle, and produced appearances of a similar nature but which he attributed to helminthoid worms. Colin (*Bull. Acad. Méd.* 1867) inoculated two sheep with bovine tubercle, but the tubercles thus resulting are not described as characteristic of the source. The mixed character of the appearances found by different observers would argue for the identity of the two diseases.

[1] *Bovine Tuberculosis in Man*, pp. 29, 30. *E.g.* pipe-shaped masses in the lung, which resemble the peri-bronchial tubercle of man; outgrowths, seen in man both in serous and mucous membranes; wedge-shaped masses, also found in man; dilated bronchi forming smooth-walled cavities, also by no means rare in the indurating phthisis of man. I would also refer to his figures in vol. iii. pp. 8, 9, and vol. iv. as common in man. Two of his cases had miliary tubercle, and were only distinguished by some of the peculiarities now mentioned.

[2] Baumgarten, *Zeitsch. klin. Med.* 1885, vol. ix. and separate publication.

[3] See *ante*, p. 92.

[4] *Micro-organisms and Disease*, also *Rep. Med. Off. Privy Council*, 1883, vol. xiii.

[5] See *ante*, note 2, p. 140. For inoculation and feeding see Autrecht (*Path. Mitth.* i. 44), who obtained identical results in rabbits by each process, with both human and bovine tubercle. Visœur and Chauveau (*Bull. Acad. Méd.* 1874) found ordinary tubercle in cats fed with the products of bovine tuberculosis. Orth (Virchow's *Archiv*, lxxvi. 237) failed to produce tubercle in rabbits by feeding with human tubercle, but succeeded with bovine, and remarks on the greater resemblance of the results to the disease than of the latter. He also found giant-cells conspicuous, and likewise the kidney-affection remarked by Klein. Note also that he had affections of the choroid, the iris,

finally Klebs and others have made the converse demonstration that inoculation of heifers with human tubercle has produced in these animals the bovine variety.[1]

The results of cultivation of tubercular tissues have given rise to considerable discussion as regards the organisms with which the production of tubercle is associated, and the question cannot yet be said to be finally settled.

Klebs, who, after Villemin, was one of the first to assert the belief that tubercle originated in a specific virus, regarded these organisms as belonging to the order of micrococci and termed the infecting agent 'Monas tuberculosum,' but he has since maintained that the infecting agent consists of a granular material, in which the rods described by Koch are found.[2] Zürn, Buhl, Aufrecht, and others had described micrococci in tubercle[3] and Schüller[4] has figured them in the tubercular growths of animals infected by inoculation with cultivated fluids. Toussaint[5] also cultivated a micrococcus which apparently produced tubercle by inoculation. Koch, on the other hand, by dry fractional cultivation, has concluded that the infective agent is a bacillus; that it, when inoculated, produces tubercle, and that it is almost universally present in pathological products which give rise to tubercle in this manner (although there are some exceptions to this, to which I shall hereafter allude). A similar bacillus was discovered almost simultaneously and independently by Baumgarten, and has been described by Aufrecht as co-existing with micrococci. The demonstration of its infective qualities after cultivation was, however, first given by Koch.[6]

The proof of the specificity of this bacillus depends, therefore, as Stricker has pointed out,[7] on the following points :—

(1) On its general existence in tubercle.

(2) On its complete isolation, and the demonstration that it differs from all other micro-organisms.

(3) On the proof that among micro-organisms it alone can reproduce tubercle.

The first point may be regarded as being almost conclusively established, although it is not universally demonstrable, and products of a tubercular nature exist, which will produce tubercle by inoculation, in which the bacillus cannot be found. This may be due either to imperfect observation, or, as has been maintained by Koch and Baumgarten, to the fact that the spores of bacilli may be present in these bodies.[8]

---

the brain, and the testicle. Cf. also Baumgarten, *Berliner klin. Woch.* 1880, and *Zeitsch. klin. med.* 1885. Koch's researches with the cultivated bacilli showed the same result. See also, for other references on feeding, Johne, *Geschichte der Tuberculose*; many of these have been inaccessible to me.

[1] Klebs, Virchow's *Archiv*, vol. xlix.; human tubercle affected the peritoneum in a calf. Günther and Harms, *Bericht Thierarzenei-Schule zu Hannover*, vol. vi. 1873; goat fed from tubercle of monkey gave evidence of bovine tubercle. This animal had also meningitis with nodules. A similar result in a goat was obtained by Bollinger; Buhl's *Mitth. aus der Path. Mitth. zu München*, 1878; see also Kitt, quoted by Johne, *Geschichte der Tuberculose*, p. 24. The original of this has been inaccessible to me. In several cases these experiments have failed; ref. Johne ib. p. 24, also Patz, *Beziehungen Tuberculose d. Menschen zur Tub. der Thiere*, 1883, quoted by Johne. In one case in the calf, human tubercle injected into the pleura was followed by granulations which contained tubercle-bacilli, but there was no appearance of bovine tubercle.

[2] Klebs, *Prager Vierteljahrsch.*, 1877. Cf. also especially *Archiv exp. Pathol.* 1880, vol. xvii. and art. 'Tuberculose' in Eulenburg's *Real-Encyclopädie wiss. Heilkunde*, Bd. xiv.

[3] For other authorities I would refer to the works of Johne and Spina (see p. 139), also to Watson Cheyne, *Practitioner*, 1883.

[4] Schüller, however (*loc. cit.* p. 76), found also rod-shaped bacteria in his cultures, but he regarded them as composed of round forms.

[5] Toussaint, *Comptes Rendus*, 1881; Malassez and Vignal (*Archiv. de Physiol. Norm. et Path.* 1883, 3rd sér. vol. ii.) found no bacilli in the subcutaneous tubercle of a child dying of tubercular meningitis. This, inoculated into guinea-pigs, gave tubercle, which showed zoogloeic masses of micrococci, and this appearance was repeated up to the fifth series of re-inoculations. After this, bacilli appeared in the tubercles produced by succeeding inoculations. They also inoculated material obtained from this tubercle by dry culture, with the same result, but they do not positively state whether the organisms found after dry culture of the original tubercle corresponded with those produced by inoculation, although, in the latter, bacilli appeared at the third re-inoculation. (Refer to Klein on Fallacies.) See also Reinstadler, *Archiv exp. Pathol.* 1879, vol. xi. It may be recalled that Grohe (*Berliner klin. Woch.* 1870) produced a generalised disease resembling tubercle by injections of *Penicillium glaucum* and *Aspergillus glaucus*, and in the nodules thus produced he found fungi. Wolff also (Virchow's *Archiv*, vol. lxvii.), by injecting putrid 'Pasteur's fluid,' produced destruction of the lung and diffuse growth in the liver, but these were probably pyæmic.

[6] Koch, *Berliner klin. Woch.* 1882, No. 15, April 10; Baumgarten, *Centralblatt med. Wissensch.* April 15, Nov. 15 and 19; Aufrecht, *Path. Mittheilungen*, 1881; *Deutsche med. Woch.* 1882; *Centralblatt med. Wissensch.* 1882.

[7] *Path. Infects.-Krankh.* 180. I have stated the case in somewhat different terms.

[8] On absence of bacilli in infective material, cf. Koch; *Mitth. k.k. Gesundheitsamt.* ii. 17; Baumgarten, *Zeitsch. klin. Med.* 1885, ix. 105. Koch's observations on lupus show that the bacilli may be extremely few in number. König (*Tuberculose der Knochen und Gelenke*, 1884, pp. 27 and 13) says that bacilli are often wanting in typical cases of tuberculosis of bones and joints, and that

The complete isolation by Koch's method is as yet a subject of discussion, but it may be regarded as approximately obtained.[1] The absolute distinction of the bacillus from other organisms rests on its mode of growth, its microscopical character, and its chemical reactions. The first of these appears to separate it from putrefactive organisms, but on its size and characters some diversity of opinion still exists,[2] and the final test—the special reaction to aniline dyes—though at present apparently established, is one on which it may at least be desirable to await further research.[3]

The last point also, that the bacillus, as defined by Koch, is the only agent capable of producing tubercle, has been strongly supported by Baumgarten and is very generally accepted. The observations of Klebs deserve, however, further investigation,[4] but it may at least be held as proved that, whether or not the developed bacillus be the sole agent, it is capable of producing this effect after every effort to ensure purity of culture, and that Klebs' organisms may possibly only represent stages in the development. Further, in some tubercles produced by Toussaint, Watson Cheyne found that Koch's bacilli were the sole micro-organisms discoverable, and failed to produce tubercle with specimens of Toussaint's fluids from which these bacilli were absent.[5]

Results of Inoculation.—The variety of animals in which tubercles have been produced by the best test of the tubercular nature of a doubtful case is its inoculability; Stricker (*Infectionx-Krankheiten*, p. 182) shows that they are not to be found in *all* tubercles in the omentum of the same monkey, but in these he found spores which showed the characteristic colour-reaction; Koch (*Mitth. k.k. Gesundheitsamt*, ii. 22) says that spores do not colour; Klein (*Micro-organisms and Disease*, 1885, p. 125) has also stated that bacilli are not invariably to be found in young tubercles; cf. also *Rep. Med. Off. Privy Council, Local Government Board*, 1883, xiii. 180. Klein even questions whether the bacilli do not cause a poison which produces the disease independently of their presence at any particular spot. They are most abundant in caseous matter, but then they are of later formation, for sometimes they are only found in the seats of inoculation when internal organs are also affected. Watson Cheyne (*Practitioner*, 1883, i. 308) says that the bacilli are not contained in the lymphatic growths in the lung, described by Klein (see later), but only in the epithelioid growths, and that the former are therefore not tubercular. I shall allude to this question hereafter, but would only remark here that, according to Klein's observations, the lymphatic growth in the lung is the first indication of the disease produced by inoculation with tubercular matter. Baumgarten's dictum 'without bacteria no tubercle, and without tubercle no bacteria,' can only therefore be stated as an approximating truth, and the statement that the bacilli are necessary as a test of tubercle, as affirmed by Koch, *Berliner klin. Woch.* 1882, p. 228, would exclude some bodies which correspond to the other test of inoculation.

[1] Cf. Creighton and Watson Cheyne, 'Discussion on Tubercle,' *Proc. Roy. Med. and Chir. Soc.* 1885, vol. i. This question turned on the relative value of the dry method for eliminating a possible tubercular poison apart from bacilli. Klein's observations on the cultivations of organisms growing in infusions of jequirity (the poison of which is independent of organisms) shows that the poison is not easy to eliminate by the dry method. Cf. *Rep. Med. Off. Privy Council, Local Government Board*, 1883-4, xiii, 146. On other micro-organisms in the lung cf. Gaffky, *Mitth. k.k. Gesundheitsamt*, 1884, vol. ii.

[2] Koch (*Berliner klin. Woch.* and *Mitth. k.k. Gesundheitsamt*, ii, 15, 16 *et seq.*) describes them as from ·0015 mm. to ·0035 mm. ($\frac{1}{7000}$ to $\frac{1}{3000}$ inch), or from one quarter to one-half of the diameter of a human red blood-corpuscle, but sometimes they may attain the length of the whole diameter of such a corpuscle. In width they are about one-fifth this length (*Cong. Med. Wiesbaden*, 1882, p. 60). Some show beads, and others modifications of a corkscrew twisting, shapes which Koch considers distinguish them from other bacilli. They resemble the bacilli of leprosy, but are sharper and more pointed at the ends, and do not colour with Weigert's 'nuclear colouring material,' as the leprosy-bacilli do. They have molecular but not independent movements, and they form spores. Aufrecht (*Path. Mitth.* 1887, p. 42, and *Deutsche med. Woch.* 1882) described, amongst other micro-organisms in tubercle, smaller rods, short glistening bodies, whose long diameter scarcely exceeded by one-half that of the transverse diameter. Koch denies that these are the genuine bacilli, but it must be remembered that they are found in tubercle, and Aufrecht (*Congress. Inn. Med. Wiesbaden*, 1882, p. 68) points out that Baumgarten's bacilli, as drawn to scale, have a length of from one-half to twice as great as their width. Baumgarten (*Centralblatt*, 1882) described them as resembling Bacterium termo, but longer and narrower and often globular at the end, and not colouring with Weigert's solution. Watson Cheyne (*Practitioner*, 1883, i. 269) describes the longest as about $\frac{1}{1000}$ inch and in width from $\frac{1}{8}$ to $\frac{1}{6}$ of this length, more or less rounded at their ends, beaded, generally straight but sometimes curved. He does not mention the corkscrew-like appearance described by Koch. For some further general remarks on this subject, see also Koch, *Deutsche med. Woch.* 1883.

[3] That the methods of colouring, and the views entertained respecting them, have undergone considerable change, see Watson Cheyne, *Practitioner*, 1883, and Baumgarten, *Zeitsch. klin. Med.* 1885, vol. ix. Through all, however, with some exceptions, the constancy and peculiarity of the mode of staining of the tubercle-bacilli has obtained. Koch (*Mitth. k.k. Gesundheitsamt*, ii. 12, 13) states that he does not regard the colour-test as absolute, and admits that other bacteria may be found hereafter possessing the same characteristics, but holds that the bacteria possess other vital properties which distinguish them. He has shown that some spores in the intestine have the same colour-reactions. Klein, also (*Rep. Med. Off. Privy Council*, 1883-4, p. 178), has found micrococci in urine with the same reaction, but did not produce tubercle by their inoculation. Stricker, however, points out that this essentially depends on one point, viz. the resistance of the bacilli thus coloured to the action of nitric acid, which, however, he appears to consider may be shared by other substances, and further that, as Spina has shown, the bacilli of putrefaction acquire this property of resisting nitric acid by digestion in solutions of tannin. It is, as Stricker remarks, still questionable whether other external conditions may not equally have this influence. The colour-test of the bacilli may be regarded as practically established, but their specificity, in the sense of an unchanged uniformity of propagation, is a point on which it appears to the author yet early to pronounce an opinion on the evidence before us.

[4] Klebs, *loc. cit.*

[5] On a case in which micrococci were found, together with bacilli, in miliary tuberculosis, see Koch, *Mitth. k.k.*

inoculation is very considerable. Guinea-pigs are the creatures in which the process is most successful; they are even more susceptible than rabbits. Carnivora are the least so, but tubercles have been produced in dogs and cats. They have also been produced in monkeys, pigs, sheep, goats, calves, a foal, mice, rats, moles, fowls, and pigeons. Koch's researches have shown that dogs, rats, and white mice resist the tubercular virus, and require larger doses for their infection, while the field-mouse is very susceptible. Hedgehogs, and also fishes and other cold-blooded animals, appear to be insusceptible of the poison. Among these animals, it is worthy of remark that some of those most susceptible to inoculation, viz. guinea-pigs[1] and rabbits, are very little liable to spontaneous tubercle. Koch says that it only occurs when they are kept with other tuberculous animals, and Baumgarten only saw three instances in between three hundred and four hundred post-mortems.[2]

In describing the appearances observed, I have to state that since I published my own account of these, further and elaborate investigations have been made on this subject by Burdon-Sanderson,[3] Klein,[4] Hering,[5] and more recently by Baumgarten,[6] and I have had in many particulars to supplement my own observations by theirs, as well as by those of other authors to whom I shall have to allude. It may be stated that in a large proportion of cases, where subcutaneous inoculation is practised, a local production of granulations of a tubercular nature is observed. In the eye and the serous membranes this is constant when the inoculation is effectual.

Eye.—In the eye, Baumgarten's recent observations may be taken as a type of the process. If the cornea only be wounded, this shows the first changes. If the injection be made into the anterior chamber, tubercle of the iris follows. As the process may be watched throughout in the iris, I shall follow Baumgarten's description.[7]

After the introduction of the infective material into the anterior chamber through the cornea, the wound of the latter closes. Within the next forty-eight hours a multiplication of bacilli is observed; they penetrate the tract of the wound, invade the fixed cells of the iris and cornea, and are also seen free in the intercellular substance, and within the ciliary processes, the ciliary body, and also the sphincter and dilator of the iris, but they are densest in the neighbourhood of the wound. No indications of other micro-organisms are seen, and the bacilli are free, not enclosed in migratory cells, as Koch believed. By the sixth day, the cells of the tissue commence to show changes, and accumulations of epithelial cells occur in spots where the bacilli are densest. By the fourteenth day, tubercular masses are formed, partly consisting of epithelial cells and partly resembling Virchow's typical figure of lymphoid cells, but the tubercle-formation here is always associated with the presence of bacilli. The first alteration in the cells commences with nuclear changes and enlargement of the fixed cells of the iris and cornea, of the connective-tissue cells and the endothelium of the iris and vessels, and of the epithelial cells on the posterior surface of the iris. The nuclear changes commence with 'karyokinesis and karyomitosis,'[8] which proceed to

Gesundheitsamt, ii. 26. Koch thinks some mixed infection was present here. Cf. also Watson Cheyne, *loc. cit.* p. 295.

[1] Klein (*Rep. Med. Off. Privy Council to Local Government Board*, 1888-4, p. 182) has found that pregnant guinea-pigs resist inoculation. Villemin observed that rabbits were more susceptible to bovine than to human tubercle (*Etudes*, p. 538). This is confirmed by Klein, who finds also (*Rep. Med Off.* 1883-4, pp. 127-185, and also *Rep.*, 1884-5) that both by feeding and by inoculation there is a difference between guinea-pigs and rabbits with respect to human tubercle and bovine tuberculosis. Both are more quickly affected by the latter, but guinea-pigs are easily and extensively affected by human tubercle, while rabbits resist this and are considerably affected by bovine tubercle, which in them also affects the kidneys more commonly than in guinea-pigs. Koch, (*Mitth.k.k.Gesundheitsamt*, ii. 44) speaks of tubercle of the kidneys as being generally more common, after infection, in rabbits than in guinea-pigs, but makes no distinction as to the material employed. Baumgarten (*Tuberkel und Tuberkulose*, p. 80) speaks of the cortical substance of the rabbit's kidney as presenting some peculiarities.

[2] Baumgarten, *Berliner klin. Woch.* 1880; Koch, *ib.* 1882. Koch states that in these cases it always commences in the lungs and bronchial glands. In the lungs there are single large caseous masses, passing into cavities. Koch has reported several cases of this nature. Favre (*Gaz. Méd.* 1854, p. 418) has described spontaneous tubercle of the guinea-pig in the liver, spleen, and mesenteric glands; cf. also Goujon, quoted by Burdon-Sanderson. *Eleventh Rep. Med. Off. Privy Council*, 1868, p. 137; Günther and Harms, *Jahresb. Thierarzneischule*, Hannover, 1873, vol. vi.; likewise Köster, Kuge, and Bernhardt, quoted by Hering, *Exp. Studien Tuberculose*, pp. 14, 15.

[3] *Tenth and Eleventh Rep. Med. Off. Privy Council*, 1867-8. The result of the first series of Burdon-Sanderson's observations was published by him (*Path. Soc. Trans.* 1867) a few weeks prior to the publication of my own.

[4] Klein, *The Anatomy of the Lymphatic System*, 1875.

[5] Hering. *Studien über Tuberculose*, Berlin. 1878.

[6] Baumgarten, *Zeitsch. klin. Med.* 1885, vol. ix.; also as a separate publication, *Tuberkel und Tuberculose*.

[7] Baumgarten refers to a paper by Hänssell, Von Gräfe's *Archiv f. Oph.* vol. xxv.

[8] Terms referring to alterations in the fibrillar texture of the nuclei; cf. Klein's *Elements of Histology*, for

division and multiplication of the cells, giving rise to masses of an epithelioid character derived entirely from this process of division, and which are advanced by the ninth day. Baumgarten insists that migratory cells take no part in the first formation of these cell-masses.

Bacilli may be found in small cells undergoing these changes, but when they are abundant in a cell, this shows no tendency to division. The epithelioid cells frequently show multiple nuclei, but giant-cells are not produced, except after inoculation with bovine tuberculosis.

The next change is the formation of a reticulum between the tubercle-cells, which Baumgarten says may be seen in frozen specimens, and is not, therefore, an artificial product, due, as some have believed, to hardening agents. In the centre of the mass this intercellular substance is less apparent. It is not constituted by processes from the cells, which remain everywhere round. The bacilli are most abundant in the centre of the mass, the periphery becomes encapsuled by a flattening of the external layer of cells as well as of those of the surrounding tissue. With the encapsuling, the cell-multiplication in these masses diminishes, but leucocytes increase. The latter come from the blood-vessels: they do not show multiplication except in isolated instances, but tend to break down. Baumgarten asserts that the epithelioid cells of tubercle are derived from the fixed cells of the tissue.

Although the growth of the bacilli appears to be arrested by the encapsuling of the periphery, it continues in the centre, and at the same time the invasion of leucocytes proceeds until the mass presents the characters of Virchow's small-celled tubercle.[1] The epithelioid structures, however, remain at first distinct, except in the centre, where they are masked by the increase of leucocytes and bacilli, and after a time they are obscured generally by leucocytes throughout the tubercle. In the leucocytes no bacilli are present, although these are found in the interior of the epithelioid cells.

The caseation of the tubercle commences with shrivelling of the leucocytes, whose nuclei have divided until they present the characters of pus-cells. They then break down, while their nuclei lose their power of taking up colouring matter, but they do not constitute abscesses. The epithelioid elements undergo a similar change, and fuse together into shapeless masses in which bacilli multiply. At first, as Weigert has described, the cheesy mass resembles in its reactions a coagulated albuminous substance, but it finally liquefies—a process which is preceded by a fibrinous exudation on the anterior surface of the iris.

Baumgarten states that giant-cells are formed in the iris only when the inoculation has been with the products of bovine tuberculosis. He does not regard them as indicating any specificity[2] or difference in the form of tuberculosis, but attributes them to the slighter infecting power of the agent, and its comparative paucity in bacilli, in consequence of which the process is less acute, and the division of the epithelioid cells is less rapid. This is borne out by the fact that giant-cells are more abundant in the more chronic processes of human tubercle, and in those conditions in which the number of bacilli is small or their infective power is weakened. He denies that the giant-cells arise from fusion, and attributes the peripheral arrangement of the nuclei in them, which distinguishes these bodies in tubercle from most others of a similar nature but different origin, to the presence of bacilli in their centre, there being, as Koch has stated,[3] a certain degree of antagonism between the positions of bacilli and of the nuclei.

In the cornea, the process varies in details according to its intensity, and modifications are caused by the presence of the wound. When the extension is watched from the iris in cases of medium intensity, the bacilli are seen to spread through the layers of the cornea, followed by an epithelioid growth, arising from the cornea-cells; this forms typical tubercle-masses, undergoing the same changes, including encapsuling, as are observed in the iris. In many cases, however, an invasion of leucocytes takes place early and obscures this growth. The invasion occurs in the first place by cells derived from the conjunctiva at the margin, also from vessels of new formation extending from the sclerotic. Baumgarten denies that these migratory cells undergo multiplication, or take any part in the formation of the epithelioid cells, and states that the fixed cells of the tissue are those in which the growth of the tubercle first commences. In some cases, in

---

various references and figures, also Flemming, *Archiv microscop. Anat.* vols. xvi. xviii. xxiii. xxiv.; also his work, *Kern- und Zelltheilung*, 1882. Baumgarten appears to find this process almost constant.

[1] See *ante*, p. 83.

[2] Creighton (*Bovine Tuberculosis*) regards the giant-cells as one of the indications of a specific character in bovine tuberculosis. Cf. *ante*, note 2, p. 144, on the susceptibility of rabbits to bovine tubercle.

[3] Koch, *Mitth. k.k. Gesundheitsamt.* ii. 16.

that situation, the process is much retarded, and the formation of granulation-tissue may precede that of the tubercle. The bacilli subsequently penetrate this granulation-tissue and induce tubercle-formation in it.

The Peritoneum.—The peritoneum was chosen by Klebs[1] as the seat of his inoculations, and his observations have been repeated by Burdon-Sanderson, Klein and Kiener,[2] and also by Cohnheim and Fränkel.[3] With some differences to be hereafter alluded to, the results obtained by injection of tubercle into the abdominal cavity resemble closely those found when the inoculation is performed in other parts. In a few cases, as observed by Cohnheim and Fränkel, a circumscribed abscess forms, from which the tubercular granulations extend in radiating lines. In the majority of instances, however, a disseminated tuberculosis is produced, affecting the omentum, the mesentery, the *centrum tendineum* of the diaphragm, and the peritoneal covering of the abdominal viscera; but in the guinea-pig when a large amount of infective fluid is injected, the omentum may form a solid mass resembling an enlarged and caseous lymphatic gland.[4] In a considerable number of cases there is but little exudation.[5] In some instances, however, ascites is present, probably due, as Lebert believed, to the impaired circulation in the liver.[6] The nodules are usually of a small size, miliary, not exceeding a pin's-head or a millet-seed, and semi-transparent, but they may attain considerable dimensions and become caseous masses (which, in some cases observed by Koch, consisted largely or almost entirely of bacilli[7]), and they are frequently associated with caseation of the mesenteric glands. In some cases, when the injection is made into the pleura, they appear as villous growths, and a similar appearance has been observed in the peritoneum.[8]

There has been considerable discussion concerning the precise seat of the tubercles in the peritoneum. In my original observations I noticed them around the vessels, commencing in the perivascular sheath, and extending thence to the surrounding tissue, and I also observed them originating independently of the blood-vessels.[9] Burdon-Sanderson had previously noted their connection with the vessels, but believed that their seat was external to the adventitia, and was in the connective tissue, which, loaded with fat-cells, surrounds this structure, and he subsequently found that they arose, not from the adventitia of arteries, but from the adenoid tissue surrounding the veins.[10] Kiener, however, has stated that when they surround capillaries, they originate from the endothelium of these. Burdon-Sanderson[11] observed that the newly-formed tissue was highly vascular, and Kiener noticed the formation of new vessels as part of the process.

All observers had remarked that a growth of nodules occurred independently of the blood-vessels,[12] and an important advance was made by Klebs[13] in recognising that they were formed from the endothelium of the lymphatics. The cells became enlarged and also germinated, sometimes forming giant-cells and sometimes masses of small cells covered by the superficial endothelium[14] which commonly isolated, situated on one side of the vessel or sometimes surrounding it, and occupying the whole or a portion of its wall. He appears (p. 800) to have recognised, as an independent mode of growth, that described by Burdon-Sanderson as commencing in the adipose tissue external to the artery. Klebs (Virchow's *Archiv*, xliv. 288) describes them in the perivascular sheath, which he says has a lymphatic structure, but the bulk of the tubercle appeared to be external to this. He quotes Colin as describing a perivascular growth of omental tubercle. (Colin's observations are in *Gazette Méd. de Paris*, 1867; also in the *Bull. Acad. Méd.* 1867, and *Union Médicale*, 1868)

---

[1] Klebs, Virchow's *Archiv*, vol. xliv.
[2] Kiener, *Archiv Physiol. Norm. et Path.* 1880, 2nd ser. T. vii. Cf. also Hippolyte Martin, *ib.* 1881, 2nd ser. vol. viii., and also *Rech. Anat. Path. Tubercle.*
[3] Cohnheim and Fränkel, Virchow's *Archiv*, vol. xlv.
[4] Koch, *Mitth. k.k. Gesundheitsamt*, ii. 71. A similar appearance, after feeding, is recorded by Orth, Virchow's *Archiv*, vol. lxxvi. p. 231. See also Villemin, *Études sur la Tuberculose*, 561, and Von Waldenburg, *Die Tuberculose*, p. 395. Koch describes these cheesy masses as crowded with bacilli.
[5] Cf. especially Klebs' experiments. Koch (*loc. cit.* p. 71) says that exudation is rare in the peritoneum of guinea-pigs, though common in dogs and cats. In the pleura of the guinea-pig, however, he found large fluid exudations.
[6] Lebert and Wyss, Virchow's *Archiv*, vol. xl.
[7] Koch, *Berliner klin. Woch.* 1882, vols. ix. xii.
[8] Concerning the omentum, see Klein, *Anatomy of Lymphatic System*, i. 79, 80; for the pleura, *ib.* part ii. p. 40; for the peritoneum, Kiener, *loc. cit.*; also Bollinger, Duhl's *Mitth. Path. Institut München*, 1878, p. 200. A scrofulous gland (human), injected into the peritoneal cavity of a goat, produced villous growths exactly like those seen in bovine tuberculosis.
[9] Compare *Lect. Coll. Phys.* pl. iii. figs. 1-3.
[10] *Tenth Rep. Med. Off. Privy Council*, 1867, p. 127, and *Eleventh Rep. ib.* 1868, p. 109. This refers to secondary granulations. Kiener describes them as
[11] Burdon-Sanderson, *Eleventh Rep. Med. Off. Privy Council*, 1868, p. 122. Cf. also Klein. *loc. cit.* part i. p. 81.
[12] Kiener noticed that the nodules occasionally formed around nerves. This may probably be explained by the fact observed by Klein, that nerves in the peritoneum are sometimes invaginated in lymphatics.
[13] Klebs, Virchow's *Archiv*, vol. xlii.
[14] Burdon-Sanderson (*Eleventh Rep. Med. Off. Privy Council*, p. 119) has figured epithelium covering a tubercular nodule. Baumgarten describes it also as at first unchanged, though later undergoing atrophy. Kiener states that the nodules subsequently penetrate this covering. There is still some ambiguity about the use of the term 'epithelium.' Schäfer prefers to retain that of 'epithelium' with the same significance as 'endothelium' for the super-

Martin and Kiener state may be brushed unchanged from the tubercular nodule beneath. Burdon-Sanderson disputed Klebs's view, and stated that the growth in the peritoneum arose from masses of adenoid tissue normally existing in the omentum. Klein has shown that, though nodules resembling follicular tissue are found in the omentum and peritoneum, there are other groups of cell-structures in the connective-tissue ground-substance, which cannot be included in this category, and that the formation of the tubercular granulations occurs in various ways. During the process, germination occurs in the endothelium of the stomata and pseudo-stomata, and extends to that lining the lymphatic capillaries of which the latter are the opening. At the same time, the peri- and endo-lymphangeal nodules and cords, normally existing in the tissue, show an increase both of their branched cells and also of their lymphatic cells, and the outgrowths from these may form secondary cords and nodules covered with germinating endothelium. Growth also occurs in the branched cells of the connective tissue ('matrix,' Klein). Some of these enlarge, and may form 'myeloplaxes' or large multi-nucleated cells, while others become vacuolated and either change into lymphatic vessels, or elongate to form blood-vessels. There is thus a new formation both of blood and lymphatic vessels. Kiener's description corresponds in this respect with Klein's in the statement that the tubercle forms from the connective-tissue cells, from masses of lymphatic cells nominally existing in the tissue, and from the fat-cells.

Klein has further observed that in tuberculisation produced by direct injection into the peritoneum, the first change observed is the germination of the endothelium of the stomata and pseudo-stomata, whereas, when the tuberculosis of the peritoneum occurs as part of a constitutional affection, this is only seen subsequently to changes in the other elements of the tissue.

Baumgarten[1] has described the process as beginning by the migration of bacilli into the fixed connective-tissue cells and also into the basis-substance of the omentum. With this commences 'karyomitosis' of these cells and of the endothelium of the capillaries. The epithelioid cells form from the changes in and proliferation of the fixed cells, and giant-cells are observed if the inoculation has been with bovine tubercle.[2] Penetration of lymphoid cells and white corpuscles into the tubercular nodule, and subsequent caseation, occur later, and in a manner similar to that observed by him in the iris. It is well to remember, however, in relation to the agency of bacilli, that the peritoneum is one of the seats where extensive tuberculisation may occur without the recognisable presence of these organisms.[3]

Subcutaneous inoculations tend to produce, in rabbits, a cheesy pus, probably from the admixture of septic products. In other cases, however, and also in the guinea-pig, it is not uncommon to find a local subcutaneous production of granulations identical in their essential characters with those found in other parts.[4] They vary in size from less than a poppy-seed to that of a hemp-seed. Some are semi-transparent throughout, others are altogether yellow and opaque. Some are yellow in the centre, but with a semi-transparent margin. Large nodules, the size of a pea, caseous in some parts, indurated in others, are also met with, and present a striking resemblance to changed lymphatic glands. The granulations also form conglomerate masses. The larger nodules and masses are commonly found near the seat of injury. The smaller granulations are scattered around these, and sometimes extend to the neighbouring lymphatic glands, around which they are grouped in masses of variable size. Some of these masses appear to soften into a caseous semi-fluid material.

In addition to the granulations, cords of induration are seen, extending to variable depths and for variable distances through the subcutaneous and muscular tissue. They may be firm and semi-transparent, but their central portions are often caseous. Sometimes they form varicose

---

ficial cells covering a serous membrane. Cf. Quain and Sharpey's *Anatomy*, 8th ed. 1876, p. 48.

[1] *Zeitsch. klin. Med.* vols. ix. x. Sep. Pub. p. 112.

[2] It must be remembered that Klebs (*loc. cit.*) observed giant-cells from inoculation with human tubercle. Klein also observed 'myeloplaxes,' but he does not state the nature of the material used. Frerichs (*Beiträge zur Lehre Tuberculose*, Marburg, 1882) injecting human phthisical sputa into a rabbit's peritoneum, obtained giant-cells.

[3] Stricker, *Allg. Path. Infections-Krankheiten*, p. 132 ; Klein, *Rep. Med. Off. Local Government Board*, 1888-4,

xiii. 180, obs. vii.—bacilli very scanty in tubercle of omentum.

[4] See *Lect. Coll. Phys.* pl. i. figs. 6 and 7. The local subcutaneous production of tubercle-granulations was described by Villemin, *Etudes sur la Tuberculose*, p. 594 ; also by Lebert, Virchow's *Archiv*, xl. 557 and by Burdon-Sanderson, *Eleventh Rep. Med. Off. Privy Council*, 1868, Langhans (*Ueebertragbarkeit Tuberculose auf Kaninchen*, Habilitations-schrift, Marburg, 1867) inoculated under the conjunctiva. Here pp. 39-40 he found also small granulations. See also Chauveau, quoted by Lépine, *Pneumonic Caseuse*, p. 78.

dilatations reaching to the lymphatic glands; sometimes cords extend from the cheesy lymphatic glands into the surrounding tissue.[1]

The structure of these granulations shows in their centre a mass of closely pressed cells of which the nuclei alone are visible. More peripherally, these cells are found to lie in the meshes of a finely fibrillated tissue, and each space, as Burdon-Sanderson has described, may contain two or more cells. In some places also these meshes may contain single cells, thus resembling the 'cytogenic tissue' of His. Burdon-Sanderson has stated that the meshes become wide at the periphery, where they enclose a greater number of cells than in the central parts.

The cells at the centre, as I have stated, are small and densely packed. They vary from $\frac{1}{7000}$ to $\frac{1}{6000}$ of an inch in diameter. Those at the periphery are larger, and vary from $\frac{1}{7000}$ to $\frac{1}{5000}$ inch, and many have double nuclei. They are epithelioid in character, as was noticed by Lebert.[2] The nuclei are tolerably uniform, varying from $\frac{1}{30000}$ to $\frac{1}{25000}$ of an inch. Their outline is sharp and well-defined, and their contents glistening and refractive. The larger cells are sometimes finely granular.

Throughout the granulations many of the cells, and also the nuclei, are seen in various stages of fatty degeneration. The fat is sometimes in drops, sometimes in a finely molecular form. This change is most common towards the centre of the granulations, but it is also seen in cells irregularly scattered through the adjacent tissue. In the granulations under the conjunctiva (after inoculation with human tubercle), Langhans noticed physalides and giant-cells.

In some of these granulations, and also in their neighbourhood, there may be occasionally observed peculiar strings of rows or cells and nuclei. Sometimes cells, sometimes apparently only nuclei, are visible. The cells are of the type of the smaller round kind. The row or string appears to be bound by a limiting membrane. The diameter of these rows is twice or three times that of a capillary. They have no fibrous investment like a vein, no muscular coat like an artery. Their appearance suggests that they are lymphatics distended by a growth of cells.[3]

Burdon-Sanderson has described other granulations in the loose connective tissue between the muscular and tendinous layers, which he regards as different in character from the foregoing, and of an inflammatory nature, indicated by the larger size of the cells, and their obvious development from connective-tissue corpuscles, together with the absence of reticulum.

Direct injection into the veins produces a generalised disease, chiefly affecting the lung. Injection into the joints also produces local tuberculosis, which may become generalised, and Schüller has found that after injection into the blood, either of tubercular matter or of culture from this, an injury to a joint is capable of localising a tubercular process in the injured part, closely resembling the scrofulous and tubercular joint-disease that occurs spontaneously in man—including the gelatinous swelling of the synovial membrane and the formation of caseous masses in the bones. The tubercular growths were characterised by epithelioid cells and giant-cells, but the latter were variable in number and appearance.[4]

The chief secondary affections observed are in the lymphatic glands, the lungs, liver, spleen, kidneys, intestines, and serous membranes. Many other secondary affections have been met with, some of a tubercular nature, others less distinctive, but akin to those of scrofula. Among the former may be mentioned tubercle of the choroid (from subcutaneous inoculation and feeding), of the meninges, the testicle, and in some cases of the bones[5] and uterus.[6] Von Waldenburg described

---

[1] See *Lect. Coll. Phys.* pl. i. fig. 7.
[2] *Ib.* pl. iii. fig. 7. In my description, I stated that these parts resembled the elementary structure of a lymphatic gland. Burdon-Sanderson considers the comparison imperfect, as the fibres are coarser and contain groups of cells. He failed to find the structure which I have figured.
[3] *Ib.* pl. iii. fig. 6. Burdon-Sanderson has figured these cells, *Rep. Med. Off. Privy Council*, 1868, vol. vii.
[4] For further details I must refer to Schüller's work, *Experimentelle und histologische Untersuchungen über scrofulöse und tuberculöse Gelenkleiden*, Stuttgart, 1880.
[5] CHOROID: Cohnheim and Fränkel. Virchow's *Archiv*, xlv. 218. Orth (Virchow's *Archiv*, lxxvi. 233) speaks of them as frequent in the choroid, and as having occurred once in the iris (experiments with feeding.) See also Von Waldenburg, *Die Tuberculose*, p. 334. MENINGES: Günther and Harms, *Bericht Thierarzeneischule zu Hannover*, 1873, p. 57. Orth (*loc. cit.*) found two cases of tubercle of the brain. TESTICLE: Orth, *loc. cit.* BONES—Ribs: Villemin, *Rech. sur la Tuberculose*, p. 587.—Periosteum of Orbit: Von Waldenburg, *Die Tuberculose*, p. 312; Caries, *ib.* p. 275 (this was by injection with non-tubercular material). Hering (*Studien über Tuberculose*, p. 55) caries of vertebræ. Baumgarten speaks of it as common.
[6] I met with this in two cases. The interior of the uterus was filled with caseous matter, and tubercular granulations existed in the sub-mucous and intertubular tissues.—*Lect. Coll. Phys.* p. 17.

peculiar skin affections and also keratitis. His cases of this nature resulted from apparent infection with indifferent substances; but, as Hering obtained similar results from inoculations with tubercle, it is probable that Von Waldenburg's cases arose from accidental infection in the manner before suggested.[1]

Of the *lymphatic glands*, it may be stated that those are almost invariably affected which lie in the direct tract of the lymph-current proceeding from the seat of local infection. Thus, in the eye, the submaxillary and cervical glands suffer, and in subcutaneous inoculations a similar rule is observed. It was also noted by Klebs that, in experiments with feeding, the mesenteric glands suffered to a predominant degree. The affection of the glands is usually also proportioned, in distribution and degree, to that of the organs to which they stand in physiological relation; but some exceptions occur, as I have myself observed, in which a generalised affection of a large proportion of the glands occurs, without any such apparent connection.[2]

The glands affected present a great increase in size; they may be found forty to fifty times their natural weight, and may be five or six times their natural dimensions.[3] The enlargement is also shown by the apparent multiplication of glands where none are naturally discoverable. The early changes appear occasionally to consist in a vascular swelling, and this may at once pass into suppuration.[4] Burdon-Sanderson observed that suppuration was found in glands adjacent to subcutaneous abscesses, but that it did not occur in the internal glands, or in those situated subcutaneously, unless in proximity to such abscesses.

In advanced stages they are found on section to be indurated, and to present a glistening, homogeneous, quasi-cartilaginous appearance, showing very little distinction between the cortical and medullary portions. Through them are scattered specks, lines, or streaks of caseous degeneration, which may form masses the size of a pea,[5] and these masses may soften into a creamy, diffluent material. The enlargement appears to take place by a thickening of the capsule, within which fresh growth of glandular tissue occurs.[6] Baumgarten has described[7] the changes in the cervical lymphatics in the earliest moment of secondary infection from the eye, as consisting, in the first place, of the finest specks of a yellowish-grey colour in the cortical substance, which otherwise presents the normal appearance. These specks enlarge, and become slightly prominent whitish nodules, which increase in size and number with the swelling of the gland, and show caseous change in their centre. From the cortical, they gradually invade the medullary substance, and in both regions, by confluence, they form large cheesy masses. These masses are at first hard and firm, so that the gland has been said to resemble a 'fresh potato,' but later they break down into a soft cheesy mass. Baumgarten believes that the mesenteric glands are infected in some cases directly from the blood, and in such cases the medullary substance is primarily affected, the variation being due to the difference in the channel by which the infection reaches the gland, the peripheral parts suffering first when this occurs through the lymph-current.

The histology of the process in the glands after inoculation has been also most fully described by the same observer. In the earliest stages, bacilli are found free in the lacunæ of the reticulum, but predominantly in the fixed cells of this structure, and also in the cells of the capillary walls. They are not found in the lymphatic corpuscles. With invasion of the bacilli, there commences a proliferation of the fixed cells of the reticulum, out of which masses of epithelioid cells are formed. These are either round or cubical, star-shaped or spindle-shaped. In the latter case their processes pass into the trabeculæ of the reticulum. Bacilli are found in their interior, and the white granulations in the cortex are formed of these accumulations of epithelioid cells. Multiplication does not occur in the lymphatic corpuscles, which gradually disappear with the increase of the epithelioid cells. These latter also show multiplication of their nuclei, and by

---

[1] See Von Waldenburg's *Die Tuberculose*, pp. 800-364. Hering (*Studien über Tuberculose*, p. 55) observed a skin disease resembling lupus, inflammation of the eye, ulceration of the cornea, and also periostitis, pericarditis, and endocarditis. (It is probable that these latter were septic.)
[2] See Villemin, *Etudes sur la Tuberculose*, p. 548; Von Waldenburg, *Die Tuberculose*, pp. 334, 343.
[3] Burdon-Sanderson, *Tenth Rep. Med. Off. Privy Council*, p. 118.
[4] Hering, *Studien über die Tuberculose*, p. 19.
[5] *Lect. Coll. Phys.* pl. i. fig. 5.
[6] Burdon-Sanderson, *Eleventh Rep. Med. Off. Privy Council*, p. 103.
[7] *Zeitsch. klin. Med.* and also *Tuberkel und Tuberculose*, pp. 58, 64, 68. He calls attention to the fact that changes of a purely histological character may sometimes be found when none are visible without the use of the microscope, and therefore remarks that statements of purely local effects resulting from inoculation must be received with reserve; note p. 58.

this process giant-cells are formed. These are constant after inoculation with bovine tubercle, and occur also when the effects produced by ordinary tubercle are retarded, either by the mode of injection or by early extirpation of the bulb of the eye.[1] In the later stages of the tubercular change there is a large increase of the white blood-corpuscles, but a complete transformation of the growth into small-celled tubercle does not occur, inasmuch as caseation takes place early, and the epithelioid cells lose their nuclei and become changed to scales, which do not imbibe colouring matter.[2] The fibroid change has been described by Burdon-Sanderson as commencing in the septa and extending to the alveoli ('follicles,' Klein), and affecting all the medullary cords and the lymph-sinuses. In the follicles, the reticulum thickens, so that a fine network of threads becomes converted into one of transparent cords, while in the sinuses there appears to be a new formation of fibre-tissue traversing these in irregular bands. Larger cells than those normally present are found in the interstices of these cords and bands.[3]

Spleen.—The affection of the spleen, which is almost constant, resembles very closely that of the lymphatic glands.[4] The organ enlarges greatly,[5] sometimes without any appreciable change of structure.[6] In the majority of cases it presents granulations and other changes.[7]

The granulations are often prominent on the external surface, forming rounded masses, sometimes miliary and transparent, sometimes opaque. On section, the appearances are more varied. Semi-transparent firm granulations are seen, singly or in groups, or similar granulations are found which have cheesy centres. In other instances the granulations, which are about twice the size of the normal Malpighian bodies, have a whitish appearance, and are agglomerated into racemose groups.

There are, in addition, areas of a clear, glistening, firm, semi-transparent tissue, resembling those found in the lymphatic glands, and hereafter to be described in the liver. In some instances, areas of caseous change may be found, dry, friable, and opaque. They are not distinctly limited from the surrounding tissue, and are not surrounded by any zone of injection. I have also found, in some instances, areas of the size of a hazel-nut composed of a diffluent softened amorphous material.[8] Haemorrhagic extravasations are only occasionally met with.[9]

Baumgarten describes the process in the spleen, like that in the lymphatic glands, as commencing with the penetration of bacilli into the tissue-cells, and the formation of tubercles as commencing both in the Malpighian corpuscles and also in the pulp and trabeculae. He describes the early stages as consisting in a production of epithelioid and giant-cells in all these parts, similar to the change which he describes in the lymphatic glands; he believes that a secondary infiltration of leucocytes occurs.

The later stages have been fully described by Burdon-Sanderson[10] as consisting of an increase of the reticulum, producing an adenoid growth akin to that seen in the lymphatic glands, and which, as I have observed, may pass into similar fibroid changes.

Lung.—The affection of the lung has been minutely described by a large number of observers. It is the most common of the secondary affections, but it may also be produced primarily by inhalation of a spray containing tubercular matters, both in the form of the sputa of phthisical patients, and of solid tubercle from the lymphatic glands and other parts rubbed up with water, or of a cultivation from these materials, and also by the direct injection of such material into the trachea.

---

[1] Hering (*Experimentelle Studien über Tuberculose* p. 57) found giant-cells in the glands after inoculation with human tubercle.

[2] Baumgarten points out that his description differs from that given by Schüppel of spontaneous tubercle of the glands, inasmuch as Schüppel thought that the epithelioid cells and giant-cells are derived from small cells, while Baumgarten believes that they arise from the proliferation of the cells of the reticulum.

[3] *Eleventh Rep. Med. Off. Privy Council.* 1868. Cornil and Ranvier (*Manuel Hist. Pathol.* i, 054) believe that the fibroid change extends from the blood-vessels.

[4] Burdon-Sanderson, *Eleventh Rep. Med. Off. Privy Council,* p. 104; Baumgarten, *loc. cit.*

[5] Burdon-Sanderson (*Tenth Rep. Med. Off.* p. 124) says that the normal size of the spleen in the guinea-pig is about half an inch long, and the normal weight half a gramme to a gramme. He met with one two inches long. I measured one 2¼ inches long, 1½ broad and ⅜ an inch thick. The weight of two given by Burdon-Sanderson was 9½ grammes and 8 grammes.

[6] Burdon-Sanderson (*Tenth Rep.* p. 125) says that this occurred in nine out of twenty-one; in all but two, however, granulations were present.

[7] See *Lect. Coll. Phys.* pl. i. figs. 2 and 3. See also Koch, *Mitth. k.k. Gesundheitsamt,* fig. 53.

[8] Koch (*loc. cit,* p. 44) says that though the spleen in the guinea-pig undergoes an extensive coagulation-necrosis, it does not caseate. I think this statement too general. Burdon-Sanderson met with calcareous changes after inoculation with human tubercle. Orth (Virchow's *Archiv,* lxxvi. p. 232) found them after inoculation with bovine tubercle.

[9] Burdon-Sanderson, *loc. cit.*; Koch, *loc. cit.*

[10] Burdon-Sanderson, *Tenth Rep.* p. 126; *Eleventh Rep.* p. 105.

A considerable number of experiments have been made of the last-named class.[1] A large proportion of failures have occurred in the hands of some observers, both by inhalation and tracheal injection, and the relative amount of success has varied considerably; in some instances it has been constant. It has, however, been relatively much greater with inhalation than with injection into the trachea.[2] Non-tubercular material and disinfected sputa have failed to produce similar results.[3]

The effect, in all the successful cases, has been the production of appearances in the lung which are practically identical with those found in tubercular disease in man, and have also very closely corresponded to those produced by inoculation. Grey granulations were frequent, diffuse caseations and infiltrations have also been found, and, in a few rare cases, cavities have been formed. The changes found have not presented any marked differences whether the materials introduced have been tubercular substances, or phthisical sputa, or cultivations. The appearances, moreover, have varied but little in different animals, although in rabbits there is apparently a somewhat greater tendency to caseation than in dogs. In two instances, sheep thus affected showed changes akin to those seen in bovine tuberculosis.[4] In these experiments, with the exception of those by Koch, there is a predominant tendency to limitation of the disease to the lungs, and a frequent absence of secondary affections; those that are recorded are often of a doubtful nature. Koch, on the other hand, by inhalation of cultivated bacilli, usually obtained secondary affections of the liver and spleen in animals living more than twenty-eight days, but in previous experiments secondary affections were absent, both by inhalation and by tracheal injection.[5]

The changes in the lungs, ensuing after secondary infection, consist mainly of three classes:—

---

[1] INHALATION: Tappeiner, Virchow's *Archiv*, vols. lxxiv. lxxxii.; Schottelius, Virchow's *Archiv*, vol. lxxxii.; Berthran, *Deutsches Archiv klin. Med.* vol. xxvi.; Deichselbaum, *Centralblatt med. Wissensch.* 1882. Frerichs, together with Vahle, Frerichs' *Beiträge Lehre Tuberculose*, 1882, and Vahle, *Beiträge Lehre Inhalations-Tuberculose*, Diss. Marburg, 1881; Veraguth, *Arch. exp. Pathol.* 1883, vol. xvii.; Giboux (air expired by phthisical persons) *Comptes Rendus Acad. Sciences*, 1882; Koch, *Mitth. k.k. Gesundheitsamt*, vol. ii. INJECTION INTO TRACHEA: Reinstädler, *Archiv exp. Pathol.* vol. xi.; Schüller, *ib.*; Küssner, *Deutsche med. Woch.* 1883; Poten, *Exp. Untersuch. Lungenschwindsucht*, Diss. Göttingen, 1883; Schäffer, *Verbreitung Tuberculose in den Lungen*, Diss. Berlin, 1884. (To the following I have not been able to obtain access: Lippl and also Schweniger, *Ber. d. 56sten Naturforscher-Versammlung München*; Balagh, quoted by Spina, *Tuberculose*, p. 68. Poten, Reinstadler, and Schäffer also injected directly into the lung, by means of a hypodermic syringe introduced through the thoracic wall, with very similar results.

[2] Thus, in cases where tubercular materials were used by inhalation, there have been, exclusive of Koch's experiments, sixty-one animals used (thirty-three dogs, four goats, twenty-four rabbits), and of these, forty-nine were found to have tubercle, 19 per cent. escaping. Veraguth was the least successful, chiefly with rabbits. Goats were affected in all the experiments. Tappeiner, Weichselbaum, Berthener and Frerichs (chiefly on dogs) were all successful. Koch, in twenty-six cases (rabbits, guinea-pigs, rats and mice) succeeded in all. Of thirty-one cases of tracheal injection (four dogs and twenty-seven rabbits or guinea-pigs) only nineteen succeeded (or failures 36 per cent.). Küssner, however, states that all his experiments of this nature were successful. (His data do not admit of numerical analysis.)

[3] Schottelius believed that non-tubercular substances, when thus introduced into the lung, could produce tubercle, but the changes thus produced appear to have been more of the nature of lobular pneumonia. Küssner produced pneumonia breaking down into cavities by injection of non-tubercular sputa, but somewhat similar results have followed division of the vagi, when the affection has been shown by Frey to be due to the passage of saliva into the lungs.

[4] Thus, apart from Koch's observations, in thirty-four dogs, chiefly infected by inhalation, there were appearances either described as grey granulations, peribronchial granulations, or miliary tubercle, in thirty-two. In thirteen they are the only kind of granulations described. In one, desquamative pneumonia was found alone. In one, 'miliary catarrhal pneumonia.' In sixteen, caseous changes were also present, and in seven, infiltration and miliary pneumonia. In twenty-one rabbits, grey granulations or bodies of this class (see above) existed in thirteen, alone (?) in five, caseous change in fifteen, alone in four. Infiltrations, with grey granulations in three, without in one. Miliary pneumonia alone (early stages) in four. Vahle (*loc. cit.* p. 53) has noticed the predominance of caseous change in rabbits by this process. The statement applies to rabbits generally (see later). In two goats (Veraguth), the nodules were large, with excess of fibroid tissue and calcification, and abundant giant-cells. In one, living 150 days, cavities were found. In the omentum of one were large calcified glands. In one goat, Bertheau found peribronchial and alveolar granulations with the structure of tubercle. Of three guinea-pigs, all had grey (?) tubercles. Cavities were found in two dogs (Tappeiner), in one rabbit (two more by Küssner), and in one goat. As regards the material employed, there are only six cases, apart from Küssner's and Koch's, where cultivations were employed, and these embrace two out of the four cases where, in rabbits, caseation was found without grey granulations, showing that the effects in the others were not due to the sputa as such. In three guinea-pigs they corresponded to the changes usually found. Koch describes the changes as more essentially alveolar, and the nodules as wanting sharp definition. This is confirmed by the observations of some authors on the early stages of inhalation-tubercle, but others describe peribronchial growths and granulations. I have classed the peribronchial as 'grey,' since they usually have this character. Baumgarten (*Zeitsch. klin. Med.* ix. 271) says that injection of bacilli into the trachea produces diffuse caseous pneumonia. It must be remembered that the early stages of the secondary affections of the lung, after subcutaneous inoculation, have been described by some writers as pneumonic (Burdon-Sanderson, Hering.)

[5] Thus, out of thirty-six inhalation-experiments (thirty-three dogs, three rabbits) there were secondary affections only in sixteen, and in thirteen only of these was there a secondary affection of more than one organ

granulations and nodules, diffuse infiltrations, diffuse caseous changes and cavities. The three last are all comparatively rare. The nodules and granulations are most abundant towards the surface of the lung, but they are also found, though less extensively, in the deeper parts. They are comparatively equally numerous in all parts of the lung, not showing any preponderant tendency to affect the apex.[1] They are, for the most part, semi-transparent, 'iron grey' in colour (Burdon-Sanderson), firm, or even hard, and intimately connected with the pulmonary tissue. They vary in size from scarcely visible specks to a pin's head, a poppy, a millet, or a hemp seed. The larger nodules are commonly caseous in their centres, with a semi-transparent margin. Before the caseous change has occurred, they are slightly prominent; after this has set in they are depressed in the centre (Burdon-Sanderson). The smaller nodules are usually semi-transparent throughout. Sometimes, however, very minute granules may be found of a yellow colour. These are chiefly met with in the rabbit, and in this animal they may sometimes be found, in very early stages (ten days), white and soft.[2] In shape they may be rounded or irregular. They are also sometimes found conical in form, with the base at the periphery of the lung.[3] The granulations may be isolated, or confluent in larger and smaller groups. In some cases they may present a distinctly racemose appearance.[4] Occasionally, when thus clustered together, an appearance of a fibrous network is seen running between the individual granulations, similar to that which is not unfrequently observed in the human lung. A large proportion of the granulations are found to be cheesy in their centres, and the caseous material may be found occasionally softened to potential cavities.[5] In rare instances, cavities of larger size may be found, apparently due to the softening of groups of granulations, but more commonly to that of tracts which have probably been larger areas of caseous infiltration.[6] The nodules are seated in the peribronchial and perivascular sheaths, affecting both arteries and veins, and they are also found in the pulmonary tissue apparently unconnected with either of the foregoing.

Klein is of opinion that the earliest change occurs in the perivascular sheaths both of the pulmonary artery and vein, though appearing first in the former.[7] In these, thickenings take place, which are rounded on transverse section and cord-like on longitudinal section, though nodular masses or swellings may also be found in the course of the vessels.[8] Growth also occurs in the endothelium of the pulmonary artery, so that the interior of the vessel may be lined by layers of cells narrowing its cavity, while the wall is laminated by lymphoid and epithelioid cells infiltrated into its structure.[9] The nuclei of the capillary walls of the alveoli also participate in this change.[10] This growth obliterates the capillaries, as is shown by the non-penetration of injection, their course being marked only by lines of nuclei, or, as Klein has described them, by nucleated threads. The obliteration of the capillaries may extend for a considerable distance beyond the apparent area occupied by the tubercle. In the sheaths of the vessels the growth is described by Klein as a filling of the perivascular lymphatics with lymphoid cells (which he regards as being for the most part elongated blood-corpuscles) between which a reticulum subsequently forms and constitutes an adenoid tissue (endolymphangeal). In some cases, however, an extension takes place into the neighbouring tissue by a growth of a similar kind surrounding the lymphatic vessels (perilymphangeal).

The *peribronchial growths* have a structure very similar to the periarterial. Burdon-Sanderson describes them as originating on the exterior of the smallest bronchi in masses of adenoid tissue,

---

in addition to the lung. Out of these thirteen, eleven are stated by Weichselbaum to have had the kidneys, bronchial and mesenteric glands affected. In seventeen cases of tracheal injection (one dog, thirteen rabbits, three guinea-pigs) there were secondary affections in nine, but only in three of more than one organ. Küssner obtained none. In one case by Poten, after injection into the lungs, these organs escaped and the liver was affected.

[1] Martin (*Revue de Médecine*, 1882, ii. 915) describes an instance of caseous pneumonia in the rabbit, passing into excavation, which commenced at the base; (peritoneal inoculation).

[2] Cheesy, cf. Villemin's *Etudes*, pp. 538-5; Von Waldenburg, *Die Tuberculose*, pp. 298, 331; white and soft, *ib.* p. 255.

[3] Burdon-Sanderson, *Rep. Med. Off. Privy Council*, 1867, x. 119; Klein, *Anatomy Lymphatic System*, ii. 52.

[4] Lebert and Wyss, Virchow's *Archiv*, xl. 562.

[5] Burdon-Sanderson, *Tenth Rep. Med. Off. Privy Council*; Lebert. Virchow's *Archiv*, vol. xli.

[6] Villemin, *Etudes*, p. 538; Kiener, *Bull. Soc. Med. Hôp.* 1881; injection into veins; affection limited to lungs. Martin. *Rev. de. Méd.* 1882, ii. 915; Hering, *Exp. Studien über Tuberculose.* pp. 19, 20, 55. See also notes on direct introduction by the trachea, when cavities appear to be more frequent.

[7] Klein, *loc. cit.* pp. 55, 60.

[8] *Lect. Coll. Phys.* pl. ii. figs. 2 and 3.

[9] Klein, *loc. cit.* p. 61. Baumgarten (*Tuberkel und Tuberculose*, p. 76) describes the early structure of their changes as being chiefly epithelioid.

[10] *Lect. Coll. Phys.* pl. ii. figs. 2, 5, and 6.

which lie outside the tube, in the loose cellular tissue between it and the adjacent artery. In the larger tubes they lie within the bronchial sheath.¹ Klein describes them as ovoid, and thus distinguishes them from the cord-like masses of periarterial growth, though they may occasionally assume the latter form.² They originate in collections of adenoid tissue normally existing in this part, which Klein describes as a perilymphangeal growth, and which are identical with lymph-follicles. In the smallest bronchi, they may pass between the muscular and mucous coats.

In the process of tuberculisation, these masses of tissue increase in size, and tend, in the larger bronchi, to become confluent; but they maintain a well-defined outline, and the chief change consists in a hyperplasia,³ mingled, however, with larger epithelial cells derived from the fixed cells by a process of division.⁴ Burdon-Sanderson states that the mucous membrane of the bronchi, around which this growth exists, may be comparatively unaffected.⁵ The growth may, however, extend into the submucous tissue,⁶ and after inoculation a stripping of the epithelium has been seen by Schüller.⁷ Direct injection into the trachea has, in some cases, been followed by ulceration;⁸ occasionally by polypoid growths of the mucous membrane.⁹

There is some difference of opinion with regard to the mode of the origin of nodules which are found in the *lung-tissue*. Burdon-Sanderson considered that the alveolar tissue is invaded from the peribronchial growth. Klein denies this, and states that the process commences around the arteries and thence extends to the alveolar walls, that in some cases the growth may be limited to the perivascular sheaths, and that the lung affection may be advanced before the peribronchial growths appear. I cannot but believe that extension occurs from both structures.¹⁰ I am disposed also to believe that the nodules may develop in the tissue, independently of either of the foregoing modes of origin. There is much evidence that, in very early stages, islets may be found, chiefly of a pneumonic character,¹¹ and this fact, together with that already alluded to (that the capillaries of the alveoli are implicated at an early period), would appear to show that the lung-tissue may be primarily affected.¹²

The most characteristic feature in this process is the thickening of the alveolar walls, which may proceed to the complete obliteration of the alveolar cavities.¹³ This growth extends irregularly, and hence these nodules are less definite in shape than those situated in the walls of the bronchi and blood-vessels. Commencing also sometimes as a lobular pneumonia, the nodules may assume the conical form described by Klein. Two sets of changes are, however, present, viz. a filling of the alveoli with epithelioid cells, and a thickening of their walls; and the two processes advance together, though one may predominate over the other, and the alveolar thickening may, in some parts, appear in advance of the epithelioid proliferation, while in others the latter may be the chief change observed.¹⁴

---

¹ The recognition of the smaller nodules as a natural appearance is due to Burdon-Sanderson (*Eleventh Rep. Med. Off. Privy Council* 1868, p. 101). The larger ones had been described by Kölliker. In my lecture (*Coll. Phys.*) I had described this origin of the granulations, but I had understood Kölliker's description to apply to all the tubes. Cf. his *Gewebelehre*, p. 508.
² Klein, *Anatomy Lymphatic System*, Part II. pp. 21, 53.
³ Klein (*loc. cit.* p. 50) points out that the peribronchial growths are naturally more vascular than those which arise in the arterial sheath, as the former are normally provided with blood-vessels. He doubts whether vessels of new formation are found in the latter.
⁴ Baumgarten (*Tuberkel und Tuberculose*, pp. 76, 77) questions whether the unstriated muscular fibres of the vessels and bronchi may not participate in the production of these. Epithelioid cells in the bronchial wall were first described by Friedländer (Virchow's *Archiv*, 1876, lxviii. 350) as a part of 'desquamative pneumonia,' and termed by him 'atypical epithelial.' Cf. also Orth. Virchow's *Archiv*, lxxvi. 229.
⁵ Burdon Sanderson, *Tenth Rep. Med. Off. Privy Council*, p. 121.
⁶ Schüller, *Exp. Untersuch. tub. Gelenkleiden*, p. 123; Reinstadler, *Arch. exp. Pathol.* xi. 118; Frerichs, *Beiträge Lehre Tuberculose*, p. 132.
⁷ Schüller, *loc. cit.*
⁸ Poten, *Exp. Untersuch.* p. 46; Schäffer, *Tuberculose in den Lungen*, p. 27.
⁹ Vahle, *loc. cit.* p. 20.
¹⁰ See *Lect. Coll. Phys.* Pl. II. figs. 1 and 2. I venture to express this opinion, although I have had no opportunity of reinvestigating this point, and my drawings were made before any discussion arose respecting it. Extension from peribronchial growth to the alveolar structure is described by Reinstadler, *Arch. exp. Path.* xi. 118. Cf. also Vahle, *loc. cit.* p. 23; Schäffer, *loc. cit.* p. 12.
¹¹ Langhans, *Uebertragbarkeit der Tuberculose auf Kaninchen*, Habilitations-Schrift, Marburg, p. 31; Hering, *loc. cit.*; Veraguth, *loc. cit.*; Vahle, *loc. cit.* pp 19 and 22.
¹² Baumgarten's descriptions (*Tuberkel und Tuberculose*) would appear to show that he regards the change in the lung-tissue as the first and the chief, and that the peribronchial and perivascular growths are less marked. Klein states that the perivascular growths may be the only change present (*Anatomy Lymphatic System*, ii. 60).
¹³ *Lect. Coll. Phys.* Pl II. figs. 1, 2, and 4.
¹⁴ Baumgarten (*loc. cit.* p. 76) states that thickening of the walls does not occur without the filling of the alveolar cavities. This is true of the mass, as a whole, but the former may be in excess of the latter: Langhans had made a similar observation, *loc. cit.* pp. 19, 20.

x

The growth in the lung-tissue was described by Burdon-Sanderson[1] as commencing in the nuclei of the interstitial stroma of the alveolar wall. Baumgarten describes it as beginning simultaneously in the nuclei of the pulmonary capillaries and in the alveolar epithelium, which are penetrated by bacilli and immediately commence to show increase in size and multiplication.[2] To the latter is due the filling of the alveoli; to the former, a thickening of the wall with epithelioid cells, the elastic tissue remaining unaltered.[3] A similar change occurs in the walls of the smallest bronchioles, the interior of which becomes blocked with epithelial cells, and into these, later, the growth penetrates.

Klein describes the growth of the alveolar wall as assuming the form of a lymphoid tissue, and consisting of cords formed of lymphatics and plugged with lymphoid cells, which gradually assume an adenoid type with a reticulum.[4] This description corresponds, but with ore precise details, to that given by most other authors, and represents, according to Baumgarten the later stages of the process, the transformation of the epithelioid into the lymphoid growth being observable in different stages. Giant-cells, chiefly derived from the epithelial cells, are found in the interior of the alveoli.[5] Schüppel has observed large polynucleated cells in the peribronchial and perivascular growths.[6]

There are some discrepancies in the statements made respecting the caseation of these nodules. Klein believes that it only rarely affects the perivascular and periarterial growths. Watson Cheyne[7] describes it as chiefly affecting the epithelioid cells filling the alveoli, and that only in these are the bacilli found in the early stages. He regards the bacilli as diagnostic of tubercle, and therefore necessarily excludes from this category the perivascular growth which Klein describes as being in some cases the earliest stage of the process. It is evident that both the epithelioid and the small-celled growths are stages of the same process, and that this cannot be divided histologically into the inflammatory and the tubercular, and also that caseation may attack both the perivascular and the peribronchial growths,[8] although perhaps with greater variety than in the case of the alveolar masses. Watson Cheyne and Baumgarten have both described an excessive accumulation of bacilli in the caseous parts, which commences in the centres of the nodules and gradually extends in area.

Diffuse infiltrations, both of the grey and of the caseous type, are also found. The former may assume the characters of a simple pneumonic infiltration, and may occasionally caseate without any other change having been observed.[9] The grey infiltration has, however, been associated with thickening of the alveolar walls, similar to that described in the nodules,[10] and from the extent and smoothness of surface it appears very doubtful whether this change is due only to the confluence of granulations, or whether it is not a diffuse process akin to the grey infiltration in man.

Diffuse caseous infiltration has also been observed, both after ordinary subcutaneous inoculation and after infection by inhalation, and presents a structure very similar to the foregoing, except that the cell-elements have to a great extent disappeared.[11]

The intestines, like the lungs, may be affected, either secondarily by subcutaneous inoculations, or

---

[1] Burdon-Sanderson, *Tenth Rep. Med. Off. Privy Council*, 1867, p. 120. Baumgarten also admits these as a source of growth.
[2] Baumgarten, *Tuberkel und Tuberculose*, p. 73 et seq.
[3] Burdon-Sanderson, *Tenth Rep. Med. Off. Privy Council*, p. 121; Baumgarten, *loc. cit.* p. 83.
[4] Langhans (*loc. cit.*) described large cells as well as small-celled growth in the thickened alveolar walls. Ref. also Lebert, Friedländer, Schäfer, Poten, Schüppel, Hering, Martin, and others for the small-celled growth.
[5] Langhans, *loc. cit.*; Klein, *loc. cit.*; Baumgarten, *loc. cit.*; Veragath, *Archiv exp. Pathol.* vol. xvii. Langhans doubted whether they did not also exist in the walls of the alveoli. Baumgarten states that they are most common after inoculation with bovine tubercle, but others have found them produced by human tubercle.
[6] Schüppel, *loc. cit.* p. 128; Vahle (*loc. cit.* p. 21) has also described them in peribronchial growths, but his description leaves some doubt whether they were not seated in the pulmonary tissue.
[7] *Practitioner*, 1883, xxx. 308 et seq. Cheyne states that the bacilli may penetrate into the small-celled growth in the alveolar wall which surrounds the epithelioid growth in the alveoli, but he regards the latter as being typical of tubercle, though the presence of bacilli is necessary to its definition.
[8] Caseation, both of the peribronchial and of the perivascular growths, has been described by Chauveau, Lépine (*Pneumonie Caseuse*, p. 58) and by Baumgarten, (*Tuberkel und Tuberculose*, pp. 81-2.) In the peribronchial growths it has also been described, but less positively, by Vahle, *loc. cit.* p. 23.
[9] Chauveau, quoted by Lépine, *Pneumonie Caseuse*, p. 59.
[10] Langhans, *loc. cit.* p. 52; Klein, *Anatomy Lymphatic System*, ii. 66; Villemin, *Etudes*, p. 542; Von Waldenburg, *Die Tuberculose*, p. 408. This form is described as 'Desquamative Pneumonia' by many writers; cf. Schüller, *loc. cit.* p. 130; Hering, *loc. cit.* p. 19.
[11] INOCULATION: Villemin, *Etudes*, p. 533; Von Waldenburg, *Die Tuberculose*, p. 437; Hering, *loc. cit.* p. 34; Orth, *Berliner klin. Woch.* 1881. INHALATION: for authors already quoted, ref. Baumgarten, *Tuberkel und Tuberculose*, p. 79.

primarily, by feeding with tuberculous material. Baumgarten appears to deny their secondary implication, except as a rare event and only by a slight implication of the follicles; but I found tubercle of the intestine, sometimes proceeding to ulceration, in twelve out of forty-two cases in which these parts were examined by me.[1]

In the experiments with feeding, the mouth, larynx, and glandular lymphatics,[2] the abomasum in ruminants,[3] and the stomach in rabbits and guinea-pigs,[4] have been found affected with caseous change, but the greatest intensity of the morbid process is in the intestines. A general constitutional affection follows in most cases. In a few, comparatively rare, instances, the gastro-intestinal canal has escaped, and the mesenteric glands and other organs have become affected,[5] and in most instances there is also an excessive affection of the mesentery. Baumgarten has produced intestinal tuberculosis by feeding with cultivated bacilli, and he has observed that some of the bacilli pass direct into the lymphatic glands and the liver.[6] The growth apparently commences in the lymphatic follicles of the intestines,[7] but, as Baumgarten describes, the penetration of the bacilli into the surrounding tissue, including the crypts of Lieberkühn, and the submucous and muscular coat, excites growth of the fixed cells of these parts, producing nests of epithelioid cells, as were described by Orth. These become confluent, and cause extensive tubercular infiltration, which is marked in the cæcum and vermiform process, and passes, both in the solitary glands and in Peyer's patches, into caseation and ulceration. Giant-cells are found after infection with bovine tuberculosis (Orth), but Baumgarten states that they also appear when the intensity of the poison is diminished by previous partial decomposition. In all essential features the intestinal affection is identical with that of man.

The liver presents some of the most remarkable alterations observed. It is diseased, as part of the general infection, with great frequency,[8] but most markedly when inoculations are made in the peritoneum.[9]

The organ is greatly enlarged, and presents a considerable variety of appearances.[10] It may present chiefly small, grey, semi-transparent granulations, sometimes almost microscopic, scattered through the tissue.[11] In other parts these spots may be of an opaque white colour. These may be of variable size, and may attain considerable dimensions, having, on section, a finely granular surface. In addition, large tracts of the liver, in more advanced stages, are converted into a firm translucent material, which breaks with a granular fracture, and by which the liver is mapped out into irregular areas.

The extent of this growth may, at times, be such as to change the shape of the organ and to give it the appearance of a cirrhotic or hobnailed liver,[12] but it differs from this in the absence of toughness, and from the lardaceous liver, which it may also resemble, in the fact that it does not

---

[1] Baumgarten, *Tuberkel und Tuberculose*, p. 112. They have been observed by Villemin (*Etudes*, p. 535); by Von Waldenburg (*Die Tuberculose, &c.* p. 308, and also pp. 262, 263, 310, 314)—sometimes in excess of the lungs and proceeding to ulceration; also by Hering, *loc. cit.* p. 39.

[2] Orth, Virchow's *Archiv*, vol. lxxvi. The only cases in which Orth obtained positive results in rabbits were with bovine tubercle; Aufrecht (*Path. Mitth.*) obtained one success with human tubercle; Johne (*Geschichte der Tuberculose*, p. 324) gives as the general result of feeding with human tubercle in twenty-five cases, only 36 per cent. of successes; with the material from three tuberculous monkeys, all succeeded.

[3] Chauveau, *Bull. Acad. Méd.* vol. xxxiii; Günther and Harms, *Bericht Thierarzenei-Schule zu Hannover*, 1873.

[4] Orth, *loc. cit.*

[5] Klebs believes that the tubercular poison thus introduced can infect the system without attacking the gastro-intestinal canal (Virchow's *Archiv*, xliv. and xlix. 291; also article 'Tuberculose' in Eulenburg's *Real-Encyclopädie*, vol. xiv.). His own observations (*Arch. exp. Pathol.* vol. i.) confirm this view, as of five guinea-pigs thus fed, one escaped entirely, four had affection of the liver and mesenteric glands, but of these only one had intestinal affection. Confirmatory evidence is given by Gerlach (Virchow's *Archiv*, ii. 298, 305) and by Klein

and Gibbes (*Rep. Med. Off. Local Government Board*, 1885, vol. xiv.); and also by Bollinger (*Archiv. exp. Pathol.* vol. i.), who remarks that in some of these cases a condition like scrofula ensues. Not having access to many of the detailed observations on this subject, I am unable to give numerical statements; but my impression is that, in the vast majority of instances of infection in this manner, an intestinal affection occurs.

[6] *Fortschritte der Med.* 1884, p. 189; *Tuberkel und Tuberculose*, p. 113.

[7] Orth and Baumgarten, *loc. cit.* Cf. also Burdon-Sanderson, *Path. Soc. Trans.* vol. xxi., who describes early growths in the villi of the intestine in bovine animals.

[8] Baumgarten, *loc. cit.* p. 93, appears to regard the affection of the liver as less frequent than that of the kidney, but his experience of the frequency of secondary renal affections is exceptional.

[9] Koch, *Mitth. k.k. Gesundheitsamt*, ii. 44. This extensive interstitial growth in the liver, associated with a granular (tubercular?) peritonitis and almost resembling cirrhosis, has been noticed by Bastian, though with a different interpretation, *Trans. Path. Soc.* xxiv. 327.

[10] See *Lect. Coll. Phys.* pl. i. fig. 4.

[11] Hering, *Histol. und exp. Untersuch. Tuberculose*, pp. 35–39. I have also seen this. Cf. *Lect. Coll. Phys.* p. 12.

[12] Burdon-Sanderson, *Tenth Rep. Med. Off. Privy Council*, p. 12.

stain with iodine. In such parts there is no trace of natural liver-tissue, though lines of this may occasionally be seen running through it. In other parts the change appears to be interacinose, mapping out the contours of the acini. Caseous masses are also found firm and hard, but sometimes forming masses the size of a hazel-nut, with a diffluent creamy centre. Baumgarten describes the early stages of the process as consisting in the penetration of bacilli into nearly all the elements of the tissue, the liver-cells, the walls of the intra-acinose branches of the portal vein, the capillaries, the walls and epithelium of the bile-ducts, and the substance and cells of the connective tissue. In all these parts cell-growth may occur, but this may preponderate in one more than in another, and the affection may be in excess either within the acini or external to these.[1]

From the cell-growth, a production of epithelioid cells results,[2] those in the liver-tissue being distinguished by their cloudiness and cubiform shape from those originating in the capillaries or connective tissue, which are more elongated. The hepatic cells also give rise to giant-cells,[3] and the growth from the bile-ducts may produce tubes of new formation of apparently glandular tissue.[4]

Baumgarten remarks that the lymphoid growth is rare. A reticular small-celled tissue, however, is described by most writers. It is of this that the diffuse interstitial growth is for the most part composed, though it passes into fibroid change. The growth maps out the acini and invades large areas of liver-tissue, and its ultimate structure is of small cells imbedded in a reticulum.[5] As the disease advances, the trabeculae of the reticulum increase in width, until the cell-structures have largely disappeared, and the adenoid growth has been replaced by a fibrous structure.[6] It is, in part, to this growth that some of the islets of degeneration in the liver are due, and they consist only of fatty-degenerated liver-cells.[7]

Kidney.—The infective disease in the kidney has been minutely described chiefly by Baumgarten. He speaks of it as the most frequent of the secondary affections, after the lungs, an observation probably due to the animals experimented upon being rabbits. Most other observers speak of renal affections as rare.[8] It is found chiefly in the cortical substance, the pyramids being unaffected. The changes observed correspond very closely with those described by him in the liver, viz. a growth of epithelioid cells from the epithelium of the renal tubules and of the glomeruli, and also of the interstitial capillaries, forming nodules which tend to become confluent. Baumgarten states that the later stages resemble those of the lungs, and they probably include therefore the small-celled and reticulated growths described by Orth.[9]

The descriptions now given show a striking identity, in all organs, with tubercles as found in man, and such differences as exist in the opinions of some writers as to their nature, are referable chiefly to those difficulties in the definition of tubercle which I have already discussed in detail. It must be once more remarked that the formation of tubercle is a process, and that the anatomical appearances observed vary, not only in its different stages, but also with the acuteness of the process, and that it is only by considering these as a whole that we can avoid the error which must arise from too limited definitions.[10] Aufrecht[11] holds that the inoculation-disease bears more resemblance to acute tuberculosis than to the more chronic forms of phthisis met with in man. The fact, however, that in the lungs, diffuse infiltrations, both grey and caseous, and also cavities, may be occasionally found, points to a close resemblance, if not identity, between the two processes, and the fact that fibroid changes[12] are also occasionally met with in some cases, showing a tendency

---

[1] This probably explains the discrepancies on this subject between different writers. Burdon-Sanderson and I described this change as occurring for the most part external to the acini. Petroff (Virchow's *Archiv*, vol. xliv.) and Hering (*loc. cit.*) described it as within the acini. Cf. Hering's figures, pl. ii. *loc. cit.*
[2] Burdon-Sanderson (*Eleventh Rep.* p. 112) described large cells of $\frac{1}{1000}$ inch within the capillaries.
[3] Baumgarten, *loc. cit.*; Watson Cheyne, *Practitioner*, 1880, xxx. 311. Koch (*Mitth. k.k. Gesundheitsamt*, ii. 24) says that in human tubercle, bacilli are only found in the giant-cells.
[4] Burdon-Sanderson (*Eleventh Rep.* pp. 113, 114) described a growth of the epithelium of the bile-ducts, producing masses of cells. The multiplication of the liver-cells and of the bile-ducts is also described by Hering.
[5] See *Lect. Coll. Phys.* pl. iii. figs. 4 and 5.
[6] Cf. Burdon-Sanderson, *Tenth and Eleventh Reps.*; Schüller, *Exp. Untersuchungen*, p. 188; Orth, Virchow's *Archiv*, vol. lxvii. (who describes it as an interstitial hepatitis); Poten, *Exp. Untersuchungen*, p. 49.
[7] Burdon-Sanderson, *loc. cit.*
[8] Burdon-Sanderson and Koch. See *ante*, note, p. 144.
[9] Orth, Virchow's *Archiv*, vol. lxxvi.
[10] These have been fully discussed in detail by Baumgarten, *Tuberkel und Tuberculose*.
[11] Aufrecht, *Path. Mitth.* 1881. i. 49. Their identity was also denied by Friedländer, Virchow's *Archiv*, vol. lxviii.
[12] See especially Schüller, *Exp. histol. Untersuch. scroph. und tuberkulöse Gelenkleiden*, p. 203 *et seq.* Schüller gives numerous instances and details, attributing the case to inhalation of benzoate of soda and other drugs. The fibroid changes, however, were distinct.

to 'cure,' points still further to the identity of the final stages of spontaneous human and experimentally produced tubercle. The changes in the liver present the greatest diversity from those found in human tubercle, but even they are not without their analogies in the latter. The multiplicity of the disease [1] as regards the number of organs affected is, however, in connection with the anatomical character, one of the strongest proofs of the identity of the two conditions. There are few cases of tuberculosis in man which proceed to a fatal issue without the implication of more than one organ, and the chief difference between these and the infective disease in animals is one of time and rapidity. The multiplicity in the latter shows, however, as I previously stated, that the question of the nature of the disease does not merely rest on histological changes observed in different organs, it also shows that we have to deal either with a disease identical with that inoculated, or with a new and previously unknown condition.

Exceptional cases do occur, with variable frequency, where the localisation of the infective disease has, for a time at least, been limited, and this has especially been the case with the lungs.[2] A considerable proportion of the animals in which this limitation has been found have, however, been killed, and probably a longer duration of life would have led to further extension. Tubercle is, moreover, so frequently localised in man, that the occasional occurrence of this event in animals rather affords an additional argument for the identity of the two affections than shows that such cases should be regarded as different in nature.

Metzquer (*Etudes Clin. Phthisis Galop.* 1874. p. 41) thinks tubercle may be re-absorbed. He inoculated six rabbits, and one killed contained tubercles. The rest recovered. Koch (*Mitth. k.k. Gesundheitsamt*, ii. 72) met with one dog, which, after infection, became ill and recovered. He says that this is the only instance in his experience.

[1] In my own observations (*Lect. Coll. Phys.*) of 117 guinea-pigs inoculated with various materials, 58 were tubercular, 6 doubtful, and there was no result in 58. I consider, for reasons there given, that all those in which tubercle occurred had been infected with tubercle. In the 64 in which some affection was produced, 58 had three or more organs affected; of the doubtful cases three had the lungs only affected, one the spleen alone, and two the bronchial glands and spleen. The lungs were affected 59 times, the bronchial glands 58 times, the spleen 59 times, the liver 51 times, the omentum 25 (not stated in 12), intestines in 12 out of 42 cases examined, the mesenteric glands 45 times, in 2 cases the kidney, in 2 the uterus.

[2] See *ante*, p. 151. Stricker (*Path. Infections-Krankheiten*, p. 141) has given instances of local infection limited to the eyes. Lebert, after inoculation, has seen them limited to the lung. Another point of interest is that, as observed by him, young guinea-pigs may continue to grow, and may remain fat, during the development of general tuberculosis. This is exceptional; Tappeiner (Virchow's *Archiv*, vol. lxxviii.) has, however, made a similar observation on dogs.

CASES.

For other references to the Cases see the descriptions of the respective Plates.

CASE 1.

ACUTE PNEUMONIA, GREY HEPATISATION.

Plates IV. fig. 3; XXV. fig. 9.

Ref.—Acute Pneumonia, p. 17.

SUMMARY.—*M. 46. Sudden onset, with rigors, cough, and dyspnœa. On eighth day, signs of consolidation of almost the whole of the right lung; bronchial and tubular breathing; bronchitic râles throughout both lungs. Death on tenth day.—Grey pneumonic consolidation throughout right lung except at apex: bronchial mucous membrane congested in both lungs. Heart, soft. Liver, fatty. Kidneys, 'cloudy swelling.'*

JOSEPH KIRK, ætat. 46, admitted University College Hospital February 2; died February 4, 1867.

Family History.—Nothing known.

Personal History.—A labourer, working lately in a railway tunnel. Has lived well. Usually moderate in alcoholic drinks, but has occasionally drunk to excess. Has been subject to winter cough for some years past, but has otherwise had good health.

Present Illness commenced January 26. Was suddenly attacked with rigors in the evening, followed by cough and difficulty of breathing. He has kept his bed since then, until carried to the hospital.

State on Admission.—Orthopnœa. Face livid; eyes prominent; expression anxious. Alæ nasi distended, and moving with respiration. Tongue dry; lips parched; cough violent and spasmodic; sputa abundant, muco-purulent, yellowish, with a slight rusty tinge, but very tenacious. (On the following day some of the sputa acquired a tint of burnt sienna.) Chest somewhat barrel-shaped, with deep anteroposterior diameter. Heart covered by lung. Left side hyperresonant from apex to base. Right side dull throughout, except in the upper anterior region. Bronchial and tubular breathing over the whole of the right lung, except at the extreme back, where the respiration is very weak but of a bronchial character. Over the whole of the lung are heard abundant metallic and subcrepitant râles. Bronchophony is present over the whole lung. The vocal fremitus is imperceptible, owing to weakness of patient's voice. On left side, respiration harsh; abundant mucous and fine submucous râles exist over the whole of this lung. The heart-sounds are inaudible. Urine acid, faint trace of albumen. No œdema of extremities.

The temperature on admission was 102·4°; pulse 100; resp. 60. On the following day T., morning, 99·6°; P. 120; R. 54; evening: T. 100·4°; P. 120; R. 52. The pulse was very weak and irregular and occasionally intermittent. The patient gradually sank and died forty-eight hours after admission, on the ninth day of disease.

POST-MORTEM.—*Lungs:* Both adherent; adhesions of right, old and firm; those of left lung easily separated. Right lung solidified throughout, except a small portion at apex, which is loaded with a dirty ash-grey serosity. On section it is of an ashy-grey colour; surface is finely granular; tissue breaks down with great ease, and when scraped yields an ash-grey fluid. Much pigment is scattered through the lungs (see Plate IV. fig. 3). Left lung emphysematous; upper lobe œdematous. Bronchi everywhere deeply congested.

Heart.—Tissue flabby, soft, and granular when torn. Some dilatation of tricuspid valve. Mitral and aortic valves healthy. Right side filled with large clot.

Liver slightly fatty, soft; weighs 5 lbs.

Kidneys very soft; section opaque, in condition of 'cloudy swelling.' *Spleen* soft.

Stomach.—Mucous membrane swollen, softened, covered with thick layers of mucus; solitary glands enlarged.

MICROSCOPIC EXAMINATION of this lung shows the alveoli filled with cells of the types seen in XXV. 9. On scraping, the preponderating character is that seen in XXV. 2, in which there are at places appearances as if some of the rounded cells are derivatives from the reticulum. Some alveoli are entirely filled with small round cells like those in XXV. 3. The interlobular and peribronchial tissue is in some parts loaded with cells, but there is no thickening of the alveolar walls.

CASE 2.

PNEUMONIA, SUPPURATION.

Plate II.

Ref.—Acute Pneumonia, p. 18.

From a drawing by Sir Robert Carswell; University College Museum, No. 46. Catalogue C. b. 306. The following is Sir R. Carswell's description:—

PERIPNEUMONY.—'LOUIS GERAIN, aged 66, mar-
'chand, came to "La Charité" on May 21, 1829.
'He had coughed more or less for a period of five
'years; the respiration has been more or less op-

'pressed when walking up an ascent. The cough
'has increased, accompanied with viscid, pituitous
'and mucous sputa. Respiration heard over the
'whole chest. Pulsation of the heart dull. No
'fever.—(8oz. of blood from the arm.)
 '*22nd.*—Complains of deep-seated pain in the
'right side; expectoration of viscid dullish-green
'matter; much oppressed; pulse frequent; deep-
'seated dull crepitation in the right side.
 '*23rd.*—The pain and difficulty of respiration con-
'tinued, when he was again bled to 12 oz. In the
'evening the sputa were viscid, yellowish, and tinged
'with blood, and the oppression continued the same.
'The blood drawn in the morning was covered with
'the buffy coat. The fever is considerable, crepitation
'is heard in the right side throughout a great ex-
'tent, but not at the top of the chest. A small
'degree of râle, sibilant, is also heard.—(Sinapisms
'to the legs.)
 '*24th.*—Very weak, and much more oppressed;
'tongue covered with dirty-grey clammy mucus.—
'(21 leeches to the epigastrium, an emulsion con-
'taining senega, a potion with two grains of squill,
'two blisters to the legs.)
 '*26th.*—Much worse, hardly able to speak. The
'tongue is attached to the roof of the palate by
'viscid dark-brown mucus. Two blisters were
'ordered to the thighs, but the patient died about
'mid-day.
 '*INSPECTION.*—*Head* not opened. *Thorax:* The
'left lung presented only slight congestion of the
'posterior part. The right was extensively diseased.
'The middle and inferior lobes felt hard, did not
'crepitate when pressed, and the pleura covering
'these was lined with recent false membranes.
'When the lobes were divided, they presented a
'yellowish-grey colour, tinged with red, proving a
'solid compact granular mass, in which the bronchia
'and blood-vessels were hardly to be seen, here and
'there marked with streaks of black pulmonary
'matter. When pressed, a considerable quantity of
'serosity oozed out, mixed in some points with pus.
'The diaphragmatic portion of the inferior lobe was
'engorged with blood and rather soft. The upper
'lobe was congested and contained a considerable
'quantity of serosity.
 'The mucous membrane of the bronchia was very
'red, and swollen a little. *Heart*, enlarged through-
'out and slightly hypertrophied. The mucous mem-
'brane of the stomach was congested.'

CASE 3.

CHRONIC PNEUMONIA. SYPHILIS.

Plates IV. fig. 1; XLII. fig. 6; XLIII. fig. 4.

Ref.—Phthisis, pp. 67, 104; Syphilitic Dis., p. 126.

SUMMARY, F. 55. *Abdominal pain and hæmoptysis, seven years before death. During last year, cough
and emaciation. Indications of previous syphilis.
Evidence of consolidation and retractation in the
upper half of right lung. No pyrexia. Great improvement for a time, then acute symptoms and death
immediately after re-admission to hospital. Duration
of symptoms fifteen months.*—*Right lung, upper part
transformed into cicatricial fibroid tissue containing*

*cavities; the middle part infiltrated with grey exu-
dation.*

ELIZABETH HAWKINS, æt. 55, a widow, admitted
University College Hospital, October 21, 1867.

Family History.—Father and mother dead; cause
unknown. One sister died after three years' illness
with cough. Several other sisters and brothers dead;
causes unknown.

Personal History.—Never pregnant. Menstruation ceased at 47. Has had bad health for years.
Subject to severe abdominal pains, for which she was
treated with benefit eleven years ago in the Hospital
for Women, Soho. Some years ago, brought up, on
several occasions, about a table-spoonful of blackened
frothy blood, but she had no cough at the time.
Breath has been getting short for the past seven
years. Cough has existed only for twelve months,
and has grown worse of late. Since attacked by
cough she has suffered in her eyesight.

State on Admission.—Considerable emaciation;
nails incurvated. Skin cool. Cicatrix of old ulceration on chest. Eczematous patch on left ala nasi.
Pupils small and irregularly contracted, as if from
past iritis. Right cornea cloudy at outer margin,
and somewhat throughout. General conjunctivitis
of both eyes; intolerance of light. Frequent spasmodic cough, which at times causes vomiting. Sputa
innumulated and muco-purulent; thorax narrow.
Flattening in infraclavicular regions, especially
marked on right side, where it extends to the fourth
rib. Expansion on right side almost nil, on left
side very imperfect. Respiration predominantly abdominal.

Right Lung: absolute want of pulmonary resonance
throughout front and axilla. Tubular note between
second and fourth ribs in the infraclavicular region,
and between the third and fourth ribs in the axilla.
Back, absolute dulness to lower third of scapula.
Respiration under clavicle cavernous, with metallic
râles; coarse bubbling râles persist to fifth rib, below
which respiration is suppressed. Tubular metallic
breathing in upper axilla; harsh blowing in mid-
axilla; suppressed below. In back, diffused blowing
breathing in supra-spinous fossæ; amphoric breathing in infra-spinous fossa; harsh blowing at lower
part of scapular region; normal at base, with
numerous bubbling râles. Vocal resonance pec-
toriloquous in the infra-clavicular and upper axillary
regions; exaggerated throughout upper scapular
region, and bronchophonic opposite spine.

Left Lung: resonance very deficient in front
but still somewhat pulmonary, especially under
clavicle. Left axilla, note tympanitic, but short and
imperfect. Back is hyper-resonant, except in supra-
spinous and infraspinous fossæ, where it is dull.
Respiration harsh over left front and axilla, and also
in back except opposite spine of scapula, where it is
bronchial. Vocal resonance also exaggerated at the
last-named spot; not elsewhere.

Heart's impulse indistinguishable; sounds normal. Liver-dulness three fingers' breadth below
false ribs. Tongue thinly furred; appetite good.

In the subsequent progress of the case she suffered
much at times during the first part of her stay in
hospital from abdominal pain, and occasional vomiting, which, however, improved. The urine varied
in specific gravity from 1010 to 1020. It only once
contained a trace of albumen. There was no pyrexia

throughout.[1] The cough gradually improved; and the sputa, which were thick, tenacious, and puriform, diminished, and at last became small in amount. The râles almost entirely disappeared from the chest, and she was discharged much relieved on December 13. She was re-admitted on February 12, in a state of acute dyspnœa, and died in a few hours.

POST-MORTEM. — *Larynx:* Mucous membrane rough, granular, not ulcerated.

Lungs.—Bronchi intensely congested throughout. Right lung; whole of apex converted into a firm, semi-cartilaginous mass of dense, pigmented, cicatricial tissue, in which ramify dilated bronchi, whose lining membrane is deeply injected. Some cavities also are found, traversed by bands. There is very little pulmonary tissue remaining in this lobe. Through it are scattered patches of indurated granulations, firm, pigmented, and passing here and there into cheesy change. The middle and lower lobes are adherent. The whole of the middle lobe, and the upper two-thirds of the lower lobe, are infiltrated with a very firm, reddish-grey exudation, which is finely granular (IV. 1). In it the bronchi are dilated, but it shows no signs of softening. The lower third of the lower lobe is dense, but still crepitant. The left lung, from base to apex, is free from any form of consolidation.

Liver.—Section, nutmeg in appearance; puckered deeply with cicatrices (syphilitic); tissue otherwise soft. The interlobular spaces are enlarged, milky in appearance, of an opaque yellowish-white colour, which, on microscopic examination, was found to depend on an amorphous albuminoid deposit. (Qy. lardaceous).

Spleen.—An intensely marked specimen of the 'sago spleen'; the Malpighian bodies much enlarged and stain deeply with iodine.

Kidneys.—Nodulated and puckered, in one spot a cicatrix. Cortical substance contracted and firm; Malpighian bodies prominent, but few in number.

Stomach.— Congested; otherwise healthy.

Intestines.—Mucous membrane roughened as if granular, like coarse velvet or sand-paper. On microscopic examination large tracts of the epithelium were found changed, and having the amorphous glistening appearance of lardaceous disease, with disappearance of their nuclei.

Heart.—Pericardium, visceral and parietal, covered with recent lymph. Thickening of mitral valve. Much atheroma in the aorta.

THE MICROSCOPIC APPEARANCES which are most common in this lung are those seen in XLII. 6, viz.: great thickening of the walls of the alveoli with fibroid tissue, which is for the most part fibrillated, but in many places (not here represented) passes into broad bands of sclerotic tissue, like XLI. 1 (*Carr*), and XLII. 1 (*Attwood*), and in places the indurated tissue is traversed by large and still pervious bloodvessels. In the midst of this are seen the alveoli filled with epithelial products and pyoid cells, which are in parts replaced by a dense small-celled growth. Where the fibroid growth is less advanced, it can be seen to originate in a small-celled growth in the alveolar walls, like XXXVII. 6 and 7 (*Griffin*).

[1] The temperature chart was accidentally destroyed, but my own recollection and the assurance, at the time, of my resident clinical assistant, confirm this statement.

XXXIX. 3 (*Gardiner*), and it proceeds in a course of fibre-formation like XLI. 7 (*Coppin*). This small-celled growth sometimes forms nodules (miliary) projecting into the cavities of the alveoli. Sometimes it forms thickenings in the arteries similar to those seen in the arteries of the brain (see XLII. 7, *aa*). Nodules of induration are also seen, singly or in groups, commencing like XXXIX. 5 and 7 (*Overall* and *Unwin*), passing into the densest masses of homogeneous sclerosis like XLI. 1 and 3 (*Carr*), XLI. 5 (*Roberts*), and by processes similar to those described in these cases. Great numbers of giant-cells exist among these sclerosed nodules; they are sometimes central, sometimes peripheral, and are of the types of XXXII. 6, 7, 10, and XXXIII. 11. Much perivascular and peribronchial thickening exists throughout these specimens. It is commonly fibroid, homogeneously sclerotic, but in a few places can be seen to be proceeding by means of a small-celled growth.

CASE 4.

ACUTE BRONCHO-PNEUMONIA.

Plates V. fig. 3; XXVI. figs. 1–4.

Ref.—Catarrhal Pneumonia, pp. 23, 27.

SUMMARY.—*M. 1. A rickety child. Acute symptoms; diarrhœa, cough, fever, dyspnœa. Bronchitic râles through both lungs, with dulness and crepitation at the bases. High pyrexia of remitting type. Duration five weeks.—Bronchi filled with puriform secretion. Pneumonic consolidation at right base, with collapse at both bases and anterior margins. Spots of lobular pneumonia, some breaking down, were abundantly scattered through both lungs.*

JOHN TANNER, ætat. 1 year; admitted University College Hospital, September 10, 1880; died October 10, 1880.

Family History.—The youngest of five children; three are living and in good health; one, the fourth, has already died of bronchitis. Parents both living; in poor circumstances, even for the labouring class. No hereditary predisposition known. Patient has had no previous illnesses; has been suckled by mother up to present time.

Present Illness.—Commenced a week before admission. The child became feverish, lost appetite, and had diarrhœa; stools slimy and green; cough commenced with the fever; vomited with cough.

State on Admission.—Fairly well nourished. Some enlargement of ends of long bones (rickety); has cut all incisor teeth; anterior fontanelle widely open. Skin hot; dryness alternates with perspirations. No marked lividity, but considerable pallor. Hair silky; eyelashes long; some down on cheeks and back.

Respiratory System.—Breathes with difficulty; is propped up in bed, alæ nasi working; respirations 44 per minute; some wheezing. Retraction of lower ribs, epigastrium, and supnasternal notch, with inspiration. Upper part of chest resonant. Dulness both bases, laterally and posteriorly, especially at the right. Breath-sounds exaggerated above, at the bases accompanied by much crepitation. Moist râles are heard throughout both lungs. Tongue furred. Diarrhœa, with green stools.

The child continued in the same state and improved but little under treatment; occasional partial improvement took place in the physical signs and in the general state, but relapse speedily occurred. Diarrhœa was frequent, and there was occasional vomiting. The patient finally died exhausted, in spite of stimulants and of cold packing.

The temperature was high throughout nearly the whole of the illness, and was only partially and very temporarily reduced by the cold packing. On admission it was 103·6°, and it reached 104° on the next day, and continued high, with scarcely any remissions. The cold pack reduced it to 101°, but it rose immediately after to 104·6°, and continued not lower than 102·6° in a cold pack renewed every hour and a half, and subsequently repeated every twenty minutes. After 72 hours it fell to 99·4°, and remained below 102° during seven days, with only one exacerbation to 108°. During this period there were regular daily remissions to a temperature varying from 99° to 100°, and exacerbations varying from 100° to 102°; after this the temperature again rose, reaching repeatedly 104° and on one occasion 105·6°, with regular daily marked remissions to 99·2°, 99·8°, 100° and 101°; the usual minimum being between 99° and 100°; these remissions occurring sometimes in the evening. During the first two days of this second rise, the temperature remained persistently above 103°. During the last four days of life, the temperature gradually rose to 105·6°, none of the remissions being less than 101·6°.

The pulse was persistently rapid, varying from 140 to 160. The respirations varied from 44 to 72.

POST-MORTEM.—*Lungs:* Both are extensively collapsed at the bases and also at the anterior margins. Both apices over-distended, markedly emphysematous, though even here are some spots of collapse. Over the base of the right lung, there is a limited patch of lymph on the pulmonary pleura; otherwise the pleura are unaffected. Bronchi loaded with fluid creamy pus down to the finest ramifications that can be followed with the scissors. They are dilated throughout, but the dilatation becomes more marked in the smaller branches, the cut orifices of which are gaping, with thickening walls, while many small globular cavities, with a similar condition of wall, and filled with puriform liquid, are scattered thickly through the pulmonary tissue. These are most numerous at the bases, but they exist also in the upper part of the lungs. The more cylindrical dilatations of the tubes exist equally in all parts of the lung. The lining membrane of the tubes is thickened, intensely vascular, and softened. At the right base, beneath the spot of inflamed pleura, is a patch of reddish-grey pneumonic consolidation. Scattered thickly throughout both lungs, but most numerous at the bases, are two sets of changes (V. 3.) The first of these are little yellow, softened spots, varying from one-eighth to a quarter of an inch in diameter, scarcely prominent, and breaking down into a semi-fluid débris, which differs from the collections of pus found in the globular dilatations of the bronchi, and leaves, when evacuated, small cavities in the pulmonary tissue. Besides these there are similar spots, solid and firmer in consistence, but breaking down easily under pressure, finely granular on section (V. 3, *a*). These vary in colour from a reddish-yellow to a dull reddish-grey or a dull red, and are scarcely prominent; in some places they are situated in the midst of highly injected tissue, others are in the collapsed tissue, while some are in the emphysematous portions. They vary in size from a hemp-seed to a split pea, and tend in parts to become confluent, but when they do so no special racemose shape is assumed by them, but they form patches of irregular size and form, and may occupy areas of a quarter of an inch to an inch on superficial section. The collapsed parts are dull bluish-red, small and glistening on section, and resistant, except where invaded by pneumonic change. In some places they are markedly œdematous, much bloody serosity flowing from them. They are traversed by dilated bronchi as before described. Nothing special was found in the other organs.

MICROSCOPICAL EXAMINATION of the nodules found in the lung shows, in the more diffuse tracts, the alveolar tissue almost entirely filled with large epithelial cells like XXV. 8. Sections of the firmer nodules, situated under the pleura, show that the pneumonia is essentially lobular (see XXVI. 1 and 2), and that the alveoli, bronchioles, and alveolar passages are crowded with epithelial-like cells in various stages of disintegration. This distension of the lobule, when single, causes, apparently by compression, collapse of the adjacent tissue, as seen in XXVI. 1, *bb*, in which, however, some epithelial proliferation also occurs. The larger masses are formed by a confluence of such nodules (as seen in XXVI. 2). The alveolar walls are unaffected by any considerable nuclear growth, though a few enlarged nuclei may occasionally be seen in them (see XXVI. 4,) but there is no multiplication of these, or any thickening of the alveolar wall by new growth, and throughout, the capillaries may still be seen distended with blood. The cells by which the alveoli are distended are, for the most part, large round cells of the epithelial type (see XXVI. 3 and 4), but some leucocytes may be seen among these (as in fig. 3). Many of the cells contain blood-pigment, and they are for the most part finely granular, but in some instances coarsely so. These lobules, especially when confluent, tend to break down into débris: the epithelial cells become increasingly granular, they lose their defined outlines, and fuse into a homogeneous mass. These areas, such as XXVI. 1, appear in most cases to soften *en masse* without any antecedent suppuration, the walls of the alveoli breaking down into débris of a finely granular character. In a few places there is nuclear growth around the bronchioles and blood-vessels, and also some in the interlobular septa. No distinct reticulum can, however, be seen here, and, as already stated, the alveolar walls are free from the growth.

CASE 5.

ACUTE ULCERATING AND SUPPURATING PNEUMONIA.

Plates V. fig. 5 ; XXXV. fig. 7.

Ref.—Phthisis, pp. 119, 121.

SUMMARY.—*F. 31. Severe bronchitis a year before the sudden onset of acute symptoms, which occurred two months before death; cough, shivering, fever. Afterwards, sudden exacerbation; purulent expectoration and profuse sweating. Signs of consolidation at the apices and fine râles throughout both lungs. Diarrhœa with intestinal hæmorrhage. Death twelve days after last relapse. Temperature, moderately raised at first, gradually fell.—Bronchi inflamed and ulcerated, surrounded by greyish-red granular consolidation. Apex of right lung fibroid. A few granulations. Inflammation of small intestine.*

SARAH BROWN, ætat. 31, admitted University College Hospital under Dr. Reynolds, February 4, 1865; died February 11.

Family History.—Father died at 70, not subject to any chest affection. Mother delicate, but condition of chest not known; died, ætat. 40, in childbed. Patient was youngest of ten brothers and sisters, all dead but herself, causes of their death unknown.

Personal History.—No previous illnesses. Has lived almost constantly in London, as a domestic servant (general servant and cook), since 17. Has always had sufficient food. Menstruated at 14 or 15, has always been perfectly regular.

Present Illness.—In 1863, went to service at Tunbridge Wells. January 1864, after being nine months at Tunbridge Wells, caught a violent cold, had bronchitis, and was laid up in the infirmary there from the end of January until March. Recovered perfectly, returned to London, and was quite well during the whole of the summer of 1864. She continued well and free from cough until December 23, 1864, when she got a severe chill, had pains in limbs, shivering, and was feverish. Cough commenced at once, but without expectoration, such as is now present, until February 1, 1865. Continued at work as a domestic servant throughout January, but felt breath very short when she went up stairs. On February 1st she became suddenly worse, in consequence, it was thought, of a fresh chill; fever increased, breath became very short, and expectoration commenced. Has lost flesh and appetite during past six weeks, and has sweated at night since February 1. Menstruation has been regular, but for the last three or four months has been pale and scanty.

State on Admission.—Light red hair; light brown eyes; fair complexion; fingers slightly clubbed; skin hot; skin now dry, but perspires profusely at night. Face and lips livid; orthopnœa; respiration panting, 44; alæ nasi expand with inspiration. Pulse 148, small but equal. Frequent cough, with copious, confluent, thick, greenish, homogeneous expectoration, streaked with a dirty brown, and, in some places, with brighter red; under microscope, nothing can be seen but pus-corpuscles and mucus-corpuscles, some of which are pigmented.

Physical Examination.—Some flattening under both clavicles. Right infraclavicular region dull to third rib, below this right front and axilla resonant. Left infraclavicular, hyperresonant but not amphoric. Rest of left front resonant. Both supra-spinous fossæ deficient in resonance, especially the left; percussion of back interfered with by blister between shoulders. At right apex, front and back, respiration bronchial, with loud sibilant and sonorous râles, mingled with fine bubbling râles. These râles of both kinds are heard over the whole of the side, anteriorly and posteriorly. Vocal resonance exaggerated under right clavicle; pectoriloquy. Left apex, respiration hollow blowing, with coarse râles; at left base râles have a metallic quality. The dulness increased under the left clavicle during the ensuing week, and also, to a less degree, on the right side. (There was no material change in the quality

of the râles). Tongue covered with thick brownish fur, and red at tip and edges, with red papillæ. Has had diarrhœa severely for a week; was disturbed six or seven times last night. Has been very sick, but no nausea at present; no abdominal pain. Has been liable to slight attacks of diarrhœa when in ordinary good health, but not severe or frequent or of long duration.

The diarrhœa continued unchecked, in spite of treatment, and on two days she passed three or four dark tarry stools, and also some fluid blood, and she became delirious at night. Exhaustion increased, the cough was almost incessant, and the sputa became diffluent, homogeneous, and greenish-yellow in tinge. She died, exhausted, on February 11.

The clinical clerk's report of the urine has been omitted in the case-book, but it is believed to have been free from albumen. Her temperature shows a course so strikingly resembling that of acute pneumonia, fatal in the stage of collapse and defervescence, that I give the record entire.

Date	MORNING			EVENING		
	Temp.	Pulse	Resp.	Temp.	Pulse	Resp.
Feb. 4	—	—	—	103·6	152	48
5	102·2	150	48	101	152	48
6	102	144	44	101	144	56
7	100·8	120	44	99·4	152	52
8	99·6	140	48	98	144	44
9	98	144	52	98·2	144	56
10	96	136	56	96	132	66

Death at 7 A.M. on the following morning.

The temperatures (9.30 A.M. and 9.30 P.M.) were almost all taken when the patient was sitting up in bed.

POST-MORTEM: *6 hours after death.*—Chest flattened laterally and much enlarged. Liver projects four-and-a-half inches below margins of 7th and 8th ribs. On opening body, a very offensive odour is observed from the intestines.

Lungs.—Left: Upper lobe emphysematous, contains only a few small hard nodules, which when cut across, have a whitish centre surrounded by pigmented induration-matter. In the lower lobe the bronchi are filled with a very tenacious mucus. They are intensely injected, and the surface of the mucous membrane is rough and uneven. In some places, distinct ulcerations can be seen in those of the third and fourth divisions, passing, in some spots into small deep excavations, capable of holding a hemp-seed or a split pea. Such bronchi are imbedded in areas of solidified tissue (V. 5), with a granular surface, greyish-red in colour, dotted with yellow and whitish spots, in the centre of which there is often a small cavity communicating with the bronchi. Some of these cavities coalesce in places, and form rugged excavations. These areas may be from one to three inches in diameter; there are several such in the lung. The tissue between them is crepitant, yielding much grumous serosity. No grey granulations, nor any distinct tubercular granulations, can be found in this lobe.

Right Lung, strongly adherent to parietal pleura. The pleura at the apex is much thickened, and when cut into, several sinuous cavities, are seen traversed by bands and trabeculæ. The rest of the tissue is fibroid, of semi-cartilaginous firmness, and contains cheesy spots. Below this, in emphysematous tissue, are numerous nodules of induration, fibroid, pigmented, and puckered; in the centre of some is a white milky fluid. These spots, when incised longitudinally, are found to be bronchi with thickened walls, surrounded by indurated pulmonary tissue. Similar nodules are scattered throughout the lung. The lower lobe contains considerable recent pneumonic tracts, like those described in the left lung, and the bronchi exhibit similar changes. Smaller spots are found in this lung, presenting granulations of cheesy greyish matter surrounded by induration.

The *bronchial glands* are free from visible tubercle.

Heart healthy.

Liver fatty, much hepatic congestion.

Kidneys congested, indurated, cortical substance too narrow. Some cloudy swelling.

Spleen small, firm.

Stomach covered with tenacious mucus. Mucous membrane somewhat thickened, and presents a good deal of fine injection.

Intestines.—First part of jejunum contains a large patch of hæmorrhagic injection. Solitary glands and Brünner's glands enlarged, but no enlargement of Peyer's patches. In ileum, intense hæmorrhagic injection of mucous membrane, with submucous extravasations into villi and valvulæ conniventes, presenting a typical picture of muco-enteritis. Mucous membrane swollen, softened, and cloudy-looking; not a trace of tubercle visible. Injection diminishes in the last six inches of the ileum, and is only slightly marked in the ileo-cæcal valve and in the cæcum, though the solitary glands are much enlarged in this region. The colon shows scarcely any trace of inflammatory action.

MICROSCOPICAL EXAMINATION. Tracts of fibroid change are numerous. The chief and most characteristic alteration, pervading nearly all parts of the lung where the affection is recent, is a dense infiltration of the walls of the alveoli with a small-celled nuclear growth, which in places almost completely obliterates their cavity. In the alveoli not thus obliterated, large cells of the epithelial type remain. The variations in appearance of different parts which are produced by these changes are identical with those seen in XXXVIII. 6 (*Ellsom*), XXXVII. 7 (*Griffin*), XXX. 5 (*Polley*), XXXIX. 3 (*Gardiner*), and in a few places like XXXVIII. 1 (*Henshaw*). The small-celled growth forms in some parts small nodules and masses; but these are rare and quite exceptional; when present they are for the most part outgrowths of the alveolar thickening, but in a few they apparently arise from the filling of the alveoli with nuclear growth instead of with epithelial cells. In one place such a nodule is seen extending from the sheath of a bronchus.

Areas of pneumonic change are frequent and extensive, where the thickening of the walls with small-celled growth is less pronounced or is only commencing. The interior of the alveoli in these parts is sometimes crowded with epithelial cells and leucocytes, but in some places these are less numerous, and the air-cells are chiefly filled by an amorphous exudation, in which are a few enlarged epithelial cells and some hyaline large mucous corpuscles, as in XXXVIII. 4 (*Henshaw*).

Areas of destruction, like XXXVIII. 3 (*Henshaw*), are also seen. This destructive process, in which all the cell-elements of the tissue vanish, does not appear to be preceded by the dense small-celled infiltration of the alveolar walls just described, since their outlines remain unthickened; but in the parts where it is proceeding there appears to be an abortive commencement of the same growth in their floor. No epithelial cells are visible, and the whole is occupied by small nuclei and occasionally by small cells, between which, however, no reticulum is visible. These are smaller than pus-cells, and the form does not resemble suppuration, but suggests the idea that the vitality of the tissue perishes in the first acute formation of a small-celled growth, similar to that which, when proceeding in a less intense manner, persists to the extent of thickening the walls. Areas of a destructive pneumonia of the suppurative type are also observed (see XXXV. 7). These resemble in their main features those described in the cases of *Brodrick* and *Smith* (*18* and *28*). The tissue contains remains of epithelial cells, but it is also infiltrated with pus-cells, and cells of the size of pus-cells, but without nuclei. The epithelial-like cells are the least numerous, and the breaking down of the tissue appears to be due to the predominance of the latter. They fuse into an amorphous débris, in the formation of which the elastic fibres also disappear, and no appearance of small-celled or nuclear growth is seen in these areas, though it is found in others immediately adjacent.

Periarterial and peribronchial small-celled growths abound throughout these lungs. The latter are not unfrequently associated with suppuration, and in some cases, the character of the infiltration of the bronchial walls is suppurative rather than tubercular, but the two appear to pass into one another. No giant-cells are seen in these lungs.

COMMENTARY.—This is a case essentially of the 'acute desquamative pneumonia' of Buhl (see p. 39), which he says may run an acute course like croupous pneumonia. There had evidently been a previous attack, probably of the same character. Desquamative pneumonia is so rare without tubercles, that it may be held to be essentially a tubercular form.

CASE 6.
ACUTE TUBERCLE.

Plates VI., XXVIII., figs. 6–10, and XXX. fig. 5.

SUMMARY.—*M. 6. Family history of phthisis. Loss of appetite and headache, commenced three months before death, and was followed by cough and muco-purulent expectoration, and by signs of consolidation in the lungs, chiefly in the upper parts. Considerable pyrexia.—Tubercular granulations in pleura. Both lungs crammed with small granulations and larger firm nodules, in places confluent into tracts of cheesy aspect, unsoftened: some were surrounded by grey pneumonic infiltration. Tubercular granulations in peritoneum, liver, spleen, &c.*

JOHN H. POLLEY, ætat. 6, admitted University College Hospital January 25, died February 16, 1868.

Family History (given by child's mother).—Father was 'paralysed' three years ago, but recovered. Father and mother now both healthy. Three of his father's brothers died of phthisis: one sister died of 'abscess of the lung' at the age of 15 months: one brother and sister still living and healthy.

Personal History.—Had measles when eight months old; chicken-pox when fifteen months old; whooping cough in the winter of 1866-7. Father's house dry, but situation confined. Has never had good appetite.

Present Illness commenced in November 1869, with anorexia and headache, so that he was forced to leave school. Cough commenced in beginning of January 1868, and has since then been attended with much expectoration. Never had hæmoptysis. Has had occasional pain in left side. Has lost much flesh. Appetite very bad and bowels irregular. Headache has only been occasional. Has been under treatment as an out-patient at the Hospital for Sick Children before admission here.

State on Admission.—Great emaciation and marked anæmia. Teeth regular, one molar decayed. Fingers clubbed, nails incurved. Skin hot to hand. Breathing hurried, but can lie in any position with ease. Cough frequent, with mucoid expectoration mingled with puriform matter. Chest pigeon-breasted in moderate degree. Sternum and costal cartilages prominent as a whole: some thickening of ends of costal cartilages.

Physical Examination.—Percussion: both fronts very imperfect resonance, fifth rib in left axilla dull below fifth rib. The right upper back absolutely dull; the left gave imperfect resonance. Both bases posteriorly were very hyperresonant. The respiration was high-pitched blowing in both supra-spinous fossæ, and tubular in the interscapular regions. It was also harsh blowing in both infraclavicular regions. Fine moist râles were heard over the whole of both lungs, back and front, even over the duller areas; at the bases sonorous sounds were mingled with the moist râles.

Heart's position and sounds normal. Liver dulness extended superiorly to fifth rib in mammary line, and inferiorly to two and a half fingers' breadth below false ribs. Spleen enlarged, and could be felt below false ribs. Abdomen tense and tympanitic; bowels confined. Tongue furred. No marked thirst. Urine throughout varied in sp. gr. from 1015 to 1020.

The child gradually sank without fresh symptoms, and died on February 16, 1868. Dyspnœa was prominent throughout; the respirations ranging from 44 to 68; the pulse from 120 to 152. His mean pulse-respiration ratio was, for the morning, $2\frac{3}{5}$: 1; for the evening $2\frac{7}{15}$: 1. The highest pulse-respiration ratio was P. 152; R. 44 ($3\frac{1}{2}$: 1); morning, the lowest was P. 120; R. 68 ($1\frac{3}{4}$: 1), evening. His mean morning temperature in fifteen observations was 101·1°, the lowest being 99·8°, the highest 103·4°. The mean evening temperature in thirteen observations was 102°, the highest being 103·6°, the lowest 100°. The average exacerbation from morning to evening in seven observations was 1·8°, the greatest being 3·2°, the lowest 0·6°. The average remission from morning to evening in six observations was 1·8°, the greatest being 3·6°, the lowest 0·2°. Remissions from morning to evening were observed on three days; mean 1·2°, maximum 0·7°. Exacerbations occurred from evening to morning on four days; mean 0·6°, maximum 1·2°, minimum 0·3°.

Post-mortem.—*Lungs:* No adhesions, but parietal pleura thickly covered with fine granulations, without any exudation, thickening, or congestion. Some emphysema of both lungs at anterior borders. The external surfaces of both lungs studded thickly with granulations, flattened, all appearing firm and semi-cartilaginous (VI. 2). The centre of some is more opaque, but having a bluish-grey tinge: in a few the centres are yellowish. The granulations vary in size from a pin's point to a hemp-seed. Even under the pleura they tend to increase into masses, around the circumference of which granulations are sprinkled, giving the groups an irregular racemose appearance; around these there is much congestion. When cut into, these are found to correspond to larger masses more deeply seated.

On section both lungs are filled from apex to base, and almost equally with solid nodules, varying in size from a split pea to a bean. These are firm and dry-looking, dense, hard, and very resisting (VI. 1). No appearance of softening anywhere except in a few small cavities at the apices. The colour of these masses is of a dull greenish-white. Between them, in emphysematous and highly congested lung-tissue, are granulations of all sizes, from a millet-seed and upwards, having the same appearance, all firm and nowhere softening.

In several places in both lungs, the conglomerate masses form large tracts occupying considerable areas, of a yellowish caseous appearance, firm and resisting but granular, and in some places manifestly composed of separate nodules. They show no appearance of softening, but in the centre of one is a spot rather more caseous than the rest. Some of these nodules are surrounded by a zone of grey pneumonic infiltration. The mucous membrane of the bronchi is pale. Here and there some fusiform dilatations are seen. In some places the bronchial wall is perforated by tubercles penetrating from the lung.

The *bronchial glands* are enlarged, intensely cheesy, a little pigmented, and of a homogeneous yellow tint.

Abdomen.—No effusion in peritoneal cavity, but the peritoneum (especially the omentum) is covered thickly with small yellowish-white bodies, varying in size from a pin's point to a millet-seed. On section most of these are cheesy and soft. The mesenteric glands are large, yellowish-white in colour, cheesy, and friable on section.

Intestines.—Numerous ulcers tending to encircle the intestine and having thickened edges, exist in both small and large intestine. Others of the same character are found both in the cæcum and in the large intestine.

Liver.—Gall-bladder full of clear transparent bile; ductus communis pressed upon by enlarged and cheesy glands. Both can only be evacuated into duodenum by strong pressure. Liver studded everywhere on surface and in substance with granulations, which vary in size from a millet to a hemp seed. Some of the larger ones are cheesy; the smaller ones are semi-transparent; many are bile-stained (VI. 4.)

Spleen much enlarged, measures $5\frac{1}{2}$ in. by $3\frac{1}{2}$ in. by 2 in., and weighs $6\frac{1}{2}$ oz. Its tissue is very firm, and is riddled throughout with cheesy masses, varying in size from a pea to a bean, opaque, very resistant, not at all friable. In several places large tracts are occupied by dense cheesy matter (*see* VI. 5 and 6). There are a number of cheesy masses near the hilus, and one of these appears to represent a supernumerary spleen filled with tubercle. Supra-renal capsules healthy.

Kidneys.—Both contain masses under the capsules and in the pyramids, cheesy, but not softening; pelves free, except a small uric acid calculus in one of the calyces of right kidney.

Heart and great vessels, *Brain*, and *Testicles* free.

MICROSCOPIC APPEARANCES.—Distinct isolated small-celled growths, constituting granulations of the purely tubercular type, are comparatively rare in these lungs: a few are, however, seen. The chief changes are pneumonic, combined with a reticular growth in the walls of the alveoli and alveolar passages, and these extend over considerable areas and are very little circumscribed. The main type of these, in an early stage, is shown in XXX. 5, where the alveoli are seen filled with epithelial cells of variable size, some of them being multinuclear. Their walls are thickened with a small-celled growth imbedded in a reticulum. Many variations are found in this process, producing appearances like XXXVII. 6 and 7 (*Griffin*), and also like XXXVII. 1 (*Griffin*) (where the reticular growth is seen proceeding in the floor of an alveolus), and like XXXIX. 3 (*Gardiner*). The lobular or infundibular type is well marked in some places, like XXVIII. 1, 2, 3, but these are less common: where they are found, the interior of the alveoli and alveolar passages are seen filled with epithelial cells as described in *Coombes* (Case 7), while the walls are thickened by the small-celled reticular growth. Some of these pyramidal nodules are purely epithelial, and side by side with them are others precisely similar, except that they are partly composed of a small-celled growth in the manner last described. In some places the interstitial thickening of the alveolar walls has taken place through very large areas, as seen in XXVIII. 9 and 10; and identical in appearance with XXXVIII, 1 (*Henshaw*). Many of these tracts are intensely pigmented.

Caseation takes place acutely in large diffuse areas, as seen in XXVIII. 6, where the outlines of the alveoli are maintained, their interior being filled with amorphous débris. In other places, where probably a reticular growth has previously occupied the whole structure, the resulting caseation appears in the form of a granular but finely fibrillated mass, as seen in XXVIII. 8, and resembling also XLIII. 5 (*Heath*). In other parts, where the caseation retains the lobular form, the remains of the dilated extremities of the infundibular and alveolar passages may be traced, resembling XL. 4 (*Heath*). When the lobular form is retained in these caseous masses it is sometimes on a large scale; occasionally it is bounded by the interlobular septa, but in other places rounded masses of caseation appear, in which the demarcation is not distinct. In some places the pyramidal (infundibular) masses of catarrhal pneumonic infiltration can be seen passing into caseation, and in these it may be observed that a small-celled reticular growth, in the floor and walls of the alveoli, precedes this change, the catarrhal epithelial cells disappearing and becoming replaced by the small-celled growth.

CASE 7.

ACUTE TUBERCLE.

Plates VIII. figs. 2 and 5; XXVIII. 4; XXX. figs. 3 and 4; XXXIV. 1.

SUMMARY.—*M. 13. Ill-fed, of phthisical family. Lung-symptoms developed rapidly, with considerable remitting pyrexia, sweating, and diarrhœa. There were signs of consolidation at the apices, and abundant râles through both lungs.—The lungs contained abundant discrete tubercles, some caseating and breaking down. In the right lung there was an embolic infarct. The intestines presented tubercular ulceration.*

ALFRED COOMBES, ætat. 13, admitted University College Hospital, under Dr. Reynolds, April 10; died April 26, 1867.

Family History.—Both parents living. Father, 55, a printer, has had a cough for six or seven years attended by much expectoration and occasional hæmoptysis. Paternal grandmother consumptive. Mother, 48; no chest affection known in her family. Patient is one of eight children, four of whom are dead; one brother died at 18, cause unknown; one died of head affection; one of some chest affection; one from whooping-cough.

Personal History.—Has had measles at 2, whooping cough at 4, and scarlatina when very young. He worked since 10 years old in printing office from 8 A.M. to 8 P.M., but occupation of late has been to drag a truck in the streets. This involved pressure on the epigastrium, and patient suffered from nausea. Has lived badly, and has seldom had meat more than once a week. Has been liable to take cold for some years past, but has never been laid by before present illness.

Present Illness commenced two months ago. Patient returned home complaining of epigastric pain; he then had rigors; his strength failed suddenly, and cough supervened a few days later. He had slight hæmoptysis soon after invasion of illness.

State on Admission.—Fair hair; long eyelashes; teeth good, enamel thin; fingers long and taper, nails incurvated, but not to a considerable degree. Marked anæmia and considerable emaciation, flushes easily. Lips dry and cracked, skin hot, perspiration profuse at times. Some enlargement of lymphatic glands in neck.

Considerable dyspnœa, with expansion of alæ nasi. Cough at first not very frequent, but increased after admission. Sputa at first scanty; became after a few days glairy and tenacious; for the most part semi-transparent, containing a few white specks; the amount increased to about 4oz. in the twenty-four hours. During the last four days of life they contained blood, intimately intermingled, but they never assumed a rusty tinge.

Physical Signs.—Chest naturally well formed, with wide costal angles. Both infra-clavicular regions flattened, and clavicles prominent. Expansion defective under clavicles, good at bases. On percussion, there is dulness at both apices in front to the third rib; behind, on the right side, to the spine of the scapula; on the left side, to the middle of the scapula. Both bases hyperresonant. Respiration in back almost masked by coarse bubbling râles which are heard over the whole back; it is bronchial in the left supra-spinous fossa, blowing at the bases. In front also the respiration is only heard indistinctly, through the abundant râles which exist everywhere; it is somewhat tubular under left clavicle, where the râles are more abundant and more metallic than under right clavicle. Vocal resonance exaggerated in right infra-clavicular and left supra-spinous regions. Tongue covered with thin fur, having a tendency to become dry, Thirst very marked. Diarrhœa present; three or four loose actions daily. No pain or tenderness in abdomen. He gradually sank and died sixteen days after admission.

The temperature was constantly pyrexial, the maximum being 104° on one occasion. The mean morning temperature (7 observations) was 100·2.° The mean evening temperature (6 observations) was 103·6°. The evening temperature was always higher than the morning. The average of the exacerbations from morning to evening was 3·1°, the greatest being 4·2°, the smallest being 1·4°. The average of the remissions from evening to morning was 3·3°, the greatest being 4·4°, and the lowest 2°. The temperature was thus of a markedly remitting type. The pulse ranged at 120; the respiration at 40; but the number of the observations is limited.

POST-MORTEM.— Right lung riddled with tubercles from apex to base; all are scattered, none confluent. There is not a trace to be seen of racemose agglomeration. The granulations vary much in character.

(A) Some are semi-transparent; none of these exceed a poppy-seed in size, and all dimensions can be traced to almost invisible specks, not larger than a pin's point. In some of the larger granulations of this class, an opaque cheesy spot can be seen in the centre, the circumference being still semi-transparent (see VIII. 2 and 5).

(B) In other portions of the lung are granulations of a dead opaque white, not prominent, larger than the foregoing but not exceeding a hemp-seed in size. They are all scattered singly and do not form conglomerate masses. Some have caseous spots in their centres, but others, apparently without having undergone this change, are broken into puriform débris. Portions of the lung in which these occur are riddled with small cavities, none of which exceed the size of a pea, and most of them do not exceed that of a hemp-seed. The granulations and their characters in the left lung are precisely similar to those in the right. In this lung, however, there is a large infarct at the base. Tubercles are thickly scattered throughout the area thus occupied. A branch of the pulmonary artery leading to it is found obstructed by a clot (probably proceeding from a thrombus in the heart).

Heart.—Right ventricle contains a fibrinous coagulum, ragged and irregular. Valves healthy.

The Intestine contains numerous tubercular ulcers, with a ragged floor, in which are cheesy masses, and with tubercular thickening of their margins.

Kidneys.—Through both, grey granulations are thickly scattered. There are numerous grey granulations on the surface of the liver, not in the rest of the peritoneal cavity. The other organs are healthy.

MICROSCOPIC APPEARANCES.—Four main changes are observed in these lungs:—(A) Granulations composed of variable proportions of small-celled and epithelial growth. (B) Peribronchial and perivascular thickening with small-celled growth. (C) Areas of interstitial thickening with small-celled growth. (D) Lobules of pneumonia, in some places isolated, and in others becoming confluent in diffused areas.

(A) These granulations are essentially round in the majority of cases. They are, however, seen in some parts to have a peribronchial origin, arising in these in the terminal bronchioles (*see* XXVIII. 4 *a*). In others immediately adjacent (see same fig.) they occupy the whole of single alveoli. In many places, however, they have a more or less pyramidal form, showing that they are constituted out of an entire infundibulum, and resemble XXVIII. 1, 2, 3. Some of these infundibular masses are almost entirely fibroid and pigmented, showing that they are of old formation. In almost all places in which they are found, there exists also a direct extension of the small celled growth into the walls of the adjacent alveoli, causing a thickening of these, and this change is occasionally attended with much pigmentation (*see* XXVIII. 4, *cc.*) The fully-formed granulations contain variable proportions of epithelial and small-celled growth. The epithelial growth is manifestly that resulting from the alveolar lining, and in such tubercles as result from the implication of several alveoli (transverse section of an infundibulum) the epithelial cells are seen to be centrally placed in the midst of masses of a reticulated small-celled formation (*see* XXX. 3 and 4, and description). In the centres of these granulations, the epithelial cells have commonly disappeared, and have been replaced by small round pyoid nuclei (?), finely granular, and evidently breaking down (XXX. 3 and 4, *a a*), and these fuse into an amorphous caseous mass in which the remains of elastic fibres may be seen undergoing disintegration (XXX. 3, *b*). The small-celled growth, here as elsewhere, is imbedded in reticulum. This is sometimes amorphous and glistening, sometimes fibrillated. (The fibrillation has been somewhat exaggerated in the engraving.) In some parts this small-celled growth is seen to be pigmented (XXX. 4, *e*). Here and there, masses of epithelial cells may be seen undergoing fusion, and remains of bronchioles, filled with remains of epithelial débris, may be seen in some parts (XXX. 4, *d d*). The proportion of epithelial small-celled growth varies much in different specimens, and in the whiter and softer forms of granulation the epithelial cells are considerably in excess, and sometimes appear to form a large proportion of the whole.

(B) Both the peribronchial and perivascular growths are numerous and extensive.

(C) The areas of interstitial thickening resemble those seen in XXVIII. 9, 10 (*Polley*), XXXVIII. 1 (*Henshaw*), and XXXVIII. 6 (*Ellsom*).

(D) Pneumonia occurs in some places in an exquisitely infundibular form, resembling the bronchopneumonia of measles and the catarrhal pneumonia of childhood. It differs, however, from the latter by the fact that caseation appears in the floor of the infundibula thus affected, and this caseation is preceded by a small-celled growth. In some of these places giant-cells may be seen in the reticular growth in the centres of the alveoli, but they are not common.

The epithelial proliferation resembles that seen in XXVI. 7 (*Ellsom*) and XXX. 5 (*Polley*). In many places it is apparent that the softer nodules arise from a small-celled growth taking place in the walls of infundibula and alveoli in which a catarrhal epithelial proliferation has occurred, and these subsequently caseate or undergo fibroid transformation. In some instances the latter change may be traced in nodules which seem to have had a pneumonic origin, or in which the first process was that of epithelial desquamation.

CASE 8.

SUPPURATION OF GLANDS. TUBERCULOSIS.

Plates XXIX., XXX. fig. 9; XXXI. figs. 1–6; XXXII. figs. 1 and 6.

SUMMARY.—*F. S. Suppurating glands in the neck. Slight lung-symptoms and pyrexia, at first remitting. Enlargement of liver; slight distension of abdomen. Acute cerebral symptoms (convulsions, &c.).—Miliary tubercle in lungs. Tubercular peritonitis; fatty liver; caseation of mesenteric glands; degenerating tubercles in kidneys. Tubercular meningitis. Suppuration of cervical and inguinal glands.*

SARAH SHIMMICK, ætat. 8 years, admitted University College Hospital, October 18, 1880; discharged November 15, re-admitted January 17, 1881, and died March 2.

Family History.—Father labourer, now 47, healthy. Mother 44, chest delicate. No miscarriages. Parents had been married 18 years at birth of patient, who is the seventh out of eight children, six of whom are living. The eldest (a daughter) had a delicate chest; another (a son) has had inflammation of the lungs; one has died from small-pox, another from convulsions.

Personal History.—Patient has been well-fed and clothed; house dry and without bad smells. Had measles when 2½. Has been liable to partial attacks of unconsciousness passing into delirium during the past year; the last of these occurred three months before admission.

Present Illness began three months ago. She lost appetite and grew thin. A lump appeared in left side of neck two months ago, which has gradually increased up to present time.

State on Admission.—Strength fair. Tolerably well nourished. Skin pallid, but no marked anæmia. No eruptions. Hair dark and fine; eyelashes thick and long; downy hair on shoulders and back, but to a less degree on cheeks. Long bones slight and thin. Intelligence good. Chest alar, long, narrow, lower ribs oblique; shoulders prominent forwards; infraclavicular and mammary regions flat. Teeth decayed in left lower jaw. A large mass of glands existed on left side of neck, extending from the submaxillary gland to the parotid, and into the anterior and posterior triangles. They were painful. No other glands affected.

The swelling on the left side of the neck increased and became soft and fluctuating. The glands on the right subsequently enlarged. The fluctuating mass on the left side was opened by incision, letting out pus, and was subsequently treated antiseptically. The temperature, previously raised, fell to 99°, and the discharge diminishing, the child was made an out-patient.

On re-admission in January into a surgical ward, a soft fluctuating mass was found in the middle line of the neck below the cricoid cartilage, bounded on each side by the sterno-mastoid muscles, superficial, and giving no dulness over the manubrium sterni. Behind right sterno-mastoid was another oval swelling, distinctly fluctuating, the skin over it being natural in appearance. At its lower border were masses of enlarged glands, and other enlarged glands could be felt beneath the right sterno-mastoid. In the left posterior triangle was another swelling, which fluctuated. The skin over this was reddened. The glands at the angle of the left jaw were much enlarged and were tender. A sinus existed behind the left angle of the jaw. Lungs and other organs still apparently healthy. The fluctuating swellings were opened, drained by horse-hair setons, and dressed antiseptically. The discharge continued, moderate in quantity and healthy, for the succeeding month, but the child remained persistently feverish, lost flesh and appetite, although she presented no other complications until a fortnight before her death.

On February 16, 1881, she was re-transferred to medical side. Some dulness was found at left apex and in left lower mammary region. Respiration-sounds harsh. Sibilant râles in both lungs, and a few mucoid râles in left lung, both at base and apex. Resp. 40, pulse 140. Liver extending nearly to umbilicus and tender on pressure; surface smooth; edge fairly sharp and defined. Spleen did not extend below false ribs. Abdomen somewhat distended, but uniformly so, and chiefly in the hypochondriac regions. No tenderness except over the liver. No dulness or fluctuation in flanks. Stools solid, but very pale. Appetite deficient; no vomiting.

On February 25, patient became drowsy and continued so during the next two days, but could be roused. Ophthalmoscopic examination showed in the right eye a normal disk, but a little to the inner side was a bright, highly refracting area with well-defined edges, and apparently slightly raised from the surface. A little below the disc there was a diffused pale area. Left eye nothing abnormal. A small ulcer was seen on right cornea, with streaks of hyperæmia extending from it. Two days later the stupor passed into unconsciousness. No paralysis or loss of reflex action. A flush of hyperæmia appeared on the right side of the face, exactly limited at the middle line, and extending from the roots of the hair to the middle of the chin on this side of the head, and limited to it. Profuse perspiration occurred at the same time. Three hours later the patient had a convulsive attack consisting of twitching of both arms and legs, and of the right orbicularis palpebrarum. Both pupils were dilated, the right excessively so, and more than the left. The fits recurred at short intervals; some were limited to the right side of the body. The hyperæmia and sweating on the right side of the head disappeared, but were renewed at intervals, and extended to the right side of the body generally. Consciousness partially returned on the following day, and both arms could be moved. There was no return of convulsions, but partial consciousness alternated with a comatose state for three days after the first appearance of cerebral symptoms. During this time the respiration and pulse grew more rapid (resp. 60, pulse 170) until the patient's death on March 2). A rise of temperature to 105·2° preceded death by a few hours.

Temperature.—During her first stay in hospital the patient was persistently feverish, but to a moderate degree, and during some part of all days the temperature exceeded 99°. Usually a rise commenced from 8 A.M. to 8 P.M. and on most days did not exceed 100° to 101°. Exceptions, however, occurred in which the temperature reached 102° to 103°, these higher temperatures being noted in both antemeridian and in the post-meridian hours. Subnormal temperatures (96·4° to 97·4°) occurred with considerable frequency, being sometimes met with at 8 A.M. sometimes at 11 P.M. (more commonly at the latter hour), and in the majority of the observations the temperature at 8 A.M. was observed to be above the normal, sometimes reaching 102° or 103°.

The second and complete operation of opening the abscesses had little effect on the temperature after the first twenty-four hours, when it was subnormal throughout the greater part of the day. For fourteen days subsequently, temperatures prevailed almost identical in degree and course with those previously described. After this the pyrexia was more continuous throughout the day, the remissions being less marked, and the range higher, temperatures of 102° and 103° occurring on most days; 104·8° being reached on one occasion, three weeks before death. The day before death the temperature, as already stated, rose to 105·8°.

The *pulse* was rapid throughout. During the first stay in hospital it never fell below 112, and varied between this and 130. Subsequently it varied from 120 to 150, rising two days before death to 176. The rate of *respiration*, which on admission was usually from 20 to 30, gradually increased in frequency to 40, 50, and 60, but the increase did not always correspond with the pulse.

POST-MORTEM, *fourteen hours after death.*—Rigor mortis slight. Subcutaneous fat almost absent. *Thorax*: no effusion in pleura. The lungs were thickly crowded, throughout and uniformly, with small semi-transparent granulations. These were for the most part scattered, but here and there they occurred in groups, though these were not of the racemose type. The granulations were so thickly scattered that hardly a quarter of an inch of the surface of any section was free from them. Scarcely any exceeded the size of a poppy-seed, and from this size they diminished to the smallest specks visible to the naked eye. They all projected above the cut surface and were glistening, semi-transparent, greyish in colour, and each was surrounded by a zone of hyperæmia. There was little or no opacity or caseation to be observed in any of them, and no softening into cavities. They projected from under the pleura, and here and there appeared to invade and pass into the membrane, which was otherwise unaffected. The lungs were very hyperæmic. Some spots of collapse, which could be easily inflated, existed at both bases. No other form of consolidation, or other abnormal appearances, existed in the lungs.

Larynx healthy.

Heart healthy.

Abdomen.—The visceral and parietal folds of peritoneum were adherent, and in these adhesions were fine granulations. Similar adhesions also existed over the surface of the liver. The mesenteric glands had universally caseated, and had broken down into soft or semi-fluid masses, but none of these had ruptured or perforated.

Stomach and *Intestines* healthy.

The *Liver* was much enlarged: weight 42 oz. Its section was of a pale yellow colour, greasy to the feel, and the tissue was found, on microscopic examination, to be intensely fatty.

Spleen soft, otherwise normal.

Kidney contained numerous small semi-transparent granulations of the size of mustard-seeds. These, in some places, had a distinctly yellow tint, and a few were found larger in size and softened into a thick, yellow, semi-fluid material.

Brain.—Dura mater normal. The membranes on the upper surface were sticky, and adherent to the brain-tissue. The convolutions were flattened. A quantity of yellowish lymph covered the base of the brain, extending into the fissures between the convolutions of the cerebrum and cerebellum. In this lymph, and also imbedded in the pia mater, were innumerable small fine semi-transparent granulations of the size of a poppy-seed. Ventricles distended with clear fluid,—from 4 to 5 oz. The fornix and corpus callosum were softened and almost diffluent.

Glands.—Almost all the cervical glands were found to be suppurating, as also were the inguinal glands. There was also found a small post-pharyngeal abscess.

Eye.—In the left a white spot was found near the disc in the same position as seen during life.

For microscopic appearances of the lungs see description of Plates XXIX.; XXX. 9; XXXI. 1 to 6; XXXII. 1 and 6.

CASE 9.

ACUTE TUBERCULISATION. CASEATION OF GLANDS.
(*Not illustrated.*)

SUMMARY.—*M. 26. Tubercular inheritance. Onset of cough nine months before death, followed by progressive weakness and night-sweats. Five months later, signs of a large pleural effusion on the left side, and of slight changes at the right apex. Temperature normal. Paracentesis (serous fluid) was followed by pyrexia, reaccumulation, and prostration. Second paracentesis; fluid purulent and offensive. Hectic fever and exhaustion.—Left lung collapsed, and contained a few granulations: these were abundant in the right lung. The mediastinal glands were enlarged and caseated. Recent pericarditis. Liver cirrhotic and tubercular. Retro-peritoneal glands and suprarenal bodies enlarged.*

ALFRED VICK, ætat. 26, admitted University College Hospital, Feb. 5; died June 18th, 1869.

Family History.—Father died aged 60, patient thinks of some chest affection. Mother died of paralysis. One brother died of 'water on the brain.' one sister died of consumption. One sister living has 'scrofulous' affection of the scalp. Two cousins died of consumption.

Personal History.—Has always lived well. Had gonorrhœa three years ago, and afterwards enlargement of glands in groin, sores on the tongue, and loss of hair.

Present Illness.—Dated by patient from July 1868, when his tongue again became sore. In September, a bad cough commenced, occurring in paroxysms, and

CASE 9 (VICK)

attended with much thick yellow expectoration. The cough ceased in November, but he has grown continually weaker. Has had profuse nocturnal perspirations. No diarrhœa. Never had hæmoptysis.

State on Admission.—Anæmia marked, emaciation moderate. No nodes discoverable. Tongue sore, ulcerated at edges; papillæ red at tip and edges. Urine 1020; free from albumen. Liver enlarged; reaching, in mammary region, from 5th rib to three fingers' breadth below false ribs. Spleen not to be felt in abdomen. Cough troublesome, without expectoration.

Physical Signs.—Left side bulged throughout: intercostal spaces immoveable and flattened. Measurement at level of nipple L. 16⅜ inch : R. 16¾ inch. Whole left side less resonant, except between 2nd and 4th ribs in the infraclavicular region, where a tubular note was occasionally, but not always, obtained, and in the upper scapular region, where a high-pitched but imperfect pulmonary note existed. The respiration sounds, vocal fremitus, and vocal resonance were suppressed in the lower half of the left lung. In the upper part there was bronchial breathing, with friction front and back, and the vocal resonance was bronchophonic in the mid-scapular region. The right infra-clavicular region gave imperfect resonance, with weak breathing. Over the rest of this side respiration was exaggerated. The heart's apex beat a little to the right of the ensiform cartilage; the dulness extended to the right border of the sternum.

He remained in the same state until March 16th, when the enlargement of the left side was found to have slightly increased, being at nipple R. 17 inch, L. 17¾ inch, and two inches below nipple R. 17 inch L. 17¼ inch. Paracentesis was performed, and eight ounces of clear, dark sherry-coloured fluid was withdrawn. The percussion resonance became tubular to 5th rib in mammary region, and 6th rib in axilla ; and imperfect resonance existed in the back to the angle of the scapula. Below these levels there was absolute dulness. Weak blowing breathing was heard over the resonant area, attended by friction, but the vocal resonance was audible to the extreme base. The heart beat at the ensiform cartilage.

The fluid gradually re-accumulated, displacing the heart to the right of the sternum. The whole left side became dull up to the clavicle. The right side was resonant throughout and without any râles. The cough was frequent, hacking, with a moderate amount of fluid, aërated, scarcely puriform, bronchitic sputa. There was much sense of dyspnœa. The tongue was red and irritable, but there was no diarrhœa. Profuse perspiration occurred from time to time. He lost much flesh ; the pallor and anæmia increased ; and he passed into a state of threatening collapse. The sputa had become nummulated and puriform. On May 1st, there was a trace of albumen in the urine; which had a sp. gr. of 1032. The dyspnœa having become severe, he was tapped by Mr. Berkeley Hill in the 5th and 6th interspaces, left side (giving exit to 7·4 oz. of fluid), and a drainage-tube was inserted. The fluid first escaping was grumous, puriform, and intensely fœtid; later a clear straw-coloured serum escaped, but this was followed (in course of the same day) by a puriform fluid.

The immediate effect of the tapping was great relief, cessation of cough and expectoration, and cessation of night sweats. The sputa continued puriform, but generally of bronchitic type. During the subsequent days subcutaneous emphysema formed around the wound and extended to the scrotum, but gradually disappeared. The expectoration continued mainly mucoid. The discharge was maintained free, with the exception of an arrest on one occasion during a few days : but it was frequently offensive and became excessively so at the last, though the cavity of the chest was washed out with carbolic acid. Bed-sores formed, and the patient sank and died on June 18.

The *Temperature*, though at first not taken very regularly, showed an absence of pyrexia on admission and up to the 17th of March, the date of his first tapping. (It was taken daily during this period, but only on ten days in both morning and evening.) The temperature never reached 100° and only on three occasions exceeded 99°. After the first tapping the patient became continuously pyrexial, and continued so until May 3, but the temperature never rose above 101·4°. After the second tapping and establishment of free drainage, it fell slightly for ten days, not exceeding 99·6°. After this he remained slightly feverish until his death. On one occasion only did the temperature reach 103°, and on two other days 102·6° and 102·4°, but on the majority of days it varied from 99° to 101°. Very few subnormal temperatures occurred. The *Pulse* was rapid throughout, always exceeding 100° and increasing to 140° towards the close of life.

POST-MORTEM.—Left lobe of liver projects five inches below ensiform cartilage, and three inches below cartilage of eighth rib, right side Right lobe projects three inches below cartilage of tenth rib. Left pleura covered by ichorous lymph, thickened, softened, and sloughing in parts. No tubercle observed.

Left Lung adherent to spine, to pericardium, and to the chest-wall in clavicular and infra-clavicular regions. It is totally collapsed and carnified, except at the apex, where there is still some crepitant tissue, which floats in water even after pressure. In this lung there are a few recent grey granulations, scanty at the apex, but somewhat more in number at the base. The tissue of the lung is much pigmented, but there is no pneumonic or other consolidation.

Right Lung.—Bronchi intensely congested and covered with a thick, opaque, blood-stained mucus. Throughout the whole of this lung there are grey granulations, semi-transparent, but pigmented, gelatinous-looking but firm, although not very firm. They vary in size from a pin's-head to a poppy-seed, and they occur singly or in racemose groups. They are almost equally scattered through the whole lung ; if anything, they are rather more numerous at the base than at the apex. The pleural surface is thickly studded with them. The lung-tissue is intensely injected in parts, and it is infiltrated by a grey, finely granular, dull purple exudation, but nearly all parts of the lung float in water.

Larynx and *Trachea* healthy.

Pericardium universally adherent to heart by recent lymph, which is thick, flaky, and gelatinous, though firm. *Heart* healthy.

Glands.—The lymphatic glands of the posterior mediastinum, and especially those at the root of the left lung, present a medullary section and have numerous caseous spots scattered through their substance. Some, however, are simply enlarged without

z

caseation, while others are indurated and have undergone much caseous change. There is great thickening of the cellular tissue in the anterior mediastinum, where the glands are also enlarged and fused together, forming masses as large as a bantam's egg. They have undergone extensive caseous change, which in some places is passing into cretification. The bronchial glands of the right lung have also undergone similar cretification.

Liver cirrhotic, with great induration. It is also studded with grey granulations (tubercular), both throughout its substance and also under the peritoneal covering.

Stomach.—Solitary glands much enlarged and in many places eroded.

Intestines.—Enlargement of solitary glands throughout. In many places these have a caseous centre and are surrounded by a zone of injection. There is a good deal of congestion in some parts of the intestine.

Omentum and *Peritoneum* healthy. *Mesenteric glands* unchanged. Retro-peritoneal glands are enlarged, forming large masses. They are indurated, opaque, and cheesy, like the mediastinal glands.

Spleen healthy.

Supra-renal Capsules.—Right enlarged to nearly four times its natural size. It is almost entirely converted into caseous matter, scarcely any glandsubstance remaining. Left enlarged to about twice its natural size. It is cheesy in scattered spots, some of which attain the size of a filbert.

Kidneys.—Right, healthy. Left presents some grey granulations scattered in its substance.

COMMENTARY.—This case affords one of the best instances with which I am acquainted in support of the opinion that acute tuberculisation is the result of the absorption of caseous matter. The course of the case, on this theory, would be pleurisy, caseation of mediastinal lymphatics, and secondary acute tuberculisation of the lung on the unaffected side. If, however, the granulations in the lung are a disease of a different nature from the affection of the lymphatics, we have to recognise that the caseation of the mediastinal lymphatic glands was not the sole manifestation of this form of disease in the body, but that the retro-peritoneal glands and the suprarenal capsules were similarly affected. We have then a multiple caseous disease, affecting three parts and two different sets of organs. What is this disease? I believe the answer must be that it also is tubercular, and that the lung-affection was only a secondary manifestation of the same nature. It must be remembered that the patient had an hereditary tendency to 'scrofulous' and tubercular affections.

I regret that the notes are not more explicit on the condition of the pleura on the affected side. Writing from memory, I believe no trace of tubercle could be found in it, but it appears to me highly probable that the pleural affection was also tubercular, and that it may have even been secondary to that of the mediastinal glands. In respect to this, another point requires notice, viz. that cretification was present both in the bronchial glands of the right lung, and also in the glands of the anterior mediastinum. It would appear probable that these may have suffered from caseous change at a date prior to the fatal illness, which was only of nine months' duration (judging from the cough which probably indicated the commencement of the pleurisy), or eleven months from July 1868. It is not, as far as I am aware, clearly known how long a period is requisite for the cretification of glands, but if their condition dated from his present illness, either the gland affection and the pleurisy must have been almost simultaneous, or, what seems more probable, the former must have preceded the latter.

Another point of great interest in this case is that in a pleurisy that was probably *ab initio* tubercular, there was very slight and sometimes no pyrexia until paracentesis had been performed. Although the notes do not state the fact, I have no doubt but that the operation was performed with Thompson's cannula, opening under water, and that every precaution was taken to exclude air. Septic infection, however, occurred after the operation, and from this time fever was present. Even then the fever was not high, and was in no respect characteristic of acute tuberculosis, nor did it present any notable peculiarities. I think it most improbable that the caseation throughout the body was the result of this septic infection. It would be almost a new fact in the history of septic infection for such a sequence to be demonstrated.

CASE. 10.

TUBERCULOSIS. PLEURISY.

Plate XXXIX. fig. 7.

Ref.—Phthisis, p. 97.

SUMMARY.—*M. 49. After an attack of gout, a month before death, pain came on in the left side, with great dyspnœa, prostration, and tenacious puriform expectoration. There were signs of effusion into the left pleural cavity, and of some pleurisy and consolidation on the right side.—Right lung hyperæmic; left compressed by fluid. Each contains numerous granulations, grouped and pigmented ; some fibroid change in the right lung, with a cheesy mass and small cavity at the apex. Tubercular granulations in the liver.*

GEORGE UNWIN, ætat. 49, admitted University College Hospital November 2; died November 8, 1868.

Personal History.—(He was suffering from acute dyspnœa, and his history was therefore imperfectly taken.) Has repeatedly suffered from gout. Was attacked three weeks ago by gout in both ankles. Shortly afterwards there was sudden severe pain in left side, but patient was only laid up for a few days. He returned to, and continued at work until October 30, when he suffered from a great aggravation of the pain and dyspnœa, attended by great weakness.

State on Admission.—A fairly nourished man of good muscular development. He had orthopnœa, and was cyanosed, breathing rapidly (48). Expectoration on the first two days was in isolated and not rusty pellets ; it became confluent, homogeneous, puriform and tenacious on the third day, and a few rusty sputa were seen during three days, increasing in number on the fifth day from admission, when the puriform character became less apparent. The left side was bulged, measuring 18½ inches at level of nipple, the right being 17½. It was absolutely dull below the 3rd rib in front, throughout the axilla, and below the upper third of the scapula posteriorly. Respiration, vocal fremitus, and vocal resonance were all weakened at the upper confines of the dulness, suppressed below; ægophony existed at the level of the dulness in the back. The right apex was resonant: the base was dull below the 5th rib in front, 6th rib, axilla, and below the apex of the scapula posteriorly. On the next day this had increased to the middle third of the scapula. In the right back there was bronchial breathing, with coarse râles over the upper part of the dull area, diminished breath-sound in the lower part, and coarse friction over the right front.

The heart beat at the ensiform cartilage: not to right of sternum: could not be felt on left side. Sounds weak. No murmur. The urine was free from albumen. No œdema of extremities. His temperature on admission was 101·4°, pulse 20, respiration 48. On the fifth day after admission the temperature fell to normal, and the dulness at the right base diminished. The dyspnœa also improved, and he appeared better for a few hours. The dyspnœa, however, increased suddenly and rapidly, and he died on November 8.

POST-MORTEM.—Large effusion of clear serosity in left pleura. Right lung adherent.

Larynx.—Slight superficial ulceration on under surface of epiglottis; rest of larynx and trachea healthy.

Lungs.—Bronchus of right filled with tenacious mucus. Tissue of lung loaded with serosity; base excessively hyperæmic. Lungs emphysematous. At the posterior part of the apex are nodules of induration of fibro-cartilaginous hardness. Near them is a cheesy mass the size of a walnut, which, when removed, leads into an irregular cavity. Below this the lung-tissue is filled with softish white granulations, forming, for the most part, racemose groups which have not undergone caseous change. In other places, small caseous granulations are connected by bands and strings of fibrous tissue which ramify between them. The granulations are all very much pigmented, as is also the pulmonary tissue surrounding them. They are scattered in groups in all parts, from the apex to the base, and the amount of lung occupied by them is very considerable. Fibroid change tends to occur in strings and bands, passing not only between groups of granulations, but between single granulations scattered through the pulmonary tissue. Some of the larger granulations, the size of a hemp-seed, where isolated, have a caseous and cup-shaped depression in their centre, and when cut into are found to communicate directly with the bronchi, as in the case of *Overall (Case 27)*. The appearances in this lung so exactly correspond with those of *Overall (see X. 8, 9, 10, and description)* that I have omitted a drawing made to illustrate them.

Left lung adherent at apex: collapsed throughout, except at apex, which is still crepitant. It is studded throughout with granulations precisely similar to those found in the opposite lung. The bronchial glands are large, indurated, and pigmented. They are filled with small granulations thickly scattered through the tissue. The granulations are firm and have a whitish hue.

Heart large, weighs 13 oz. Large adherent clots, formed shortly before death, are found in both right auricle and ventricle. Some thickening of mitral valve. Wall of left ventricle is ⅜ of an inch thick. Muscular tissue softer than natural.

Liver weighs 67 oz., capsule separates easily. Tissue mottled with granulations, which are irregularly dispersed throughout its substance. They vary in size from a hemp-seed to the minutest specks. The smallest are semi-transparent; the largest are opaque, not cheesy. In some places they coalesce into tracts of some size. They are evidently situated between the acini, but press very irregularly upon these.

Kidneys.—Indurated: present a few small granulations, grey and semi-transparent. *Spleen* soft; no enlargement of Malpighian bodies.

Stomach.—Mucous membrane more opaque than natural; contains a few follicular ulcerations.

Intestines.—Much congested. Solitary glands enlarged throughout both small and large intestine, no ulceration.

MICROSCOPIC CHARACTERS.— The appearances found in these lungs are the following :—

A. Areas of caseous pneumonia.

B. Areas of suppurative pneumonia mingled with the former.

C. Diffuse infiltrations of small-celled growth.

D. Nodules of small-celled reticular growth.

E. Nodules of intermingled small-celled and epithelial growth, passing in some cases into induration, in others into caseation.

F. Some peribronchial and perivascular thickening.

§ A. The areas of caseous pneumonia are not numerous or extensive. They are diffuse in some places, in others circumscribed by thickened interlobular septa. They originate in processes of thickening of the alveolar walls by a small-celled growth, in the manner described in *Griffin (Case 1⁰)*, and *Lloyd (Case 23)*.

§ B. Portions are found in the areas of caseous pneumonia where all structure has disappeared except the framework of elastic tissue, and where the final result is an appearance similar to XXXV. 5 *(Smith)*, but where all appearance of suppuration is absent. It may, therefore, be questioned whether, in some instances, destructive changes of this nature may not occur without suppuration, and be caused solely by the disintegration of the cellular elements.

§ C. Diffuse small-celled growth occur, either like XXXVIII. 8 *(Hall)*, XL. 2 *(Heath)*, or more commonly in the form of alveolar thickenings like XXXVII. 2, 6, and 7, and XXXVI. 2 *(Griffin)*. The latter are found adjacent to, and merging into, masses of caseation, which therefore probably proceed from them.

§ D. Nodules of small-celled growth, without admixture of other elements, are occasionally found. In many cases they commence purely in the alveolar texture.

§ E. Nodules of intermingled small-celled and epithelial growth, in various stages of transformation, are the most common objects in these lungs. They occur either singly or in groups, and may, in the latter form, occupy large areas. Their most common type is seen in XXXIX. 7. Single nodules, like *a* in this figure vary, from $\frac{1}{50}$ to $\frac{1}{15}$ or even $\frac{1}{3}$ of an inch. The most common size is about $\frac{1}{25}$ inch. In their earlier stages they commence with a variable amount of epithelial growth, like XXXVII. 5 *(Griffin)*.

Many, however, resemble XXXIV. 1 (*Acute Tubercle*), and XI. 1 and 3 (*Heath*); others are found with giant-cells, epithelial cells, and small-celled growth intermingled, and caseating in their centres as in XXXIX. 7, and like XXXII. 7 (*Smith*). In others, giant-cells are absent in the centre and are only seen at the periphery.

The margin of all these nodules is composed of concentrically arranged rows of fusiform cells and fibres, with small round cells and nuclei intermingled. Beyond this again is usually a dense small-celled growth. Scattered giant-cells surround many of these nodules and also the masses of caseous pneumonia. Caseation usually begins in the centres of the nodules, and advances until the zone last described is reached. In the latter, especially when caseation has occurred, there is often much pigmentation. In others there is induration, and the formation of a sclerotic tissue resembling XLI. 3 and 5 (*Carr* and *Roberts*), commencing in the centre, may be variously intermingled with spots of caseation in different parts of the same nodule.

§ F. Peribronchial small-celled growth, diffused longitudinally in the sheaths of the bronchi, is occasionally met with, but is not common. No ulceration of the bronchi is found. Perivascular small-celled growth also occurs, but usually the walls of the vessels are thickened with an almost homogeneous fibroid thickening.

The *Bronchial Glands* present dense masses of cells, which in some places are seen to be undergoing a fibroid change similar to those of the lungs. In fact, such tracts present features almost identical in appearance with those seen in the lungs.

The *Liver* presents masses of small-celled growth, which is present also as a diffuse infiltration. The former tends to pass into cheesy change, and in some places there is much pigment. The larger part of the liver is, however, cirrhotic.

CASE 11.

Tuberculosis; Tubercular Peritonitis.

Plate XXXI. fig. 8.

Ref.—Phthisis, p. 96.

Summary.—*M. 45. Symptoms, for a year or two, of slight emphysema and bronchitis, with enlargement of the liver. Increasing dyspnœa, which finally became intense, and ended in death after 36 hours.— General tuberculosis ; intense tubercular peritonitis ; fatty liver. Granulations in lungs, some old, with induration. Dilatation of bronchi. Old and recent pleurisy.*

George Beale, ætat. 45, admitted University College Hospital July 11, 1871.

Personal History.— A groom in gentleman's service ; has followed this occupation all his life. Regular in his habits ; drinks rather largely of beer, but comparatively little of spirits. Always well-fed and well-clothed. House said to be damp, but situation open.

Family History.—Father and mother both living and healthy. No known history of phthisis. Has had three children, all living and healthy. Previous health good, no illnesses ; has not had syphilis.

Present Illness.—Consulted Dr. Fox in July 1870 ; complained of pain in right side of chest. Liver (?) dulness was found to extend from 4th rib to three fingers' breadth below edges of false ribs in mammary line, and to 9th rib in back ; an edge could be felt hard and somewhat nodulated. Some dyspnœa and sibilant râles in chest. Strength and appetite had failed. Bowels costive. No albuminuria. Heart healthy. Diagnosis then made was emphysema and slight bronchitis with enlarged liver, probably cirrhosis (see, however, the post-mortem). He consulted Dr. Fox two or three times at intervals, before admission to hospital, where he finally applied in consequence of rapid increase of the dyspnœa and weakness.

State on Admission.—Some cyanosis. Moderate emaciation. Complained of pain in right side. Dyspnœa on exertion. Pulse 102 ; resp. 28 ; temp. 100^5. Dry cough without expectoration.

Chest, good resonance, both sides. Sonorous and sibilant râles, mingled with a few coarse moist râles, over whole chest. Heart unduly covered by lung ; no murmur. Below margin of thorax on right side, what seemed to be the liver (see below) was felt for three inches in mammary line ; edge hard and resistant, somewhat nodulated. Appetite defective ; much thirst ; bowels regular.

On the night of his admission he had an attack of paroxysmal dyspnœa, relieved by inhalation of chloroform. This recurred on the following night, and was unrelieved by remedies. The patient continued to suffer uninterruptedly and intensely from dyspnœa during the ensuing twenty-four hours ; he became increasingly cyanosed, and died on the next evening.

Post-mortem.— General old adhesions of both lungs to chest-wall in upper and anterior portions. In the middle third of the lungs, recent adhesions ; those on the right side contained numerous grey granulations, but none were found on the left side. About a pint of yellow, turbid fluid was found in each pleural cavity, and there was much recent flocculent lymph in the left.

Right lung : apex contained a few small cavities ; which collectively might contain a walnut. Around these were deeply pigmented indurated tissue, mingled with emphysema, in which were some indurated nodules.

The whole upper lobe was deeply pigmented, and contained indurated granulations, some tracts of fibroid induration, and some recent pneumonic consolidation in patches. The lung was densely infiltrated with glistening, firm, grey granulations in deeply pigmented tissue. In some places these granulations were collected into racemose groups with much pigmentation, and were passing into fibroid change. In others they were single and scattered through the pigmented tissue. In a few places they were undergoing caseous change, but this was not common. The granulations were all small ; the greater number did not exceed a poppy-seed in size, and many were not larger than pins' points, but prominent above the surrounding tissue.

Left lung : marked emphysema. No cavities. It was crowded with granulations, similar to those seen in the other lung. The tissue was much pigmented and congested in places. In a few spots the granulations formed groups, with caseous matter in their centres, but this appearance was rare.

The bronchi in both lungs showed in places moderate fusiform dilatations; mucous membrane hyperæmic; no other change.

Bronchial Glands indurated, and deeply pigmented; otherwise unchanged.

Larynx and *Trachea*: mucous follicles enlarged. No grey granulations.

Heart large; white patch covering the greater part of the anterior surface of the ventricles; no recent pericarditis. Coagula in pulmonary artery and in pulmonary and systemic veins, which were apparently formed *post mortem* and did not fill vessels. Valves healthy.

Abdomen.—Liver visible for about an inch below false ribs; a large thickened mass of plastic matter, of about two inches' vertical depth, adhered to its free border. It was nearly an inch in thickness, wedge-shaped, and covered with granulations. On section, it presented only a uniform mass of thickened lymph, with very little vascularity. To it were adherent coils of intestine, matted together into a thickened mass, studded with fine granulations. The intestines were everywhere adherent to the abdominal wall, and massed together by dense adhesions, studded with fine semi-transparent granulations. The coats of the intestines were thickened. The omentum was thickened, adherent to the intestines, and filled with grey granulations. No fluid in the abdominal cavity. The mesenteric glands were swollen, and showed numerous grey granulations on section, but no cheesy masses.

Intestines.—The mucous membrane contained numerous ecchymoses. A few scattered ulcerations of the solitary glands are seen in the small intestine; none elsewhere.

Liver fatty. No tubercles seen under capsule, but a few are found in its substance.

Spleen not materially enlarged; weight 4½ ounces. Tissue soft. No tubercles seen in it.

Kidneys contain some scattered granulations; tissue otherwise healthy. Pelves and calyces healthy.

THE MICROSCOPIC APPEARANCES of this lung present the following characteristics:—

§ A. Nodules of various characters, viz.

(1) Nodules of small-celled growth, consisting of groups of alveoli, each containing a giant-cell, and resembling XXXI. 1 (*Shimmick*). The nodules are intensely fibrillated, with broad-banded fibres, containing the remains of nuclear growth, in which no giant-cells are visible. They resemble XLIII. 2 and XLI. 7 (*Coppin*). In some of these, however, partial caseation has occurred, and giant-cells are also present. Such nodules are almost identical in appearance with XXXI. 3 (*Shimmick*).

(2) Nodules where the fibrillation is passing into sclerosed tissue, like XL. 2 (*Carr*), and tracts where groups of these nodules are passing into masses of broad-banded fibres among which are remains of nuclei and of epithelial cells, like XLI. 1 (*Carr*), XLII. 1 (*Attwood*).

§ B. Tracts, like XXVIII. 2 and 7 (*Acute Tubercle*), of small-celled growth, surrounding alveoli which still retain their form, and the centres of which contain a variable proportion of epithelial cells. Some of these also form distinct nodules; these are very numerous, and some are identical with XXXVII. 5 (*Griffin*).

§ C. Large areas are also occupied by diffuse small-celled growth, mingled with epithelial cells, like XXXVIII. 8 (*Hall*), and XL. 2 (*Heath*).

§ D. Nodules and also diffused areas of mingled small-celled and epithelial growth, like XXXVII. 2 and 3 (*Griffin*).

§ E. Caseation occurs both in nodular and diffuse forms. The nodular forms are sometimes of the granular fibrillated character seen in XXXVII. 9 (*Henshaw*), and XLIII. 5 (*Heath*). In others a combination of caseation with fibrillar change may be seen co-existing, the caseation invading the fibrillation, as in XXXI. 3 (*Shimmick*). Other nodular forms resemble XXXV. 4 (*Smith*), where the small-celled growth is seen passing into caseation, and is surrounded by fibro-nucleated tissue, among which are the remains of alveoli occupied by a small-celled growth. Again, in other places, the small-celled growth is disappearing, and the caseation is occurring in nodules in a fibrillar structure, like XXXIX. 5 (*Overall*), and XL. 3 (*Heath*). In other places nodules of complete caseation are found, almost identical with XXXVI. 1 and 2 (*Griffin*) and having apparently a similar origin in the destruction of a mingled epithelial and small-celled growth, the former being replaced by the latter antecedently to this change.

§ F. Caseation in the more diffuse forms is found like XXVIII. 6 and 8 (*Acute Tubercle*), but more commonly like the latter (fig. 8) of the fibrillar type, thus reproducing in the diffuse form what has been already described in the nodular (§ E). Other areas of caseation resemble XXXVI. 3, and XXXVII. 4 (*Griffin*), where the caseation takes place in nodules of small-celled growth in the midst of pneumonic areas.

§ G. Pneumonic areas of limited extent are seen, like XXXVIII. 2 and 4, (*Henshaw*), but they are for the most part invaded by a small-celled growth, as already described (§ B).

§ H. Perivascular and peribronchial thickening with small-celled growth is common.

CASE 12.

ACUTE TUBERCULAR PNEUMONIA.

Plates VII. fig. 1; XXXIX. fig. 4.

Ref.—Phthisis, p. 96.

SUMMARY.—*F. 44. A chill four weeks after confinement. Three weeks later was pyrexial, prostrate, sweating, with signs of consolidation and excavation at both apices. Mucous and crepitant rales throughout lungs; considerable persistent pyrexia. Increasing exhaustion, and death four weeks later, seven weeks after the chill.—Reddish-grey pneumonic infiltration scattered through both lungs, with numerous cavities, firm or softening nodules of caseation, and ill-defined grey granulations.*

CATHERINE PRICE, ætat. 33, admitted under Dr. Reynolds, January 18, 1868; died July 13, 1868.

Family History.—Father died from inflammation of the chest: mother living, healthy.

CASE 12 (PRICE)

Personal History.— Married; has had three children, two stillborn. Her last confinement was seven weeks ago.

Present Illness.— Three weeks ago, got wet through; a severe cold ensued, with sense of weakness and pains in the limbs.

On admission, complained of thirst and of frontal headache. She was pyrexial, and suffered much from perspirations, the skin being at times covered with sudamina. Physical signs showed consolidation at both apices, front and back, most marked in the right. There were signs of excavation at the right apex, and also in the right midscapular region. General disseminated moist râles throughout both lungs, passing into fine crepitation at different spots in the back.

She had no diarrhœa. The urine was free from albumen. She suffered much from dyspnœa, was persistently feverish, and died of acute exhaustion a month after admission.

Her *temperature* was high throughout, and during the first days after her admission the prostration excited suspicions of typhoid. The pyrexia approached a uniform type, the mean temperature being—morning 102·1°, evening 102·4°. The highest morning temperature was 102·2°, the lowest 99·6°. It ranged commonly between 101·5° and 103°. The highest evening temperature was 103·6°, the lowest was 99·4°, the usual range was between 102° and 103°. The mean of the remissions from evening to morning was 1·3°; the maximum being 4, and the least 0·4°. The most common were between 1 and 2°. The mean exacerbation from morning to evening was 1·8°, the greatest being 3·8°, and the least 0·6°; the most common were between 0·5° and 2°. Exacerbations from morning to evening, and remissions from morning to evening (inverse type), were not common. Exacerbations from evening to morning occurred on nine occasions; their mean was 1·2°; the greatest being 1·8°, and the least 0·1°. Remissions from morning to evening occurred on two occasions; their mean was 1·2°, the greatest being 3·4°, and the least 0·4°. The pulse, except on two occasions, invariably exceeded 120, and repeatedly reached 130 and 140. The respirations, except on one occasion (28), ranged above 30, and occasionally reached 50 and even 60.

POST-MORTEM.— *Lungs:* thick yellow fluid in moderate amount in both pleuræ; right, 5 oz.; left, 3 oz. Right lung firmly adherent at apex, no adhesions of left lung. Both lungs present much emphysema, particularly at the apices. Portions of them are infiltrated with a reddish-grey pneumonic exudation. The remaining tissue is, for the most part, hyperæmic and very œdematous. Both lungs contain numerous cavities, scattered through the tissue and also through the pneumonic infiltration. They also contain caseous nodules, from the size of a hemp-seed to that of a split pea, firm in some parts, in others softening into cavities (VII. 1, *a*). Many of these are irregular in their outline, and pigmented in their centre; they are not racemose. There are also numerous grey and more transparent nodules, but these are not so firm or so rounded and defined in outline as the ordinary grey granulations. They are variable in size; some are as small as a pin's point. They are all somewhat soft, and have a granular surface on section (VII. 1, *c*). The tissue surrounding both forms of granulation is intensely congested. The larger caseous granulations soften into small excavations, and larger cavities are numerous, tending to the globular shape, and communicating with dilated bronchi, into which the granulations have softened and excavated, the mucous membrane being abruptly cut off. Some of these cavities contain caseous matter in their floor (VII. 1, *b*).

Liver.— Hyperæmic in patches, in other parts pale; feels greasy.

Spleen medium-sized, soft, and pulpy. Other organs healthy.

MICROSCOPIC EXAMINATION.—The larger proportion of the destructive processes and of the nodules and granulations in this lung are of the pneumonic type. They may be thus classified:—

A. Tracts of nodules of caseating pneumonia.
B. Tracts of diffuse small-celled growth.
C. Tracts of great interstitial thickening of the walls of the alveoli with small-celled growth.
D. Agglomerated masses of small-celled growth of the type of miliary tubercles.
E. Tracts of peribronchial growth, but without ulceration.
F. Perivascular small-celled growth.

§ A. The areas of caseating pneumonia resemble those seen in XXVIII. 6 and 8 (*Acute Tubercle*), XXXVI. 4 (*Griffin*), XXXVIII. 3 (*Henshaw*), and XLIII. 5 (*Heath*). They originate for the most part in areas like XXXVII. 2 (*Henshaw*), to which is added an intra-alveolar small-celled growth, which passes rapidly into caseation by processes akin to that seen in XXXVII. 6 (*Griffin*). Some of these areas, in breaking down, pass at their margins into suppuration. They progress until they are bounded by the larger interlobular septa, which are thickened, and often they form large, rounded masses. In other parts the nodular masses of caseating pneumonia are formed by the confluence of nodules, as seen in XXXIX. 4. These represent alveoli, or ultimate pulmonary lobules, akin to those seen in XXVIII. 7. The centre of these is occupied by a mingled epithelial and small-celled growth, passing into caseation, which is again surrounded by a dense, small-celled growth in the walls of the alveoli and ultimate bronchioles. The whole finally passes into caseation. Areas resembling XXXVIII. 3 are produced in some places by the destructive disintegration of these masses. Some nodules very closely resemble XXXVIII. 7 (*Hall*), and various gradations can be traced between them and XL. 1 and 3 (*Heath*). When these nodules are found in a state of caseation they are occasionally surrounded by giant-cells like of the type of those seen in XXXII. 10, and XXXIII. 10.

In other parts, these destructive processes are seen to commence by a mingled epithelial and small-celled growth like XL. 6 (*Heath*), but proceeding diffusely. These are variously intermingled with, and pass into, tracts like XXXIX. 2 (*J. Thomas*), and all possible variations are discoverable in the relative proportions of mingled epithelial and small-celled growth. When the destruction of the cell-growth is nearly complete, the changes bear in parts a resemblance to XXXVII. 3 (*Griffin*).

§ B. Tracts of diffuse small-celled infiltration, with or without the intermingling of alveoli, occupied by epithelial-like cells, and resembling XXXVIII. 8 (*Hall*) and XL. 2 (*Heath*), are common. Some of these cells appear to pass into large caseating areas. Giant-cells are found in and around them.

§ C. The tracts of interstitial thickening of the alveolar wall resemble those seen in XXXVIII. 1. (*Henshaw*), and XXVIII. 10 (*Acute Tubercle*). These, in some places, contain much pigment, both in the granular and in the crystalline forms.

§ D. The agglomerated masses of small-celled growth have also the characters of that seen in miliary tubercles, but they are not very numerous.

§ E. The tracts of peribronchial growth rarely lead to ulceration. In some places bronchi may be found filled with inspissated secretion, but without ulceration.

The nodules in this lung are evidently not of bronchial but of pneumonic origin.

CASE 13.
DIABETIC PHTHISIS.

SUMMARY.—*M. 19. Inherited tendency to diabetes. Thirst and polyuria for two years. Much sugar in urine. Three months before death merely general defect of resonance on right side, and moist râles at left base. Then followed signs of slowly increasing consolidation in lower part of right lung, and at the middle of the left; cough and sputa slight. Trifling evening pyrexia; steady emaciation.—Apices normal; opaque white granulations, tending to aggregate, throughout lower two-thirds of right lung, in a grey pneumonic infiltration at the base, where also cavities existed.*

ALFRED BROOM, ætat. 19; admitted University College Hospital October 10, 1870; died January 9, 1871.

Family History.—Mother and one maternal aunt died of diabetes. One sister suffers from nervous debility, no hereditary tendency to chest affection or other diseases known.

Occupation and Personal History.—A greengrocer. Has had no illnesses prior to present.

Present Illness commenced two years ago. First noticed excessive thirst, attended by weakness, and frequency of micturition. Was temporarily benefited by treatment in St. Mary's Hospital, but has relapsed. No cough or hæmoptysis before admission.

State on Admission.—Skin dry and harsh, but he perspires at night. A spot of pityriasis on left elbow. Marked anæmia. Much thirst. Appetite maintained. Bowels open twice daily; motions hard. Tongue raw and glazed. Breath offensive, but with a sweet odour. Mouth and fauces dry. No nausea or vomiting. No complaint of indigestion.

Physical Signs.—On admission, the house-physician noted some general defect of resonance on the left side; none distinct on the right. Moist râles were heard in the lower part of right back on the left side. Respiration weak. Heart natural.

During the month of November, dulness appeared at both bases, chiefly at the right, where the respiration became tubular, attended with subcrepitant râles and whispering pectoriloquy, the apex being hyperresonant. There were also advancing signs of consolidation in the middle regions of the left axilla and back, attended by moist râles, coarse and fine. These signs continued to extend in area until the patient's death. He had throughout but little cough; the sputa were moderate in amount, and sometimes absent.

His urine varied from 236 ounces to 150 ounces during the first three weeks of his stay in hospital; the amount subsequently varied from 110 to 80 ounces. The quantity of sugar passed varied from 6244 grains to 2880 grains in the twenty-four hours. A trace of albumen appeared towards the close of life. He lost 20lbs. in weight from November 2 to January 9 (from 106½ lbs. to 86½ lbs.). His temperature records are somewhat imperfect, but occasional observations throughout his stay in hospital showed that he was commonly febrile in the evening, the temperature varying from 100° to 102°. In the morning the temperature was often subnormal, viz. 97°. The pulse, on admission 78, rose to 100 and 120. The respiration, at first 14, varied later from 20 to 28.

POST-MORTEM.—*Right Lung*: Upper lobe emphysematous and entirely free from morbid change. Middle lobe studded with opaque, white, soft granulations, some of which are becoming caseous in their centres. They are confluent in some places, forming racemose masses of irregular outline, in which the separate granulations are still distinct. The granulations project from the surface of the section. The lower lobe presents more advanced changes, increasing in intensity from above downwards. The upper part is intensely hyperæmic, and in this hyperæmic tissue are patches of grey infiltration, not prominent. The surface is uniform, slightly granular, greyish-white on section, not very friable. Whitish caseating granulations, like those in the middle lobe, are also seen here. Lower down, the grey infiltration is nearly uniform, but through it are scattered cheesy masses, and groups of caseous granulations are also found. Along the base and free borders, irregular caseous masses are likewise seen. Cavities exist, especially in the middle part of this lobe, lined by necrotising caseous material, not truly gangrenous.

Left Lung.—In the lower part of the middle lobe, tracts are found of pneumonic infiltration, similar to those of the opposite lung. Isolated opaque granulations are also scattered through it, and these in parts become confluent and cheesy. The lower lobe is entirely free from all change.

Larynx healthy. *Trachea* intensely injected; glands very prominent; a few small superficial ulcerations in mucous membrane. The *Bronchi* are injected, but otherwise unchanged, except where they open into ulcerating cavities in the right lung. *Bronchial glands* swollen, intensely hyperæmic, with a soft medullary appearance. Scattered through their tissue are numerous granulations, varying in size from a pin's head to a pin's point; the granulations are opaque, white, and soft.

Intestines.—Enlargement of solitary glands at lower end of ileum; several exhibit commencing ulceration; one ulcer is the size of a hemp-seed, with thickened edges and cheesy floor.

Kidneys hyperæmic.

Brain.—Some opacity of membranes at base. No other morbid change. Nothing abnormal to naked eye in *liver*, *pancreas*, *spleen*, or *heart*.

MICROSCOPIC APPEARANCES.—The histological changes in this lung are as follows:—

§ A. Pneumonic areas like XXXVIII. 2 and 4 (*Henshaw*). In some places, the alveoli are filled with greatly enlarged epithelial cells, like XXVI. 7

(*Ellsom*), some containing two or more nuclei; others finely granular.

§ B. Areas of infiltration of the alveolar walls with a small-celled growth like XXXVII. 6 and 7 (*Griffin*), and XXXVIII. 8 (*Hall*), which in some parts proceeds to a dense thickening, producing a honeycombed appearance like XXVIII. 10 (*Polley*) and XXXVIII. 1 (*Henshaw*). In these cases the alveoli mostly contain large cells, but in the walls of some a dense small-celled growth is proceeding to their complete occlusion.

§ C. The general character is the prevalence of a mingled epithelial and small-celled growth, producing areas, sometimes nodular, and sometimes more diffused, like XXVIII. 2, 7, and XXIX. 6 (*Acute Tubercle*), and these, in some parts, proceed until nothing is visible but dense masses of small-celled growth, in some of which the outlines of the alveoli can still be traced, their interior being filled with the growth.

§ D. Caseation occurs, sometimes in nodules like XXXIX. 4 (*Price*), sometimes in more diffuse areas, like XXVIII. 6 (*Polley*). It tends to assume the lobular form where circumscribed by thickened masses of interlobular tissue. In some places this caseation takes place directly in masses, as described above. In other places, in more distinctly pneumonic areas, it can be traced to the replacement of the epithelium by a small-celled growth proceeding in the floors of the infundibula and alveoli, in nodular shapes or in diffused areas—a process identical with that seen in XXXVII. 1, 2 (*Griffin*). In these is apparently a direct caseation of the pneumonic areas, without the intervention of the denser small-celled growth, but in most instances the latter precedes the caseation, which takes place in nodules and areas like XXVIII. 6 (*Acute Tubercle*).

There are no giant-cells discoverable in this lung. Their absence is probably due to the acuteness of the process. Peribronchial small-celled growth is abundant, and occurs occasionally in large nodular masses, extending into the interior of the tube (cf. XLIII. 6—*Brown*).

CASE 14.

DIABETIC PHTHISIS.

Plate VII. fig. 2.

The lung, of which this plate presents an illustration, was given me in 1867 by one of my colleague's assistants, as having been just taken from a diabetic patient dying in University College Hospital. I regret that at the time I omitted to make a memorandum to enable me to identify the case.

The apex was entirely occupied by a soft, yellow, cheesy infiltration, finely granular on section, and breaking down into numerous cavities, so that the whole surface looks cribriform. In the neighbourhood of this is a uniform, smooth, grey, pneumonic infiltration, through which are scattered masses of variable size. Below this the tissue is studded with yellow nodules, also granular on section, without any grey margin, but here and there surrounded by pigment. These granulations have a slight tendency in some places to form irregular racemose masses, but for the most part they coalesce into larger tracts of the same cheesy infiltration.

The separate granulations tend readily to break down, and they then form excavations, filled with a dirty-yellow fluid, and these, with spots of softening material, forming small cavities, are here scattered through the tissue. At the bases and edges are tracts infiltrated with the same cheesy matter as is seen in the apices (VII. 2 *a a*), and having also a cribriform appearance, due, in part, to the infiltration occurring in an emphysematous tissue.

MICROSCOPIC EXAMINATION.—The chief features of this lung are:—

A. Extensive pneumonic areas, some with large epithelial cells, like XXVI. 7 (*Ellsom*), while others are small-celled like XXV. 8.

B. Interspersed among these are masses of small-celled growth like XXXVIII. 8 (*Hall*), and XL. 2 (*Heath*). Among these are caseating areas, some being diffuse like XXXVI. 4 (*Griffin*), XXVIII. 6 (*Polley*, *Acute Tubercle*), and others circumscribed like XXXVI. 3 (*Griffin*) and XXXVIII. 8 (*Henshaw*).

Dense solid masses of small-celled growth fill the alveoli, and replace the epithelium which has disappeared; much perivascular and peribronchial small-celled growth is also seen; in some of these masses micrococci are visible.

CASE 15.

TUBERCULISATION AND TUBERCULAR PNEUMONIA.

Plate VII., fig. 3.

Ref.—Syphilitic Disease, p. 127.

SUMMARY.—*M. 26. Probable tubercular inheritance. Weakness, cough and occasional hæmoptysis during six months: then more considerable hæmorrhage occurred, and signs of consolidation and excavation were found at both apices. Persistent moderate pyrexia.—Fibroid induration at each apex, containing cheesy spots, irregular cavities, and numerous granulations, for the most part grouped. Opaque, yellow nodules thickly scattered through the lower lobes.*

WILLIAM SCARROW, ætat. 26: admitted University College Hospital April 28, died May 2, 1868.

Family History.—Unknown, except that mother and two sisters died young.

Occupation and Habits.—Working chemist; has lived well; has been temperate and has had a healthy residence.

Previous Diseases.—Had a chancre three years ago; took mercury, lost hair one year ago, but this grew again. Never had sore-throat or skin eruption.

Present Illness commenced August 1867. No apparent cause; felt unwell and was treated for liver disorder and dyspepsia. This was followed by cough, and later by hæmoptysis. First hæmorrhage was a few clots. He had, at same time, night perspirations. Cough continued during winter. In March got a chill; this was followed by larger hæmorrhages, from half a pint to a pint on two separate occasions.

State on Admission.—Great anæmia and emaciation: nails incurvated. Skin hot: perspires at night. Granular pharyngitis. Has nausea and loss of appetite, which have persisted since beginning of attack. No diarrhœa or tenderness in abdomen. Tongue red, glazed, fissured. Breathes hurriedly, but is not conscious of dyspnœa. Sputa muco-purulent, isolated nummulated pellets, profuse; urine free from albumen.

Chest naturally fairly formed: costal angles wide; flattening under both clavicles. Signs of consolidation and excavation at both apices. Bases hyperresonant, but with râles. Heart healthy. He was feverish during his stay in hospital, the maximum temperature being 102·8° (evening), the minimum (morning) being 99·5°. The maximum pulse was 132, the minimum 120. The maximum number of respirations was 58, the minimum 82.

POST-MORTEM.— Cavities in both apices numerous, intercommunicating, and situated in an iron-grey indurated tissue, mostly fibrous and deeply pigmented, in which are scattered cheesy spots. Below this, other parts of both apices, which are still fibrous, are crammed with granulations, forming dense solid masses of racemose form, deeply pigmented, opaque in their centres. These masses occupy large tracts of tissue. The lower lobes (VII. 3) are crammed with opaque yellowish nodules, scattered in highly congested tissue, which for the most part is emphysematous. The nodules are frequently single, but are often also in clusters, forming mucomose masses of the size of a pea and upwards. These are, however, composed of smaller granules, diminishing in size from a poppy-seed to a mere speck. In a few places these masses have formed small cavities of the size of a pin's head. In a few places there is a little firm pneumonic infiltration, yellowish-grey, and finely granular. Granulations are thickly scattered on the pleura. Both lungs are affected in a precisely similar manner.

The Intestine presents extensive ulceration. Some of the ulcers have thickened edges and granulations in the floor; in others this character is not apparent. Some of the solitary glands are distended with a milky fluid, which, when evacuated, leaves a cavity in which no trace of tubercular formation is visible. The other organs are healthy.

MICROSCOPIC EXAMINATION of this lung was limited to the nodular masses. They were seen to be of three kinds.

A. Peribronchial, small-celled growth, like XXXIV. 5, and XLII. 5.

B. Nodular masses like XXIX. 6 (*Acute Tubercle*), XXXIV. 1 (*Coombes*), XXXVIII. 8 (*Henshaw*), and like XLI. 1 (*Heath*), with varied gradations in the amount of epithelial proliferation and alveolar small-celled growth.

C. Lobular nodules like XXVIII. 2 (*Acute Tubercle*). Some of them contain giant-cells of the types of XXXII. 4, and XXXIII. 2 and 11.

There are, in addition, numerous nodular masses of caseation, surrounded by small-celled growth, and bounded by thickened interlobular tissue, like XXVIII. 6 and 8, and XXXVII. 3. These are the result of processes like that seen in XXXVII. 1 and 2 (*Griffin*), and also of the confluence of nodules like XXXVII. 5 (*Griffin*), or are due to the caseation of areas and nodules like XXXIV. 1 (*Coombes*), in the midst of many of which giant-cells can be seen. A few nodular masses entirely composed of small-celled growth are found, but this growth is for the most part combined with epithelial proliferation, either in nodules, or in more diffuse areas like XXXVII. 6 and 7 (*Griffin*).

CASE 16.

ACUTE TUBERCULAR PNEUMONIA.

Plates VIII. figs. 1, 4, and 6; XXXI. fig. 7; and XXXVIII. figs. 1, 2, 3, 4.

SUMMARY.—*M. 20. Phthisical inheritance. Sub-acute lung-symptoms. Signs of consolidation at both apices; repeated hæmoptysis; evidence of irregular extension of consolidation through lungs, especially at bases; considerable pyrexia. Duration of definite symptoms about three months—Degenerating granulations through lungs, in part aggregated; irregular cavities in right apex, and grey infiltration in left upper lobe.*

WILLIAM HENSHAW, ætat. 20, admitted University College Hospital under Dr. Reynolds, February 25; died March 15, 1867.

Family History.—Father living, aged 54, healthy. No chest affection in father's family. Mother died of phthisis, ætat. 41. Has been one of a family of fifteen, twelve brothers and three sisters. One sister and two brothers have died, one of chest affection, the other two of unknown causes.

Personal History.—Occupation, smith's labourer. Has been well until shortly before present illness; has drunk freely of both beer and spirits, and has smoked much. Never had syphilis or any other illness before present.

Present Illness.—Had a cough a month before Christmas, which got quite well. At Christmas was out of work and not living well: left off a warm jersey and his cough returned. Shortly afterwards he went by sea to Newcastle, insufficiently provided with clothes, and got wet; his cough increased; and he had a sharp pain in left side. He had rigors occasionally during illness. Expectoration, which had been very slight in previous attack, returned immediately, at first white and frothy, afterwards thicker, with solid lumps. Hæmoptysis occurred on day before admission, to extent of four to five ounces, of a bright red colour. Appetite has always been good, but for the past year he has had dyspeptic symptoms. Epigastric pain after food. Heartburn, bad taste in mouth; a feeling of nausea in the morning, but has never vomited.

State on Admission.—Moderate anæmia; no marked dyspnœa. No marked wasting. Skin hot; no perspiration. Chest well-formed. Physical signs of consolidation at both apices, with coarse and fine râles. Slight dulness at right base, with fine râles: friction in left lower axillary region. Heart in natural position. Urine free from albumen; no diarrhœa.

The hæmoptysis, which commenced the day before admission, continued at short intervals until a few days before death. It was at times profuse, and on one occasion, after taking an emetic dose of ipecacuanha, he brought up a pint of blood. All remedies tried, including large doses of gallic acid, the mineral acids, turpentine, acetate of lead, and inhalations of spray of tinct. ferri perchloridi, were ineffectual. In the intervals of the hæmoptysis, the sputa were frothy, viscid, and tenacious. Râles appeared over the whole left side, and the left base gradually became dull. Some patches of percussion dulness, attended by moist râles, also appeared in the left back. Prostration, cyanosis, and anæmia

A A

increased rapidly. He suffered from dyspnœa and at times from faintness. The skin was at times pungently hot, at times perspiring; sordes appeared on the lips; and he sank and died on March 15.

The temperature throughout his stay in hospital was continuously pyrexial—a non-febrile temperature (97·6°) was only twice observed—on the morning after admission, and after a considerable hæmorrhage. The large subsequent hæmorrhages certainly did not reduce the temperature below a febrile standard, though temperatures of 99·6° and 99·2° were each once observed in the morning. The mean morning temperature in sixteen observations was 100·4°, the maximum (once only) being 105·2°. The mean ordinary morning temperature ranged from 100° to 101·5°. The mean evening temperature, in thirteen observations, was 101·6°, the highest being 102·6°, the lowest 100·2°. The mean ordinary evening temperatures ranged from 101° to 102°. The fever followed the regular course of attaining the highest degree in the evening; on two occasions only was there a rise from evening to morning, and on only one was there a fall observed from morning to evening. The mean exacerbation from morning to evening was 1·24°, the highest being 2·6° and the lowest 0·2°. The mean remission from evening to morning was 1·5°, the greatest being 3·6°, the lowest 0·2°, the majority ranging from 1° to 2°.

POST-MORTEM.—*Larynx:* mucous glands prominent; no tubercle.

Lungs.—Both adherent; the right universally, the left only at apex. The lungs meet in middle line, bases of both emphysematous. Bronchi of both contain thick mucus, but there is more in right than in left; mucous membrane pale; no marked congestion anywhere. No trace of tuberculisation in bronchi, but some tubes in the apex of the left lung pass into irregular cavities. Some bronchi in left lung of fourth division have their walls thickened and indurated.

Right lung: tissue of apex indurated, dense, fibrous, containing some encapsuled cheesy nodules. Below this is an irregular sinuous cavity, lined with cheesy masses, and communicating directly with bronchi of the second division. The tissue of this lung, from apex to base, is riddled with granulations, soft and of variable size. Some are extremely small and tend to semi-transparence (VIII. 1, *a*); most, however, are soft and opaque, but not caseous. They tend to agglomerate in groups of a racemose character, sometimes occupying considerable areas, the surface of which, on section, is finely granular (VIII.1,*cc*, and 6). The granulations of which these are composed are for the most part larger and coarser than grey granulations. Most of them are soft, and break down easily under the finger; in many places they do not stand out prominently, but blend insensibly with the surrounding tissue, while in other places they have irregular serrated margins. The smallest granulations are softer and more opaque than typical grey granulations, and are easily detached from the lung. In portions of the lung which apparently have been emphysematous, the confluence of the granulations gives rise to opaque granular masses, in which small spots are breaking down and give to the whole an irregular, worm-eaten appearance (VIII. 4). Gradations between these and the granular racemose masses can be seen in different parts.

Left Lung: apex puckered and contracted like the right; contains a few caseous nodules. Immediately below this the lung-tissue is infiltrated with an opaque, greyish exudation, granular and friable, but in the mass firm. Patches and spots of this character, assuming an irregular, lobular form, are scattered through the upper lobe. Through the whole of the lower lobe are scattered granulations similar to those of opposite lung, varying in size from a pin's point to nodules of the size of a pea, which are formed by the agglomeration of the smaller granulations. They are for the most part surrounded by a zone of congestion: and are less prominent than typical grey granulations, their outline is also more irregular and less defined. Although some have a certain semi-transparency, they are for the most part opaque. A few between are grey, semi-transparent, and stand out prominently.

Bronchial Glands swollen and opaque, do not contain any visible tubercle.

Heart, Liver, Spleen, Kidneys, Supra-renal Capsules, and Testicles healthy.

Stomach: mucous membrane excessively opaque, white, not softened. Numerous erosions of variable size, not exceeding a hemp-seed; some are covered with an ash-grey slough, which, when separated, leaves a small cavity. Hæmorrhagic spots are seen in other parts of the mucous membrane.

Intestines: duodenum much congested. Upper part of ileum contains much mucus, and the fine congestion extends throughout it. Petechiæ and ecchymoses at lower end of ileum. Over one Peyer's patch there is exceedingly fine congestion, but this is not general. A cheesy spot, the size of a pin's point, is found in one of Peyer's patches. Cœcum free. Mesenteric glands free.

THE MICROSCOPIC APPEARANCES in these lungs are the following:—

A. Pneumonic infiltration, both with large epithelial proliferation, and also with amorphous exudation matter, in which a few cells are imbedded.

B. Similar tracts attended by great thickening of the alveolar walls by small-celled growth.

C. Tracts of small-celled infiltration mingled with epithelial proliferation.

D. Tracts of pneumonic infiltration interspersed with spots of caseation.

E. Distinct nodules of small-celled growth.

F. Nodules of caseation.

G. Peribronchial and perivascular infiltration with small-celled growth.

§ A. The areas of pneumonic infiltration are of two kinds. In some places the alveoli are entirely filled with large epithelial cells resembling XXVI. 7, and XXXVIII. 5 (*Ellsom*).

In large tracts, however, the alveoli are filled with an amorphous and finely granular exudation-matter, in which a few large epithelial cells are imbedded, as seen in XXXVIII. 2 and 4, where it is probable that the exudation matter was of a mucoid character, coagulated by chromic acid. In the walls of most of these, nuclear proliferation is seen advancing (XXXVIII. 4, *aa*, and 2, *cc*) which in some places proceeds to denser masses (2, *a*).

§ B. This infiltration at times produces great thickening of the walls, and where it has apparently taken place in an emphysematous structure, it produces a honeycombed appearance, as seen in Coloured

Plate VIII. 3. The microscopic appearances of this part are seen in XXXVIII. 1, and they resemble also those seen in XXVIII. 9 and 10 (*Polley, Acute Tubercle*). In other places, appearances occur identical with those seen in XXXVIII. 6 and 7 (*Griffin*) and XXXIX. 1, 2 and 3 (*Lloyd, Thomas, and Gardiner*).

§ C. In other places this small-celled infiltration advances, until the whole tissue is more or less uniformly solidified by its progress, producing appearances like XXVIII. 3 (*Acute Tubercle*). In some parts this is mingled with epithelial proliferation in alveoli which are not yet completely occluded, and appearances are then produced resembling XXXVIII. 8 (*Hall*) and XL. 2 (*Heath*).

§ D. Spots of caseation occur in the midst of the pneumonic areas, resembling those seen in XXXVI. 3 and XXXVII. 4 (*Griffin*). The processes by which this caseation occurs resemble that described in Griffin's case (see p. 185). Small-celled growth forms in the walls and floors of the alveoli, as seen in XL. 6 (*Heath*) and XXXVII. 1 and 2 (*Griffin*); they pass finally into changes like those seen in XXXVI. 2 (*Griffin*) and XXXIX. 1 (*Lloyd*). These changes not unfrequently assume the nodular form, and thus caseation in these parts is preceded by a small-celled growth, either diffuse or nodular, in the walls of the alveoli.

§ E. Nodules of small-celled growth are of two kinds. The larger number have a variable amount of epithelium mingled with their structure, and the most common type is that seen in XXX. 2 (*Acute Tubercle*). Some, however, resemble XXX. 1 (*Acute Tubercle*), and consist almost entirely of a small-celled growth imbedded in a reticulum. Many of the nodules can be seen to have a lobular formation, and to consist of groups of terminal infundibula filled with epithelium, while in the walls of the alveoli and alveolar passages, a small-celled growth is proceeding, as in XXVII. 1 and 2 (*Acute Tubercle*), and where, in some places, the epithelium is entirely replaced by a small-celled growth. Variations in the amount of epithelium give rise to other appearances in these nodules, some of which resemble XXXVII. 5 (*Griffin*), and XXXIX. 7 (*Unwin*). These nodules caseate by a process seen in XXXIX. 1. The epithelium disappears, and the caseation is seen to proceed in the midst of a reticulated small-celled growth, the caseation invading the reticulum, as well as the nuclei and cells imbedded in it.

§ F. Caseation, as previously described, takes place both in diffuse areas like XXVIII. 6 and 8 (*Acute Tubercle*) and also in nodules. The latter may consist only of entirely amorphous débris, or may show merely wasted puriform cells, like XXXVI. 1 and 2 (*Griffin*), or the cell-structure may have entirely disappeared and a granular fibrillated structure, sometimes much pigmented, may alone remain, as seen in XXVIII. 8 (*Polley, Acute Tubercle*), and XLIII. (*Heath*).

§ G. Peribronchial small-celled growths are abundant in these lungs. They resemble XLII. 5 (*Smith*) and XLIII. 6 (*Brown*). In some places a submucous infiltration is seen extending for a considerable distance, with very little change in the epithelium. In others the growth in the bronchial sheaths forms small round masses, one of which measured $\tfrac{1}{50}$ inch diameter. Perivascular infiltration is also seen.

CASE 17.

ACUTE DESTRUCTIVE PNEUMONIA.

Plates IX. figs. 1, 2; XXVI. fig. 7; XXXVIII. figs. 5 and 6.

Ref.—Phthisis, p. 106.

SUMMARY.—*M. 42. Intemperate. Sudden invasion after exposure to cold; admitted seven days later, suffering from 'delirium tremens,' with signs of pleuro-pneumonia at the left base, some defective resonance at both apices, general bronchitic râles, and muco-purulent expectoration. Imperfect recovery, and five months later a relapse after fresh exposure: cough offensive; blood-stained sputa; signs of consolidation throughout right lung and in middle of left; slight continuous fever; increasing prostration; death at the end of the second week.—Throughout right lung, and in lower half of left, a dull grey infiltration in irregular tracts, with raccmose caseous spots, softening; gangrenous odour; a cavity at the right apex. Inflammation and ulceration of larynx.*

T. ELLSOM. Male; ætat. 42. Cheesemonger's porter. Admitted May 13, 1867. Discharged, relieved, in July; readmitted November 25, and died November 30, 1867.

Family History.—Father died of heart-disease, aged 67. One sister died, ætat. 19, of lung-disease.

Personal History.—Patient has seven children, all living and healthy. He has for years drunk to excess. Has long been subject to a cough in foggy weather.

Present Illness.—Invasion attributed to long exposure to cold on previous day; went to bed well, awoke with pain in left side and much cough, unattended with expectoration. He became feverish and continued so up to admission.

On Admission he was febrile, and presented symptoms of delirium tremens, which lasted some days. Dulness on percussion existed at both apices in front, and some dulness at the right base. Blowing breathing existed over the left apex, and coarse friction over the whole of the left base. Abundant moist rhonchus existed at both bases; sibilant and sonorous râles were present in both lungs. The sputa were throughout muco-purulent. The urine was free from albumen and sugar; its specific gravity, at first high, became low during convalescence (1020 to 1010).

The patient remained in hospital until the middle of July. No notes exist of his state when discharged, but he appears to have been convalescent and able to work. Readmitted November 25, stating that he had been well until ten days ago, when he got a fresh cold. His cough increased and was attended with blood-stained sputa. He has pain in the side, weakness, headache, and anorexia.

The skin was hot; the face flushed. The breath had a faintly gangrenous odour, which persisted until his death on November 30. He had frequent cough, with grumous, confluent, watery, offensive, blood-stained sputa. Dulness existed throughout the right side, front and back, except over a limited area at the right base. The left apex was resonant, but there was some dulness in the mid-scapular region, which, within three days, extended into the inframammary region.

There was high-pitched bronchial breathing under the right clavicle, with fine crepitation, tubular breathing, and metallic râles at the third interspace. Tubular breathing, with metallic râles, was heard at the base, front and back.

On the left side the respiration was harsh, with sonorous râles. The respiration over the dull area in the left back was bronchial. It became weak in the mammary region as the dulness extended there. The heart was natural in position and sounds.

The urine had an average specific gravity of 1020, and contained urates. There was no diarrhœa. Great prostration was present from the first, and the patient sank rapidly.

No notes have been preserved of the temperature during first period of his stay in hospital. On his readmission he was continuously febrile till death, but his temperature only reached 101·6° on two occasions. It once fell to 99·6°; otherwise it ranged from 100° to 101.° His pulse varied from 96 to 112, his respiration from 32 to 44.

POST-MORTEM.—Right lung firmly adherent throughout; left lung only by loose bands. Much hyperæmia of left pulmonary pleura.

Larynx.—Arytenoid and thyroid cartilages ossified. Mucous membrane swollen, injected, opaque, here and there finely granular. Much ulceration on the vocal cords.

Bronchial and *Post-tracheal Glands* swollen, cloudy, opaque, without visible tubercle.

Right Lung.—Bronchi highly injected; equally so in all lobes. No ulceration or dilatation. Upper and middle lobes adherent together. They are both infiltrated with a dull grey exudation. The tissue thus infiltrated is firm, uniform, and smooth on section, but when scraped, it shows a finely granular surface, though not nearly to the same degree as is observed in acute pneumonia. This infiltration is scattered in irregular tracts (IX. 2, *a*) through these lobes, with some congested but crepitant tissue intervening.

At the extreme apex is a cavity capable of holding a walnut, with sloughing walls. In the lower part of the upper lobe, are patches undergoing acute cheesy metamorphosis (IX. 1). This occurs in clustered spots of a dirty yellowish-grey colour, forming racemose groups, which, in some places, are so completely softened that when they are cut into, a cavity is left. A gangrenous odour pervades all this portion of the lung. The upper part of the lower lobe is in a similar condition.

Left Lung.—Apex loaded with spumous serosity. Lower part of upper lobe is infiltrated with the same grey pneumonic exudation above described. The infiltration occurs in patches among still sound pulmonary tissue. Some parts that appear infiltrated float in water, but sink after strong pressure. The section of some of these is uniform, smooth, and glistening; in others it is somewhat granular. Softening is observed to be commencing in some patches more distinctly granular than the rest, which are surrounded by a zone of intense injection. The lower lobe shows a similar lobular infiltration, associated with more active congestion of the pulmonary tissue. Here also spots of caseous matter, breaking down into cavities, are scattered thickly through the lung. The whole of the lobe has a sickly gangrenous odour.

Heart.—Some atheroma of aorta. Some thickening of free edge of mitral valve, and slightly so of tricuspid.

Liver pale, soft, opaque, fatty in patches; capsule separates easily.

Stomach hyperæmic. Mucous membrane soft, opaque. *Intestines* hyperæmic. No tubercle. *Spleen* very small, opaque, soft. *Kidneys* congested.

MICROSCOPIC APPEARANCES in the lungs were as follows:—

A. Large tracts of pneumonic infiltration, in some places without thickening of the alveolar walls, but in several places attended by this change, and passing in many parts into diffuse suppuration.

B. Nodular masses of small-celled growth, passing into caseation.

C. Diffuse areas of small-celled growth, passing into caseation.

D. Peri-bronchial and peri-vascular thickening; the former passing in many places into ulceration.

E. Large tracts of fibroid thickening.

§ A. The pneumonic tracts are variously characterised.

(1) Extensive areas present appearances like that seen in XXVI. 7, where the alveoli and alveolar passages are filled with large epithelial-like cells, sometimes showing multiplication of their nuclei, and finely granular. In many places of this nature the walls show no signs of small-celled infiltration. This infiltration occurs, however, in other parts, as in XXXVIII. 5, where the small-celled growth is seen to pass into the interior of the alveoli. In other places the alveoli are filled with an amorphous exudation, in which only a few epithelial cells are scattered, like XXXVIII. 2 and 4 (*Henshaw*).

(2) Considerable tracts present the appearance of a diffuse suppuration resembling XXXV. 1 and 2 (*Brodrick*), and stages may be observed like XXXV. 6 (*Smith*), where this apparent suppurative change is produced by the formation, in the floors of the alveoli, of a small-celled growth which replaces the epithelial proliferation, and apparently softens and breaks down.

(3) In other places small-celled growth forms in the alveolar walls, which become thickened, and tracts are produced like XXXVIII. 8 (*Hall*), in which the small-celled growth is mingled with the epithelial formation, the latter still showing traces of its origin in the alveoli. Intermediate stages are also seen, like XXXVII. 6 and 7 (*Griffin*) and XXXIX. 2 and 3 (*Thomas* and *Gardiner*). In many places the inter-alveolar thickening extends over large areas, giving rise to appearances like XXVIII. 9 and 10 (*Polley*), XXXVIII. 1 (*Henshaw*). It is also seen surrounding the bronchioles and inter-alveolar passages, the epithelium of which then becomes 'cuboid' in form, as seen in XXXVIII. 6.

§ B. Nodular masses of small-celled growth are seen, breaking down in their centres, like XXX. 2 (*Coombes*). These masses are evidently in some places formed out of lobular thickenings of the alveolar walls, like those seen in XL. 1 and 8 (*Heath*), and, like the latter, they pass into caseation.

§ C. Diffuse areas of caseation, like XXVIII. 6 and 8 (*Polley*), and like XXXVI. 3, 4, and 5 (*Griffin*), and others like XXXVIII. 9, are also seen. They proceed from a small-celled growth invading the alveolar wall, and the direct passage of epithelial proliferation into caseation is nowhere seen.

§ D. Large tracts of induration occur, in some places of peribronchial origin. In the larger proportion, however, they arise from a fibroid change in the small-celled growth in the alveolar walls, and produce appearances resembling XLI. 1 (*Carr*). In other parts the origin in small-celled growth is not apparent, and we have alveoli still filled with epithelial cells of seemingly pneumonic origin, while their walls are thickened by a fibroid growth like XLII. 6 (*Hawkins*). In some, again, the fibroid change is seen to be proceeding in the floors of the alveoli, mingled with a small-celled growth like XLI. 7 (*Coppin*).

COMMENTARY.—The invasion in this case much resembled acute pneumonia, but differed from it in the general dissemination of râles, and in the slowness of convalescence. I regret that I was unable to take notes of the patient before he was discharged. It appears, however, extremely probable that the pneumonia never resolved. This is shown, I think, by the fibroid changes found in some parts. It is also probable that the disseminated râles, heard in different parts of the lung on his first admission, were due to tubercle (lobular pneumonia passing into induration, and caseation). The whole series of changes in the lung were not, however, those of chronic pneumonia which passes into induration. Here the tendency was distinctly to breaking down and softening, a tendency probably existing *ab initio*, but undergoing an acute exacerbation on his second attack. This softening and breaking down was due to caseation following an interstitial growth. The cavities, where found, were for the most part the result of this process, although in one place the pneumonic infiltration appeared capable of undergoing acute softening, probably of a gangrenous character. The relapse of pneumonia, which was very likely an extension of the first attack, appears to have induced this process, in consequence of the patient's exhausted vitality. It may be noted that in this case also the larynx was affected.

CASE 18.

TUBERCULAR SUPPURATING PNEUMONIA.

Plates XIII. fig. 3 and 4; XXXV. figs. 1, 2, and 3.

Ref.—Phthisis, pp. 119, 121; Syphilitic Disease, p. 127.

SUMMARY.—*M. 43. Syphilis three years before death. Cough for many years, increasing three months before admission. Laryngitis: purulent expectoration, hæmoptysis. Signs of consolidation and excavation at left apex and of consolidation at base and at right apex, with excavation in upper part. Persistent moderate pyrexia. Ulceration of larynx. Induration at apex: granulations, indurated and caseating, scattered through both lungs, with old pneumonic infiltration in places, partly puriform. Cavities at left apex.*

JOHN BRODRICK, ætat. 43, admitted University College Hospital in January, and died February 15, 1865.

Family History.—Father died, ætat. 60, of some chest affection. No other known instance of lung disease in family.

Personal History.—A bricklayer's labourer: a native of Ireland; has had abundant food, but has drunk excessively.

Previous Illness.—Has had the epidemic diseases of childhood, also an attack of fever when ætat. 9. Had syphilis in November 1862. In February 1863 he came under me as an out-patient with aphonia, sore-throat, psoriasis guttata, and dulness under the left clavicle. He took bichloride of mercury and recovered, and has had no return of the sore-throat or skin eruption up to the present time. He has, however, had morning cough and slight expectoration for the last four or five years (perhaps even prior to the syphilis).

Present Illness.—His cough has increased during three months. He had been out of work, with insufficient food and clothing, especially at night. His cough grew suddenly worse on January 8, and the expectoration became profuse, clear, and frothy, occasionally mixed with blood in small quantities. Had been confined to bed for past fourteen days.

Symptoms.—Emaciation, great weakness, tremor of hands: lividity of nose and lips. Some orthopnœa. Skin perspiring. Tongue red, with a creamy fur peeling off. No diarrhœa. Urine free from albumen. Heart healthy. Pulse occasionally intermitting. Has pain in throat and on swallowing, and some pain behind sternum. Voice reduced to a hoarse whisper. Considerable congestion of epiglottis and of both vocal cords. A patch of exudation on cartilages of Santorini and Wrisberg. Expectoration profuse, with diffluent pellets of yellowish puriform matter, some of them pigmented. The sputa became increasingly diffluent and puriform, and he had a large hæmoptysis about a fortnight before his death.

Physical Signs.—Chest well-formed, with wide costal angles. There were signs of consolidation and excavation at the left apex, front and back, and of consolidation at the left base. The right apex gave signs of consolidation posteriorly. There was also a limited area of consolidation at the base. The right front and axilla, at first hyperresonant, became gradually more dull; coarse râles were heard from time to time in both lungs, but became especially marked in the right front and the left base. Sibilant and sonorous râles were also heard in both lungs. From time to time the respiratory murmur and the vocal resonance became almost suppressed in the left back; vocal fremitus, however, persisted. He died on February 15, 1865.

The pulse varied from 150 to 96, the ordinary ratio being between 100 to 120. The respirations varied from 36 to 60. They were almost invariably over 40. He was persistently feverish during the whole of his stay in hospital, a normal temperature being only observed on one occasion. The mean morning temperature in twenty-seven observations was 101°; the mean evening temperature was 101·3°. The highest temperature was 103°, observed on two different days, in the morning and evening respectively. The mean exacerbation from evening to morning on twelve occasions was 1·1°; the highest being 2·4°, and the lowest 0·2°. The mean remission from morning to evening was 0·9°, the highest being 1·8°, and the lowest 0·2°. On no less than nine days the morning temperature was equal to that of either the preceding or succeeding evening. Exacerbations from evening to morning occurred on seven days, and remissions from morning to evening on eight days. The highest of these exacerbations was 1·2°, the lowest 0·2°, the mean being 0·8°, the highest of the remissions from morning to evening was 2°, the lowest 0·4°, the mean being 0·9°. On several occasions a progressive ascent or a progressive fall appeared during thirty-six hours, thus disturbing in both directions the normal course of morning and evening temperatures.

POST-MORTEM.—Both lungs firmly adherent to parietal pleura. On right side, among the adhesions (which are very firm and dense), is found a calcified nodule. On left side, the adhesions are looser and contain numerous granulations. Epiglottis thickened and indurated: on each side its lateral borders are scooped out into a deep excavated ulcer with thickened edges, clean cut and very firm and resistant. Cords healthy. Arytenoid and thyroid cartilages calcified.

Left lung.—The apex is entirely occupied by dense, indurated, cicatricial tissue, of almost cartilaginous firmness and deeply pigmented (XIII. 3). In this are bronchi that have undergone dilatation, for the most part sacculated (*b b*). The mucous membrane is intensely congested. Nodules of fibroid induration exist also throughout this lobe, varying in size from a hazel-nut to a walnut, semi-cartilaginous and deeply pigmented. They are composed of firm granulations, which are resistant like cartilage, and firmer in the more central portions of these nodules than at their periphery. Some of the latter (in the outer zone) are opaque, yellowish-white, and much softer than those at the centre. They are not, however, caseous, and there is no appearance of softening in any of them. Isolated, indurated, semi-transparent granulations are also scattered through the tissue. In other parts of this lobe are groups of softer granulations, which, by their agglomeration, form nodules. In some places these granulations are quite soft. Small cavities have here and there formed in the larger masses thus constituted; in others, larger cavities may be observed to be in process of formation, and at places a communication with the bronchi is already established. Some of these nodular masses, though soft, are situated in the midst of indurated and pigmented tissue (*a*); probably they formed in patches of lung which remained unaffected during the process which indurated the adjacent tissue (see Microscopic Description, § A). In the middle third of this lobe, groups of caseous granulations are situated in the midst of densely indurated tissue. Grey granulations are also scattered among them.

The base of the lower lobe is largely occupied by a dirty-greenish, soft, almost liquid, puriform, pneumonic exudation, breaking down with great readiness (XIII. 4, *b*). Some parts are thus entirely infiltrated, sinking in water without pressure. In this tissue ramify bronchi ulcerating into the surrounding exudation (*c c*), and presenting a striking resemblance to the appearance observed in *S. Brown* (*Case 5*, p. 162, Plate V. fig. 5). In this tissue, and in fact partly composing it, are soft granulations, scarcely prominent, but granular in section, varying in size from a rape-seed to a hemp-seed or larger, and sometimes uniting to constitute large tracts of a yellowish-grey colour, breaking down completely under pressure. Most of these have a central depression, and some are softening in the centre (XIII.

4, *a b*) and communicating with the bronchial tubes (*c c*). They have, in many places, an irregular outline, as if composed of smaller granulations, and some of them tend to occur in groups. Higher up, and where this pulmonary tissue is not thus infiltrated, are groups of very soft granulations. Some of these break down into a milky juice on pressure, others do not. In some places these soft granulations occur around puckered and contracted tissue (Microscopic Description, § B).

The right lung presents appearances very similar to those observed in the left. The apex posteriorly is indurated and pigmented, and contains dilated bronchi, and also some cavities, within which are cheesy nodules and masses of cretaceous matter. The middle and lower lobes present pneumonic infiltration, precisely similar to that described in the left lung, in which the bronchi are irregularly dilated and in some places ulcerated. The solidified portions have a dirty ash-grey colour, in which are scattered round spots of a deeper tint and more greenish hue, appearing on section to represent the cut orifices of bronchi (Microscopic Description, § C). The bronchial and mediastinal glands are enlarged, indurated, and almost gristly in consistence, but not otherwise affected.

Kidneys somewhat indurated.

Liver has, near the surface, two or three cheesy nodules, otherwise healthy.

Heart, Supra-renal Capsule, Spleen, mucous membrane of *Stomach* and *Intestines, Mesenteric Glands,* all healthy.

MICROSCOPIC EXAMINATION.—*Left lung:* In the part below the apex, where nodules are scattered through partially infiltrated tissue, various appearances are seen.

§ A. (1) Large tracts (represented by XXXV. 1, 2, and 3, *see* description of figures) in which the tissue is breaking down in a process of acute suppuration. It is infiltrated throughout with cells resembling pus-cells, measuring from $\frac{1}{7000}$ to $\frac{1}{3500}$ inch. Some contain proliferating nuclei. No large epithelial cells are to be seen in these parts. The cells lie in some places in dense groups; in others they are imbedded in the meshes of a fibrinous reticulum of the character of that seen in acute pneumonia (fibrinous exudation), but in many places the alveolar walls are denuded of their epithelium, and the tissue is seen to be infiltrated with granules in a manner similar to that seen in XXXV. 5 (*Smith*).

(2) Tracts of dense epithelial proliferation mingled with small-celled growth, like XXXVIII. 8 (*Hall*), and others where, in addition to this, there is a dense nuclear infiltration of the wall of the alveoli, like XXXVII. 7 (*Griffin*), XXXIX. 3 (*Gardiner*). In the alveoli of such tracts, large hyaline cells can be seen, not imbedded in meshes, but floating free in the interior. Further, some of the tracts, breaking down, closely resemble those in XXVIII. 8 (*Polley*), and XXXVIII. 3 (*Henshaw*).

(3) In addition to these appearances, there are numerous nodules of induration, with an amorphous or caseous indurated centre, surrounded by a zone of small-celled growth, as in XXXIX. 7 (*Unwin*), XXXIX. 4 (*Price*), XLI. 3 (*Carr*). In these tracts, a few giant-cells can be seen, of the pigmented type. They are, however, infrequent, and none can be found

in the pneumonic parts of this lung. Other tracts of dense nuclear infiltration can be observed, like XL. 2 (*Heath*), in which the nodular formation is absent. These show no signs of breaking down, and are altogether distinct and different from the suppurating processes before described.

In some parts, suppuration can be seen in the interior of the bronchi. Their walls are then usually infiltrated with a small-celled growth, and nodular masses of nuclear formation appear in the peribronchial sheath. Ulceration from within is also observed in limited areas of this wall.

§ B. In the tracts described above with a reference to B, the appearances seen resemble those above described, except that the suppurative destruction of the lung is less distinct, and the bulk of the change consists of desquamative pneumonia with alveolar thickening like XXVI. 7 (*Ellsom*), passing into forms like XXXVII. 5 and 6 (*Griffin*). With these are found dense nuclear infiltration of the tissue, and also a few nodular growths, peribronchial, in some places periarterial, and in some parts there is also great fibroid thickening of the tissue.

§ C. *Right lung.* The appearances in the pneumonic portions of this lung resemble very closely those described in the others, except that nodular masses are not found. The predominant characters are two: tracts of suppurative pneumonia like those before described, and large tracts of caseating or necrotising pneumonia like XXXVI. 4 (*Griffin*), and XXXVIII. 3 (*Henshaw*), and XXVIII. 8 (*Polley*). Diffuse nuclear growth, like that before described (§ B), is largely prevalent, and in many parts there is desquamative pneumonia, with thickening of the alveolar walls, like XXXVIII. 4 (*Henshaw*) and XXXVII. 6 (*Griffin*). Some tracts of dense fibroid growth also occur, and in places there are periarterial and peribronchial nuclear growths.

COMMENTARY.—The conclusion to be drawn from this case appears to be that the acutely destructive pneumonic process, which formed the larger proportion of the area of recent disease, was superadded to older disease of a tubercular type. In many places the destructive processes were identical with those seen in the acute tubercular pneumonias, but in others the ordinary epithelial proliferation ('Desquamative Pneumonia') passes into suppuration, and in this change, destruction of the pulmonary tissue rapidly ensues.

CASE 19.

CHRONIC INDURATING AND CASEATING TUBERCULAR PNEUMONIA.

Plates X. figs. 1, 2, 3, 4; XXXVI., XXXVII.

Ref.—Phthisis, p. 119; Syphilitic Disease, p. 127.

SUMMARY.—*M. 41. No phthisical heredity. Intemperate. Three years before death, severe cough commenced after a chill, and continued, varying in degree. Two years afterwards, hæmorrhage from stomach or lungs; three months later, another chill, followed by pain in left side, blood-stained sputa, variable fever, occasional rigors, dyspepsia and diarrhœa. Anæmia with slight icteric tint: nightsweats, dyspnœa,cough with muco-purulent expectoration. Signs of consolidation in upper half of right lung, and also, in slighter degree, at left apex, and of cavities in both. Persistent pyrexia.—Lungs presented firm pigmented induration at the apices, with grey pneumonic consolidation in the rest of the upper lobes, and small cavities, with cheesy granulations in their walls. Reddish pneumonic infiltration at the bases. Numerous grey nodules, isolated and confluent, with caseous spots in them, softening into small cavities.*

WALTER GRIFFIN, aged 41; admitted University College Hospital April 1, died August 14, 1868.

Family History.—No known predisposition to phthisis. Father and mother both living at advanced ages; brothers and sisters all living and well, except one sister who is short of breath. Collateral relations not recorded. Some tendency to rheumatism in the family.

Occupation and Habits.—Traveller: formerly a paper-stainer, and used to suffer from the dust of emerald green. Doubtful whether residences healthy. Has lived well: has taken considerable quantities of rum. Born in Berkshire and lived in London since ætat. 18.

Previous Illness.—Has had diseases of childhood, also both typhus and typhoid fevers. Is reported to have broken a blood-vessel from a fall, ætat. 15. and 'bled from nose, ears, and mouth': was, however, very strong and robust until present illness.

Present Illness.—Three years ago, got wet through, and remained all night in wet clothes; this caused a severe cough, attended by copious yellow expectoration. He recovered, and has been comparatively well in the interval, but has had cough, more or less, ever since (for two or three years) without any appreciable expectoration. Twelve months ago brought up suddenly a quart of thick black matter (Qy. hæmoptysis or hæmatemesis). In November 1867 he again got a severe wetting; this was followed by pain in the left side, and by blood-stained sputa. Since then he has been repeatedly feverish, has felt skin hot, and has had occasional rigors and pains in different parts of his body. The appetite has failed, with flatulent distension and diarrhœa.

State on Admission.—Earthy tint of skin; extremely anæmic, but somewhat icteric. Muscular power deficient; hands tremulous. Distinct but not excessive emaciation. Finger-ends clubbed, nails incurvated. Perspires much, especially at night. Dyspnœa on slight exertion. Sputa profuse, mucopurulent, diffluent. Tongue clean; appetite better. No diarrhœa at present.

Physical Examination.—Chest naturally well-formed, costal angle wide. Right infra-mammary region somewhat contracted. Very deficient general expansion. Consolidation in right lung about as low as fifth rib in front and lower border of scapula posteriorly. The right lower axillary region was also dull. The left apex was less extensively consolidated than the right. There was tympanitic resonance anteriorly in front, but absolute dulness in the upper scapular region. There was also consolidation at the base. Râles were heard from time to time at the bases. A faint systolic murmur existed over the heart. The urine had throughout a sp. gr. varying from 1016 to 1025. It was free from albumen and sugar, but frequently deposited lithates.

The physical signs varied but little until his death. He lost 19 lbs. weight from May 1 to July 15. Diarrhœa returned during the last month of his stay in hospital, and he gradually sank.

He was persistently feverish during his stay in hospital, normal temperatures being observed only once on mornings and evenings respectively. The mean morning temperature was 101·1°, highest 103·2°, lowest 98°. The usual morning temperatures ranged from 100° to 101·5°. The mean evening temperature was 101·4°, highest 103·2°, lowest 98·4°. The mean of the exacerbations from morning to evening was 1·3°, highest 2·2°, lowest 0·6°. The mean of the remissions from evening to morning was 1·3°, highest 2·4°, lowest 0·6°. Remissions from morning to evening took place in four days; exacerbations from evening to morning on five days. The mean of the former was 0·7°, highest 2°, lowest 0·1°. The mean of the latter was 0·8°, highest 1·8°, lowest 0·1°. A nearly equal temperature was repeatedly observed on the morning and evening. The morning pulse varied from 84 to 11; the evening pulse from 80 to 108. The respirations varied from 34 to 40, not exceeding the latter. The mean pulse-respiration ratio was 2·4 : 1, highest 3 : 1, lowest 2 : 1.

POST-MORTEM.—Both lungs partially but firmly adherent to chest-walls, most so at apex. *Larynx* and *Trachea* healthy.

Lungs.—Bronchi show some fusiform dilatations, but not to any marked extent. The *right lung* was reserved for injection. The destructive changes in it were almost identical with those described in the other. *Left lung* (X. 1-4): Apex emphysematous anteriorly, and the emphysema extends through the anterior margin of the upper lobe. Posteriorly, the apex is consolidated. In the upper part, this consolidation is very firm, indurated, and much pigmented. This passes into a grey pneumonic exudation, which occupies nearly the whole of the remainder of the upper lobe, but is mingled with spots of reddish pneumonic infiltration (see figures). Here and there, patches of crepitant tissue, apparently in part invaded by the pneumonic process, are scattered through this part of the lung. A cavity exists within half an inch of the apex, capable of holding a walnut, lined by a false membrane, and in the walls of the cavity are numerous cheesy granulations. Immediately below this, in the indurated tissue, small cavities are thickly scattered. The grey and reddish pneumonic infiltrations are also riddled with cavities, which appear to originate from the softening of little cheesy nodules, scarcely larger than a poppy-seed, though some attain the size of a hemp-seed (X. 1 and 4, *a a*). (The smallest specks are not here figured.) They are scattered thickly through the consolidated tissue, and are mingled with, and appear to be produced by, the caseous degeneration of small grey granulations scarcely larger than pins' heads.

These caseous masses also become confluent in the pneumonic bases. Some are of the size of a hemp-seed on section; others are smaller. They are in many cases surrounded, and delimited from the pneumonic bases, by a zone of congestion, but in some places they are surrounded by a zone of pigmentation. Some of these spots, which are softening, appear, when cut into, to communicate with bronchi, and, if followed by a bristle, are found to open into sinuous ulcerations, bounded by caseous matter, in which, however, no bronchial wall is discoverable (see X. 4 *bb*). In some places, unaffected bronchi may be found opening into them (4, *b*). When these ulcerations form larger cavities, caseous granulations can be found in their walls (3 and 4. *c*). Thickened vessels, still pervious, may occasionally be found crossing their floors. Through the emphysomatous border of the upper lobe are scattered nodular masses: softish, semi-transparent, varying in size from a poppy-seed to a hemp-seed, confluent in places and then becoming caseous in their centres: in others entirely converted into cheesy nodules, in which softening and excavation are commencing. The lower lobe contains, in its upper part, a reddish pneumonic infiltration, and lower down some isolated nodules of grey infiltration. In both of these, caseous changes occur (2 *b* and 4), commencing apparently in little specks which become confluent and soften. In other places the grey infiltration becomes indurated and pigmented. Scattered through the non-consolidated tissue of this lobe, there are also the same semi-transparent softish nodules, passing into caseous change, which were described in the upper lobe. Some of these nodules appear like a grey pneumonia, soft and granular.

Bronchial glands enlarged, swollen, hyperæmic; in parts semi-transparent, in parts cloudy; nowhere cheesy.

Heart.—Muscular fibre somewhat soft; some thickening of free edge of tricuspid valve.

Kidneys opaque, cloudy, otherwise healthy.

Liver distinctly waxy. Some portal congestion: does not stain with iodine: some fatty degeneration in outer zone of acini, waxy in middle zone. *Spleen* healthy.

Stomach.—Mucous membrane thickened and indurated. Much grey pigmentation at pyloric end.

Intestine has a waxy look. Some enlargement of solitary gland in small intestine. Cæcum presents some superficial ulceration, without thickening of edges, and apparently some abrasion of mucous membrane, having a quasi-diphtheritic appearance. The same process is seen in colon. It appears to be preceded by a uniform infiltrated thickening of the mucous membrane in spots.

MICROSCOPIC CHARACTERS.—The following are the chief characteristics.

A. Pneumonic infiltration in various forms, but presenting prominently a destructive character.
B. Tuberculo-pneumonic masses of lobular type.
C. Areas of infiltration with a small-celled growth.
D. Ulceration and suppuration of the bronchi.
E. Perivascular and peribronchial changes and areas of fibroid thickening.

§ A. The pneumonic changes are the most extensive and varied. The predominant character is the infiltration of large tracts with a pneumonia which has proved almost entirely destructive, all traces of cells having disappeared; leaving only a fibrillated granular tissue, as shown in XXXVI. 4 and 5, and like XXXVIII. 2 (*Henshaw*), XXXV. 1 and 5 (*Brodrick* and *Smith*), XXVIII. 6 and 8 (*Polley*), *Acute Tubercle*).

(1) The areas of destructive change represented in XXXVI. 4, and resembling XXXVIII. 2 (*Henshaw*), and XXVIII. 6 and 8 (*Acute Tubercle*), may be traced at their margins to be proceeding by means

of a more or less complete filling of the alveoli with large epithelial cells (which sometimes contain two or more nuclei) in a manner similar to that seen in XXXVIII. 4 (*Henshaw*), and which is seen more highly magnified in XXXVII. 5 and 6. Simultaneously with the epithelial proliferation, a rapid growth of nuclei and small cells invades the alveolar wall, which is thereby thickened, and the alveolar space is narrowed, the capillaries being destroyed, while in some places this new growth projects in masses into the interior of the alveoli (XXXVII. 7). This growth does not, as a rule, proceed to a considerable degree, but the tissues appear to perish early from the obstruction of the capillaries, combined, in all probability, with the intensity of the inflammatory process. The differences between the appearances seen in XXXVI. 4, and XXXVIII. 3, is due to the relative amount of epithelial proliferation filling the alveoli. Where this is considerable, dense masses like the former are produced: when this is less, a change occurs like that seen in XXXVII. 1, 2, and 3; the thickening of the wall is inconsiderable, but a nuclear growth invades the whole of the capillaries in the wall of the alveolus; the epithelium disappears, and the whole passes later into a granulo-molecular detritus. Every gradation can be seen between these two forms of change. In some preparations, side by side, may be seen alveoli with epithelial proliferation, and others where there are few epithelial cells, but a network of round and of retiform nuclei, tracing the lines of the obliterated capillaries as in XXXVII. 1 and 2.

(2) Areas occupied by destructive detritus, like XXXVI. 5, are very numerous. They are characterised by the preservation of the elastic fibres marking out the walls of the vesicles, while the interior of these is entirely occupied by an amorphous detritus. Such areas may be either diffuse or circumscribed. They are distinguished by the absence of thickening in the alveolar walls, and appear to owe their origin to two processes. When diffuse they are commonly found associated at their margins with changes similar to those seen in XXXV. 1, 5, and 7 (*Birdrick, Smith*, and *S. A. Brown*) of 'suppurative pneumonia,' and the process of the passage of leucocytes into an amorphous débris may be often traced in these parts. In a few places they appear to result from changes akin to those previously described under (1), and A small-celled growth appears in the walls of the alveoli and invades the capillaries, but this, instead of proceeding to thickening of the walls, passes into amorphous granular disintegration. In other places, where 'lobular,' these areas result from changes next to be described.

(3) Lobular destructive changes resembling XXXVI. 1, 2, and 3, and XXXVII. 4, are found in all parts of these specimens. They occur in the midst of extensive small-celled infiltrations, and also in the midst of pneumonic areas where no degeneration is as yet apparent. They seem to originate in various ways. In some places they arise from destructive changes like those described under (1) and (2), extending until the whole of a group of lobules has been invaded, and the nodule thus formed is bounded by the the thickened tissue of the larger interlobular septa. The appearance thus produced is of a lobular mass resembling XXXVIII. 3 (*Henshaw*) and XXVIII. 6 and 8 (*Acute Tubercle*). In XXXVI. 1 and 2 there are illustrations of this process, which appears in the main to approximate closely to the suppurative type. Thickening is seen proceeding in XXXVI. 3, where the portions *a a a* resemble XXXVI. 5, and in part are like XXXVIII. 3 (*Henshaw*), while at *c c* are parts like XXXVII. 2.

In some places the mass of amorphous débris, or of degenerating leucocytes, bounded only by a zone of thickened fibroid tissue, strongly suggests that they might have resulted from the filling of bronchial tubes with inspissated secretion, and that the walls of these have subsequently undergone ulceration and suppuration. This appearance is very closely simulated in XXXVII. 4, but examination of these parts with higher powers shows that there are, throughout the islets, the remains of pulmonary tissue, as seen in XXXVI. 1, which therefore proves their pneumonic origin.

Some of these circumscribed nodules, passing into detritus, have an origin like that seen in XXXVII 2. Others, which have undergone a greater amount of cell-growth before cascation has occurred, resemble the nodules of XL. 1 (*Heath*), where a process of epithelial filling of the alveoli and thickening of their walls is proceeding in lobular areas. Another series is found like XXXV. 4 (*Smith*), but passing into more complete granular débris. Some of these by coalescence form elongated masses, which strongly suggest the appearance of thickening originating in bronchi, but show, in their interior, traces of a pulmonary structure, although occasionally, by the mode of their juxtaposition, even an appearance of the branching of a tube is simulated. Another, and very common form of growth, out of which they appear to originate, is what may be described as tubercular pneumonic nodules, like that seen in XXXVII. 5, where a mixed epithelial and small-celled growth is simultaneously invading the lobule, and also passes rapidly into granular detritus (caseation).

§ B. Tuberculo-pneumonic masses, as described in the preceding section, are the most common form in which tubercle appears in these lungs. Isolated nodules, composed only of small-celled growth, are comparatively rare, though in a few spots, in sections otherwise resembling XXXVII. 2, isolated alveoli, or a limited group of alveoli, may be so filled with a reticulated and small-celled growth as to present a perfect microscopic resemblance to the smallest form of miliary tubercle. It is, however, more common to find the reticulated small-celled growth in irregular masses in the inter-alveolar, peribronchial, and interlobular tissue.

In general, however, the nodules, when not of the destructive pneumonic types before described, resemble those figured in XXXVII. 5. In these a mingled epithelial and small-celled growth simultaneously occurs in variable proportion, but the latter predominates, and the nodules tend to pass early into caseation and detritus. Hence epithelial-like formation is almost constantly to be found in those which have not yet undergone destructive metamorphosis.

The formation of these nodules appears to be from lobular changes which, in their earlier stages, resemble XXXVII. 1. As the small-celled growth progresses, appearances are sometimes produced like those seen in XL. 1 and 3 (*Heath*), and in some preparations of this kind, the caseation can be seen commencing in the centre. A few giant-cells of the type of those found in connection with bronchioles (and resembling XXXII. 4 and 11), may be occasionally found at the margins of these nodules.

§ C. In a few spots large areas can be found completely infiltrated with a small-celled reticulated growth, as in XXXVI. 4. In some of these, all appearance of alveolar structure has disappeared and the infiltration is almost uniform : in other places, remains of the alveoli are still apparent, as in XXXVIII. 8 (*Holl*). Such parts are often intensely pigmented, and in some the pigment appears in crystalline forms. Pigment is also found abundantly in places where small-celled growth appears in the walls of the alveoli, together with epithelial proliferation in their interior (*see* XXXVII. 7).

§ D. Perivascular and peribronchial growths assume forms identical with those already described.

CASE 20.
CASEATING TUBERCULAR PNEUMONIA.

Plates VII. 4 ; XX. 2 ; XXXIX. 2.

Ref.—Phthisis, p. 119.

SUMMARY.—*M. 33. Intemperate. Suffered for six months from cough, purulent expectoration, weakness and swelling of feet. The liver was enlarged. There were signs of consolidation and excavation in the upper part of each lung. Persistent remitting pyrexia. Extensive ulceration of larynx and trachea. In the upper half of each lung was grey pneumonic infiltration ; through both, groups of granulations were scattered ; the apex of the right was fibroid.*

JOHN THOMAS, ætat. 33, admitted University College Hospital June 15th, 1869 ; died June 28th, 1869.

Family history indefinite : no history of phthisis. Father a drunkard.

Occupation and Habits.—A shoemaker, has lived fifteen years in London ; has lived well : habitually indulged in excess of alcohol for last fifteen years and has had delirium tremens. Has had syphilis and gonorrhœa. Has been subject to morning sickness.

Present Illness began five months ago, without assignable cause, but patient had been much exposed to the weather. The first symptom was cough ; he felt very ill, and unable to continue his work, and was confined to his bed. Has had swelling of feet and ankles.

State on Admission.—Anæmia ; emaciation ; cyanosis, with look of distress. Œdema of feet. Some ascites. Urine scanty ; sp. gr. varied from 1012 to 1018 : repeatedly examined, it contained neither albumen nor sugar. Liver large, extending from 6th rib to two fingers' breadth below false ribs. Heart's apex indistinct, covered by lung, no murmurs. Frequent cough : expectoration copious, tenacious, and mostly puriform. Pain in the chest and dyspnœa. Chest barrel-shaped ; expansion small. Superficial veins prominent. There were physical signs of consolidation with excavation at both apices, and also of consolidation in the mid-scapular regions, accompanied everywhere by coarse bubbling râles. Diarrhœa set in, prostration increased, and the patient died June 28.

The Temperature was persistently pyrexial, of a remitting type. The mean morning temperature was 101·1° ; the mean evening temperature was 101·5°. The highest morning temperature was 102° ; the lowest (one occasion only) 99° ; it was generally over 101°. The highest evening temperature was 103·2° ; the lowest (one occasion only) 98° ; in a large proportion it reached or exceeded 102°. The mean exacerbation from morning to evening was 0·9°, the greatest 1·8°, the least 0·4°. The mean of the remissions from evening to morning was 1°, the greatest being 2·2°, and the least 0·2°. On two occasions the morning temperature was higher than the succeeding evening (0·2°). On one occasion it was higher than the preceding evening (0·6°). The *Pulse* was invariably above 120, with a maximum frequency of 141. The *Respirations* were commonly 36, and never less than this, increasing occasionally to 40 and even to 48.

POST-MORTEM.— *Larynx and Trachea* : Both vocal cords thickened and ulcerated ; the ulcer on the right cord has a thick everted edge. The mucous membrane of the sacculi laryngis and false vocal cords is also thickened. Mucous membrane of trachea almost entirely eroded, only small islets of deeply congested membrane being left amid serpiginous ulcers (see XX. 2). The edges of the ulcers in the trachea are irregular and ragged, but not thickened. The ulceration extends to the bronchial tubes in the right lung, but does not reach beyond the first division : in the left lung it passes into the third and fourth divisions, and in the upper lobe it penetrates even further, the bronchial mucous membrane being apparently almost entirely destroyed.

Left Lung.—The upper lobe is entirely solidified by a grey pneumonic infiltration (VII. 4, *a a*) riddled with sinuous irregular cavities (*c c*). They are filled with puriform matter, and in their walls are caseous fragments of granulations. Throughout the grey infiltration are scattered irregular caseous masses (*b b*), and groups of granulations forming racemose masses. These are in some places whitish, in others yellow and softening, and their softening produces potential cavities. The upper two-thirds of the inferior lobe is in a similar condition. The lower part is in a state of intense congestion, with isolated granulations scattered through it.

Right Lung.—The apex is indurated, fibroid, and pigmented. Below this is a grey infiltration with softening of caseous masses, and racemose granulations, similar to those seen in the opposite lung. In the lower lobe also, thickly scattered throughout it, are racemose groups of granulations.

The post-tracheal lymphatic glands are indurated and pigmented ; they contain cheesy and some cretaceous spots. *The bronchial glands* are in some places swollen, in others indurated, and they contain cheesy masses, which in some places have softened ; in others there is cretaceous matter.

Liver large, weighs fully 5 lbs. 8 oz.
Kidneys indurated. *Spleen* somewhat large, otherwise healthy.

Stomach.—Mucous membrane much congested, thickened at pyloric end.

Intestines.—Solitary glands enlarged throughout the whole intestine, and in some places ulcerated. Peyer's patches ulcerated ; ulcers extend in transverse diameter of intestine, and have thickened edges. Ulcers with the same character are seen in the large intestine.

No enlargement of *mesenteric glands*; a few granulations seen in them.

The MICROSCOPIC CHARACTERS in this lung are like those of *Lloyd* and *Griffin* (Cases 22 and 19).

A. Diffuse pneumonic infiltration of the type of XXXVIII. 2 and 4 (*Henshaw*).

B.* Areas of destructive pneumonia like XXXVIII. 3 (*Henshaw*), and XXXVI. 4, 5 (*Griffin*).

C. Suppurative areas, sometimes widely extended, like XXXV. 1 and 5 (*Brodrick* and *Smith*).

D. Nodular, and E diffuse, small-celled growth.

F. Tracts of induration.

G. Perivascular and peribronchial growth.

§§ A and B. These destructive areas, variously intermingled, tend to assume round circumscribed forms, which in some parts pass insensibly into the processes by which they arise, but in other places extend until they are bounded by the interlobular septa. The mode of their production is mainly by the thickening of the alveolar walls with a small-celled growth, while the epithelium perishes and passes, in their interior, into an amorphous granular mass (see XXXIX. 2). Large areas become thus occupied, but at times the whole tissue so affected appears to pass into a state of suppuration. The small-celled growth has lost its solidity: the reticular structure has disappeared, and the cells, closely crowded, are spherical and sometimes nucleated, imbedded in a material which appears as if it had been originally fluid (see XXXV. 1—*Brodrick*).

§ C. Masses of small-celled reticular growth, forming rounded nodules, sometimes distinctly originating in alveoli, both conglomerate and single, having all the characters of miliary tubercle, and, at their margins, resembling XXX. 3 (*Coombes, Acute Tubercle*).

§ D. Diffuse, small-celled growth, reticulate in character, like XXXVIII. 8 (*Hall*); but areas of this structure are not numerous.

§ E. Tracts of induration, where, in combination with the foregoing, bands of thickened fibres extend across the alveolar structures, like XLI. 7 (*Coppin*).

§ F. Perivascular growth is abundant, but peribronchial growth is less apparent, and no forms of bronchial ulceration are to be found in the specimens prepared. It is somewhat remarkable that, as contrasted with the lungs of *Lloyd* (*Case 23*), no giant-cells were found in the preparations.

CASE 21.

CHRONIC PHTHISIS. PNEUMONIC INFILTRATION.

Plate IX. fig. 3.

This figure was taken from a case of chronic phthisis (*Gowling*), with cavities at the apices, and in which the upper parts of the lungs were entirely converted into a fibroid tissue. Nodules of induration, and groups of indurated and caseous granulations, existed in the lower lobes, which were also the seat of a grey, firm, pneumonic infiltration (see figure).

The chief MICROSCOPIC APPEARANCES were :—

A. Extensive pneumonic tracts, filled with very large epithelial cells, and without thickening of the alveolar walls, like XXVI. 7 (*Ellsom*).

B. Tracts where the alveoli were filled with amorphous exudation-matter (mucoid), like XXXVIII. 2 and 4 (*Henshaw*).

C. Areas of considerable extent, where great thickening of the alveolar walls had occurred, like XXVIII. 9, 10 (*Polley, Acute Tubercle*), and also reproducing appearances like XXXVII. 6 and 7 (*Griffin*), and XXXIX. 2 and 3 (*Thomas and Gardiner*).

D. Areas of small-celled growth, proceeding in the floor of the infundibula and passing into caseation, like XXXIX. 4 (*Price*), and also occurring in a diffuse form, mingled with epithelial proliferation, like XXXVIII. 8 (*Hall*), and XL. 2 (*Heath*).

E. Peribronchial and perivascular small-celled growth was abundant in many places.

CASE 22.

ACUTE CASEATING TUBERCULAR PNEUMONIA.

Plates XI. and XXXIX. fig. 3.

Ref.—Phthisis, p. 119 ; Syphilitic Disease, p. 127.

SUMMARY.—*M. 28. Intemperate. Sudden onset ; cough and expectoration. Three months later, signs of consolidation in the upper part of each lung and at the right base, and of excavation at apices ; moist rales throughout. Extreme emaciation, hectic, moderate pyrexia, diarrhœa. Death a week after admission.—Caseous ulceration of larynx. Caseous nodules in lungs, breaking down into cavities ; in parts, more diffuse grey pneumonic consolidation. Enlargement and ulceration of the solitary glands of the intestine.*

T. GARDINER, ætat. 28. Compositor ; admitted University College Hospital November 27, died December 6, 1867.

Family History.—No phthisis known.

Personal History.—Has drunk freely at times. Has had a chancre, and three years ago had sore-throat. No skin eruption.

Present Illness began suddenly, three months ago ; attributed by patient to a wetting some weeks previously. First symptom was cough with frothy expectoration. There had been loss of flesh ever since the cough began. No hæmoptysis. No previous chest affection.

Physical Signs.—Chest well-formed. On the right side there was evidence of consolidation at the apex anteriorly as low as the 3rd rib, and posteriorly through the upper half of the scapular region : reaching also into the upper axilla. There was imperfect resonance in patches throughout the mid-scapular and interscapular regions, and evidence of absolute consolidation at the base posteriorly in its outer half. The infra-axillary and infra-mammary regions were dull below the 6th and 5th ribs respectively. There were signs of extensive excavation at the right apex, and there was bronchial breathing, with coarse metallic râles, over the consolidated areas at the base, in front and behind. In the left apex the physical signs showed consolidation posteriorly throughout the scapular regions, and in the upper axilla to the 5th rib ; in the infra-clavicular to the 3rd rib. There was no dulness at the base. Coarse moist râles existed through the whole of this lung, but there were no signs of excavation at the apex. The chest was well-formed. The heart was natural. The urine was free from albumen. There was extreme emaciation and hectic; diarrhœa set in, and he died on the 8th day after admission.

He was continuously febrile. The mean morning temperature was 101·1°, the highest being 102·6°, the lowest 99°. The mean evening temperature was 102·3°, the highest being 103°, the lowest 100·2°. The mean of the exacerbations from morning to evening was 1·4°, the highest being 3°, and the lowest 0·2°. The mean of the remissions from morning to evening was 2°, the highest being 2·8°, the lowest 0·2°. No remissions were observed from morning to evening, but exacerbations occurred on two days from evening to morning; the greatest was 1·4°, the least 0·6° (mean 1°). The pulse, always above 120, varied between this and 142. The respirations varied from 32 to 40. The pulse-respiration ratio varied from 3·5 : 1 to 2·6 : 1.

POST-MORTEM.—*Larynx*: The epiglottis is thickened, and there are granulations on the lower surface; the edge is irregularly notched. Both vocal cords are ulcerated deeply at anterior angle. The ulcerations rest on a cheesy base extending through the thickness of the mucous membrane. Some small superficial ulcerations are scattered over the trachea; the whole mucous membrane is intensely injected.

Lungs.—Both are loosely adherent by scattered bands. In the *left lung* the bronchi of lower lobe present some fusiform dilatations, chiefly in the second divisions; the smaller branches are less affected. The apex is occupied by nodules, varying in size from a walnut to a horse-bean, all very soft, yellowish-grey in colour, here and there pigmented, and composed of finer soft granulations, having in the main a yellowish-white colour. The larger masses are more uniform on the surface, and they are softer than the smaller ones. They are distinctly circumscribed from the surrounding tissue. In places they break down into irregular cavities. One, at the extreme apex, is seen covered only by a thin layer of pleura, apparently on the point of sloughing (see XI. 2). The greater part of the apex is occupied by these masses; some non-infiltrated pulmonary tissue, however, intervenes between them, and is loaded with serosity.

The anterior margin is occupied by a grey exudation, infiltrated, but not uniformly, through an emphysematous tissue. This infiltration is homogeneous, glistening, uniform on section, and scarcely granular. In it, and also in the emphysematous tissue, are yellow masses, similar to those described at the apex, softening into small cavities, with which this part of the lung is riddled. The yellow masses are sharply defined from the pneumonic infiltration, and they have at the margin a racemose appearance, as if made up of little granules like those described at the apex. They also are pigmented.

The same grey infiltration extends inwards at the part of the lung corresponding to the upper axillary and scapular regions; and in this infiltration nodules of yellow matter of various sizes are seen, separated by a distinct line of demarcation from the surrounding tissue. They are also abundant in parts where the pneumonic infiltration exists. In many parts they have softened into small cavities. One cavity, in the axillary portion, is of the size of a Brazil nut: it has a cheesy sloughing base, but no granulations are seen in its floor. The lower lobe is intensely congested and is loaded with serosity. It is occupied by smaller nodules, of the size of a hemp-seed, which, at the extreme margin, are conglomerated into masses similar to those seen at the apex, but for the most part these granulations are only scattered singly or in groups through this part of lung. The yellow nodules of the size of a hemp-seed are seen, on minute examination, to be again formed by the agglomeration of smaller granules of the size of a poppy-seed, which gradually coalesce. The larger granulations stand out prominently from the surface of the lung and are very soft. Their section is smooth.

The *right lung* (XI. 1) also shows some dilatations of the bronchi. The apex is occupied with large nodular masses of the size of a Maltese orange, similar to those observed in the other lung. The upper half of the lung is almost entirely occupied by these masses. Between them is either a grey pneumonic infiltration or emphysematous congested tissue, loaded with serosity. The extreme base presents the same yellow granules and nodules lying in a tissue entirely consolidated. There is a large cavity in the upper lobe, with a dirty-grey sloughing floor, and others of smaller size and similar characters are scattered through the upper two-thirds of this lung. The tissue beneath this sloughing floor is intensely hyperæmic, and is occupied by the same grey pneumonic infiltration. There are no ordinary grey granulations of tubercle in either lung.

Heart healthy, with the exception of some thickening on the mitral valve.

Liver, Spleen, and *Kidneys* present no abnormal appearances.

Stomach : mucous membrane thickened, especially near pylorus. *Intestines.* Injection commencing in jejunum and increasing throughout ileum. This injection is particularly marked around Peyer's patches. One small spot of ulceration is seen just above the ileo-cœcal valve. The solitary glands are enlarged throughout the small intestine, and in some of Peyer's patches, single follicles are enlarged. In the large intestine, the solitary glands are enlarged, and two are ulcerated. The ulceration does not rest on a caseous base.

MICROSCOPIC EXAMINATION. — The destructive processes in this lung are of several types.

A. Large areas of acutely caseating pneumonia.
B. Large areas of suppurative pneumonia.
C. Nodules of mingled pneumonic and small-celled growth passing into caseation, and tending to become confluent.
D. Nodules of small-celled growth.
E. Diffuse small-celled growth.
F. Peribronchial and perivascular small-celled growth.

§ A. The areas of acutely caseating pneumonia resemble those seen in XXXVIII. 3 (*Henshaw*), XXXVI. 4 (*Griffin*), and XXVIII. 6 and 8 (*Polley*). They commence apparently in an inflammatory process, in which the alveoli are filled either with an amorphous mucous exudation like XXXVIII. 4 (*Henshaw*), or with enlarged epithelial cells like XXVI. 7 (*Ellsom*). The process of caseation, as seen at the margins of the masses in which it is proceeding, is apparently induced essentially by the small-celled growth in the walls of the alveoli, and a destruction of capillaries, but the precise mode in which this process occurs produces several variations in appearance and character. The predominant type resembles that seen in XXXVII. 1, 2, 3, and 6 (*Griffin*), and XL. 6 (*Heath*), such variations as occur being due to the greater or less amount of small-celled growth in proportion to the epithelial proliferation. When the small-celled growth is extensive, considerable thickening of the alveolar walls takes place antecedent to the caseation, as in XXXIX. 3. When this is less extensive, the granular disintegration takes place at an earlier stage, as in XXXVII. 3, *Griffin*. These tracts and masses are also formed in parts out of processes similar to those described in § E.

The caseous areas are sometimes diffused over considerable spaces; in other parts they are circumscribed and bounded by thickened interlobular septa, and then they form lobular masses. In the latter case, they sometimes consist only of an amorphous granular homogeneous débris, enclosed in spaces marked out by lines of fibres (also granular), which represent the remains of the alveolar walls.

§ B. Suppurative areas may, like the foregoing, be either diffuse or circumscribed. When diffuse they resemble the forms seen in XXXV. 1, 2, 3, 5, and 7 (*Brodrick*, *Smith*, and *S. Brown*). Areas like XL. 4 (*Heath*) are also seen. When circumscribed they have the appearances seen in XXXVI. 1, 2, 3, and 5 (*Griffin*), and occasionally like XXXIX. 1 (*Lloyd*). They arise from a round-celled growth, taking the place of the small-celled growth seen in XXXVIII. 2 (*Henshaw*). The whole tissue becomes infiltrated in this manner with densely packed round cells, most of which have the character and appearance of pus-cells or white blood-corpuscles, while others, non-nucleated, are of the class of 'pyoid bodies,' but, as a rule, they are without any interposed reticulum. They all pass rapidly into disintegration, like XXXV. 2 and 5 (*Smith* and *Brodrick*), or when in circumscribed areas, like XXXVI. 1, 2, and 5 (*Griffin*). Quasi-suppurative areas are very extensive in these lungs. They pass insensibly into, and are mingled in various forms with, the caseating masses before described, and they also pass into various types of diffusesmall-celled interstitial growth.

§ C. Nodules of mingled small-celled and epithelial growth are also common. They likewise tend to form caseous masses, which, by their confluence, may occupy large areas. Their types are various. Some (and these are the most common) resemble XXXVII. 5 (*Griffin*), and XXXVIII. 7 (*Hall*). Changes like XXXVII. 2 (*Griffin*) are also found in nodular masses passing at the centres into caseation. Nodules are also found like XL. 3, and XLIII. 5 (*Heath*), likewise undergoing granular disintegration. Variations and intermediate stages between these and XXXV. 4 (*Smith*), and XXXIX. 5 (*Overall*), may also be found. In some places thickening of the reticulum and fibres has proceeded to a greater extent before caseation occurs, and then it appears in the form of a granular disintegration in the midst of nodules having the structure of XLI. 2 (*Carr*) and XLI. 7 (*Coppin*).

§ D. Nodules entirely, or almost entirely, composed of small-celled growth, with intervening reticular structure, also occur. Some are like XLI. 6 (*Cox*), but a considerable proportion are like XXX. 1 and 2 (*Acute Tubercle*). Gradations can be seen between these and others like XXXVII. 5 (*Griffin*). In some cases, nodules of small-celled growth of this nature, forming 'miliary tubercles,' may be found completely filling the alveoli. In others, buds and projections extend into the cavities of the alveoli from the growth in their walls (see XXXIX. 3). These nodules also pass into caseation, which commences in their centres.

§ E. Diffuse small-celled growth is common over large areas. It is found variously intermingled with epithelial proliferation in the interior of the alveoli, and has characters seen in XXXVIII. 8 (*Hall*), XL. 2 (*Heath*), XL. 4 (*Heath*), and XXXVII. 2 (*Griffin*). All these forms are found passing into diffuse or circumscribed granular disintegration (caseation), and produce tracts like XXXVIII. 3 (*Henshaw*), and XXXVI. 4 (*Griffin*). In some parts, where the section passes perpendicularly in the long axis of the bronchioles, the small-celled infiltration appears in the walls of these as well as in those of the pulmonary infundibula. Caseation, suppuration, and in a few spots fibroid induration, appear to arise indiscriminately out of this change. Giant-cells are numerous in the vicinity of nearly all the caseating parts, most so around the nodular forms § C and § D. They are of the types of XXXII. 4, 5, 9, 10 c, and XXXIII. 1, 3 c, 6, and 11. In some places they surround the caseating masses, as in XXXII. 7, while in others they are found singly. In a few spots they are of the types of XXXII. 5 and 9, in the midst of nodules described in § C.

§ F. Peribronchial growth in the walls of the larger bronchi, attended in a few spots with ulceration, is not uncommon, but it is not the source of the greater part of the destructive changes found in this lung. Periarterial growth is also found, and in some places extends to the adjacent alveolar walls.

The bulk of the destructive changes in this lung are induced by a pneumonia which either caseates or suppurates, the latter process sometimes inducing the former, which, however, generally occurs without its intervention. The processes by which caseation are induced are various; all concur in one common feature, viz. the growth of nuclei in the walls of the capillaries and of the alveoli, by which the vascular circulation is arrested, and the same is probably true of the lymphatics.

Microscopical examination of the enlarged follicles in the intestine showed an infiltration of the submucous tissue with a small-celled growth, identical with that found in other instances of phthisical (tubercular?) ulceration of these parts.

COMMENTARY.—The following points appear to deserve especial attention in this case. The acute course, apparently little more than three months, and yet ending in extreme caseation in both lungs. Ordinary pneumonia does not, within this period, produce caseation either so intense as was seen here, or so acutely destructive, except in cases of abscess and gangrene. This process was essentially different from that of abscess.

The process was not, however, limited to the lungs. In the larynx there was ulceration with a caseous floor, and in the intestines there was enlargement of the lymphatic follicles, passing here and there into ulceration. The laryngeal disease appeared to the naked eye to be of the same nature as the pulmonary. The question may therefore be asked:

If the theory be correct that the lung-affection was a 'caseous pneumonia,' distinct in its essential nature from all the tubercular affections, of what nature is the laryngeal affection? Is it also an independent inflammation, or a secondary 'caseous laryngitis'? If secondary, can caseous inflammations, besides being infective in the production of tubercle, be also infective in the production of secondary caseous inflammations in distant organs? Or, finally, are the diseases of the larynx and intestine of the same nature as that of the lung, or are they different?

I think that the tubercular nature of the caseous pneumonia is shown in this case by the character of the changes in the interstitial tissue, and that the laryngeal and intestinal affections were only part of a general disease, finding its first manifestation in the lung, but subsequently attacking—and probably by blood-infection—other parts. The small caseous granulations (out of which the large masses were apparently formed in most instances) are, I believe, to be regarded as the analogues, and as having, in this case, precisely the same pathological signification as the grey granulations which are observed in other and less acute cases of phthisis, but which here were entirely absent to the naked eye. The explanation of the caseous appearance of the granulations is, I think, that already given, viz. that it is due to the amount of pneumonia present, and to the acuteness of the destructive process, when once the circulation has been arrested by the small-celled growth.

How the disease was acquired in this case must remain open to doubt. The nature of his occupation affords a not improbable explanation.

CASE 23.
CASEATING TUBERCULAR PNEUMONIA.

Plates XII., XXXIII. figs. 2, 5, and 6; and XXXIX. fig. 1.

Ref.—Phthisis, p. 104. Syphilitic Disease, p. 127.

SUMMARY.—*F. 27. Duration of symptoms fourteen weeks. Sudden onset after a chill. Cough and purulent expectoration. Two weeks before death there were signs of consolidation and excavation at both apices, and throughout right lung. Diarrhœa; pyrexia moderate.—In both lungs, especially in the right, were extensive tracts of grey pneumonic consolidation with irregular yellow nodules, both breaking down into sinuous cavities, lined with membrane and caseated material. Smaller nodules and granulations were scattered through the unconsolidated parts. Tubercular ulceration of the small intestine.*

JANE LLOYD, ætat. 27, admitted into University College Hospital, April 15, died April 30, 1867.

Family History.— Father died of bronchitis, ætat. 52. Mother living and in good health. One brother died of fever. Has had two sisters, both living—one healthy, the other delicate.

Personal History.—Has had the exanthemata in childhood, also small-pox, and an attack of rheumatic fever two years ago. Menstruation commenced at 14. Married at 16; has had one miscarriage and one child, who is healthy.

Present Illness began three months ago. Caught a violent cold, followed by cough; at first it was unattended by expectoration, but lately this has become profuse. No large hæmoptysis, but streaks of blood have occasionally appeared in the sputa. Voice has been hoarse without intermission for past two months; for some time the catamenia have ceased. Bowels have been relaxed since commencement of illness. Appetite has failed, and she has lost flesh considerably, and has had to keep her bed, occasionally but not constantly, owing to weakness.

State on Admission.—Considerable anæmia. Marked but not excessive emaciation. Skin hot. Deep cicatrices in both groins. Pain behind sternum. Respiration accelerated; cough frequent with abundant thick and opaque, green, non-aërated sputa. Voice hoarse. Appetite defective. The physical signs were those of extensive consolidation at both apices, with excavation and still more extensive consolidation in the right lung. Diarrhœa existed from time to time, and she sank exhausted a fortnight after admission. Her temperature was not taken with regularity. The evening temperature occasionally reached 102°; the morning temperature occasionally 101·5°; on a few occasions the morning temperature was normal, but as a rule it ranged from 99° to 100°.

POST-MORTEM.—*Lungs: right* generally adherent. It is almost solid throughout, large tracts being occupied by a finely granular, ashy-grey exudation, which, however, is redder in parts (*see* Plate XII.) Throughout this infiltration are scattered yellow masses which on section do not project above the level of the surrounding infiltration. They are irregular in size, varying from a millet-seed to a hazelnut, but their shape is very irregular and their outline is sinuous. They are apparently imbedded in the surrounding infiltration (Plate XII. *a, a*). In some places (*b*), these tracts can be seen softening into excavations which occasionally progress by the breaking down of caseous tracts of considerable size; finally they form irregular and sinuous cavities (*d, d*), surrounded by caseous walls, in which ragged nodules of caseous matter still exist. The cavities, lined with a dirty ash-grey membrane, in which are caseous nodules and the remains of vessels, are thickly scattered through all parts of the lung. In such portions of the tissue between the excavations as are not infiltrated with the pneumonic exudation before described, are yellow-grey nodules, in size from a millet-seed to a hemp-seed, sometimes agglomerated into large racemose groups. They are all soft, and have a granular section; their margins are irregular, with fine granulations extending into the surrounding tissue. In other places these granulations are whitish in colour; they occur singly and in groups, and in some places are surrounded by a semi-transparent pigmented zone, while others of a similar kind are situated in an area of infiltration.

The *left* lung presents appearances almost identical with those of the right, but the pneumonic infiltration is less extensive.

MICROSCOPIC EXAMINATION.—The characteristics of these lungs are chiefly these:—

A. Large tracts of pneumonic change.
B. Masses, either circumscribed or diffuse, of acutely destructive pneumonia.
C. Areas of small-celled infiltration.
D. Perivascular and peribronchial infiltration, with ulceration and destruction of the bronchial walls.

§ A. The pneumonic infiltration is chiefly of the types of XXXVIII. 2 and 4 (*Henshaw*) and XXVI. 7 (*Ellsom*). The alveoli are either filled with large epithelial-like cells, or contain these more sparingly scattered in the midst of an amorphous and finely granular exudation (mucin). The walls, in some places, show a slight degree of nuclear growth, like XXXVII. 4 (*Griffin*), but large areas of this are not visible.

§ D. Masses of destructive pneumonia occur in the midst of areas of the diffuse kind last described. They resemble XXXVIII. 3 (*Henshaw*), XXXVII. 4 (*Griffin*), XXVIII. 8 (*Polley*), and XL. 4 (*Heath*). These destructive areas are for the most part formed by processes akin to XXXVII. 6 (*Griffin*), and also to XXVIII. 7 (*Polley*, *Acute Tubercle*). The epithelium perishes early within the alveoli, while a small-celled growth invades the wall, but also perishes before any notable thickening has occurred. Other areas, however, are akin to the suppurative destructive alveolitis seen in XXXVI. 5 (*Griffin*) and XXXV. 5 (*Smith*). Both of these forms of nodules are often distinctly circumscribed, and even when this is not the case, they form rounded masses, more or less defined from the pneumonic area by which they are surrounded. At the margins, however, evidence exists of the earlier stages in which they originate; and they are distinctly of the forms of XXXVIII. 3 (*Henshaw*), and apparently originate like XXVIII. 7 (*Polley*). They are often surrounded by a series of giant-cells, similar in distribution to those seen in XXXII. 7 (*Smith*), and in some instances by a zone of small-celled infiltration (see XXXIX. 1). In other cases the necrotic areas originate in processes resembling XL. 1 and 3 (*Heath*), where interstitial growth proceeds to a greater extent before caseation occurs. In some of the alveoli, during this stage, giant-cells may be frequently seen, but they are not constant. Transitional forms between these and XXXVII. 2 (*Griffin*), and XXXVIII. 8 (*Hall*), may also be occasionally observed.

All these pneumonic areas tend to soften and break down in their centres, and they are undoubtedly the origin of the greater part of the excavations found in these lungs.

§ C. Small-celled infiltrations are not very extensive in this lung. They do, however, occur in forms like XL. 2 (*Heath*), and also mingled with pneumonic products like XXXVIII. 8 (*Hall*). In some places they agglomerate in dense, rounded masses having all the characters of miliary tubercle, and resembling XXXV. 6 (*Smith*) and XLI. 6 (*Cox*).

§ D. Perivascular infiltration with small-celled growth is not uncommon. Peribronchial infiltration, with subsequent ulceration, occurs in a few spots, but is comparatively infrequent compared with the destructive pneumonic processes previously described.

CASE 24.

ACUTE PHTHISIS; CASEATING TUBERCULAR PNEUMONIA.

Plates XIV. fig. 2 ; XXXVIII. figs. 7, 8, 9, and 10.

Ref.—Phthisis, p. 94 ; Syphilitic Disease, p. 127.

SUMMARY.—*F. 23. For twelve months before death, cough, progressive emaciation, and, later,* occasional *hæmoptysis. During the last three weeks of life, considerable persistent pyrexia and great exhaustion. Signs of consolidation and excavation in the upper parts of both lungs, with general imperfect resonance except at the bases.—Grey pneumonic infiltration in upper and middle parts of both lungs ; caseous masses at apices, numerous cavities, some with smooth and some with sloughing walls ; in lower lobes small opaque agglomerated granulations. Enlargement and ulceration of follicular glands of intestine.*

MARGARET HALL, ætat. 23, married ; admitted University College Hospital March 20; died April 13, 1868.

Family History.—See that of *Mary Corney* (*Case 25*), whose sister she is.

Personal History.—Worked in manufactory of percussion caps before marriage. Married about three years. Has not lived well of late. Has one child, born fourteen months ago. Good health, with exception of infantile diseases, up to date of present illness, which commenced about two months after birth of child, with cough ; began abruptly, without apparent cause. Since then she has grown progressively weaker, and the cough has increased in severity. Three months ago she had a considerable hæmoptysis (one pint), and hæmoptysis has occurred to a less degree on several subsequent occasions. She has grown rapidly weaker of late.

State on Admission.—Extreme anæmia, but lips cyanotic and hectic flush on cheeks. Looks very ill and emaciated. Fingers taper ; ends slightly clubbed. Cough frequent ; expectoration copious, of dense masses of greenish-yellow colour.

Chest fairly well-formed. Distinct flattening in both infra-clavicular regions, especially on left side. Signs of absolute consolidation and excavation at both apices, front and back. General deficiency of pulmonary resonance over both lungs, except at bases, where there is hyperresonance. Blowing and bronchial breathing, mingled with metallic râles, is heard over greater part of upper portions of both lungs. Some coarse râles also heard at bases.

Nausea after food. No diarrhœa. Excessive thirst. Tongue red, covered with thin, dry fur. Voice natural ; no pain on swallowing. Urine, except on one occasion, free from albumen. She sank rapidly, and died on April 13.

The respiration was rapid throughout, varying from 34 to 64. The pulse varied from 112 to 148. The pulse-respiration ratio varied from 1 : 2¾ (morning) to 1 : 1¼ evening. The mean morning temperature, in seventeen observations, was 102·2°. The mean evening temperature, in nine observations, was 103·3°. The morning temperature on three occasions reached 104° ; on four occasions ranged from 103° to 104° ; on five occasions from 101° to 102° ; on three occasions from 101° to 102° ; and on three from 100° to 101°. It never fell either to normal or to subnormal. The evening temperature was on all occasions between 103° and 104². The mean exacerbation from morning to evening in seven observations was 1·2°, the maximum being 2·2° and the minimum 0·4°. The mean remission from evening to morning, in six observations, was 1°, the highest being 1·6° and the lowest 0·3°. Exacerbations from evening to morning were observed on two occasions, the highest being 1° and the lowest 0·2°.

One remission from morning to evening of 0·4° is recorded.

Post-mortem.—Lungs: Both lungs firmly adherent throughout. *Right lung:* At the posterior part of the apex is a firm and fibrous tract of limited extent. Below this, the whole of upper and middle lobes are infiltrated with a grey pneumonia, which passes at the apex into solid masses of cheesy matter. Both of these lobes are riddled with cavities, containing softened cheesy material capable of being washed out with water. Some cavities communicate with one another; others do not. Their walls are lined with a dirty ash-grey membrane, smooth and glistening, in which no granulations are seen. In the upper part of the lower lobe is a similar infiltration, uniform above and passing below into isolated nodules, composed of small granulations agglomerated together, soft but not cheesy, semi-opaque, and greyish-white in colour, which are thickly scattered through an emphysematous tissue.

Left lung.—Appearance similar to that of right. It contains numerous cavities, filled with a dirty puriform matter, lined with a yellow sloughing material. The cavities are surrounded by a semi-transparent grey infiltration (XIV. 2, *a a*), which occupies the greater part of the upper lobe. In it are caseous masses, which present various stages of softening into cavities (*b d*). Below this (*c*) is an infiltration, in part semi-transparent, without any granular look of the surface, but passing into a semi-opaque consolidation, which again passes gradually into an injected and emphysematous tissue. In this emphysematous tissue, soft, isolated granulations are seen, and in some parts there are nodular patches, of a dry, firm, opaque appearance, and distinctly granular surface.

Larynx healthy.

Intestines.—Solitary glands of ileum much enlarged. A little lower, they are seen to be opaque and cheesy, and are surrounded by a zone of injection. Still lower, Peyer's patches are dotted over with small milk-white spots, which, near the end of the ileum, are replaced by spots of punctiform ulceration.

Stomach intensely catarrhal.

Kidneys cloudy.

Liver presents early stage of lardaceous disease.

The Microscopic Appearances in these lungs are the following:—

A. Large areas of pneumonic infiltration, characterised by the alveoli being filled with very large epithelial cells.

B. Large areas of caseous pneumonia.

C. Areas of suppurative or destructive pneumonia.

D. Diffuse small-celled growth.

E. Nodules of small-celled growth.

F. Nodules of mingled epithelial and small-celled growth undergoing caseation.

G. Perivascular and peribronchial small-celled growth; the latter occasionally passing into ulceration.

§ A. Areas of pneumonia, distinguished by the size of the epithelial cells filling the alveoli, are found abundantly throughout these lungs. They occur in places without manifest thickening of the walls, like XXVI. 7 (*Ellsom*). In other places nuclear growths are seen forming in the walls. The epithelial cells (see XXXVIII. 8, *a a*) are large, increasing from $\frac{1}{1000}$ to $\frac{1}{500}$ inch in diameter. Many of them contain two, and frequently three, or even four nuclei. The contents of the cells are, for the most part, homogeneous and transparent. The tracts tend to pass insensibly into the areas of caseous and suppurating destructive process next to be described, but only through the various intermediate changes.

§ B. The areas of caseous pneumonia resemble XXXVIII. 9, and are also like XXXVI. 4 and 5 (*Griffin*), and XXVIII. 6 and 8 (*Polley, Acute Tubercle*). They occur in a diffuse and also in a circumscribed form. In the latter, they resemble XXXVI. 1 (*Griffin*). In both they appear to originate from changes akin to those described in Griffin (*Case 19*), by the growth of nuclei in the alveolar wall, like XXXVII. 2 and 6. In some places they are preceded by a large-celled epithelial formation, but, as at the margins where caseation is proceeding, the epithelial cells disappear and are mingled with a gradually increasing small-celled growth. In other places the epithelial formation is less abundant, and the small-celled growth predominates.

§ C. The areas of suppuration resemble those seen in XXXV. 1 (*Drodrick*). They pass into completely destructive changes, like XXXV. 5 (*Smith*). The processes by which they occur resemble those described in these instances (*Cases 18 and 28*).

§ D. Diffuse areas of small-celled growth are very abundant. They are seen in XXXVIII. 8, and resemble XL. 2 (*Heath*). In other parts, large tracts are found, like XXXVII. 6 and 7 (*Griffin*), XXXIX. 2 and 3 (*J. Thomas* and *Gardiner*). In some parts, they enclose alveoli containing large epithelial cells: in others, the alveolar structure has disappeared; in others, again, they produce great thickening of the walls of the alveoli and narrowing of their cavities, similar to XXXVIII. 1 (*Henshaw*), and XXVIII. 9 and 10 (*Polley, Acute Tubercle*).

§ E. Nodules of small-celled growth are seen, in some places originating like XL. 1 and 3 (*Heath*), and in others growing into dense masses, in which only the small-celled reticulated structure is apparent, like XXX. 1 (*Acute Tubercle*). In others, a growth like XXXVII. 7 (*Griffin*) extends in one part of the wall of the alveoli, forming a quasi-rounded mass.

§ F. Nodules of mingled epithelial and small-celled growth are common. Some resemble XXXVIII. 7 and also XXXVII. 5 (*Griffin*). Others, which are numerous, arise from changes like XXXVII. 2 (*Griffin*) assuming the nodular form. All these pass, apparently with great rapidity, into caseous change, and form circumscribed nodules of detritus, surrounded by a pigmented thickened wall, like XXXIX. 7 (*Curwin*); XXXIX. 5 (*Overall*); XLIII. 5 (*Heath*), and in some places like XXXII. 7 (*Smith*).

Giant-cells are occasionally seen round these nodules, and also round the masses of caseating pneumonia. They are not numerous in these lungs. When present, they are for the most part of the types of XXXII. 10, *a*; and XXXIII. 11. The destructive processes in this lung are by the caseation of large tracts, through the formation of small-celled growth in the alveolar walls, and also by the coalescence of nodular growths (§ F) with larger areas of destruction

CASE 25.

CHRONIC PHTHISIS; INDURATING TUBERCULAR PNEUMONIA.

Plate XIV. fig. 1.

SUMMARY.—F, 17. *Family tendency to phthisis. Chronic cough for several years; 2 years before death, signs of consolidation in upper part of each lung and of excavation in left. Temperature slightly raised. Three months before death, the signs of consolidation had increased in the left lung, and those of excavation had appeared at the right apex. Cough frequent; sputa tenacious. Pyrexia moderate but almost continuous.—Left lung adherent, extremely contracted: both lungs contain large cavities, separated by fibroid tissue, in which (and also in the remaining pulmonary tissue of the lower lobes) were cheesy nodules and tracts, together with grey granulations.*

MARY CORNEY, ætat. 17, single; admitted into University College Hospital under Sir William Jenner, November 13th, 1865; died February, 1866.

Family History.—Father and mother both living and healthy; have had four children; one died ætat. 3; a sister died of phthisis before patient, and another sister died here subsequently of acute phthisis (Case 24, Mrs. Hall).

Personal History.—Has worked in close room for some years, crowded with other workers. Catamenia appeared last Christmas and have been regular since. Appetite has been bad for years; and patient has been subject to coughs, for which she has been repeatedly an out-patient of the hospital. She has had a continuous cough all the last summer, and lately had a sharp pain diffused over the left side. She was known to me as a phthisical out-patient for some years before her admission, but I have no record of her physical signs.

State on Admission.—A puny, ill-nourished girl, who looked younger than her real age. Dyspnœa after talking, with action of alæ nasi. Pulse 96, Respiration 60. Chest very small; deep anteroposterior, narrow transverse diameter; lower regions contracted; left infraclavicular region flattened; extraordinary movements greatly in excess. There were physical signs of consolidation in both apices, front and back. In the left these extended through the greater part of the front, and at the back to below the spine of the scapula. In the right, there was consolidation to nearly the middle of the scapula. There were also signs of excavation at the left apex. Both bases were hyperresonant, but moist râles were heard to the extreme left base, and friction also was present there. The sputa were mucoid and frothy.

The temperature varied from 99° morning, to 100° evening, and on one occasion reached 103° in the evening, but gradually subsided. The urine was free from albumen.

The râles in the chest diminished, but had not entirely ceased when she left the hospital on January 8, 1866.

She remained at home, occasionally attending as an out-patient, and taking cod-liver oil, until October 1867, when an aggravation of her illness brought her again to the hospital. There was then considerable anæmia. Breathing was rapid, pulse 100, resp. 52. The signs of consolidation had increased very little in the right lung, but there were indications of a cavity there. The signs of excavation had increased in area in the left apex, and those of consolidation had also advanced, occupying the greater part of the anterior and axillary regions on this side, and leaving only a small area of pulmonary resonance in the middle third of the back. Bubbling râles were also heard in the lower portions of the lung. The cough was frequent. The sputa were tenacious, nummulated, mingled with masses like grains of rice.

The heart's sounds were healthy, except for accentuation of the second sound at the base. The urine was free from albumen. The appetite was bad, but there was no diarrhœa.

She gradually grew weaker, and left the hospital at her own desire, at the end of January, and died shortly afterwards at home.

Her temperature, during her stay in hospital, was almost continuously febrile; 103·4° was reached on two occasions, once in the morning and once in the evening. The mean morning temperature in 74 days was 98·9°. The mean evening temperature, in 68 observations (days), was 99·5°. Temperatures between 98° and 97° were observed occasionally both in the morning and evening. The maximum remission from evening to morning was from 4° to 5°. The mean of 17 observations was 1-2°, but in 27 per cent. of these the remissions did not exceed 1° and in 81 per cent. they did not exceed 2°. Exacerbations from morning to evening were recorded on 15 days; the maximum was from 2° to 3°, 59 per cent. were under 1°; 86 per cent. were under 2°. Exacerbations from evening to morning occurred on 8 days; the maximum was from 2° to 3°, the mean 1°; in 50 per cent. they were less than 1°, in 87 per cent. they were less than 2°. Remissions from morning to evening were recorded on 11 days. In none did these exceed 2°, and in 63 per cent. they were under 1°.

POST-MORTEM.—The organs removed after death presented the following appearances.

Larynx and *Trachea* healthy. Glands at lower end of trachea slightly enlarged.

Lungs.—Left firmly adherent throughout. Some recent lymph at base of right lung.

Left lung contracted to little more than a quarter of the normal size, surrounded by a dense capsule of thickened pleura. There is scarcely any pulmonary tissue left in this lung, except in a portion of the lower lobe. The tissue is otherwise dense and solid, with fibroid structure. The shrunken upper lobe is almost entirely occupied by two cavities, each capable of holding a Maltese orange. They have evidently been formed by ulceration, and they contain cheesy masses in their floor. One or two smaller ones of a similar nature are seen in the lower lobes. Nodules of cheesy matter are found scattered throughout the lower lobes, some softening into cavities. The walls of the bronchi, passing into the densely indurated tissue, are much thickened. In some parts the bronchi are dilated. No trace of grey granulations or of recent tubercle is to be found in the lung.

The right lung has its apex occupied by a dense fibrous tissue, in which caseous nodules are thickly scattered, and in which dilated bronchi are seen. There is also here a large mass of soft caseous material. Immediately below this there is a cavity, the size of a Maltese orange. In the rest of this lobe, the tissue of which is emphysematous, are scattered isolated grey granulations, which also occur in indurated groups and patches. The lower half of the inferior lobe (XIV. 1) is occupied by a pneumonic infiltration, reddish in places, but for the most part grey, and finely granular. It presents similar induration and granulation. Bronchial glands pigmented, and in some places softened in their interior into a grumous débris.

Intestines.—Small intestine free from ulceration. No enlargement of solitary or of agminated glands. Tubercular ulceration in cæcum.

Liver fatty. *Spleen* soft and pulpy.

Kidneys healthy to naked eye.

Heart.—Wall of right ventricle thickened; measures ⅜ inch ; tissue much indurated.

The preparation of this lung was unfortunately lost, so that I am unable to describe the histological appearance. I have, however, thought it best to introduce the figure and the description as illustrating the difference of the pulmonary affection in two sisters, the companion figures in this plate being from the lung of her sister (*Hall, Case 24*), who died of acute pneumonic phthisis.

CASE 26.

CHRONIC PHTHISIS; INDURATING TUBERCULISATION.

Plates X. figs. 5, 6 ; XL. figs. 1 to 6 ; XLIII. fig. 5.

Ref.—Phthisis, pp. 64, 95, 97.

SUMMARY.—*F. 36. No known inheritance. Pleurisy and rheumatism twelve and three years before ; the last time with hæmoptysis. Cough, weakness, and hæmoptysis developed nine months before death, with dyspnœa and night sweats. Signs of consolidation and excavation in upper half of right lung, and at apex of left ; bronchitic râles. Continuous but moderate pyrexia.—Right lung, in upper part, a series of very large cavities lined with congested membrane and surrounded by indurated lungtissue : lower portion partly fibroid, partly solid from recent pneumonia and containing granulations and larger cheesy nodules. Left lung presented tracts of fibroid change in upper part, some emphysema, a few cavities and granulations. Tubercular ulceration of small intestine. ' Sago spleen.' Localised pelvic peritonitis.*

ESTHER HEATH, ætat. 36, unmarried, admitted University College Hospital April 18, and died August 21, 1868.

Family History.—No hereditary predisposition to phthisis known. Mother died in childbed. Father living, ætat. 59 : suffers at times from 'rheumatic gout.'

Personal History.—Has been in early life in domestic service ; for last six years a dressmaker. Has always lived in healthy houses, and has had sufficient food and clothing. Abstemious from alcohol, but has drunk much strong tea.

Previous Illness.—Had scarlatina and dropsy, with some lung complication, when ætat. 11. Twelve years ago, ætat. 24, she had typhus (typhoid ?) fever, with jaundice and bronchitis, followed by rheumatic fever and pleurisy ; was in St. Mary's Hospital during three months and was discharged cured, but has not been strong since. Three years ago had 'inflammation of the kidneys,' rheumatism, and double pleurisy, followed by abscesses over the ischia on both sides ; recovered, but about this time had hæmoptysis, scarlet-coloured and frothy, which continued for some days—brought up in all about a teacupful. No return until present illness.

Present Illness began November 1867 (six months ago). Had been much exposed to cold and wet in walking to and from her place of business, and remained on one occasion in wet clothes. She first noticed cough, with great soreness behind the sternum, followed by dyspnœa. Has repeatedly spat blood (in small quantities) during the last six months. She has lost strength, and the dyspnœa has increased. The appetite has become capricious, and there has been occasional vomiting. She has had two attacks of diarrhœa, has lost much flesh, and has perspired profusely. Menstruation has been regular until the last two months ; since then the catamenia have not appeared.

State on Admission. Pallid : anæmia distinct, but not excessive. Cyanosis to moderate degree. Considerable wasting. Ends of fingers clubbed and nails incurvated. Skin pungently hot, perspires much at night. Some enlarged and painful glands in right axilla ; others slightly enlarged but not painful in left axilla. Cough frequent : expectoration copious, in dense nummulated masses.

Chest well-formed : some flattening under both clavicles. The physical signs were those of consolidation of the whole of the right apex, extending posteriorly to the lower border of the scapula, and anteriorly to the 4th rib. Over the greater part of this area there were signs of excavation. The base also was dull, with weak breathing. Moist râles were heard over the whole lung. The left apex also gave evidence of consolidation with some excavation. The axillary and postero-inferior regions on this side were hyperresonant. The respiration here was exaggerated, but attended by friction and sonorous râles. The heart's position and sounds were normal.

The urine was free throughout from albumen and sugar, but at times deposited lithates.

There was much thirst, anæmia, heartburn, occasional epigastric pain, and flatulence. The bowels were for the most part regular, but she suffered occasionally from diarrhœa. She continued to lose strength, and died on August 21, 1868.

The Temperature was seldom high. The mean of sixty-nine morning observations was 100·7°, that of thirteen evening observations was 101·5°. The fever was, however, almost continuous. The morning temperature was only on two occasions below 99°, and only on twelve below 100°. On thirty-one, out of sixty-nine days, it exceeded 101°, reaching 102° on six days and 103° on two days.

The evening temperature, taken less frequently, always exceeded 101° (except on two occasions, when it was 100°) ; 103·2° was observed once, and 102° twice. No subnormal temperatures were observed. The mean of the exacerbations from morning to evening was 0·8°, the maximum being 1·3°, the minimum 0·2°. The mean of the remissions from evening to morning was 1·1°, the maximum being 2·7° and the minimum 0·4°. On two occasions the temperature fell from morning to evening by 0·2° and 0·4°. On two occasions exacerbations occurred from the evening to the following morning of 1° and 0·2°.

The morning pulse varied from 152 to 92, with a mean of 106; the evening pulse varied from 100 to 126. The respirations varied from 22 to 36.

POST-MORTEM twelve hours after death.—Enlarged glands in anterior mediastinum. Heart displaced, lying almost entirely to right of middle line. Pericardium almost universally adherent. Right lung strongly adherent throughout to the chest-wall and to the pericardium. Left lung emphysematous at anterior margin; moderately adherent.

Larynx free from ulceration.

Lungs.—Bronchi open in right lung into a series of cavities at the apex, which occupy nearly the whole of the upper lobe, and extend into the middle lobe. The cavities, the largest of which is capable of holding an orange, are irregular, sinuous, and crossed in all directions by bands. They are lined by a highly-injected and deeply ecchymosed false membrane, in which lie cheesy nodules. The walls, in many cases, consist of little but thickened pleura and indurated pulmonary tissue. The remains of the lung between the cavities consist of indurated pulmonary tissue, deeply pigmented and traversed by ulcerated bronchi. In this tissue are seen some caseous masses, and some nodules of induration. Of the lower lobe, in which also are some cavities, the upper portion is consolidated in part by a semi-cartilaginous, fibroid, pigmented induration, and in part by a more recent pneumonic infiltration. Below this, the lung is emphysematous, traversed by tracts of iron-grey, indurated tissue, in which are interspersed nodules, single and in racemose groups, surrounded by a zone of pigment, which can be seen in many parts to be undergoing a fibroid change (X. 5). These granulations and masses of granulations are scattered throughout this part of the lung. Mingled with these are large isolated cheesy nodules, which vary in size, many of them attaining that of a pea, and are surrounded by a zone of indurated tissue, which is deeply pigmented. These masses are also seen interspersed among the smaller indurated granulations situated in the midst of indurated tissue (*see* X. 5 and 6). In this tissue are also some large, soft, and semi-transparent granulations (recent pneumonic granulations). Some of these become confluent, and there are in addition tracts of limited areas of a grey pneumonic infiltration.

The left lung is highly emphysematous at the base and anterior border. In the upper lobe there are large tracts of fibroid change, through which are scattered small granulations, both indurated and caseous, similar to those observed in the right lung. Some semi-transparent granulations are also scattered through this tissue. In the midst of these are a few cavities lined by a highly injected false membrane, similar to those seen in the right lung, but none larger than a walnut. In the emphysematous tissue of the lower lobe are some large, soft, semi-transparent granulations, similar to those seen in the base of the other lung. The bronchi of this lung are very extensively ulcerated into small cavities.

Heart.—Muscular tissue pale, evidently fatty. Flaps of tricuspid valve are shortened and somewhat thickened. Flaps of mitral valve much puckered and shortened, with many granulations on surface; aortic valves healthy.

Liver weighs 4 lbs. 6 ozs.; fatty; capsule separates easily; tissue does not stain with iodine.

Stomach.—Mucous membrane presents a few aphthous ulcerations.

Intestines.—Mucous membrane of lower end of ileum thickened, presenting numerous scattered superficial ulcerations, aphthous in appearance, and not connected with the follicular structures. Close to ileo-cæcal valve there are numerous ulcerations of tubercular type, having everted edges and a tubercular floor. Colon throughout much pigmented and thickened, covered with scattered serpiginous ulcers, which tend to run in lines along the longitudinal bands. These ulcers have clean-cut edges, and for the most part are not thickened; a few, however, are seen with thickened edges. Mucous membrane of intestines does not stain with iodine.

Spleen, distinctly waxy; well-marked 'sago' characters; stains markedly with iodine.

Kidneys. Paler than natural, firm. Throughout the tissue are numerous opaque spots of dead white colour, evidently fatty degeneration. Malpighian bodies very distinct. Tissue has a waxy tint, but does not stain with iodine.

Peritoneum.—In Douglas's space there is localised peritonitis, and about two drachms of pus are collected. This inflammation does not appear to extend to any adjacent viscera, and the rectum is unaffected.

THE MICROSCOPIC APPEARANCES found in this lung are the following:—

A. Tracts of pneumonic infiltration, not numerous.

B. Nodules and areas of destructive pneumonia.

C. Nodules of caseation.

D. Nodules of mingled pneumonic and small-celled growth.

E. Nodular masses of small-celled growth.

F. Diffuse areas of small-celled infiltration, both with and without epithelial growth in the interior of alveoli.

G. Nodules and tracts of fibroid growth.

H. Peribronchial and perivascular growth.

§ A. Simple pneumonic infiltration does not form a large proportion of the changes found on microscopic examination of these lungs. When present it is of the type like XXXVIII. 8 (*Hall*), and XXX. 8, (*Acute Tubercle*).

§ B. Nodules and areas of destructive pneumonia form a large proportion of the changes, mingled, however, with those hereafter to be described. They are figured in XL. 4. The outlines of the alveoli and bronchioles remain, but their interior is occupied by cell-débris, or by only a fibrillated structure, resembling that seen in XXXVIII. 3 (*Henshaw*), and in XXXV. 5 (*Smith*). Stages intermediate between these and also akin to XXXVI. 4 and 5 (*Griffin*), are not unfrequent, showing that these are produced by a process analogous to that by which the more rapid forms of caseating pneumonia originate. They can further be traced to such changes as are figured in XL. 1, 2, and 3, by which a small-celled growth invades the alveolar wall; and the difference between these and the acute form of caseating pneumonia apparently depends on the fact that in the former a larger amount of fibroid and fibro-nucleated growth occurs in the alveolar walls and in the interlobular tissue, prior to caseation, than in the latter, in which the necrobiotic change takes place more rapidly. These areas may be diffuse or circumscribed. In the former they are variously mingled with nodules of induration and caseation next to be described. When circumscribed they form round masses, bounded by the thickened interlobular cellular tissue.

§ C. Nodules of caseation, shown in XL. 3, and also like XLII. 5, XXXII. 7, and XXXV. 4 (*Smith*), XXXIX. 5 (*Overall*), and XXXIX. 7 (*Unwin*), are abundant. They are variously intermingled with nodules of induration. Their origin will be considered hereafter.

§§ D, E, and F. The most characteristic and abundant change in these lungs is, however, a small-celled growth invading the alveolar walls, as figured in XL. 1, 2, and 3. It occurs in nodules more or less circumscribed by thickened interlobular tissue, as in fig. 1, where it represents a limitation to pulmonary lobules. These nodules in some places are almost identical with XXXIV. 1 (*Coombes : Acute Tubercle*), or the growth is diffused through large areas, as in XL. 2 and 3. The cells in it are partly fusiform, but it chiefly consists of small round cells and nuclei, imbedded in many places in a distinct reticulum, and resembling that seen in XXXVII. 7 (*Griffin*) and XXXIX. 8 (*Gardiner*). The alveoli contain large epithelial cells (XL. 1 and 2, *a a,*) and bronchioles similarly surrounded may also be observed (*d d*, fig. 1), but both these and the alveoli are gradually invaded and obliterated by the small-celled growth. Injection does not penetrate these areas. The small-celled infiltration becomes, in some places, almost homogeneous, all other traces of pulmonary structure having disappeared, as in XXXVI. 4, *b b* (*Griffin*). In other parts it forms isolated masses (miliary) growing in the walls of the alveoli. Nodules of mingled epithelial and small-celled growth, like XXXVII. 5 (*Griffin*) are also seen, and all variations in type between these and XL. 1 may be observed.

The changes which these two formations undergo are in two directions, caseation and induration.

Caseation occurs either in nodules, as before described, or of the type of XL. 4, and XLIII. 5. The origin of the latter has been already described (*see above*). Caseous nodules are also seen (in XL. 3) to originate from lobular forms of perialveolar small-celled growth, like XL. 2 ; and other nodules, of the type of XXXII. 7, XXXV. 4 (*Smith*), and XXXIX. 7 (*Unwin*), are seen to arise in the same manner. All these forms of caseation tend to become more or less intermingled. In some places areas like XL. 4 are interspersed among nodules like those last described, and intermediate forms between the two types are not infrequent. In some places the diffuse caseation may be seen to arise from changes like that seen in XL. 6, where the epithelium has been entirely replaced by a growth of small cells, partly fusiform and partly round, in the walls of the alveoli. Much pigment attends this change, and indeed it is abundant throughout these lungs.

§ G. Nodules and areas of fibroid growth also arise out of the perialveolar thickening. The nodular forms resemble XLI. 1 and 3 (*Carr*), and XLI. 5 (*Roberts*). Others, also retaining the nodular form, indurate in bands, with round cells in their meshes like XLI. 7 (*Coppin*). These various nodules of induration arise from the masses of perivalveolar small-celled growth already described, and in some cases the fibroid thickening is mingled, in parts of those nodules, with caseation. In other parts there is an extensive fibroid perialveolar thickening, but accompanied by intra-alveolar epithelial proliferation, like XLII. 6 (*Hawkins*)

Giant-cells are seen in abundance throughout these specimens. In a few places they exist in the centre of lobules, forming apparently in the alveoli, and of the types of XXXII. 5 and 10. They are more common around the nodules, and are then of types seen in XXXIII. 6 and 11. Some are found scattered in different parts of the specimens without any special relation to the nodules. The type of XXXIII. 10 is also reproduced.

§ H. Periarterial and peribronchial thickening is met with frequently. In both places it occurs predominantly in the shape of fibroid change, but small-celled growth is also met with. No bronchial ulceration is observed.

It is thus seen that most of the nodular masses in these lungs are formed from a perialveolar growth, passing into caseation, and surrounded by zones of induration. They do not represent sections of bronchi, or merely peribronchial thickening, but they are formed out of the pulmonary tissue. The caseous masses in their centres result either from the caseation of confluent nodules, or from that of the pulmonary tissue, as in XLIII. 5, and the zones of induration surrounding them, as seen in X. 5 and 6, are areas of induration either of the alveolar or of the interlobular tissue.

CASE 27.

INDURATING AND CASEATING TUBERCULAR PNEUMONIA.

Plates X. figs. 7-10 ; XXXIX. figs. 5, 6 ; XL. fig, 9 ; XLIII. fig. 3.

Ref.—Phthisis, pp. 94, 97.

SUMMARY.—*M. 38. Hæmoptysis two years before death, repeated eighteen months later, when the temperature was slightly raised, and there were signs of consolidation at both apices, and of slight excavation at left. The latter afterwards became more distinct, but the pyrexia ceased. A month before death high fever was present, and there were signs of more extensive consolidation and excavation at both apices.—The upper parts of both lungs were indurated, and contained cavities, and also nodules, caseous and cretaceous. Granulations, many in racemose aggregations, were scattered through both lungs. There was tubercular ulceration of intestines.*

JAMES OVERALL, ætat. 38, admitted University College Hospital May 27, 1868, sent to Eastbourne and Walton July and September ; re-admitted in October, and died November 4, 1868.

Family History.—Father died, aged 50, from the rupture of a blood-vessel, having been previously a strong, healthy man. Mother died, aged 72 ; cause unknown. The whole of patient's brothers and sisters, eleven in number, died under 25, but patient believes that they did not suffer from pulmonary disease. Collateral relations not recorded. Has three healthy children. Some of his children have died in infancy.

Occupation and Habits.—An organ-builder ; has lived well and temperately.

Previous Health.—Scarlet fever in childhood. Typhus (?) fever ætat. 15. No severe illness since.

CASE 27 (OVERALL)

Has been subject to colds and coughs for some years.

Present Illness.—Dated by patient from eighteen months ago. Had a severe cold, and while straining at work, he ruptured a blood-vessel, and brought up more than a pint of bright florid blood; was only laid by for ten days; returned to work, and continued pretty well until February 1867, when, after exposure, his cough became worse. He lost flesh, but improved under treatment by ol. morrhuæ and quinine, and continued better until May 28, 1868, when he was again attacked with profuse hæmoptysis, bringing up large quantities of blood, which, he stated, exceeded a pint on four successive days. The hæmoptysis had continued until shortly before admission.

State on Admission.—Prostrate from hæmorrhage. Moderate emaciation; marked anæmia. He had blood-stained expectoration at first; when the blood disappeared the sputa were mucoid, glairy, tenacious, and purulent in streaks, moderately abundant. The amount of pus increased, but the sputa never became excessive, and even near the close of life consisted only of a few glairy tenacious pellets.

The urine contained neither albumen nor sugar. There were one or two attacks of diarrhœa in the later periods of his life, but this was not constant. The appetite was fairly maintained, and there was no sickness. He got wet and chilled at Eastbourne, and returned thinner. Rallied again, and was sent to Walton, where he became feverish and rapidly lost strength. There was slight pyrexia during his stay in hospital until June 30, but the evening temperatures were not taken regularly. The morning temperatures were almost invariably febrile, the maximum, however, being only 100°. During a few days which he spent in hospital in September, both morning and evening temperatures were non-febrile. On his return in October, he was highly febrile, the evening maximum being 108° and the minimum 102°: the morning maximum being 102° and the minimum 101°. The pulse and respiration, which, at his first admission, had not exceeded respectively 100 and 20, and fell as low as P. 84, R. 16, had risen on his final admission to P. 120, R. 80; with a minimum of P. 112, R. 20.

Physical Signs, taken after subsidence of hæmorrhage. Consolidation both apices, most on left side: doubtful signs of cavity at left apex, only 'moist crackling' at right apex: bases free.

On August 24 the signs of a cavity had become quite distinct under the left clavicle. In October the dulness at the apices had increased in extent; signs of excavation had become distinct at the right apex: coarse metallic râles were heard scattered in various spots through the left lung. The heart's sounds were healthy.

POST-MORTEM.—*Lungs:* Both intensely emphysematous in lower lobes; over whole lower portion of right lung are large emphysematous bladders. Both lungs are firmly adherent at the apices, which are puckered and contracted. Right lung reserved for injection. *Left lung:* bronchi show fusiform dilatations both in the upper and the lower lobes. No ulceration or tubercle in the bronchi. At apex of lung, where tissue is puckered, there are numerous cavities, containing caseous, and in some places cretaceous nodules, and surrounded by indurated fibroid tissue. Some of the bronchi leading to these cavities contain cretaceous matter. Some are completely obliterated, and converted into fibro-cartilaginous cords in which little nodules of cretaceous matter are seen. (X. 8, *a a*, 10, *b d*). Some of the obliterated bronchi have lines of granulations forming groups on their external surface. Some of these granulations, which vary in size and are occasionally as small as pins' points, form apparently part of the wall of the thickened bronchus.

Below this are numerous granulations scattered through the tissue, varying in size and appearance. In some of the larger ones, there is, in the centre, a puckered dimpled depression, these are harder and have a more yellow tint (X. 9, *e e*); in some no central depression can be seen. Others similar, in some instances semi-transparent and in others pigmented, tend to form racemose groups. These racemose groups are deeply pigmented, and the individual granulations have much pigmented tissue interwoven between them. In the larger masses there are also enclosed caseous nodules. Lines of fibroid tissue also pass between single granulations. The granulations are thickly scattered, singly and in groups, throughout the whole lower lobe of this lung. The middle portion is occupied by a greyish-red pneumonic infiltration; part of this is dense and airless; part, however, still floats in water but sinks after pressure. Throughout this area granulations are also seen, scattered and in groups, with the characters last described.

The *right lung*, after injection, is found to be intensely emphysematous and to have numerous cavities at the apex, larger than those of the left, but few exceeding the size of a walnut. Some of them have cheesy nodules in their floors. Some communicate directly with large bronchi. Lines of thickened bronchi can also be traced in this lung, and on cutting some of these open, granulations can be seen penetrating into the interior of the cavity, but only on one side. In some places the thickening round the bronchus can be seen to extend irregularly into the adjacent pulmonary tissue (*see* X. 7). In other places, groups of smaller racemose granulations surround the larger masses, as if branches of smaller bronchi had undergone the same change as those next above them in size. In the emphysematous tissue, the granulations are on the whole larger than elsewhere. Some of them are solid throughout, and consist of an opaque but firm material, while the contents of others are more cheesy. Some are seen distinctly to be dilated bronchi, with a thickened wall and soft contents, the dilatation being remarkable in the presence of so much thickening, for the inner surface is uniform and presents no appearance of ulceration (X. 7, *a a*). In other tubes it is more irregular, as if ulceration had occurred.

The *Bronchial Glands* are indurated and pigmented, but not cheesy. *Larynx* healthy.

Liver fatty. *Spleen* soft.

Heart, left ventricle hypertrophied; muscular tissue has undergone fatty degeneration.

Intestine.—Ulceration at lower end of ileum with thickened everted edges; some of the ulcerations contain small granulations in their floors. A few solitary glands are enlarged and caseous. In the mesentery are some cretified glands.

MICROSCOPIC EXAMINATION of the lungs revealed the following changes:—

A. Tracts of caseating pneumonia.
B. Tracts of suppurative pneumonia.

C. Diffuse tracts of small-celled growth.
D. Nodules of small-celled growth.
E. Nodules of induration.
F. Nodules of caseation with or without induration.
G. Large tracts of fibroid induration.
H. Peribronchial and perivascular growth.

§ A. The tracts of caseating pneumonia resemble those seen in XXXVIII. 3 (*Henshaw*), XXVIII. 8 (*Polley*), and are also like XXXVII. 3 (*Griffin*). They originate, for the most part, in a small-celled growth invading the alveolar walls, like that seen in XXXVII. 6 and 7 (*Griffin*), and XXXIX. 2 (*J. Thomas*). They are largely intermingled with nodular formations to be hereafter described, also with areas of suppurative pneumonia, and with tracts of fibroid induration. In other respects they resemble the appearances described in Henshaw, Griffin, Lloyd, Price, and Polley.

§ B. The tracts of suppurative pneumonia, which are intermingled with the former, resemble those seen in XXXV. 1, 2, 3, and 5 (*Brodrick* and *Smith*), and have their origin in processes similar to those described in those cases.

§ C. Diffuse tracts of small-celled growth, with a reticular structure, are very common. They are found alone, resembling XL. 2 (*Heath*), or variously intermingled with epithelial products, as in XXXVIII. 8 (*Hall*), or more commonly like XXXVII. 6 and 7 (*Griffin*), and extending over considerable areas. In other places they thicken the alveolar walls until appearances are produced like XXXVIII. 1 (*Henshaw*) and XXVIII. 10 (*Polley*). They tend to pass into fibroid induration in the manner hereafter to be described, as well as into tracts of caseating pneumonia.

§ D. In some places these areas of reticulated small-celled infiltration are limited to single alveoli or groups of alveoli, which are entirely occupied in this manner by a structure such as is shown in XXXIX. 6. These masses then form a structure identical with that of the typical miliary tubercle. Similar nodules occasionally form in the alveolar walls, in the interalveolar tissue, and in the walls of the bronchi. They are, however, in all respects identical with the diffuse small-celled growth before described. In preparations that have been injected, it is seen that no blood-vessels remain pervious in these infiltrations or nodules.

§§ E and F. The nodules, other than those last described, may be conveniently considered together. They are very numerous throughout these lungs. They occur singly or in groups, and form confluent masses, passing in some places into caseation, in others into induration, while in some parts both processes may be seen in combination. They originate apparently in processes similar to that seen in XXXVII. 5 (*Griffin*), XXXVIII. 7 (*Hall*), and XL. 1 and 3 (*Heath*). The centres of the alveoli in them, where these are distinguishable, contain a mingled epithelial and small-celled growth in variable proportions; the epithelial cells are often much pigmented. Others, still maintaining the nodular form, commence by a process similar to that seen in XXX. 7 (*Acute Tubercle*). It is not uncommon to see giant-cells in the centre of those in which the small-celled growth is less advanced, and sometimes a group of small alveoli may be seen, each containing a giant-cell of the types of XXXII. 8 and 9, and XXXIII. 1, 2, 3, and 4; but the nodular character of these alveolar groups is still maintained by means of the small-celled thickening surrounding the whole, a formation which strongly suggests the origin of the nodule from an individual pulmonary lobule. In other places, these alveolar formations, with small-celled growth, produce conglomerate masses, similar to XXXIX. 4 (*Price*), and XXXIX. 7 (*Unwin*), in which the alveolar walls are still marked out by circles of fibres mingled with fusiform cells and nuclei. In some, again, the mingled epithelial and small-celled growth takes place in masses of an elongated character, suggesting that the latter is mainly from the nuclei of the capillaries, as shown in XL. 9.

These nodules undergo two series of changes, variously intermingled. Some contract in their centres, and produce changes such as are seen in XXXIX. 5, *aa*, and like XXXVI. 7 (*Unwin*). In many of these, the nuclei and cells have disappeared in the granular degeneration, while the fibre and reticular growth remains, like XLIII. 5 (*Heath*). Fibroid change is almost equally common. It commences in some places in the centre of the nodules, which become nearly homogeneous, or traversed only by lines of fatty degeneration, or by spaces akin to those seen in tendon, as in XLI. 3 (*Carr*) and XLI. 5 (*C. Roberts*). In other places, where the centres are caseous, fibroid change takes place in broad bands throughout the whole of the remainder of the lobule. Nodules undergoing fibroid change also arise from those composed entirely of small-celled growth, as previously described (§ D). Groups of these nodules thus undergoing fibroid change produce areas resembling XLI. 1 (*Carr*), where the site of the confluent nodules is still marked, more or less, by their concentric arrangement, but where the whole tissue is almost entirely composed of broad bands of fibres. Many of these nodules are surrounded by zones of giant-cells, like XXXII. 7 (*Smith*).

§ G. Large tracts of fibroid induration also occur, such as are shown in XLIII. 6 (*Brown*), which, with a low power, closely resemble sections of bronchi, although the alveolar structure is still apparent under higher power; also like those of XLII. 1 (*Attwood*), and XLII. 6 (*Hawkins*), originating from the fibroid transformation of the small-celled growth, found in the alveolar walls, similar to that of XXXVII. 6 and 7 (*Griffin*).

§ H. Peribronchial and perivascular small-celled growth is also met with. The latter is uncommon; although in the greater number of specimens the vessels are found greatly thickened, it is only by fibroid transformation, and perivascular growth is found only in a few places, undergoing ulceration. Where it occurs, it is usually in the midst of areas of caseating pneumonia, and extends into them, thus causing cavities.

The formation of cavities in these lungs is almost entirely due to two processes: (*a*) the softening of areas of caseous and suppurative pneumonia, and (*b*) the softening of nodules of small-celled growth, which have undergone caseation in their centres. The naked-eye appearances strongly suggested that the cavities were due to the caseation of the contents and of the walls of the bronchi, but it was only in quite exceptional instances that this origin was discoverable. In most places it was due to changes like those described in *Griffin* and *Price*, where the pneumonic areas break down until circumscribed by thickened bands of interlobular tissue, which then, even under the microscope, may present a very close resemblance to the walls of bronchi. The large amount of fibroid change in this lung renders this appearance very common, but an examination of the margins of these caseous tracts shows, almost invariably, that they have proceeded from alveolar tissue.

Nodules such as are described in § F and § G, caseating and breaking down in their centres, with much fibroid induration in their margins, can often be found with high powers. They not infrequently occur in the midst of areas of diffuse caseous pneumonia, and also at times present a striking resemblance to bronchi, but their origin and nature can usually be ascertained by a more minute investigation of their structure. The remains of a reticulum can then be found, and in some places the centre is broken down and the caseous wall (as seen in X. 7, *aa*), is seen to be composed of a reticular small-celled growth, passing into caseation, and resembling in character that seen in XXXIX. 1 (*Lloyd*), and XLI. 6 (*Cox*).

CASE 28.
INDURATING TUBERCULAR PNEUMONIA.

Plates XIII. figs. 1 and 2; XXXII. figs. 7-9; XXXIII. figs. 1, 3, and 10; XXXV. figs. 4, 5, and 6; XLII. 5.

Ref.—Phthisis, pp. 94, 121.

SUMMARY.—*M. 40. Trifling cough for some years. Eight months before death, acute onset of severe cough with rigors, followed by progressive weakness and increasing expectoration. Seven months later, emaciation and night sweats. Signs of consolidation and excavation at each apex, greater in the left, Persistent moderate fever. Death from suffocating hæmoptysis.—The upper part of each lung was occupied by glistening, grey, indurated tissue, with caseous nodules, and their cavities, of which one, in the left, was very large, traversed by some pervious vessels, and filled with blood. Grey granulations in lower lobes.*

WILLIAM SMITH, ætat. 40, admitted University College Hospital January 19, died February 12, 1867.

Family History.—Imperfect: affords no evidence of phthisis.

Personal History.—A native of London, and has always lived here; has always been a horse-keeper. Has had gonorrhœa and syphilis. Had inflammation of lungs in childhood. Has always lived fairly well. He had no living children; his wife has had several miscarriages.

Present Illness.—Has been subject to trifling cough for some years; has not felt ill or lost in weight (12 stone) before present illness. This began in June 1866. Being heated he left off flannel waistcoat and had a rigor on same evening. This was repeated on subsequent evenings. Cough came on gradually. No hæmoptysis. His appetite failed, and in August he grew very weak, and sought advice. Expectoration commenced, thick and glutinous from the first. Has lost flesh since beginning of illness, and appetite has failed. Has been thirsty and feverish from the beginning, and his lips have felt dry and parched. Has not perspired much.

State on Admission.—A well-developed man, but emaciated; florid colour in cheeks. Great weakness. Weight 127lbs. (which fell in a fortnight to 124lbs.) Urine, slight trace of albumen. Cough with glutinous, opaque, thick, greyish-yellow sputa, not nummulated. Much perspiration at night. Chest naturally well-formed, with wide angle. Physical signs of extensive consolidation and excavation at left apex, also at right but to a less degree, and of some consolidation at right base. No diarrhœa, but appetite bad. The patient died, suffocated by a profuse hæmoptysis, on July 12.

He was persistently feverish, both morning and evening temperatures being constantly above the normal, and the fever approximating to a continuous type, but not intense in degree. The evening temperature was 100·1° (highest 101°, lowest 99·2°). The mean morning temperature was 100·4° (highest 101·6°, lowest 99·4°). The remissions from evening to morning were small, the mean being 0·5°, the greatest 0·6°, the lowest 0·4°. The exacerbations from evening to morning were also small, the mean being 0·7°, the highest 1·6°, and the lowest 0·4°. An inverse type was not infrequent, remissions occurring from morning to evening on seven days, with a mean of 0·8°, the highest being 1·4°, and the lowest 0·2°. Exacerbations took place from evening to morning on nine days, the highest being 1·6° and the lowest 0·4°. Neither the pulse nor the respiration was markedly accelerated; the pulse seldom attained 100, but was never less than 80; the respirations occasionally fell to 17, were usually more than 20, but did not exceed 28 in number.

POST-MORTEM.—Both lungs adherent at apices, left very firmly so. Left apex occupied by a large cavity, filled with blood, and from this it is evident that the fatal hæmorrhage has proceeded. It is crossed by bands and trabeculæ in all directions. Some of these are evidently vessels whose cavity is still pervious, but the source of the hæmorrhage was not discovered. The walls are otherwise for the most part smooth, and lined by a film of oxydation-matter, but cheesy nodules project here and there. The wall itself is composed of dense tissue, which, on section, is firm but has a glistening semi-transparent appearance, with cheesy nodules imbedded. Below this the whole of the rest of the upper lobe is occupied by a glistening, grey, semi-transparent tissue, very firm and resisting; uniform on section, but showing in a few places nodules of the size of a horse-bean, whitish in appearance, and a few thickened bronchi with caseous contents. Large tracts of the lung are in this condition, firm, indurated, and fibroid (XIII. 1, *e*); but where less firm, a thick sanious fluid exudes on section. Lower down it is thickly studded with whitish nodules varying in size from a horse-bean to a poppy-seed, or even to minute specks (*a a*). The larger ones are uniform at their margins, but finely granular on their cut surfaces. In some places they are becoming cheesy, and breaking down into small cavities (*bb*). The lower lobe is thickly studded with grey granulations, some semi-transparent, some pigmented, mingled with opaque white granulations, and the latter are seen softening into cavities (A in microscopic description).

Right Lung.—Apex presents a few puckered cavities. The greater part of the upper lobe is composed of the same firm, grey, semi-transparent tissue as that described in the left lung, smooth on section and not granular. In some places it is thickly mingled with cheesy masses imbedded in it. Small granulations are also seen in it, but these are not numerous. The lower lobe is studded with grey, firm, pigmented granulations.

Heart.—Two of the aortic valves adherent.

Brain, Kidneys, Stomach, Intestines, Mediastinal and *Mesenteric Glands* healthy.

Liver enlarged, weighs 5 lbs. 5 oz. Under the capsule it is covered thickly with granulations of an opaque whitish colour, none larger than a poppy-seed, and some only minute specks. They are soft, and look like little whitish masses of lymphatic cells, or like some forms of leucocythæmic liver (XIII. 2).

THE MICROSCOPIC APPEARANCES seen in this lung are the following:—

A. Tracts of pneumonia, presenting various changes of the indurating, caseating, and destructive types.

B. Areas of small-celled infiltration.

C. Nodules and granules of various characters.

D. Caseation, diffuse and circumscribed.

E. Areas of induration.

F. Peribronchial and perivascular growths.

G. Giant-cells.

§ A. The pneumonic processes in this lung are varied. In some places tracts of epithelial proliferation are seen, like XXVI. 7 (*Ellsom*), but in many places these appear to be filled with an amorphous exudation-matter, containing but few cells, like XXXVIII. 2 and 4 (*Henshaw*). Thickening of the alveolar wall, however, occurs early in many of these tracts, and gives rise to appearances to be described later (§ C and § D).

Another not uncommon appearance in these pneumonic areas is the immediate destruction of portions of the tissue by the inflammatory process, as seen in XXXV. 5. These resemble very closely the processes described in XXXV. 1 and 2 (see *Case 18 Brodrick*, p. 182). In these all cell-structure has perished, though remains of epithelium may be seen in places, and in some parts there are groups of small cells, not imbedded in a reticulum, but having the characters of pus-cells. Suppuration does not, however, appear to precede the destructive changes in the greater part of these areas; the epithelium perishes at once, without the occurrence of other growth, while the elastic fibres of the alveoli remain imbedded in a finely granular material. The process is akin to caseation, but the appearances produced differ from this in the absence of density in the granular mass. It is not unimportant to observe that these changes are not isolated, but are variously intermingled with those next to be described.

§ B. Small-celled infiltration takes place around alveoli filled with large epithelial cells like XXX. 5, 6, and 7 (*Polley, &c. Acute Tubercle*), and like XXXVII. 6 and 7 (*Griffin*). It also extends in a diffuse form, varying in extent and intensity, and sometimes intermingled with nodular and caseating masses, and reproduces appearances like XXXVIII. 2 (*Henshaw*); XXXVIII. 8 (*Hall*); XL. 2 (*Heath*); and in many places like XXXVI. 3 and XXXVII. 4 (*Griffin*). In other places it occurs in both diffuse and lobular forms, surrounding alveoli containing remains of epithelium like XXVIII. 2 and 7 (*Acute Tubercle*).

§ C. The nodules met with are sometimes composed entirely of small-celled growth, imbedded in a reticulum, and filling isolated alveoli, like XXXV. 6. Others are found of the lobular type of mingled epithelial and small-celled growth, like XXX. 2 (*Coombes, Acute Tubercle*).

The most common types, which are very numerous throughout these lungs, are shown in XXXII. 7, and XXXV. 4. Their centre is caseated, either amorphous and granular, or showing traces of a reticulum like XXXII. 7, and in some places remains of a small-celled growth, intensely pigmented, is seen in the meshes (XXXV. 4). Around this is a zone of deeper pigmentation, and beyond the latter is an area of fibroid thickening, in which nuclear growth is imbedded, and which still shows, in places, traces of alveolar formation. In this latter area, giant-cells are common (XXXII. 7). These granulations are very numerous, and form a considerable part of the changes in this lung. They apparently originate from a gradual thickening of the alveolar walls in lobules, commencing like XXXVII. 5 (*Griffin*), and extending like XL. 1 (*Heath*).

§ D. Caseation takes place in the pneumonic areas both in diffuse and lobular forms. Both of these occur in the two types—first, of amorphous débris in which traces of alveolar structure and of elastic fibre remain, as in XXXVI. 4 and 5 (*Griffin*), and XXVIII. 6 (*Polley*), and, secondly, like XXVIII. 8 (*Polley*), and XXXVIII. 3 (*Henshaw*), and XLIII. 5 (*Heath*). In the nodular forms they represent the centre or the whole of granules as seen in XXXII. 7, XXXV. 4, and also reproduce appearances like XXXIX. 7 (*Unwin*). Groups of this form, like XXXIX. 4 (*Price*), also occur. In other places, where mingled small-celled and epithelial growth has occurred, large caseous nodules are produced, like XXXVI. 1, 2, and 3 (*Griffin*).

Many of the nodules like XXXII. 7, and XXXV. 4, which have attained, by confluence, a large size, and are surrounded by much fibroid thickening, present, under low powers of the microscope, a most striking resemblance to sections of bronchi, especially where the section is longitudinal to a series of these. Their centres present, however, the remains of pulmonary structure, and a further examination shows that they arise from pneumonic lobules, as in XXXVI. 1 and 3, and like XXXVII. 4 (*Griffin*), or, more commonly, by the immediate invasion of groups of alveoli by a small-celled growth, resembling that seen in XXXIX. 7 (*Unwin*), and XL. 1 (*Heath*).

§ E. Fibroid thickening occurs in areas like XLII. 6 (*Hawkins*). Tracts of dense thickening, like XLII. 7 (*J. Brown*), are also seen. In some places these assume a nodular form, and are then seen to be proceeding by the formation, from the reticulum in the floor of the alveoli, of broad-banded fibres, in the meshes of which small cells are still imbedded, like XLI. 2 (*Carr*), and like XLI. 7 (*Coppin*). The nodules of induration have been already described.

One peculiar feature in the centre of tracts of induration consists in single alveoli and groups of alveoli being filled with an amorphous exudation-matter, in which are scattered a few single large cells devoid of nuclei (physalides), looking like large bubbles, but more transparent and glistening. These are found both at the apex (XIII. 1, *c*), and also in the lower lobes.

The areas of induration are variously interspersed

among the pneumonic areas, and also around the granules and groups of granules.

§ F. Peribronchial and perivascular thickening are both met with, but the former does not produce the amorphous masses which arise from the caseation of lobules surrounded by fibroid thickening, and in one or two places – where the bronchi, whose walls are thus thickened, are filled with a granular mass resulting from retained secretion – no trace of structure is apparent in this.

§ G. Giant-cells are numerous throughout these lungs, and they commonly appear in the middle of the alveoli. They are sometimes single; sometimes they occur in groups of alveoli (see XXXII. 8 and 9, XXXIII. 1, 3, and 10). In one specimen, each alveolus of an ultimate lobule was seen to have a giant-cell in its centre. They also form around the nodules of induration (see XXXII. 7).

Microscopic examination of the *Liver* (Coloured Pl. XIII. 2) shows that lines of lymphoid cells, sometimes massed in groups of two or three, intervene between the hepatic tubules. In some places no cells are apparent in these parts, but only lymphatics, filled with an amorphous débris. The liver-cells are enlarged and granular, and show a multiplication of their nuclei. The process is apparently identical with that of lymphangiectasis as described by Reynard, Cornil, and others in the lung.[1]

CASE 29.

INDURATING TUBERCULAR PNEUMONIA : LARYNGEAL TUBERCLE.

Plates XV. 1, XLII. fig. 7, and XLIII. 6 (Lung); XX. fig. 3, and XXXIV. figs. 2 and 3 (Larynx); XV. 2, 3, and XXXIV. 6 and 7 (Glands).

Ref.—Syphilitic Disease, p. 128.

SUMMARY.—*M. 44. Pleurisy fifteen years previously. Four months before death, a chill, followed by rigors, cough, dyspnœa, and hæmoptysis. Admitted to hospital four days before death with considerable fever, dyspnœa, cough, and muco-purulent expectoration. Signs of consolidation and excavation at both apices, and bronchitic râles on left side. Liver enlarged,—Firm, grey induration throughout middle of left lung, and upper lobe of right; cheesy nodules in both lungs, and more extensive tracts in the left. Small cavities, especially in the right apex, due to the softening of caseous nodules, and surrounded by indurated granulations, which were also scattered through the lower parts of both lungs. Larynx, tubercular granulations and ulcers. Liver fibroid and fatty.*

JAMES BROWN, ætat. 44, admitted University College Hospital August 6; died August 10, 1866.

Family History.—Father died, ætat. 87, from dropsy. Mother still living, aged 70, in good health. No history of chest affections in family. Patient has had three children; two died at birth, one born prematurely.

Personal History.—Occupation a traveller, walking his round, but not especially exposed to wet. Small-pox when young. Had a chancre sixteen years ago, but has not had secondary symptoms. Fifteen years ago had a sharp pain in one side (cannot remember which), and was told by a medical man that he had pleurisy. Twenty-two years ago was thrown from his horse, and had right knee badly cut; was sixteen weeks in St. Bartholomew's Hospital. With these exceptions has enjoyed good health.

Present Illness.—Had a cough in the winter of 1864-5, but recovered. Three or four months ago he got wet through; shortly afterwards felt unwell, had rigors, and was laid up. Cough and difficulty of breathing came on, and he gradually became weak and unable to follow his employment; for last four months has been losing flesh. Two months ago had a slight hæmoptysis; none since.

State on Admission.—Face cyanotic. Eyes prominent and suffused. Skin hot and perspiring. Some œdema of skin of thorax; considerable dyspnœa apparent while speaking. Breath very short; movements tremulous. Pulse 120, resp. 36. No distension of jugular veins. Cough frequent; expectoration muco-purulent, tenacious: twice during his stay in hospital it became of a uniform rusty-brown for one day.

Chest well-formed, wide costal angle. Expansion very imperfect at both bases and under clavicles. Left apex dull, front and back, dulness extending to middle third of scapula. Right apex dull posteriorly; right front hyperresonant. Heart covered by lung to sixth rib. Bases hyperresonant; cavernous breathing and râles both apices. Fine moist râles over whole left side. No cardiac murmur. Urine acid, no albumen or sugar. Abdomen distended and tympanitic. Liver four inches below cartilage of eighth rib. No enlargement of spleen. The bowels were loose during whole of stay in hospital. He became very prostrate; the tongue was dry; and he sank on August 14.

The temperature was only taken on four days. It was persistently febrile, with a maximum of 103·2°. Morning temperatures of 101·2° and 102·1° were observed.

POST-MORTEM. — Cartilages of ribs calcified throughout. Glands of anterior mediastinum enlarged.

Lungs.—Some emphysema at anterior borders of both. Apex of left lung contains numerous cavities, none exceeding the size of a pea, occurring in nodules of cheesy matter, which again are surrounded by areas of finely granular pneumonic infiltration. Non-solidified portions of lung intervene between these, and are loaded with frothy serosity. The cheesy nodules here also tend to form racemose groups (XV. *b b b*). This region is traversed by bands of fibroid tissue. Below this (above, in the figure) the whole of the lower third of the upper lobe and the upper portion of the lower lobe (which are united together), are converted into a solid indurated area of semi-cartilaginous-looking tissue. It is homogeneous and of a grey tinge, except where it is traversed by lines of deeper pigmentation; the cut surface is smooth and glistening (XV. *c c*). In it, however, are some cheesy nodules, *d*, and at its lower margin some racemose granulations, from which lines of fibroid induration extend into the adjacent tissue (XV. *d*). At this margin, and extending for some distance

[1] For bibliography, see Klein, *Anatomy of the Lymphatic System*, Part 11.; also Troisier, *Sur les Lymphangites Pulmonaires*, Thèse de Paris, 1874. See also *Case 47*, Leather (Plate XXIV.)

into this indurated part, are numerous cavities, varying in size from a pea to a horse-bean. Some of these can be traced to a series of sinuous passages, and are evidently formed by the ulceration of dilated bronchi, one of which can be traced to a series of such cavities.

Below this portion are numerous clusters of granulations (XV. *a a*) about the size of a poppy-seed, disposed in racemose groups, some showing an indurated and semi-transparent centre, and with induration-matter between and around them, extending in branching lines. They are surrounded by granulations (which indeed form their margins) grey, semi-transparent, or pigmented, some caseous, others nodular, larger in size, and, as stated, forming caseous masses. These are thickly scattered throughout the remainder of the lower lobe, the tissue of which is highly congested and œdematous.

Right Lung emphysematous in anterior border of upper lobe and in posterior border of lower lobe. The whole upper lobe is consolidated throughout, except a small portion of its anterior margin. Nearly the whole of it is converted into an indurated fibroid tissue, resembling that in the middle third of the opposite lung. The upper portion of the lower lobe is occupied by a tract of caseous matter, of the size of a Tangerine orange. It is soft in consistence, has a finely-granular fracture, and presents at its margin irregular nodules of a cheesy consistence, varying in size from a hemp-seed to a pea. Numerous masses and nodules of a similar character are scattered throughout this lobe. None of them present the indurated fibroid centre seen in the other lobe, nor do they bear any resemblance to the granulations seen in the base of the opposite lung.

Bronchial Glands enlarged, deeply pigmented, and indurated. The post-tracheal glands are deeply injected; they are studded with small white nodules, and here and there with larger tracts of an irregular shape, milky-white in colour. There are also some small semi-transparent granulations in the tissue, as small as pins' points (XV. 2, *a*, and XX. 3). The nodules, the milky-white tracts, and the small granulations are scattered irregularly through the tissue, and are not limited to any one part. Some of the larger glands are both indurated and pigmented, and present tracts of a yellow colour, firm and resisting, in which is a mottling of congestion (8, *a*); these tracts have but little trace of structure in their centres, but at their circumference they present an appearance as if composed of small granulations, though the surface on section is firm and smooth (XV. 3, *b*).

The Larynx presents, at the inferior border of both vocal cords, ragged ulcerations with elevated edges, which, at the inferior border, extend somewhat deeply into the cartilages. There are several spots of these ulcerations, which in places contain cheesy matter in their floor (XX. 3, *c c*). The under surface of the epiglottis is studded with small granulations, some of which are semi-transparent and of vesicular aspect; some are caseous and passing into ulceration (XX. 3, *a*). Below the vocal cords, over the cricoid cartilage, are numerous granulations, some semi-transparent and glistening, others opaque, yellow, and caseous; some of the latter are passing into minute ulcerations (XX. 3 *a*). In the lower part of the trachea numerous lenticular ulcerations are scattered over the highly injected mucous membrane, mingled with granulations like those last described (XX. 3, *b*);

and at the bifurcation, and especially in the right branch, they are so densely massed as to occupy almost the whole of the surface.

Heart.—Some dilatation of tricuspid valve. Fatty degeneration, in patches, of the muscular tissue of both ventricles. Atheroma of posterior flap of mitral valve, and numerous patches of atheroma in aorta.

Liver large; measures 12 inches transverse diameter, 11 inches vertical, and 2½ inches greatest thickness. Capsule adherent over right lobe; section granular: tissue indurated; some fatty degeneration.

Stomach.—Mucous membrane thickened, indurated, mammillated, tough, opaque and cloudy in patches, and much congested with arborescent injection, passing here and there into minute extravasations.

Intestines.—Duodenum presents similar induration and thickening of mucous membrane. One Peyer's patch, close above ileo-cæcal valve, presents an appearance of cicatricial tissue, but without any contraction of the intestine.

Kidneys indurated, with streaks and nodules of fatty degeneration.

THE MICROSCOPIC APPEARANCES in these lungs are the following:—
A. Areas of pneumonic infiltration passing into (*a*) induration; (*b*) caseation; (*c*) destructive change.
B. Nodular masses of small-celled growth, mingled with epithelial formation, and passing either into caseation, or induration, or into both combined.
C. Nodules composed exclusively of small-celled growth.
D. Small-celled infiltration, existing either alone or combined in various degrees with epithelial proliferation in the interior of the alveoli.
E. Extensive areas of fibroid induration.
F. Perivascular and peribronchial thickening.

§ A. The pneumonic areas are distinguished by very large epithelial cells, such as have been described in the case of *Henshaw* and *Ellsom*, pp. 179 and 180. Independently of other changes they are not extensive, but are generally found passing into one of the following: (*a*) *Induration*. This takes place by means of a small-celled growth in the walls of the alveoli, similar to those seen in XXX. 5 (*Polley, Acute Tubercle*); XXXVII. 6 and 7 (*Griffin*); and XXXIX. 8 (*Gardiner*). It passes into fibroid growth, producing appearances like XLII. 1 (*Attwood*) and XLII. 6 (*Hawkins*).—(*b*) *Caseation* occurs in these pneumonic areas in parts where induration has not taken place. It is found both in diffuse and nodular forms, giving appearances like XXX. 6 and 8 (*Acute Tubercle*); XXXVI. 3, 4, and 5 (*Griffin*); and XXXVIII. 8 (*Henshaw*). It proceeds in the same manner as that described under *Griffin* (10) and *Gardiner* (22), and by a nuclear growth in the floor of the infundibula, arresting the circulation, and leading to a granular disintegration of the tissue. The lobular forms are mainly determined by the limitation of the growth by the thickened zones of perilobular tissue, and thus may be limited to single lobules, or may embrace several. Nodules of caseation also arise in the manner to be described under § B.—(*c*) *Destructive Change*. The areas where more complete destruction has taken place resemble XXXV. 1, *a a* (*Brodrick*); XXXV. 5 (*Smith*); XXXVI. 5

(*Griffin*); and XXXVIII. 3 (*Henshaw*). The epithelial and small-celled growths disappear by a granular disintegration, and only the fibroid structure is left. The processes by which this occurs are similar to those mentioned in the description of these figures.

§ B. Nodular masses are very common throughout this specimen. In their earlier stages they are chiefly of the types of XXX. 2 (*Coombes, Acute Tubercle*); XXXVII. 5 (*Griffin*); XXXVIII. 7 (*Hall*); XXXIX. 7, *ee* (*Unwin*); and XL. 1 and 6 (*Heath*). They originate in the alveolar wall and infundibulum by a small-celled growth, as seen in XXXVII. 1 and 2 (*Griffin*); and XL. 6 and 7 (*Heath and Mears*). Some also commence with a formation of giant-cells in the centre of the infundibulum, like XXXI. 1 (*Shimmick, Acute Tubercle*). These nodules pass, in some places, into caseation, like XXXIX. 7 (*Unwin*), or into groups of caseating lobules like XXXIX. 4 (*Price*). Larger lobules of caseation like XXXVI. 1 (*Griffin*) are produced by the confluence of lobules like XXXVI. 5 (*Griffin*). Other nodules of caseation resemble XXXII. 7, and XXXV. 4 (*Smith*), but each is surrounded by a dense small-celled growth, and some are like XXVIII. 7 (*Acute Tubercle*), commencing with distinct nodular masses of small-celled growth in their centres, like XXXV. 6 (*Smith*). Some of these nodules pass into induration like XL. 1 and 3 (*Carr*), and XLI. 5 (*C. Roberts*).

§ C. Small-celled nodular growths like XXX. 1 (*Polley, Acute Tubercle*), are met with. They appear in some places as outgrowths from the walls of alveoli, in which dense but diffuse small-celled proliferation is proceeding. In other places they occur in the centre of lobules, and around them are areas of epithelial pneumonic infiltration.

§ D. Diffuse small-celled infiltration is one of the most common changes in this lung. It occurs for the most part mingled with varying amounts of epithelial proliferation in the interior of the alveoli, like XXXVIII. 8 (*Hall*) and XL. 2 (*Heath*), In some places also it proceeds to thickening of the tissues, like XXVIII. 1, 9, 10 (*Acute Tubercle*) and XXXVIII. 1 (*Henshaw*). Areas of a more distinctly pneumonic type—like XXXVII. 6 (*Griffin*)—have been already described. These tracts of infiltration pass either into caseation of the type of XXXVIII. 3 (*Henshaw*), or of destructive type, like XXXV. 1 and 5 (*Brodrick* and *Smith*) and XXXVI. 5 (*Griffin*), or more commonly into the areas of induration next to be described.

§ E. The areas of induration are the most characteristic features of this lung. Some are nodular, like XLI. 1 and 3 (*Carr*) and XLI. 7 (*Coppin*). A large number are diffuse, like XLII. 1 (*Attwood*) and XLII. 6 (*Hawkins*). In many places they proceed, however, in a diffuse form, from the areas of small-celled infiltration previously described, by means of a gradual thickening of the reticulum into broad bands which enclose groups of cells in their meshes, like XLI. 1, *b, c* (*Attwood*). In some places they appear to extend into the pulmonary tissue from the perialveolar and peribronchial thickening, which is abundant here (see XLII. 7). They also occur as broad bands, representing apparently thickening of the interstitial tissue, like XLII. 7 (*d, d*). In all the latter cases there are few or no remains of epithelial cells visible, and the tissue consists of a more or less dense mass of ramifying broad-banded fibres, among which is imbedded a small-celled growth.

These indurations are variously intermingled with pneumonic areas, with and without alveolar thickening and fibroid changes, and with caseous nodules and areas of pneumonic caseation. Areas, like XXXVI. 3 and XXXVII. 4 (*Griffin*), of growth in the alveolar walls mingled with diffuse and nodular forms of caseation, are also common in the parts where induration is less marked, and are even found among the latter, giving to the whole of the structure a very complex arrangement.

Giant-cells, some of large size ($\frac{1}{450}$ inch), are very abundant both in the pneumonic and indurating areas, and also in the nodular forms. In the pneumonic areas they are seen of the types of XXXII. 1, 11; and they are found of the types of XXXII. 5, 7, 8, and 10; and also of XXXIII. 6 and 11.

Pigment is abundant throughout this lung.

§ F. Perivascular and peribronchial induration is very common. It is mostly of the fibroid type, but proceeds by a small-celled growth. No ulceration of the bronchi is seen, but inspissation of their contents is observed in some tubes with thickened walls.

Larynx.—Sections of the laryngeal mucous membrane are seen in XXXIV. 2 and 3. In places where ulceration has not commenced (fig. 3) there is observed to be a proliferation of the epithelium of the surface, and a dense small-celled growth immediately below this (see description of Plate XXXIV.), extending through the whole of the sub-mucous layer and recommencing around the mucous glands. When ulceration has already occurred (fig. 2), the accumulation of the small-celled growth in the sub-mucous tissue is seen to be denser, and to have arranged itself in quasi-nodular forms (miliary).

Glands.—The lymphatic glands show changes closely corresponding in many parts to those found in the lungs. The milky-looking spots are seen to correspond to dense accumulations of nuclei. In other parts, the trabeculae are occupied by dense masses of nuclear growth. There are in addition sclerotised areas, seen in XXXIV. 7, and elsewhere resembling XLI. 1 (*Carr, lung*); while in other places appearances are seen like XLI. 7 (*Coppin, lung*). Some of these masses of sclerotised tissue pass into caseation or granular disintegration.

CASE 30.

CHRONIC PHTHISIS. INDURATING TUBERCULISATION.

Plates XVI.; XXXIII. figs. 7 and 8; XLI. figs. 1, 2, 3, and 4.

SUMMARY.—*F. 36. Duration of marked symptoms four or five months; weakness, shortness of breath, cough, thick yellow expectoration, œdema, pallor. Signs of consolidation and excavation throughout left lung, and of consolidation at apex of left. Urine albuminous. Diarrhœa. Pyrexia for the most part absent.—Left lung consisted of a dense fibroid tissue containing numerous cavities, one occupying almost the whole apex. Dilatation and thickening of bronchi. Right lung contained a small cavity, surrounded by induration at the apex; elsewhere it contained indurated or caseating nodules with fibrous capsules. Larynx and intestine ulcerated. Liver lardaceous and fatty. Kidneys granular, and fatty degeneration. 'Sago spleen.'*

MARY ANN CARR, aged 36, admitted University College Hospital March 2, 1867; died on or about April 15, 1867.

Family History.—Imperfect; no chest affections known.

Personal History.—Born in London; lived badly in childhood; never wore flannel. Went into service in laundry at 11, and worked in ironing-room fourteen years. Menses appeared at sixteen or seventeen. Was regular up to marriage. Married at 25; has had three children; good confinements. Children are living and healthy; suckled each for nine months. Menstruation regular in intervals between lactation and pregnancies. Has been at times subject to leucorrhœa, but not profusely. Never very strong, but has not been ill or laid by till present time.

Present Illness.—Twelve months ago menses ceased suddenly without assignable cause. About this time she had moved to newly-built rooms over stables, which were very cold. She only dates her present illness from three months ago, when she became very weak and had shortness of breath. No rigors or other symptoms of acute invasion. Cough commenced two months ago; was worst at night. Expectoration from first, thick and yellow; never had hæmoptysis. Has suffered from palpitation on exertion for past twelve months. Feet and legs began to swell a fortnight before admission. Has had occasional perspirations of late, not profuse.

State on Admission.—Waxy look of face; marked anæmia; finger-ends clubbed; nails incurvated; ankles, legs, and skin of thorax pit on pressure. Dyspnœa on exertion, not at rest. Cough frequent, with moderate amount of thick yellow expectoration. Chest pigeon-breasted; flattening from fourth to seventh cartilages. Signs of consolidation in greater part of left front and back, with signs of excavation both at apex and base, anteriorly and posteriorly, and coarse râles over the whole side.

Right side generally hyperresonant, with exaggerated breathing, but some signs of consolidation at apex and mid-scapular region, and coarse râles in mammary region. Heart-sounds natural. Urine albuminous, with waxy casts. Diarrhœa was present, also retching in the morning. The patient died, exhausted, six weeks after admission.

The temperature never exceeded 99°. It was almost always normal, but on a few occasions, both morning and evening, it was subnormal.

POST-MORTEM.—*Lungs:* Left strongly adherent to thorax. The adhesions at the apex consist of dense induration-matter, from a quarter to three-quarters of an inch in thickness. The apex is entirely converted into a large cavity lined by a deeply injected false membrane. In it are a few projecting nodules, pigmented externally and cheesy in centre. The cavity is crossed by bands and trabeculæ in all directions. The lower lobe is almost entirely converted into fibrous tissue and cavities, hardly any pulmonary tissue is present. The bronchi pass into an irregularly trabeculated structure of firm fibrous consistence and deeply pigmented. The bronchi themselves are thickened, their elastic fibres are hypertrophied, and in many places they are dilated. Here and there are a few fine granulations, and a few cheesy nodules, but the whole lung is in a state of fibroid transformation.

The right lung has some loose adhesions in places. A group of these are at a dense puckered contraction in the upper lobe—over which there is much hyperæmia (XVI. 1). This is found to correspond to a cavity, the size of a Maltese orange, surrounded by indurated walls, and having the same characters as the cavities observed in the left lung. Throughout this lobe there are large tracts of fibroid induration, similar to those seen in the left, and there are also scattered firm racemose nodules (XVI. 2, *a*), indurated and pigmented, which, when seen near the surface, give this a peculiar puckered aspect. These nodules are semi-cartilaginous in hardness, and for the most part semi-transparent; a few caseous spots appear among them, but these are not common. They consist of small nodules encapsuled by a semi-cartilaginous material (XVI. 2, *b*). In some places large masses are thus seen, encapsuled externally, but caseous in their centres (XVI. 2).

One *Bronchial Gland*, in the hilus of the left lung contains a cheesy mass; otherwise the glands are unaffected. The *Larynx* and upper part of the *Trachea* contain a few small spots of ulceration. These are round, smooth-edged, not thickened, and not everted. They do not exceed a millet-seed in size, and have no evidence of tubercle in their floors.

Heart.—Some gelatinous swelling of edges of flaps of mitral and tricuspid valves. Muscular tissue healthy.

Liver large, pale; not waxy, but iodine shows faint lines of staining in course of blood-vessels: aspect that of the granular form of albuminoid degeneration.

Kidneys pale, soft, with streaks of fatty degeneration: general cloudy, granular appearance; do not stain with iodine.

Spleen typical 'sago' character, stains markedly with iodine.

Stomach healthy. *Intestines.*—Lower end of ileum presents several ulcers, with granulations and cheesy matter in their floor. Some of the solitary glands are enlarged, fluctuating, and when cut allow escape of gruel-like matter; after the escape of this an undermined ulcer is found, without tubercle or cheesy matter either in the walls or the floor. There is much ulceration in cæcum. The intestines give a brown stain with iodine in their villi.

Uterus and *Ovaries* healthy.

MICROSCOPIC APPEARANCES.—By far the larger proportion of changes in this lung consist of nodular masses of extreme fibroid change, as seen in XLI. 1 and 3. They tend to become confluent, and pass into tracts of broad-banded fibres, or into areas of almost homogeneous, fibroid-looking tissue, only interrupted by lacunæ, like the remains of the channels seen in sections of tendon. In other places, and mingled with these, are nodules, here and there caseous in their centres, and indurated in their periphery, having, beyond the zone of induration, a third outer zone of mingled small-celled and epithelial infiltration (XLI. 3 and 4). The origin of both these forms is seen to be from nodules like XXXVI. 5 (*Griffin*); or XL. 1 and 3 (*Heath*). The small-celled growth invading the alveoli passes into fibroid change, as seen in XLI. 1, *b b b*, by processes akin to those seen in XLI. 7 (*Coppin*) and XLII. 1 and 2 (*Attwood* and *Roberts*). The manner in which the change takes place is seen in XLI. 2. Broad bands form in the floor of the alveoli, and also in their walls. These have their origin from the reticulum of new-formation between the cells, and pass into broad bands until the whole become more or less homogeneous, and the cells, at first imbedded in the meshes of the reticulum, gradually disappear. In some places, remains of alveoli, instead of becoming fused in the fibroid transformation, caseate, and the two processes are thus intermingled. Groups of nodules are seen almost side by side, some in the early stage of change from a lobular pneumonia to a dense, small-celled, lobular mass, others fibroid, and others caseating to a greater or less degree. Giant-cells are common in the centres of the alveoli. They present, in early stages of the transformation, the types of XXXII. 5, 8, and 10; XXXIII. 2. Forms like XXXIII. 10 are also seen. As the fibroid change advances, the giant-cells are seen to participate in this by a thickening both of their investing substance (*mantle*), and also of the processes proceeding from them, producing changes like those seen in XXXIII. 7 and 8, and XXXII. 9. Similar cells are also seen in the periphery of the nodules of induration, but their origin and change are identical with the foregoing.

Pneumonic areas are met with rarely. When present they are associated with perialveolar small-celled growth, and pass into areas of induration like XLII. 1 (*Attwood*) and XLII. 6 (*Hawkins*). The small-celled growth tends in places to form isolated 'miliary' nodules, but these also participate only in the common fibroid change, in which they become merged and disappear.

There is considerable perivascular thickening (*see* XLI. 1, *e*), mostly of the fibroid type. In a few places it is found in an earlier stage of small-celled growth. Peribronchial thickening is also found, but to a less degree than the perivascular.

CASE 31.

TUBERCULAR INDURATION AND PNEUMONIA.

Plates XVII. figs. 1 and 3; XL. fig. 10.

SUMMARY.—M. 45. *Cough for two years, varying weakness, occasional hæmoptysis. Seven weeks before death, signs of consolidation and excavation in left, and slighter consolidation in right lung. Continuous pyrexia; diarrhœa. Extensive tracts of fibroid induration in the lungs, with a very large cavity in the left apex; grey granulations, apparently recent, passing into fibroid change; grey pneumonic infiltration. Tubercular ulceration of intestine.*

JOHN LACK, ætat. 45, domestic servant, admitted University College Hospital January 15; died March 7, 1868.

Family History.—No hereditary tendency to lung-disease known.

Personal History.—Has lived well. Has taken alcohol, somewhat, but not largely, in excess. Has had the eruptive fevers of childhood, and also gonorrhœa. Has been liable to rheumatic pains.

Present Illness.—Commenced two years ago, December 1865; attributed to chill. Began with a cough, unattended with expectoration, which continued until the spring of 1867; when he had a temporary cessation of the cough and marked improvement in general health until August 1867.

Since the latter date there has been a great and progressive increase in weakness, which continued until admission. In the spring of 1866, he was also extremely weak, and had night-perspiration. In the autumn of 1866, he had three successive attacks of hæmoptysis, and brought up about half a pint of blood altogether. For the last six weeks he has had indigestion, weight and fulness after meals, with occasional abdominal pain, nausea in the morning, and much flatulence.

State on Admission.—Extreme marasmus, great anæmia. Breath so short as to render him incapable of the slightest exertion. Arcus senilis well marked; arteries tortuous. Cough not frequent; no expectoration whatever. Chest: great flattening of left side, which measures, in semi-diameter, 1¾ inches less than right. Heart: apex in normal site; no murmur, base or apex. The left lung presents physical signs of extensive consolidation in the whole of the upper part, front and back, with a large cavity under the clavicle. Consolidation also in the axillary and mammary regions, and throughout the back, except at the extreme base, where percussion-note is hyperresonant. Right apex: hyperresonance anteriorly, and evidence of consolidation posteriorly. Hyperresonance also at right back posteriorly, below scapula. Tongue furred, much thirst; nausea occasionally; flatulence and occasional abdominal pain. The urine was free from albumen. The sp. gr. varied from 1010 to 1025.

Diarrhœa, which had existed in September, recurred in February, and he died exhausted on March 7. The temperature records are somewhat imperfect, but they show that, even in the morning he was almost continuously febrile during his stay in hospital.

POST-MORTEM.—*Larynx and Trachea* perfectly healthy.

Lungs.—The left is firmly adherent to the thoracic wall, especially at the apex, where the membranes are very thick. The right has only loose recent adhesions. Some dilatations (fusiform) of bronchi where they pass through dense fibrous tissue in both lungs. No other bronchial changes. The right apex is converted almost entirely into a dense, indurated tissue, chiefly fibrous, deeply pigmented, and yet composed of masses of indurated granulations. The granulations are more distinct at the margins, where they form groups projecting above the adjacent pulmonary tissue. In the tissue a few small cavities are present. Groups of these granulations, which form masses of the size of a pea, a bean, a walnut, or a Maltese orange, are scattered through the tissue of this lung, which is emphysematous (XVII. 1, *a*, *a*). Isolated granulations, firm, indurated, pigmented, are also seen scattered through this emphysematous tissue, and by their conglomeration they form the larger nodular masses. These granulations, whether singly or in groups, are for the most part indurated. Single, isolated granulations are also scattered thickly throughout this lung; most of them are transparent, small, glistening, and firm. Others are rather larger, greyish, whitish, or yellow, either centrally or throughout. They are, however, in most cases, firm and indurated, a few only of the yellow ones being soft. In some, a small cavity appears in the centre (1, *b*). Small cavities are also seen here and there, in the midst of the nodules of induration. Portions of lung between these masses of induration are of a bright scarlet hue, and deeply injected, (fig. 1, c, c). The lower part of the upper lobe contains an area of grey pneumonic infiltration. In this infiltration, opaque spots are seen, of variable size, from a split pea, or a hemp-seed, to a poppy-seed. They are opaque and yellow; some have softened into cavities, with a caseous floor in which no granulations are visible, and in some places larger areas of caseous infiltration are seen, which have a more granular surface (see fig. 3, c). The lower lobe contains masses and granulations similar to those described in the upper lobe.

The left lung had, in the apex, a large cavity, crossed in all directions by bands and trabeculæ, and having caseous nodules in its walls. Much of the tissue surrounding it is emphysematous. In this emphysematous tissue are firm, yellowish nodules, surrounded by a zone of semi-transparent fibroid growth. A little lower are nodules of caseous matter of the size of a hemp-seed, finely granular on section, some of which are softening into cavities. Still lower down, in similar emphysematous tissue, are thickly scattered, semi-transparent, grey granulations, most of which are isolated, but between the indurated granulations in some places pass bands of fibroid tissue which are much pigmented, giving to this part of the lung (in which the emphysematous character is still apparent) a peculiar fibroid look. The granulations are nearly all semi-transparent, but some are opaque, with a central cavity. Large tracts and large nodules also exist, composed of fibroid tissue, similar to that described in the opposite lung. They stand out prominently from the lung-tissue. This fibroid tissue is mottled with yellowish specks, and with a few yellowish streaks, and in it are a few small cavities. In the lower lobe is an area of pneumonic infiltration, somewhat similar to that seen in the opposite lung; part of it is semi-transparent, grey, and homogeneous, but small yellow specks are thickly scattered through it. Parts are yellow, finely granular, and friable (caseous), and in these latter, patches of softening are seen, breaking down into cavities. The excavations vary in size from a walnut to a pea; some are elongated and communicate with bronchi.

Heart healthy, with the exception of some opacity and slight thickening of the mitral valve.

Stomach and *duodenum* very hyperæmic; mucous membrane thickened, and roughly granular. There are a few spots of follicular ulceration. Hyperæmia also of *jejunum*. Throughout *ileum* there is extensive ulceration of Peyer's patches. Some ulcers have thickened edges, and there are minute granulations in their floor. Others have sharply punched out edges, without thickening or granulations. Extensive ulceration is also seen in the *caput cæcum coli*, and a few ulcers exist in the *colon*.

Kidneys studded with tubercular granulations; capsule thickened, tissue indurated, with shrinking of cortical substance.

Liver contains tubercular granulations. Tissue otherwise healthy. *Spleen* natural. *Mesenteric glands* indurated.

MICROSCOPIC EXAMINATION shows that the greater part of the changes in these lungs arise from perialveolar small-celled growth, diffuse or in nodules. In a few places, pneumonic changes are found, the alveoli being filled with large epithelial cells. The walls thicken with nuclear growth, and may then present extensive diffused tracts like XXXVIII. 8 (*Hall*); XXXIX. 3 (*Gardiner*); XL. 1 and 2 (*Heath*). These changes, in some places, pass into areas of extensive fibroid induration, or they caseate acutely, producing areas like XXXVI. 4 (*Griffin*) and XXXVIII. 8, 9 (*Hall*). In other parts, the caseation is of a more fibroid type, becoming finely granular like XXXVIII. 3 (*Henshaw*); and in other cases, again they pass into the destructive type of XLIII. 5 (*Heath*), while in some they simply produce large areas, with caseous centres surrounded by a zone of thickened interlobular tissue, an exaggeration in size, but presenting all the other characteristics, of the nodular form of caseation seen in XXXIX. 5 and 7 (*Overall* and *Unwin*).

Nodular changes of the lobular form are, however, the most common. They resemble for the most part those seen in XXXIX. 7 (*Unwin*)—a caseous centre surrounded by a zone of induration, or by this combined with a small-celled growth. The origin of these can be seen to be from nodules like XXXIX. 7, c, c, d (*Unwin*), which, in their earlier stages, proceed by an invasion of the lobules with small-celled growth, at first mingled with epithelial cells like XXXVII. 5 (*Griffin*), and XXXVIII. 7 (*Hall*). This is shown in XL. 10, where much pigment exists in the epithelium. The early stages of this growth resemble XXXVII. 1, a, and 2 (*Griffin*); and XL. 6 (*Heath*), where the nuclear growth invades the floor of the alveoli, and gradually replaces the epithelial formation, and they may at last proceed to miliary nodules of small-celled growth like XXX. 1 (*Acute Tubercle*). Instead of caseation, however, these nodules may pass into extensive fibroid change, producing tracts like XLI. 1 (*Carr*), or the nodules may indurate in the centre, and remain surrounded by a zone of dense nuclear growth, like XLI. 3 and 5 (*Carr* and *Roberts*). The process by which this occurs is seen to resemble those of XLI. 2 (*Carr*) and XLI. 7 (*Coppin*). The caseating and indurating processes are variously intermingled, but the types are usually distinct throughout these lungs.

Giant-cells are abundant throughout these specimens. They occur in the centres of alveoli like XXXIII. 3 and 7, and also in the peripheral zone, both of the indurating and caseous masses.

Perivascular thickening is common, chiefly of the fibroid type. Peribronchial thickening is less common, but it occurs, chiefly fibroid in type, and unattended with any evident bronchial ulceration.

COMMENTARY.—On comparing the history of this case with the *post-mortem* appearances, it should be observed in the first place that it advanced by a series of attacks with intermissions, and that death was apparently the result of two factors, viz. serious diminution of the respiratory capacity and exhaustion by diarrhœa.

The more recent changes in the lung appear to have led up to those of a more advanced kind, and the essential nature of nearly all is an evolution of grey granulations, around which pigmented fibroid tissue gradually forms, until they become merged in dense fibroid masses. There is, in addition, a certain degree of pneumonic infiltration, followed by thickening and occlusion of the alveolar walls, and leading, in some places, to rapid caseation of masses which probably originally were groups of granulations, around which the pneumonic processes occurred. It is probable that the cavity at the left apex may have been due to an attack of this nature in the autumn of 1866.

If this view of the nature and progress of the pulmonary consolidation be correct, it will be seen that, unlike some cases in which the chronic fibroid induration was due to the pneumonic exudation followed by alveolar thickening, in this instance it was due to a series of attacks of acute tuberculisation, the earlier of which were recovered from, but with fibroid change.

I am disposed to believe that this is a more common form of progressive pulmonary phthisis than is now usually accepted. It was recognised by Bayle and Laennec, but since modern theory has restricted the significance of the grey granulation, it has not had that degree of recognition which it appears to deserve. The only alternative is to term it a chronic lobular pneumonia, but this appellation would leave out of view the constitutional state which induces the chronicity, and which is best expressed by the term 'tubercular.' The infiltration of the intestines again points to a general constitutional state.

CASE 32.
Chronic Induration of Lungs.
Plate XLII. fig. 1.
Ref.—Chronic Pneumonia, p. 47.

SUMMARY.—*M. 60. Previous rheumatic gout. Palpitation and winter cough for several years. Increase of cough, with copious, greenish, offensive expectoration; pain in left side; progressive weakness and emaciation. Left side of chest dull, retracted, motionless; breathing tubular and bronchial, in places inaudible. Abundant râles in both lungs. Mitral regurgitant murmur. Duration of symptoms a year. Pyrexia slight and inconstant.—Left lung intense fibroid induration throughout, grey and black, semi-cartilaginous in consistence; a small cavity at apex. Bronchi dilated in both lungs. Pulmonary apoplexy and old pleurisy at right base.*

WILLIAM ATTWOOD, ætat. 60, admitted University College Hospital June 2; died November, 1870.

Family History.—One sister had cancer. No tendency to lung affection or other hereditary disease known.

Personal History.—A gardener's labourer; well fed and clothed. Takes two or three pints of beer daily. No spirits. House dry and airy. Five years ago had an attack of 'rheumatic gout.' Has suffered from palpitation for three years. Has had cough every winter for seven or eight years, with shortness of breath.

Present Illness dated by patient from October 1869; attributed to a wetting. It was followed by a pain in the left side of his chest, aching in limbs, thirst, and copious expectoration. He lost flesh and grew weak, and had to leave off work on December 1. The sputa became offensive two months ago. Six weeks ago he noticed streaks of blood in them.

Symptoms.—Emaciation marked; anæmia distinct; muscles wasted; ends of fingers clubbed; commencing arcus senilis. Respiration accelerated; no subjective sense of dyspnœa while lying in bed. Occasional profuse perspiration. Appetite bad. Paroxysmal cough, worse at night. He expectorated a copious amount of greenish, semi-fluid sputa, the upper part frothy, and beneath this were nodulated masses, greyish-green in colour, and having an offensive odour.

Heart: impulse diffused, extending from half an inch outside nipple-line to epigastrium. Systolic apex thrill and loud rough systolic apex-murmur, lessening in intensity towards base.

Physical Signs.—Marked general retraction of left side, especially in infra-clavicular region; expansion of this side nil. Left side absolutely dull, with great resistance, except in a limited area in left infra-clavicular region, where there is some high-pitched resonance. The respiratory sounds on the left side were tubular under the clavicle and in the upper scapular and axillary regions, and also at the extreme base, alternating, in the first-named situation, with occasional almost complete suppression. Throughout the rest of this side the respiration was bronchial or blowing. Coarse bubbling râles were heard, and coarse metallic moist râles were present from time to time in all these situations. The vocal fremitus was exaggerated throughout the side. Bronchophony was also present throughout the greater part of the side. Whispering pectoriloquy existed at the apex, front and back, and also at the base posteriorly. The right back on admission was healthy.

In September, an attack of pneumonia occurred at the right base; the patient gradually grew weaker, and died in November. Hæmoptysis occurred occasionally during the latter period of his life. The urine from time to time contained a trace of albumen.

He was only slightly feverish during the whole of this period. Sometimes, for a week at a time, the temperature only reached 99°. Then it would, for many days, range from 100° to 101°, the morning temperature being sometimes 98·4° to 99°, sometimes 100°. It only once reached 103°, and once 102°. The pulse was habitually rapid, varying from 80 to 100. The respiration was commonly from 24 to 32, occasionally reaching 36 and 40.

POST-MORTEM.—In my absence the organs were removed and placed in spirit.

Lungs.—Right much enlarged. Bronchial glands natural and small. Bronchi show, in some places, fusiform dilatations, but these are not well marked. Where they occur, they are surrounded by indurated pulmonary tissue, and in one spot, in the posterior part of the middle lobe, there is a limited area of this induration, deeply pigmented, in which the bronchi show fusiform dilatations, passing at their extremities into the globular form. In the lower lobe there is a spot of pulmonary apoplexy, occupying an area of two inches square, and, at the base, another spot of induration, covered by a greatly thickened pleura. In this area also the bronchi are found dilated.

Left lung shrunken and contracted, adherent firmly to costal pleura, and the pulmonary pleura is thickened. Bronchi universally dilated; the dilatations are fusiform for the most part, but some are markedly sacculated, and the transverse bands are much thickened; the mucous membrane is distinct. At the apex, a small excavation communicates with a bronchus. It is irregular in form, and for the most part is filled with calcareous matter. When this is taken out, the walls are fibrous and irregular. The lung-tissue surrounding it is indurated and pigmented, and covered by thickened pleura. There is no trace of ulceration discoverable in any other part of the bronchi. The lung throughout is almost entirely fibrous; in some parts, however, it is dense and firm, resembling collapsed rather than absolute fibroid change. The tissue is not traversed by bands or septa, but is solid with fibroid induration, and pigmented, the consolidation being especially marked around the dilated bronchi. The colour is greyish-black, with deeper pigmentation in places, and the indurated tissue is of semi-cartilaginous firmness.

Bronchial glands much enlarged, uniformly indurated and pigmented; they show no traces of calcareous or cheesy matter, or of tubercle.

Heart enlarged. A calcareous ring nearly surrounds attachment of mitral valve. Calcareous deposits also occur in the flaps of the valve and in the chordæ tendineæ. Aorta shows comparatively little change. Valves in right side healthy.

Kidneys indurated. *Liver* and *Spleen* healthy. The other organs were not examined.

MICROSCOPIC EXAMINATION.— In both lungs similar changes were found. They consist, for the most part, of those seen in XLII. 1.

A. Great and very general induration of large tracts of the lung with fibrous tissue, which, in many places, and especially on the left side, has almost entirely replaced the pulmonary structure. The fibroid tissue is sometimes in broad bands of sclerosis (see figure), but more commonly in wavy fibres. In some places it includes the remains of alveoli filled with epithelium, like XLII. 6 (*Hawkins*).

B. Adjacent to the former, and passing into it, is a thickening of the walls of the alveoli with a small-celled growth, like that seen in XXXVII. 7 (*Griffin*). This thickening also extends through very large areas in both lungs, where no fibroid change is apparent, and in parts it almost entirely obliterates the alveolar structure of the lung. In some parts alveoli remain empty (XLII. 1); in others they are filled with epithelium; but this is not, as a rule, much enlarged (*ibid. e*), and in some it can be seen to be replaced by a small-celled growth. In some tracts, however, pneumonic areas occur, like XXXVIII. 2 (*Henshaw*). In the fibroid areas, sections of bronchi may be seen, filled with inspissated contents, or with puriform cells (XLII. 1, *d, d*), and considerable peribronchial and perivascular thickening, chiefly fibroid, is found throughout the preparation. Bronchial ulceration is not, however, met with. The small-celled growth passes into the fibroid change by a gradual thickening of the reticulum (*e, f*), until the cells are gradually obliterated, or only a few remain enclosed in the meshes of the broader bands (*b, b-g, g*). A very few (miliary) nodules are found of the small-celled growth in isolated form and in a few places like XL. 1 (*Heath*), and imperfect attempts at the lobular form are observed. But both these, and the miliary nodules, are rare and exceptional; nearly the whole change in the lung is of the nature of that just described.[1]

[1] A paper attached to the MS. of this case contains the following memoranda for a commentary. 'Not the induration of heart-disease; not mere fibrosis. Chronic Pneumonia.'

CASE 33.

INDURATED AND PIGMENTED TUBERCULISATION.

Plates XVII. figs. 2 and 4; XLI. fig. 7;
XLIII. fig. 1 and 2.

Ref.— Phthisis, p. 97.

SUMMARY.— *M. 39. Brother phthisis. Loss of voice and cough commenced fifteen weeks before death, and was followed by enlargement of the abdomen. Nine weeks later there were signs of consolidation at both apices, and, in spots, at the bases; signs of excavation also at the right apex. Evidence of increasing ascites. Moderate continuous pyrexia, rapid exhaustion.— Ulceration of the larynx. The lungs presented dense fibroid change at the apices, with sinuous cavities in the right. Below this were grouped indurated and pigmented granulations, and in the left some yellowish-grey nodules. Liver cirrhotic and tubercular. Intestines, tubercular ulceration.*

W. H. COPPIN, ætat. 39, admitted University College Hospital July 3; died August 16, 1868.

Family History.— Father dead, cause unknown. Mother living, ætat. 75. One brother died of phthisis. Has had eight children; four living, three died of scarlatina, one of croup.

Occupation and Habits.— Warehouse porter; a native of Ireland. Has always lived well, habits temperate, residence dry and airy.

Previous Illness.— None, except typhoid fever five years ago. Never had syphilis.

Present Illness.— Only recognised by patient nine weeks before admission. First had swelling of throat, lost voice, and had a cough. After six weeks he improved. Three weeks ago was attacked with epigastric pain, soon followed by swelling of the abdomen, and of the feet and ankles. Cannot account in any way for his illness.

The Physical Signs showed consolidation at both apices, with cavities at the right, and moist sounds at the left. The bases gave also signs of consolidation in spots. Cough was not a prominent symptom. The heart was normal. The urine was free from albumen or sugar. The liver was enlarged, reaching from the 3rd rib to two fingers' breadth below false ribs; total vertical height 7 inches. There was no vomiting. The tongue was red, glazed, and irritable. The bowels are noted as regular. The abdomen was much enlarged on admission, and manifestly contained fluid; the enlargement increased subsequently. He sank exhausted, and died in a little more than a month after admission.

He was almost continuously feverish, the morning temperature being only on two occasions below 99°; the mean morning temperature was 99·7°, the maximum being 101·2°. The evening temperature was only irregularly taken; the mean was 100·5°, the maximum 101·5°, the minimum 99·5°. The data of the relative height of the morning and evening temperatures are too imperfect for comparison. The pulse ranged from 84 to 120; the respirations from 20 to 24.

POST-MORTEM.— Large amount of transparent serosity in abdomen. Omentum firmly adherent to liver, stomach, and intestines. The membrane is thickened, puckered, and covered with fine granu-

CASE 33 (COPPIN)

lations. The peritoneal surface of the intestines is also covered with fine granulations.

Larynx.—Cartilages calcified. Deep ulcerations on both vocal cords. The mucous membrane of the sacculus laryngis is swollen, and the vocal cords are thickened. Ulcerations exist in numerous spots in the trachea. Bronchi intensely congested, and show in some places fusiform dilatations.

Lungs.—Right apex riddled with sinuous cavities, lined by a highly vascular membrane situated on an ash-grey floor of dense fibroid tissue. In the walls of the cavities caseous masses still adhere. There is a little emphysema at the anterior border of the apex, otherwise the whole of the tissue intervening between these cavities, and extending for some distance beyond them, is constituted by a dense fibrous tissue, ash-grey in colour, streaked with lines, and of almost cartilaginous firmness (XVII. 2, c c). Below this is a tissue of almost equal firmness, also intensely pigmented, but evidently composed of groups of granulations fused together. In a few spots around the cavities there is a grey uniform pneumonic infiltration, which is, in places, intensely pigmented, and is very firm and hard. Lower down, the amount of crepitant pulmonary tissue increases, but in it are masses of hard, firm, pigmented, and racemose granulations. Some of these are caseous in centre. The granulations vary in size from a poppy-seed to a hemp-seed. In the emphysematous margins of the upper lobe a similar condition is found, but here the granulations are less fibrous and less pigmented. Some are showing a tendency to caseation, but all are firm, and in appearance tend to the type of the grey granulations, none being larger than a poppy-seed. Here, and also in the middle lobe, these granulations tend to form clusters, with fibrous bands intervening. A few similar masses are found in the lower lobe, but are not common there.

(The *Left Lung*, examined after injection, presented, at the apex, granulations in emphysematous tissue. The granulations formed fibroid groups and masses, like those in the opposite lung. Softer, larger, yellow masses were also found, firmer, greyer, and more irregular than the ordinary large yellow granulations. They existed chiefly in the lower edge of the upper lobe. Some also were found in the lower lobe. They were discrete, and did not form racemose masses. Groups of greyish granulations, not semi-transparent but opaque, appeared in places. They were not caseous, and were surrounded by much pigment. There was no pneumonic infiltration in this lung.)

The *Bronchial Glands* are enlarged, indurated, pigmented, and contain masses of cheesy matter scattered through grey, semi-transparent tissue. The glands in the posterior mediastinum are also enlarged. The cervical and posterior laryngeal glands are indurated, semi-transparent, and in some places have become cheesy; but they are firm, dry, and very hard, nowhere showing traces of softening.

Heart healthy.

Liver (XVI. 4) enlarged; measures 11 inches by 8, and is 2½ inches thick; it weighs 4 lbs. 2 oz. Capsule thickened and opaque. Section presents an appearance of granulations, different from those of an ordinary cirrhosed liver. They are firmer, of lighter colour, more grey, and semi-transparent. They are discrete, but with some tendency to aggregation. They vary in size from a rape to a hemp seed, and some are as small as a poppy-seed. Some of the smaller ones exactly resemble miliary tubercles, and are surrounded by a zone of injection. The hepatic tissue is in some parts intensely congested, but not specially so where the granulations in question are the most abundant. The liver, as a whole, is firm and dense, and the morbid process suggested by its aspect is that of a combination of cirrhosis and tubercle.

Kidneys large; capsule separates with some difficulty. Tissue unduly firm. No tubercle seen.

Spleen normal.

Intestines.—Tubercular ulcerations in ileum, extending in the transverse diameter of intestine, with thickened edge containing granulations of tubercle. Ulcerations also exist in the caput caecum coli, and in the first part of the colon. *Mesenteric Glands* enlarged; in part firm and of semi-cartilaginous appearance; in part simply swollen, but still firm and containing grey granulations; and in part filled with cheesy matter, which is, however, also firm.

MICROSCOPIC EXAMINATION.—The chief changes presented by this lung are fibroid, among which are interspersed patches of caseation, but the latter are less frequent than the former. Both the fibroid and the caseous changes occur in circumscribed areas (lobular), and also in the non-circumscribed (diffuse) form. The greater part of the lung is occupied by nodular forms resembling XXIX. 1; XXXIV. 1 (*Acute Tubercle*); XXXIX. 5 (*Overall*); XXVIII. 6, 7, and 8 (*Acute Tubercle*). In the early stages of these there are many variations, of which the following are the chief:—Nodules like XL. 1 (*Heath*), with a small-celled growth invading the alveolar wall, but passing into fibroid change as in XLI. 7. Nodules where the small-celled growth is denser, and intermediate in appearance between XL. 1 (*Heath*) and XXXVIII. 8 (*Hall*). Nodules like XXXIX. 4 (*Price*), but which, instead of caseating, pass into a mingled small-celled growth and fibre-growth, shown in XLIII. 3, with which much pigment is intermingled. In all these a denser, small-celled growth occurs in the walls of the alveoli, reproducing in early stages the appearance of XXXVII. 1 and 2 (*Griffin*), and when more fully developed resembling XXXIX. 5 (*Overall*). In some places this growth forms nodules which may be truly called miliary, and which pass either into caseation or into fibroid induration, the types of which are seen in XXX. 1 (*Acute Tubercle*), and XLI. 6 (*Cox*). In their further stages of induration, these nodules produce forms resembling XLIII. 1; where the remains of the alveoli may be traced in whorls of fibres, mingled with remains of small-celled growth and a few epithelial cells, the whole being deeply pigmented, and also others like XLI. 1 and 3 (*Cox*). and XLI. 5 (*Roberts*). Caseation also occurs in them, resembling XXXIX. 7 (*Unwin*), and like XXXVI. 1 and 2 (*Griffin*), and in some places diffuse forms of small-celled growth are also seen in abundance. In some, it occurs in forms intermediate between XXXVIII. 8 (*Hall*) and XL. 2 (*Heath*). These pass, in some cases, into fibroid change, in others into caseation, chiefly of the fibrillo-granular type of XXXVIII. 3 (*Henshaw*), and XLIII. 5 (*Heath*). In some cases the growth produces thickening of the walls of the alveoli like XXVIII. 10 (*Acute Tubercle*). and like XXXVII. 1 (*Henshaw*). The more common change, however, is a complete filling up of the alveoli with the dense, small-celled growth, very closely resembling XXVIII. 2 and 7 (*Acute Tubercle*); which may pass into areas of caseation like XXXVI. 4 (*Griffin*) or into fibroid areas like XLI. 7 (*Coppin*). Some tracts closely resemble XXXVII. 4 (*Griffin*), and are apparently produced in the same manner, but the difference between these processes in this case and in that of Griffin (*see* p. 185) is that the small-celled growth is denser, the cells rather smaller, and the caseous change is less acutely produced.

Giant-cells are numerous. They occur both in the centres of nodules, and in groups of alveoli where the small-celled growth is proceeding both in the nodular and in the diffuse form. They reproduce the types of XXXII. 1, 2, 3, 6, and 11. One very large one measured $\frac{1}{30}$ by $\frac{1}{40}$ inch, of the type of XXXII. 8 *h*, and others nearly equally large were also seen.

Perivascular and peribronchial thickening with both small-celled and fibroid growth, are abundant, the former more so than the latter. No bronchial ulcerations are seen, and the pulmonary changes are almost entirely alveolar in their origin and extension. The whole of this lung is intensely pigmented, as seen in XLIII. 1.

CASE 34.

Chronic Phthisis; Tubercular Induration.

Plates XVIII. 3, 4; XLI. 6.

Ref.—Phthisis, pp. 97. 116.

Summary.—*M. 27. Chronic cough and progressive weakness, during four years. No hæmoptysis. Three months before death, an acute illness of uncertain nature. Three weeks before death extreme anæmia and emaciation. Signs of consolidation through greater part of left lung, and in right lung at the apex and at spots elsewhere, of excavation at apices, extensive in right. Urine albuminous. Continuous pyrexia.—Ulceration of larynx and trachea. In both lungs indurated groups of granulations, fused into fibrous tissue at the apices; in the left this tissue is extremely dense, and surrounds extensive sinuous cavities. Tubercle of bronchial glands, pericardium, and liver. Ulceration of intestines. Albuminoid kidneys.*

H. Cox, ætat. 27, admitted University College Hospital January 15, and died February 8, 1868.

Family History.—Father and mother both living and healthy, aged respectively 66 and 60. Some of his maternal aunts have died of phthisis. One brother died of pleurisy; another, living, suffers from abscesses; and a third brother is healthy.

Previous History.—A warehouse clerk. Has lived well; very temperate in stimulants; has clothed warmly. Has always lived in London, and has inhabited the same house for eight years; situation airy, but house somewhat damp. Has had gonorrhœa, never syphilis.

Present Illness.—Cough came on gradually, without known cause, in October 1863 (four years and a quarter ago); was laid up at outset. Expectoration did not appear until some months after the commencement of the cough, and then it became profuse, but subsequently diminished. Never had hæmoptysis. Has continued to lose strength up to present time. At the end of November, 1867, had an acute febrile illness, described by him as 'spotted fever.' He was laid up for six weeks. He was feverish, occasionally delirious, and had epistaxis, blood in urine, and purple spots on the body: the spots on the limb left scabs. He had pain in the limbs, head, and spine, and much stiffness of the neck. Has still some numbness in left hand, with a sensation of 'pins and needles' in it. Was treated with lemon-juice and turpentine.

State on Admission.—Excessive anæmia and pallor; great emaciation; œdema of ankles. Headache occasionally; digestion undisturbed; no diarrhœa. Urine very copious, specific gravity varying from 1006 to 1010, albuminous. Cough frequent; expectoration abundant, muco-purulent, the mucoid character preponderating; greenish, moderately tenacious.

Chest, naturally well-formed, right costal angle smaller than left. Right infra-clavicular region flattened and deficient in expansion; no flattening elsewhere. Signs of consolidation existed in the whole upper half of the right side, extending through the upper and lower axillary, and the infra-mammary regions. The right base posteriorly gave pulmonary resonance. The left apex was also consolidated, but less so than the right. There were likewise signs of patches of consolidation in the left midscapular region, and at the base. There was evidence of extensive excavation at the right apex; slighter, but distinct, at the left. Râles also existed at both bases, coarse and bubbling at the right.

No material change occurred until his death on February 8.

He was continuously febrile during the whole of his stay in hospital. On one occasion only did the morning temperature fall to 98°, and on one evening to 99. The mean morning temperature was 100·5°, maximum 102·6°. The mean evening temperature was 101·5°, maximum 104·8°. The mean of the exacerbations from morning to evening was 1·7° (maximum 3·1°, minimum 0·2°.) The mean of the remissions from evening to morning was 2·0°. (maximum 4·0°, minimum 0·8°). Inverse types were not infrequent; remissions occurred from morning to evening on five occasions, the greatest being 1·6°, the least 0·1° (mean 1°.) Exacerbations also occurred from evening to morning on six days, the greatest being 2·6° and the least 0·2° (mean 1°). He perspired profusely at times and lost eleven pounds in weight from January 19 to February 8. The pulse varied from 120 to 142; the respirations from 28 to 44. The mean pulse-respiration ratio was 3·8.

Post-mortem.—*Larynx* and *Trachea.* Ulceration on upper surface of left vocal cord. Below the vocal cords there is very extensive ulceration, with patches of highly injected and very granular mucous membrane between the ulcers. Fine semi-transparent granulations can be seen in some places in the floor of these ulcers. Islets of granulations are seen in the whole length of the trachea, and some of these granulations extend deeply into the tissue at the bifurcation of the trachea. The ulceration has almost perforated into the posterior mediastinum, the outside of the trachea being covered with a soft fibrinous exudation, which extends through its wall into the interior, and occupies the space between the larynx and œsophagus. The ulcerations do not extend into the bronchial tubes.

Lungs.—The bronchi in the middle lobe of the

right and the lower lobes of both lungs present fusiform dilatations. In the upper lobe of the left lung, globular dilatations exist, and where passing through some pneumonic induration, the bronchi are ulcerated, and are surrounded by tracts of caseous matter. In the upper lobe of the right lung they are with difficulty traced, owing to the extensive excavation.

Right Lung.—Whole upper lobe shrunk to the size of a large orange. The pleura covering it is nearly a quarter of an inch in thickness. The whole of this lobe, where not excavated, consists of a dense pigmented fibrous tissue, of cartilaginous hardness, studded here and there with minute cheesy spots. The whole of the apex is converted into a series of sinuous cavities, and traversed by bands, in the walls of which are caseous spots and nodules. The middle and lower lobes are emphysematous. They contain nodules of fibroid structure, made up of groups of granulations, firm and indurated, some of which are grey and others pigmented, while some are caseous in their centres (XVIII. 3, *dd*). Scattered granulations, the size of poppy and millet seeds, are seen throughout this tissue, grey, firm, and not pigmented. Some also of these have caseous centres (*cc*). Masses of caseous matter, apparently formed from these nodules, also occur, and among these some dilated and ulcerating bronchioles are seen (*b*).

Left Lung.—The upper lobe is in places emphysematous, but it consists in greater part of old grey granulations, fused into a mass of fibrous tissue, each of the component granulations having a caseous centre (as in XVIII. 8, *ccc*). These form nodules and masses, between which islets of emphysematous pulmonary tissue exist. There are also tracts of glistening transparent pneumonic exudation, containing caseous nodules (XVIII. 4, *h*). In this are some dilated bronchi, ulcerating, and surrounded by a zone of caseous matter where they pass through the pneumonic infiltration (*e*). Isolated soft granulations are also seen (*d*), and dilated bronchi, whose walls are caseous (*g*), pass into dense masses of cheesy matter (*f*). The lower lobe is emphysematous; it is studded with racemose masses of indurated pigmented granulations, like those seen in the upper lobe. These masses are most abundant in the upper part of the lower lobe, where also some patches of grey pneumonic infiltration can be seen. In the lower part of this lobe isolated, firm, grey granulations are present.

Bronchial Glands.—Those at the bifurcation of the trachea, are small, contracted, and deeply pigmented; those in the posterior mediastinum are large, cloudy, and contain yellow, opaque, indurated spots, mingled with much pigment. Small granulations can here and there be seen on the cloudy floor. Some of the glands in the posterior mediastinum contain cretaceous matter. The post-tracheal glands are swollen and cloudy on section, and on this base, in some instances, grey granulations are thickly scattered. These granulations are for the most part soft. Some are passing into the cheesy state, and in some a further change to cretaceous matter is observed.

Heart.—Recent tubercular pericarditis. There is a considerable amount of fluid in the pericardium. The surface of the heart is covered with a layer of flocculent lymph, and numerous grey, semi-transparent granulations are seen, on both the visceral and the parietal pericardium. The valves are healthy.

Liver, large; weighs 12 oz.; section smooth, glistening, too friable. No reaction with iodine. Numerous granulations of tubercle in capsule and scattered throughout substance.

Kidneys, normal size, no contraction of cortical substance. Stellate veins on surface too prominent. Malpighian bodies not very prominent. Tissue albuminoid, glistening, does not stain with iodine; it passes in spots into fatty degeneration.

Spleen, normal size; no special induration or friability. Malpighian bodies very prominent. (This, however, from the description given, had evidently not attained to the condition of the 'sago spleen.')

Stomach much injected; mucous membrane at pylorus thickened and indurated. Solitary glands not distinct.

Intestines.—Ulcerations of tubercular type (circular with thickened edges and with granulations in floor) commence at upper part of ileum, and extend through the small intestine. The solitary glands are greatly enlarged, attaining the size of a hempseed, and have an opaque centre and a semi-transparent margin, which, in some cases, is firm and semi-cartilaginous. Ulcerations exist in the large intestine, almost perforating its wall.

Mesenteric Glands.—Tubercular throughout; much cheesy matter in some.

Brain.—Much thickening and opacity of membranes along the fissures of Sylvius, but not extending within the fissures. Nothing else remarkable at base. Membranes are very opaque on both sides, but separate with moderate facility. Ventricles present nothing remarkable. Rest of brain apparently healthy.

THE MICROSCOPIC APPEARANCES found in this lung are as follows:—

§ A. Areas of pneumonic infiltration like XXXVIII. 2 (*Henshaw*), in which a gradual thickening of the walls takes place by growths resembling those seen in XXX. 5 (*Acute Tubercle*) and XXXVII. 7 (*Griffin*). This also proceeds to the production of a dense tissue, in which the cavities of the alveolar passages are narrowed, resembling XXVIII. 10 (*Acute Tubercle*) and XXXVIII. 1 (*Henshaw*).

§ B. Small-celled infiltration takes place also through diffuse areas like XXXVIII. 8 (*Hull*). These tend to pass into fibroid induration like XLI. 7 (*Coppin*).

§ C. Nodular forms, both of induration and caseation, are the most common, though not the exclusive changes in this lung. In many parts they present appearances like XXXIX. 4 (*Price*). Others apparently commence like XXXVI. 5 (*Griffin*), and others again are formed like XXXIX. 7 (*Cawin*). A large number commence like XXXVI. 1 and 2 (*Griffin*), XL. 6 (*Heath*), and XL. 7 (*Mears*). In all of these, there is a progressive growth of small cells in the floor of the alveoli until the epithelium has disappeared. The nodular form is, however, maintained throughout. In other places a miliary growth of small cells, imbedded in a reticulum (as shown in XLI. 6), commences in the floor of an alveolus and thence extends to adjacent alveoli, and produces a structure like XXX. 1 (*Acute Tubercle*). These nodules caseate and commence break-down in their centres.

§ D. Nodules and areas of caseation are formed of the types both of XXVIII. 6 (*Acute Tubercle*) and also of the more fibrillar types of XXXVIII. 3

(*Henshaw*) and XLIII. 5 (*Heath*). They have their origin in changes similar to those described as occurring in the nodules, but often extending over larger areas. They also assume the nodular form, sometimes lobular, sometimes enclosing two or more lobules. Larger areas of caseation are also sometimes produced by the coalescence of single nodules. The larger and smaller areas are in these cases bounded by thickened zones of peribronchial tissue. Some of these resemble XXXVI. 1 (*Griffin*); and various forms intermediate between these and XXXIX. 1 (*Price*) are also seen. Others, commencing like XXVIII. 7 (*Acute Tubercle*), also pass in their centres into areas of caseation.

§ E. Induration proceeds in some of these nodules, producing forms like XLI. 1 (*Carr*). Giant-cells are seen but rarely—a few are found of the pigmented type, like XXXII. 7 (*Smith*).

§ F. Peribronchial and perivascular thickening occurs, both with small-celled growth, and also of the fibroid type. Ulceration of the bronchi from within is met with in a few places, but this is not common, and the destruction of the lung is almost entirely of alveolar nature and origin.

COMMENTARY.—This case presents a tolerably typical illustration of a quasi-chronic affection progressing constantly but gradually to a fatal issue. Its course was probably determined by a combination of pneumonic and tubercular processes, the latter assuming in great measure the character of indurating granulations, but passing into the caseating form. The pneumonic changes are sufficiently illustrated by the *post-mortem* report and the microscopic examination. It may be questioned whether the acute illness, occurring in the autumn before his death, was not an attack of acute tuberculisation; but of this there is no distinct proof, though the condition in which the membranes of the brain were found, *post mortem*, is unusual in a person of temperate habits at the age of this patient. The supervention of the lardaceous kidney within four years is also worthy of remark. Here also many organs were diseased. In the final stage, pericarditis occurred, attended with grey granulations.

CASE 35.

INDURATING TUBERCULISATION.

Plates XVIII. figs. 1 and 2; XXXII. fig. 10; XXXIII. figs. 9 and 11; XLI. fig. 5.

Ref.—Phthisis, p. 97.

SUMMARY.—*F. 26*. *Cough began suddenly after exposure to cold. Six months later, there were signs of consolidation at both apices, greater in the left and accompanied with those of excavation. The consolidation increased rapidly on both sides, extending through the whole of the left lung, with general bronchitic râles. Much pyrexia during the last three months of life. Death thirteen months after the onset.—Extensive induration through both lungs, due to firm masses of granulations and fibroid change about them. A large cavity at the left apex. Dilated bronchi, opening into sinuous cavities.*

CAROLINE ROBERTS, ætat. 26; admitted University College Hospital July 10, 1867. Discharged relieved in September: re-admitted October 30, 1867 died on or about February 28, 1868.

Family History.—Father alive and healthy, mother died of chest affection, called by patient 'asthma.' Has had eleven brothers and sisters. One brother only living: he suffers from cough in the winter and has done so for many years. One sister died three weeks ago. All the rest died young. causes of death unknown.

Personal History.—Has had measles, scarlatina, and whooping-cough when young. Married, and has had three children; the last was stillborn, the first two are alive and healthy. Patient was always strong and healthy until lately.

Present Illness.—Commenced in January last, when she got her feet wet and caught a severe cold. Cough began then, and has continued uninterruptedly. During first part of her illness, was engaged nursing her dying sister, and was much exposed to night air and draughts. She has grown rapidly worse during the past six weeks. The sputa, at first scanty, have become profuse, and are occasionally streaked with blood. No large hæmoptysis. Has lost strength and flesh rapidly of late, but has not kept her bed.

State on Admission.—Considerable emaciation and anæmia; night-perspirations. Cough frequent; expectoration about 4 oz. in twenty-four hours; thick, airless, and opaque, of dirty greenish tint. Much pain in left side.

Physical signs of consolidation at both apices. Extensive on left side, but only posteriorly on right. Extensive excavation at left apex.

Urine free from albumen. No discomfort from food: has had one attack of diarrhœa a short time ago; now bowels habitually regular. Tongue furred.

On re-admission, a few weeks later, the whole left side was found dull, and the consolidation at the right apex had increased. Moist râles, fine, coarse, and metallic over whole left side. Some scattered râles over right side, base and apex.

She sank gradually, and died about February 28, 1868.

The temperature, as taken during her second stay in hospital, was very variable, and during nearly two months it showed almost constantly an inverse type, the morning being nearly always higher than the evening. The morning temperatures ranged from 100° to 103°; the evening from 99° to 100°. In January it became irregular, oscillating from 99° to 108°, and once reaching 104°. Up to the time of her death, it was constantly over 100°, twice exceeded 104°, and the evening temperatures were frequently lower than the morning. The pulse never fell below 110°. It was usually about 120°, and occasionally reached 114°. The respiration was usually about 30°, ranging from this to 40°, and not falling below 25°.

POST-MORTEM.—*Lungs*: Both adherent, the left firmly so, almost universally; the right at apex. About 8 oz. of turbid fluid in right pleura.

Left Lung.—Much shrunken. Apex occupied by a cavity about the size of a small orange, but loculated by septa and irregular in shape; wall composed of dense, indurated tissue. Nearly the whole of the lung is composed of dense fibroid tissue; through this dilated bronchi pass, and these, in many places, intercommunicate so as to form a series of sinuous cavities (c c, XVIII. 1). In the pulmonary tissue remaining, which is traversed in all directions by pigmented fibroid tissue, are numerous indurated granulations (a b).

Right Lung.—The anterior portion and greater part of the base is emphysematous. The apex is indurated by semi-cartilaginous fibroid growth, almost like the left, and is traversed by cavities which, in some places, appear to proceed from dilated bronchi, but in other places have evidently resulted from ulcerations. The walls of the bronchi are everywhere much thickened, and their lining membrane is injected. Below this the tissue is extensively indurated, but not uniformly, by groups of firm, pigmented granulations, passing into and surrounded by zones and bands of fibroid induration. Some of the granulations show cheesy changes in their centre, but the prevailing character is of fibroid induration (XVIII. 2). Lower down, in the midst of emphysematous tissue, are groups of grey granulations tending to the racemose form, indurated, and surrounded by much pigment. Still lower, are scattered numerous isolated granulations having the same character; very few present caseation, but this change is more common in the lower than in the upper portions. There is considerable induration in tracts, and also much congestion throughout the tissue in this part of the lung.

Bronchial glands much enlarged, with grey infiltration.

Larynx.—Ulceration in upper surface of both vocal cords.

Intestines.—No ulcerations. *Kidneys* show some fatty degeneration. *Liver* fatty.

MICROSCOPIC EXAMINATION shows that the changes in this lung consist almost entirely of nodules of fibroid forms of induration, like those described in *Unwin, Overall, Carr,* and *Heath,* mingled, however, with caseous changes.

The fibroid nodular masses are almost identical with those seen in XLI. 1 and 3 (*Carr*). They are often intensely pigmented, and through the sclerotic centre may sometimes be seen lines of pigment, marking in places the position of capillaries (see XLI. 5, *a b*). These nodules are sometimes surrounded by a zone of thickened small-celled growth (see fig. 5), but the lobular zone of thickened fibroid tissue usually marks them very distinctly. They are, throughout this lung, very intensely pigmented. They merge into one another and form dense masses of large area.

Some nodules, instead of being indurated throughout, are caseous in their centres, like XXXIX. 7, *a* (*Unwin*), and are variously intermingled with the fibroid nodules. The origin of these nodules can be clearly traced to a small-celled infiltration of the alveolar walls in a lobular form, presenting an appearance identical with XL. 1 (*Heath*), and these may be seen side by side with nodules like XL. 3 (*Heath*), also seated in the midst of areas of dense fibroid change. Other nodules are formed identical in structure with XXXV. 4 (*Smith*), and others with XXXIX. 6 and 7 (*Overall and Unwin*), and XL. 9 (*Overall*). The transformation of these into the fibroid and caseous nodules can also be distinctly traced. Some nodules, entirely composed of small-celled growth, like XLI. 6 (*Cox*), and XXX. 1 (*Acute Tubercle*), are also seen, some caseating, others passing into fibroid change.

Areas of small-celled infiltration, sometimes of considerable extent, can be traced in the various forms represented by XXX. 5 and 6 (*Acute Tubercle*); XXXVII. 7 (*Griffin*); XXXIX. 3 (*Gardiner*); XXXVIII. 8 (*Hall*); and XL. 2 (*Heath*). These pass in some places into extensive fibroid change, in others into a fibrillar caseation like XXXVIII. 3 (*Henshaw*), XLIII. 5 (*Heath*), and in others into areas of destructive pneumonia, like XXX. 5 (*Smith*), and XXXVI. 5 (*Griffin*).

Peribronchial and perivascular thickening is met with, both fibroid. No bronchial ulceration can be seen.

Giant-cells are abundant. They are of the types seen in XXXII. 8 and 10, and XXXIII. 3, 9, and 11.

CASE 36.

INDURATING TUBERCULISATION.

Plates XIX. figs. 1 and 2; XXXIII. fig. 4;

XL. fig. 7; XLII. figs. 3 and 4.

SUMMARY.—*F. 15. Strong phthisical heredity. Chronic cough since nine, increasing, with expectoration. Four months before death, defective resonance through whole left side, with bronchial and metallic breathing and râles. On right side, resonance imperfect at the apex, with weak bronchial breathing, and abundant moist râles. Liver much enlarged.— Left lung converted into a mass of fibroid tissue containing dilated bronchi, sinuous cavities, and a few masses of granulations. Right lung emphysematous, with a large cavity at the apex and many smaller ones, and also with granulations, indurated and pigmented, grouped and contracting, or separate and grey, a few cheesy masses. Albuminoid liver, kidneys, and spleen.*

EMMA MEARS, ætat. 15, admitted University College Hospital June 8; died October 18, 1868.

Family History.—Father died of apoplexy, ætat. 35. Mother died, ætat. 45, of 'consumption.' Maternal grandmother and three of her mother's cousins have also died of 'consumption.' Has had three brothers and three sisters. One sister died when young from an abscess; one brother subject to cough, another brother and sister suffer at times from glandular enlargement in the neck.

Personal History.—Has always been well clothed, and has always had sufficient food. House confined, but dry, and has lived all her life in London.

Previous Illnesses.—Always thin, never strong; at nine years old she went into city to work, used to get her feet wet and began to cough. This obliged her to give up work, and she has never lost this cough. Six years ago attended at King's College Hospital, and two years ago at the hospital for sick children. At the last-named period, stomach became irritable. She used to vomit, and lost flesh considerably. Was sent into the country, and improved. Lately, cough has been worse. Expectoration has been thick, and of a yellow colour, ever since cough commenced. Has never had hæmoptysis. Catamenia have never appeared.

Present Illness dates from three weeks ago, as an aggravation of her previous cough and weakness. Thinks that its immediate cause was over-exertion from a long walk.

State on Admission.—Imperfectly developed. Frame exceedingly small. Considerable emaciation both of subcutaneous fat and of muscular tissues. Muscles have almost disappeared from the upper arm. Marked anæmia, and some cyanosis. Skin perspiring. Finger-ends clubbed; nails incurvated. Abdomen enlarged, owing to increased size of liver and spleen. Thorax naturally well-formed; lower axillary regions pushed outwards by enlargement of liver and spleen. Both infra-clavicular regions flattened, especially the left. Tubercular percussion-note under left clavicle, extending to fourth rib; heard also in upper axilla. The rest of left front is absolutely dull, also the whole of the left back, except a small portion near the angle of the scapula. The respiration over this lung is bronchial; in parts weak, in others, and, especially near the apex, metallic in quality. Throughout the lung there are coarse bubbling râles. Sibilant râles are also heard in parts.

Right infra-clavicular region yields 'wooden' resonance down to second rib; the rest of this front is hyperresonant, and this character continues across middle line to left border of sternum. The apex posteriorly is dull, high-pitched 'wooden' in upper third of scapular region, below this hyperresonant to 9th rib. Axilla dull only below 9th rib. Respiration under right clavicle weak, bronchial almost masked by sibilant and coarse bubbling râles; bronchial breathing is heard also at the apex posteriorly. Over the rest of this side respiration is weak, and attended by sibilant and bubbling râles.

Heart's apex indistinct, beats in 4th interspace, immediately beneath nipple. Sounds normal.

Liver dulness commences (absolute) at 5th rib in mammary region and 3rd rib on deep percussion. In axilla at 7th rib, deep at 4th rib. Inferiorly liver reaches nearly to crest of ilium, and extends across front of abdomen. A solid mass extends across the abdomen into the left hypochondrium, reaching to the cartilages of the 10th and 11th ribs, and thence extending in a pyriform shape to within an inch of a line drawn transversely from the anterior superior spinous process of the ilium. A sharp notch can be felt between the right and left portions. (This condition led to the diagnosis of an enlarged spleen meeting the enlarged liver.) Resonance exists in both lumbar regions.

Tongue free from fur; redder than natural. Much thirst. Appetite defective; suffers from nausea. Has had occasional diarrhœa before admission, but not to a marked degree, and has none now. Has pains in the abdomen.

The temperature was, for the most part, taken only in the morning. It was then frequently pyrexial, but did not exceed 102·8°. The more common temperatures ranged from 99° to 100°. The pulse varied from 96 to 120. The respirations, always accelerated, were commonly above 30, and frequently between 40 and 50.

The urine contained albumen, but sometimes only as a trace; the specific gravity varied from 1010 to 1014, and only once reached 1018.

The patient continued to sink, and died on October 13. Hæmoptysis to the extent of 4 oz. occurred three days before death.

POST-MORTEM.—The liver is found to occupy nearly the whole front of the abdomen, extending on the right side superiorly to the fourth rib, reaching on the left side beneath the false ribs to within two finger-breadths of the spinal column, and passing downwards to seven inches below the ensiform cartilage, and within five inches of the pubes.

Lungs.—*Right lung* extends downwards to fifth rib, and across middle line of sternum. Apex adherent to rib, and base to diaphragm.

Left lung (XIX. 2), everywhere adherent, and greatly retracted; measures only five inches by two inches. Thickening of pleura at apex and middle portions ⅔ inch, at base nearly ¼ inch (fig. 2. *c c c*). Tissue of nearly the whole of this lung is converted into a dense fibroid mass. Lobes indistinguishable. At apex is a sinuous cavity, some of the divisions of which reach within two inches of the base, but the greater part measures only two inches in either diameter (fig. 2, *d*). The walls are smooth, and lined by a false membrane, yellow in colour, thick and opaque, but not presenting any special granulations. The whole of the rest of this lung is composed of little else than fibroid tissue enclosing dilated bronchi (*b b*) of the first and second divisions, whose walls and lining membrane are greatly thickened and congested, but not otherwise diseased.

In the lower part of this lung, indistinct traces of pulmonary tissue may be seen, and in these parts are groups of small granulations and some cheesy nodules, surrounded by a semi-transparent zone, but these latter are not common.

Right lung for the most part in condition of hypertrophous emphysema. Adhesions of lobes together only slight. Apex dense and puckered. A large puckered spot in the upper part of lower lobe, and smaller puckerings are scattered over other portions. The larger puckerings are found to correspond to cavities, the smaller to groups of indurated granulations. At extreme apex is a cavity of the size of a Tangerine orange. It is covered by thickened pleura (fig. 1, *b b*). The walls are less smooth than those on the opposite side. It is lined by a caseating membrane, which does not, however, present any distinct granulations. The tissue of the lung generally is emphysematous, and throughout it are scattered, singly or in groups, very small firm hard granulations, most of which are still semi-transparent, very few being cheesy (fig. 1, *a a*), even where collected in racemose groups. The granulations are often smaller than those ordinarily found in such formations. The tissue of the groups is deeply pigmented, and the granulations are surrounded by zones of deep pigmentation. A few cavities are seen here and there, small in size, and opening into ulcerated bronchi. Granulations are densely grouped around these, but on the whole excavations are rare. In a few places large cheesy masses are found, surrounded by much induration, and in some places such spots are softening into pultaceous matter and forming cavities. Lung-tissue stains unduly with iodine, and the staining is more marked in the pulmonary tissue than in the groups of granulations.

Larynx and *Trachea* perfectly healthy. Stain somewhat unduly with iodine.

Heart.—Right auricle dilated; walls of right ventricle firm, crisp, not markedly thickened. Cusps of mitral valve thickened at free border; no shortening or puckering; no atheroma or opacity.

Liver weighs 6 lbs. 4 oz.; presents typical waxy change. Stains intensely with iodine. Spots of fatty degeneration are seen in parts, and in others there is a general opacity with yellow spots.

Kidneys firm, waxy, passing into opaque albuminoid; do not stain with iodine. Weight, collectively, 8 oz.

Supra-renal bodies very firm; cortical substance very pale and firm; do not stain with iodine.

Spleen comparatively soft, but has waxy look, as if this change were commencing; not enlarged; measures 5 × 3 × 1½ inches; weighs 5 oz.

Stomach.—Mucous membrane pale and thin. Solitary glands very distinct. Shows slight iodine-staining.

Intestines.—Solitary glands prominent throughout. Peyer's patches enlarged, hyperæmic: one or two show small patches of ulceration. Mucous membrane throughout small intestine is too pale and transparent, and stains unduly with iodine, especially in the prominent parts of the valvulæ conniventes. In the cæcum and first part of colon are groups of small cheesy nodules beneath the mucous membrane, surrounded by marked hyperæmia. None of them appear to have ulcerated. Solitary glands enlarged throughout colon, but mucous membrane everywhere pale except in the tracts of hyperæmia last described.

Mesenteric glands enlarged and too transparent: show no traces of tubercle: do not stain with iodine.

Tracheal glands indurated, too transparent, full of fine granulations: do not stain with iodine.

MICROSCOPIC EXAMINATION.—The most prevalent changes in this lung are as follows:—

Nodular masses of induration similar to those described in *Overall*, p. 198; *Smith*, see p. 200; *Unwin*, see p. 171; and *Carr*, see p. 204. They present all varieties of indurative and caseous change intermingled: represented in XXXII. 7 and XXXV. 4 (*Smith*), XLI. 1 and 3 (*Carr*), XLI. 5 (*Roberts*), XLI. 7 (*Coppin*), each of which has almost identical analogues in this lung.

The process by which they are formed can be further seen to be by the gradual thickening of the alveolar tissue with a small-celled growth in a lobular form, similar to that seen in XXXIX. 7 (*Unwin*). Adjacent lobules may be seen side by side, some in the early stages of the perialveolar growth, like XL. 1 and 3 (*Heath*); others presenting more fibroid change, passing, in some places, into an almost uniform fibroid tissue, and others fibroid in their margins but caseated in their centres.

The process of this invasion is seen, in XL. 7, to be taking place by means of a nuclear growth in the walls of the capillaries, the outlines of which, in the floor of the alveolus, are still distinct, while the sides are already invaded by a denser infiltration of small-celled growth, thus resembling XL. 8 (*Indurating Tubercle*), and also XL. 9 (*Overall*).

Interspersed between these, are larger areas of small-celled infiltration, like XXXVII. 7 (*Griffin*), and in other parts mingled with more or less pneumonic epithelial proliferation in the interior of the alveoli, like XXXVII. 8 (*Hall*). This small-celled growth also extends through considerable areas, narrowing the lumen of the alveoli and producing appearances similar to XXXVIII. 1 (*Henshaw*), and it also in places passes directly into fibroid induration, like that seen in XLII. 6 (*Hawkins*). The spots of caseation in this lung are almost entirely produced by the lobular nodules just described and none can be ascribed to changes in the bronchi. Nodules of small-celled growth, of the type of the smallest miliary tubercle, also occur.

Giant-cells are very abundant throughout this specimen. They are not uncommon in the centres of the alveoli and the lobules of commencing small-celled growth sometimes contain groups of these 'cells,' one being situated in the centre of each alveolus. They are for the most part of the types of XXXIII. 4 and 11. They are also found in the zones and tracts of induration.

Perivascular and peribronchial thickening are also frequent. This is most apparent in the vessels, and is commonly found in the fibroid form, the orifice of the vessel being much narrowed, and its coats uniform, fused into an almost homogeneous semicartilaginous-looking tissue, like XLII. 7, *a a* (*J. Brown*). The early stages of this can be traced to a small-celled growth in the perivascular sheath and in the coats of the vessels, as seen in XLII. 3 and 4.

The changes in this lung are almost entirely confined to those above described, and the induration is thus seen to result from alveolar changes due to a small-celled growth in their walls, and terminating in fibroid transformation, which, however, also affects the vessels and the bronchial tubes.

CASE 37.

INDURATING TUBERCULISATION.

Plate XX. fig. 1.

SUMMARY.—*M. 27. Phthisis in both parents. Occasional cough and slight hæmoptysis during four years, increasing during the last six months of life, with diarrhœa. A few days before death there were severe cough, extreme dyspnœa, copious expectoration, and considerable pyrexia, with signs of consolidation in both lungs, of excavation at the left apex, and abundant bronchial râles.* —*Tubercles and ulceration of bronchi of the left lung, with peribronchial pneumonic consolidation; yellowish granulations in fibroid tissue at the apex. Similar tissue at the right apex surrounds a series of cavities; below, the lung is crowded with racemose granulations. Ulceration of larynx. Liver tubercular. Ulceration of intestines and bladder.*

ALFRED SCHOFIELD, ætat. 27, admitted University College Hospital March 9; died March 12, 1867.

Family History.—Father died of phthisis, mother died of small-pox and suffered from consumption.

Personal History.—Entered army as drummer-boy, ætat. 15, and left army in 1865; was in India 1863-4: denies syphilis.

Present Illness began on voyage to India in 1863. Got wet through on deck, and began to cough; had repeated rigors, and thick yellow expectoration. Was sent into hospital on board, but was better on arrival in India. Cough returned when on guard at Lucknow; was sent into hospital and remained there two months. Had diarrhœa in India, and ague several times. Left India end of 1864, and was discharged in 1865. Has been a light porter since return, but has suffered much from cough, and has been in Consumption Hospital at Brompton.

Had hæmoptysis with cough on board ship. The blood was mixed with the expectoration, and he never brought up any considerable quantity. Streaks of blood have appeared in his expectoration throughout his illness. He became much worse last October, and has had diarrhœa severely of late. In October a hard swelling appeared in right testicle. Appetite has been bad, and he has suffered much from flatulence after eating.

State on Admission.—Great exhaustion, cyanosis, extreme dyspnœa, relieved by inhalation of chloroform. Frequent cough with coarse râles in throat. Expectoration copious, greenish, tenacious, mingled with blood in streaks and rusty patches. Skin pungently hot, not much perspiration. Temp. 106°, pulse 120, resp. 34.

Chest well-formed. Examination imperfect, owing to weakness of patient. Signs of consolidation over whole left lung, and at right apex and base of excavation under left clavicle. Fine and coarse râles over whole of both sides. He sank and died three days after admission.

POST-MORTEM.—*Larynx:* Commencing ulceration in upper part. This occurs in spots which are not larger than pin's heads. There are also a few scattered cheesy spots and some very small transparent specks.

Lungs.—Both adherent. One bronchus of 3rd division in the upper lobe of the right lung is found obstructed by cheesy matter, the wall being thickened around this. No dilatation of the bronchi, either in upper or lower lobes. In the bronchi of the lower lobe of the left lung are numerous ulcerations, apparently commencing in the mucous membrane (XX. 1). The membrane is eroded, and the edges of the ulcer are elevated and thickened, in some places undermined, in others cheesy (XX. 1, *a*); the ulcerated surface is of a yellowish-grey colour. Around the ulcers are cheesy nodules of the size of a poppyseed or hemp-seed, some only seen through the mucous surface, while others have broken through this, and in some of these, small openings are seen undermining the mucous membrane. These nodules in some places are clustered so thickly as to occupy almost the whole of the surface of the bronchus (XX. 1, *b*). In others, in the immediate neighbourhood, fine granulations of yellow colour and of variable size, down to pin's heads and pin's points, are scattered in the mucous membrane (XX. 1, *c*). The lung-tissue around these is for the most part occupied by a reddish pneumonic exudation, covered with minute yellow spots, and looking as if sprinkled with a yellow sand. In this are numerous orifices of bronchi, the mucous membrane of which is seen to be ulcerated. The greater part of the upper lobe of the left lung is converted into a fibrous cicatricial and deeply pigmented tissue. It is studded with cheesy granulations, and in the walls of some bronchi, where ulceration has not commenced, granulations can be seen of all sizes, from a pin's point to a poppyseed.

In the right lung the bronchi of the upper lobe lead into a series of large cavities, lined by cheesy matter, and surrounded by indurated tissue, which is entirely fibroid, and in which no trace of pulmonary tissue remains. Below this the whole of the right lung, from apex to base, is riddled with granulations clustered in racemose groups, which in some places bear the strongest resemblance to the structure of the parotid gland or pancreas. The tissue in most is indurated and deeply pigmented in the centre, while the greater number of the granulations are more or less cheesy but not softened. The intervening pulmonary tissue is emphysematous, hyperæmic, and contains islets of pneumonia.

The *Bronchial* and *Tracheal Glands* are much enlarged and softened, and contain grey opaque spots, scattered thickly through their tissue; these are as numerous in the cortical as in the medullary substance.

Heart healthy.

Liver studded with tubercular granulations, some grey and semi-transparent, others yellow and cheesy. In the centre of the middle lobe is a puckered cicatrix, which, when cut into, is found to contain some cheesy matter, and suggests a healed abscess.

Kidneys.—Left contains, at lower end of pelvis, a firm cheesy mass, with indurated tissue around. Above this are numerous fine granulations, which in some places have ulcerated. Some granulations are also seen in the substance of the kidney. Right kidney healthy.

Bladder has a spot of ulceration a quarter of an inch in diameter. Both vesiculæ seminales are filled with cheesy matter, solid and firm.

Stomach.—Mucous membrane thickened, and covered with firm mucus; it is opaque and pigmented near pylorus.

Intestines.—Duodenum much congested; Brünner's glands enlarged: some superficial ulcerations having characters of follicular ulceration. Mucous membrane of upper part of ileum pale, but ulcerations commence in upper third. They have the ordinary characters of tubercular ulcers with granulations in their floor and thickened everted edges. The ulcerations are numerous in cæcum, and extend to end of transverse colon. No tubercle in mesenteric glands. Both *Supra-renal Capsules* contain masses of cheesy matter. Right almost entirely degenerated into mingled cheesy and fibroid material.

Spleen and *Brain* healthy.

The preparations of this case put aside for examination were spoiled and could not be utilised.

CASE 38.

POTTER'S PHTHISIS.

Plates XXII. fig. 1; XLIV. figs. 5, 6, and 7.

Ref.—Disease from Inhalation of Dust, p. 56

SUMMARY.—*M. 56. Cough, expectoration, and shortness of breath for some years, increase of symptoms after severe cold, six months before death. During the last days of life, lividity, œdema, purulent expectoration, and signs of consolidation in both lungs, apex and base, with bronchial râles.—Both lungs contained numerous hard, black, fibroid masses, large and small, most numerous at the apices, and mingled with calcification. Bronchi and bronchial glands blackened.*

CHARLES BARLOW,[1] ætat. 56, admitted into North Staffordshire Infirmary, March 5; died March 8, 1867.

Is a hollow-ware presser. Has always been sober. Has suffered from winter cough and palpitation for the past seven years, and of late his breath has been short. Expectoration commenced two years ago. It was at first frothy, then became viscid, and has been purulent during the last few weeks. It has never been black; a few streaks of blood have been seen in it from time to time, but there has never been any larger hæmoptysis.

Present Illness.—Caught a severe cold last October, recovered imperfectly, and relapsed at Christmas. Has kept his bed for some weeks before admission to the infirmary.

Present State.—A pale emaciated man, with dark hair, grey eyes, and sallow complexion. Some lividity; legs swollen, and pit on pressure; abdomen slightly swollen; skin cool. Pulse, 98 jerking; Resp. 32. Cough frequent; sputa copious, purulent, confluent in masses. Chest, deep antero-posterior diameter, flattened in lateral regions. Expansion-movement defective; elevation exaggerated. Percussion-resonance defective under both clavicles, most so under right. Some diffused dulness at both bases, greater at left. Large and small coarse râles heard over whole front of chest. Expiration in right front prolonged and blowing, not on left side. Sibilant râles exist in the lower two-thirds anteriorly on right side. Coarse moist râles at left base posteriorly; a few sibilant moist râles heard at right base. Vocal resonance exaggerated at left apex and base; no bronchophony.

Cardiac dulness nearly normal: apex-beat indistinct; a coarse systolic apex-murmur is present, slightly conducted towards axilla, not towards sternum or base; second sound occasionally reduplicated at base.

Urine scanty and high-coloured, contained a trace of albumen.

He sank rapidly and died on March 8th.

POST-MORTEM.—Only small portions of heart uncovered by lung. In anterior margin of left lung, where it overlaps the heart, are numerous hard nodules.

Heart enlarged, particularly the left auricle, but right auricle also enlarged. Edges of mitral valve puckered; some puckering also of tricuspid valve. Microscopic examination shows some fatty degeneration of muscular tissue of the heart.

Lungs.—Left firmly adherent throughout pleura; emphysematous at anterior margin. Apex almost entirely solidified, and converted into firm fibroid masses, separated from one another by thin lines of condensed pulmonary tissue. These masses are about the size of walnuts, and are very hard and black. Among them are some calcified masses, which also exist, in some parts, in the centres of the fibroid blackened masses, giving them a mottled appearance. No cavity is to be found except in some places where the calcified matter breaks down under the knife. Similar masses exist scattered throughout the lung; they appear to be encapsuled in a firm fibrous tissue, but they cannot be enucleated. They are of variable size; some are no larger than a pea or hemp-seed, but all are intensely black; they stand out prominently from the cut surface of the lung, and are very resistant on section. Bronchi are intensely blackened. No ulceration anywhere. There are black striæ in the pulmonary pleura, wherever this is not adherent to the costal pleura.

The *right lung* presents appearances identical with those described in the left.

The *Bronchial Glands* at the root of the lungs are filled with black matter. One which has softened in the centre is of the size of a walnut, and contains a dark matter, not fatty, but like thick black grease. No black matter can be found within the bronchial tubes, as far as they can be traced.

Liver much congested, and has nutmeg appearance.

Kidney contracted; left contains many cysts, and, under the microscope, shows excess of fibroid tissue, and fatty degeneration of epithelium. *Stomach, Intestines,* and *Brain* healthy.

THE MICROSCOPIC APPEARANCES of this lung were only studied after immersion in spirit, and the cell-structures were therefore not easily investigated.

The indurated parts consisted mainly of two forms of fibroid formation: (a) large tracts, like XLII. 6 (*Hawkins*), but where the central cavity of the alveoli had entirely disappeared, though quasi-alveolar outlines still remained; (b) tracts like XLII. 1, b (*Attwood*), where, however, the spaces between the interlacements of the fibres were filled with pigment, having still the shape of round, ovoid, and fusiform cells, but without any definite cell-wall.

Nodular forms, such as are shown in XLIV. 6, were the most common, but other forms like XLI. 3 and 5 (*Carr and Roberts*) abounded, although they were more densely pigmented than those figured. They tended to become confluent, and to form large tracts, some of which closely resembled XLI. 1 (*Carr*), but with the addition of intense pigmentation. Other nodules were almost completely solid and fibroid (as in XLIV. 5), but these also showed an alveolar origin.

It was difficult to trace the earlier stages of these changes, partly from the mode of preparation, partly from the intense pigmentation, which rendered many tracts absolutely opaque and black. The following characteristics could, however, be made out. Pneumonic alveoli were seen, filled with enlarged epithelial cells rendered almost black with pigment. These tracts tended to a nuclear thickening of their walls, as seen in XLIV. 7, which in many places resembled XXX. 5 (*Acute Tubercle*) and XXXVII. 6 (*Griffin*). In a few places, nodular masses could be made out like XXVIII. 7 (*Acute Tubercle*). There was great periarterial and peribronchial fibroid thickening, and there were dense accumulations of pigment around the bronchi.

CASE 38A.

I append the description of the lung in another case, from a potter, in which I was prevented, by an accident to the preparation, from making a microscopic examination of the changes present.

Right lung highly emphysematous. It contains, at the apex, a large cavity filled with a thick creamy

---

[1] This case and the following have been published by Dr. Charles Parsons of Dover, in his Thesis which obtained the Gold Medal of the University of Edinburgh in 1864 'On a form of Bronchitis simulating Phthisis which is peculiar to certain branches of the Potting Trade.'

F F

pus. Throughout the lung are scattered black masses, firm on section, and are mingled with very firm white, opaque spots, projecting above the cut surface. The black masses are of an irregular shape and size; some are as large as a walnut, others as a Maltese orange. Section of the whitish masses is gritty, that of the black is smooth, and these are less elevated above the surrounding tissue than the white. The white spots are nowhere larger than millet-seeds. Several small cavities are found in the middle and lower lobes. They are all simple; some are crossed by trabeculæ, but they do not intercommunicate. The left lung has the same character, but to a less extent; near its base and root is an area three inches in diameter, filled with rough granular spots like those before described, but much more free from colouring matter.

Heart and *abdominal viscera* healthy.

This patient was a potter, ætat. 35, who inherited asthma, and had been short-breathed all his life. He had never had any severe illness, but his dyspnœa had increased much of late, and he had lost flesh greatly. The physical signs were those of emphysema, with consolidation and excavation at the apices, and disseminated moist râles throughout the lungs.

CASE 39.

MINER'S PHTHISIS.

Plate XXII. fig. 2; XLIV. fig. 3.

Dr. E. Headlam Greenhow, *Transactions of the Pathological Society*, vol. xx. p. 41, and Plates II. fig. 1; III. fig. 1.

'I am indebted to Mr. Thomas Underhill, of
' Tipton, in Staffordshire, for the specimens exhi-
' bited to the Society. They were taken from the
' body of a man aged about sixty-five, who had worked
' in a coal-mine from boyhood. At the time of his
' death he had been incapacitated from work for
' two years, during which time he had suffered from
' cough and shortness of breath, with occasional
' attacks of what was called bronchitic asthma. He
' had only come under the care of Mr. Underhill a
' month before his death, and was then much ema-
' ciated; but with the exception of dulness on per-
' cussion below the clavicles, he presented none of
' the ordinary symptoms of phthisis. About ten
' days before death he suddenly spat up a considerable
' quantity of sputum closely resembling black paint,
' and continued doing so to the amount of four or
' five ounces daily until he died. He sank at last
' very rapidly.

'The lungs, on being incised, exuded a large
' quantity of thick fluid containing amorphous black
' pigment. The spirit in which they were placed for
' preservation very soon had the appearance of being
' mixed with soot, and on boiling a portion of it with
' an equal quantity of strong nitric acid the colour
' underwent no change. Another portion, evaporated
' to dryness, left a black sooty-looking deposit upon
' the walls of the test-tube, and at the bottom of the
' tube a small amount of brownish deposit, which
' burnt with a strong smell of animal matter. The
' sooty-looking deposit, when boiled for a considerable
' time in a mixture of strong nitric and hydrochloric
' acids, underwent no perceptible change, and on being

' allowed to settle remained, in the form of minute
' black granules at the bottom of the tube.

'The upper part of the right lung had been firmly
' adherent to the parietes of the thorax posteriorly;
' it was generally of a black colour. The pleura was
' everywhere thickened, and presented in several
' places smooth yellowish-white patches, one of which
' formed a sort of hood, as it were, over the apex of
' the lung, and was about a tenth of an inch in thick-
' ness, presenting, on section, a dense white appear-
' ance. The apex of the lung was solidified into a
' firm mass, somewhat larger than a walnut, cutting
' with a smooth section, and perfectly dry, and look-
' ing, when cut across, not unlike a piece of black
' india-rubber' (XXII. 2, c). 'Immediately below this
' mass of condensed lung was a large, irregular,
' ragged cavity, containing a quantity of black pulpy
' débris, in the midst of which was a detached piece
' of lung the size of a hazel-nut. A smaller con-
' densed mass was situated at the root of the lung,
' identical in character with the larger one at the
' apex; the remainder of the lung was also perfectly
' black on section, but for the most part of a spongy
' texture. Many of the bronchial tubes appeared to
' be dilated and thickened, and their mucous surfaces
' injected; they mostly contain mucus blackened
' by intermixture with pigment. The bronchial
' glands were enlarged, dense, and perfectly black,
' and exuded, when incised, an abundance of black
' fluid, which stained everything with which it came
' in contact. The general appearance of the lung,
' when recently divided across from the apex down-
' wards, is well shown in the accompanying drawing'
' (XXII. 2), ' but the consolidated apex looks duller and
' less glistening, and the hue of the whole lung less
' perfectly black than in the fresh specimen.

'The left lung contained a solid mass occupying
' the greater part of its centre, and closely resembling
' the condensed portion at the apex of the right lung,
' being perfectly black, smooth, and dry on section,
' and presenting to the naked eye no trace of lung-
' tissue. This mass was sharply circumscribed, and
' was entirely surrounded by a layer of spongy inelas-
' tic lung-tissue, also nearly black in colour; the
' spongy layer exhibited, on section, dilated air-cells,
' and much resembled the lung-tissue of senile emphy-
' sema; scattered through this spongy portion were
' several opaque, greyish-yellow, solid nodules, from
' the size of a hemp-seed to that of a pea. The pleura
' corresponding to the solid mass was thickened, but
' moved freely over it in consequence of the layer of
' the spongy lung-tissue intervening between them.

'Sections taken from the most densely consoli-
' dated portions of either lung showed, under the
' microscope, only an abundance of black pigment
' arranged in masses and granules, greatly obscuring
' the natural tissue, which was so compressed that no
' definite normal structure could be seen in it. Sec-
' tions taken from the somewhat less dense parts of
' the mass, in the centre of the left lung, presented
' fibrous tracts, containing curved elastic fibres thickly
' studded with masses of black pigment, and repre-
' senting, probably, collapsed lung-tissue. In other
' sections, taken from the borders of the condensed
' part of the lung, the walls of the air-cells were seen
' to be considerably thickened, and to contain much
' black pigment, generally arranged in masses and
' granules, as seen in the drawing' (XLIV. 3). 'Black
' pigment is also seen, apparently contained in

'cells, lying loose in the air-cell cavities; these sections were intersected by fibrillated tracts, closely set with elongated nuclei, which in some places passed into and were continuous with the walls of the air-cells. In the spongy portion of the lung-tissue, the air-cells themselves were in many places blocked up with exudation-cells. The pleura was seen under the microscope to be much thickened; it contained a distinct layer of pigment-deposit immediately below the surface, and presented here and there, on its free surface, distinct small projections, or nodules, loaded with black pigment. Black pigment, in the form of granules, was seen under the microscope, pouring freely from sections of the lungs immersed in glycerine.

'A small portion of one of the lungs, having been first dried at a gentle heat, was incinerated in a porcelain crucible over a gas-jet for upwards of three hours, when it left nearly thirteen per cent. of ash of a yellowish-brown colour. On boiling this ash in nitro-hydrochloric acid for upwards of an hour the greater part of it dissolved, but there remained an insoluble residue, which on being exposed in a covered platinum vessel to the fumes of hydrochloric acid, was entirely dissipated. Two separate experiments gave the following proportions as the result of these processes: One hundred grains of dried lung left after complete incineration 12·92 grains of ash, and this ash on being boiled in the mixed acids left four grains of insoluble residue. Under the microscope this residue did not polarise light. The acid liquor contained abundance of iron and alumina.

'*Remarks*.—The specimens afford an unusually striking illustration of the condition of the lungs in fully developed cases of the disease known as "collier's phthisis." The history of the present case resembles in its main features that of a French millstone-maker, who died under my care in the Middlesex Hospital in the year 1865[1]; the more universal and intense discolouration of the lungs in this case being accounted for by the different atmosphere in which the man had passed his working life. The disease had, no doubt, been primarily chronic bronchitis, excited by the inhalation of grit, but, by degrees, the substance of the lungs had become affected, probably from the penetration of grit into their tissues, and the morbid condition termed by Rokitansky "interstitial pneumonia" had been induced. The formation of the consolidated masses in the lungs, and the general black pigmentation of the lung-tissue, must have been very slow processes, going on insidiously long before the man was disabled from work. His last illness appears to have arisen from an accession of pneumonia, causing the blocking up of a large portion of the still pervious air-cells with the inflammatory deposit seen on microscopical examination.'

CASE 40.

DISEASE OF LUNGS IN COPPER MINER.

Plate XLIV. fig. 4.

Dr. Greenhow, *Transactions of the Pathological Society*, vol. xx. 1869, p. 47, and Plate III. fig. 4.

[1] See 'Pathological Transactions,' vol. xvii. p. 24.

'The lung was both externally and internally of a deep black colour, and exuded when fresh a black fluid resembling Indian ink, and full of minute black granules. The pleura was somewhat thickened and opaque, and a distinct tract of black pigment was deposited in the subpleural connective tissue. The lung was dense in texture, but still contained air and just floated in water. It cut with a smooth section.

'On examination of thin sections of the lung under the microscope, the walls of the air-vesicles were seen to be thickened, and to contain numerous deposits of black pigment disposed in masses and granules. Many cells containing black granules were found lying loose in the cavities of the air-vesicles, some of them well-defined, and others apparently surrounded by granules of free pigment. The accompanying drawing by Mr. Henry Arnott' (XLIV. 4) 'represents a section of the lung as seen under the microscope. It was selected with the view of showing the arrangement of the tract of pigment in the thickened pleura.'

CASE 41.

DISEASE OF LUNG IN A FLAX-DRESSER.

Plate XLIV. figs. 1 and 2.

Dr. Greenhow, *Transactions of the Pathological Society*, vol. xx. 1869, p. 49, and Plate III. figs. 6 and 7.

'This specimen was taken from the body of a man aged 43, who died in the Leeds Infirmary under Dr. Clifford Allbutt's care in 1868. He had worked as a flax-dresser from early life, and for some time at the inferior kinds of flax, which are the most dusty. He twice discontinued his employment, for a period on each occasion of two years. During the first of these intervals he appeared to recover his health entirely, and during the second he improved very much. Being obliged to return to work in order to keep himself and his family, his pulmonary complaint on each occasion returned also, and he eventually died of it.

'POST-MORTEM.—The right lung (that exhibited) had evidently been adherent, posteriorly and laterally, to the parietes of the thorax. The pleura, where not adherent, was thickened and opaque. The anterior border of the lung was elastic and emphysematous, but with this exception the whole organ from the apex to the base was much consolidated. On making a section through the lower and more consolidated lobe, the surface of the section, for about two inches from the pleura, was granular and of a red colour, intermixed with black. Towards the centre of the lung the tissue was crepitant, and contained much more black pigment. The surface of the section in the granular part presented numerous minute orifices, which, under the microscope, were seen to consist of dilated and broken-down air-cells. This appearance was probably due to their having been emptied of the exudation with which the neighbouring air-cells were filled, by the washing of the spirit in which the specimen was kept. The walls of the air-cells appeared thickened, and contained masses of black pigment, and their cavities generally were filled up with exudation-cells, one of which contained black granules. In

'the consolidated part the branches of the pulmonary
'artery were plugged. The minuter branches of the
'bronchial tubes stood out from the surface of the
'section with unusual prominence, and appeared
'thickened. The emphysematous portion near the
'anterior margin was more deeply pigmented than
'the consolidated part. Sections taken from the
'dark crepitant portion towards the centre of the
'lung, examined under the microscope, showed abun-
'dant deposits of black pigment in the interstitial
'tissue. These deposits were usually in masses, con-
'sisting apparently of agglomerations of small
'granules; but the adjacent tissue, and even the air-
'cells, usually contained granular cells, more or less
'completely filled with black pigment in free granules
'or larger masses. The deposits of pigment in the
'lung-tissue were sometimes arranged in the form of
'tracts, which appeared to follow the course of blood-
'vessels, but more frequently the pigment seemed
'to be deposited around the minute bronchial tubes.
'The granular pigmented cells found in the air-cells
'were of various sizes, from the $\frac{1}{2500}$ to the $\frac{1}{1000}$ of
'an inch in diameter. Sometimes they lay singly,
'at others in groups of ten or twelve together, and
'were generally round, but sometimes only irre-
'gularly roundish in shape. In some of the sections,
'ciliated columnar cells, containing black pigment,
'were also found lying loose in the interstices of the
'section.

'The accompanying drawing by Mr. Henry Ar-
'nott' (XLIV. 2) 'exactly represents a section of the
'lung containing a small bronchial tube surrounded
'by masses of black pigment. The adjacent tissue
'is crowded with granular cells, many of which also
'contain pigment. Some of these pigmented cells
'were also seen lying loose in the bronchial tubes,
'but were not distinctly visible at the same focus as
'the parts represented in the drawing. A few of the
'pigmented cells, both of the round and ciliated forms
'as seen under a higher power, are also drawn to scale
'on the same paper' (XLIV. 1).

'A portion of this lung was incinerated and
'treated in the manner described in the previous
'case. The experiment yielded the following results:
'One hundred grains of dried lung left 2·609 grains
'of ash, of which 2·139 grains were dissolved by
'boiling in the acids; the insoluble residue, amount-
'ing to 0·47 of a grain, was amorphous, and entirely
'dissipated on exposure to the fumes of hydrochloric
'acid: the acid liquid contained both alumina and
'iron.'

CASE 42.

SIDEROSIS PULMONUM.

Plate XLIV. figs. 8 and 9.

Ref.—Disease from Inhalation of Dust, pp. 54, 55.

(Dr. F. A. Zenker, from vol. ii. of the *Deutsches Archiv für Klinische Medicin*, somewhat abridged from the original.)

SUMMARY.—F. 31. Occupation, colouring blotting paper with oxide of iron. Cough and shortness of breath commenced two years before death, followed by signs of bronchitis. The sputa contained red streaks. Later, there was weak breathing under the left clavicle, together with dyspnœa, œdema of limbs, ascites, and the signs of double pleural effusion.—Lungs coloured brick-red (from oxide of iron) and contained cavities with friable red and grey walls, and also numerous nodules, 'yellowish-grey with specks of red, situated on the smaller bronchi. Bronchial glands enlarged, reddened at the periphery. Kidneys indurated. Traces of past peritonitis.

'MARIE FRANK, ætat. 31, admitted into the 'Nuremberg Hospital January 19; died January 30, '1864.'

'*Previous History.*—Patient was healthy in child-
'hood, although never strong. Up to the age of 20,
'she worked in a charcoal manufactory, where she
'had fair health and never suffered from chest
'affection. She has had some children, the last two
'years ago. She has worked seven years at her
'present occupation, at which she continued until
'shortly before her death.

'(Her last occupation consisted in the prepara-
'tion of the small books of blotting-paper in which
'fine leaf-gold is kept. Four women are thus
'employed. The room where the colouring is pre-
'pared is very small. There is no special ventilation,
'but if the dust is too unpleasant the window is
'opened; if, however, this is closed, the dust is very
'thick, so that not only are walls and tables covered,
'but the air appears coloured by it, and the mouth of
'anyone not accustomed to it becomes dry in a few
'minutes. In the rooms where the binding takes
'place there is also dust, but the air can be breathed
'without difficulty. In these rooms the whole day is
'spent, and the meals are also taken without any
'preventive against the inhalation of the dust.
'The manipulation of the colouring matter consists
'in rubbing the finely pulverised powder in a dry
'state into the paper by means of felt until the paper
'is impregnated with it.)

'None of the workers, of whom inquiry was made,
'complained of suffering in the chest. Their mouths,
'however, are always filled with dust, and their saliva
'is coloured red. Arrangements exist by which they
'can clean themselves when they leave the works,
'but these appear to be seldom used. Patient had
'worked in two of these manufactories, chiefly in the
'colouring of paper. The first signs of her illness
'appeared about eighteen months ago, in obstinate
'cough and shortness of breath, but she continued
'her work up to Christmas 1863, when she was com-
'pelled to leave by shortness of breath.

'*State on Admission.*—Ill-nourished, pallid, with
'some lividity of face. Able to leave bed. No rise
'of temperature; pulse frequent and small. Nervous
'system healthy. Good appetite; some constipation;
'occasional abdominal pain. Menses regular. Re-
'spiration short. Chest well-formed; some sinking
'of the left infraclavicular region, but otherwise
'movements are equal. Heart's apex in normal site;
'dulness and sounds normal. Percussion-resonance
'everywhere equal. Some diminution of respiratory
'murmur under left clavicle. Sonorous rhonchus in
'different parts of the chest. Liver-dulness normal.
'Cough moderate, worst in the morning. Sputa
'scanty and nearly homogeneous, mucoid; in it are
'some small red streaks like blood.

'The patient's state showed very little change,
'except some improvement in the cough, until
'January 24. On this day œdema was observed in the

'feet and ankles. This extended to the legs and was
'painless. Dyspnœa and cyanosis came on, with in-
'creased dulness, diminished respiration, and ab-
'sence of vocal fremitus at the bases of the lungs, ex-
'tending quickly to the lower end of the scapula.
'Ascites appeared, but was not extreme. The sputa
'in the last days of life became puriform and nummu-
'lated. Death took place on January 30.

'POST-MORTEM.—*Heart* flabby, right ventricle
'dilated, valves normal.
'*Abdomen.*—Moderate amount of clear serum in
'abdominal cavity. Some thickening of capsules of
'liver and spleen. Numerous adhesions between the
'coils of intestines, and of these to the abdominal wall.
'In the mesentery, mesocolon, and broad ligaments,
'are numerous small spots with chalky contents.
'(Nothing could be learned regarding the history of
'this past attack of peritonitis.) *Liver* normal.
'*Spleen* flaccid and friable. *Kidneys* indurated;
'cortical substance yellow, but of normal extent.
'*Uterus* adherent to neighbouring organs. (No other
'changes of importance.)

'*Lungs.*—Clear serum in the pleural cavities.
'Both lungs covered with fibrous false membranes and
'bands. After their removal, the surface of the lung
'has an intense uniform brick-red colour; here and
'there on the red ground are black lines, marking out
'the interstices of the lobules. The fibroid thickening
'also presents, on its pleural surface, in patches of
'considerable extent, an intense brick-red colour.
'In some places, particularly on the right middle lobe,
'the surface is coarsely uneven, partly in consequence
'of the prominence of some nodules from retraction of
'their septa, and partly from nodules to be hereafter
'described.

'On section, the whole of the still remaining
'pulmonary tissue is uniformly coloured of an in-
'tense brick-red. The colour does, indeed, appear, on
'minute inspection, as a uniform, finely cellular, red
'network, in which the lobular septa in many places
'appear as fine red bands, enclosing wide polygonal
'meshes; so that, even to the naked eye, the red
'colour can be recognised as existing in the pulmonary
'tissue itself. The bronchi also contain some of the
'colouring matter, which exudes as a turbid brick-red
'fluid from the surface of the section. Throughout
'the lobes of both lungs are scattered numerous oc-
'cluded nodules. They vary from the size of a pin's
'head to a pen, or larger; the latter are of irregular
'outline. They are very tough; their section is of a
'yellowish-grey colour, sprinkled with specks of a brick-
'red, and to a less degree with black spots. While some
'of these nodules appear on section to be uniformly
'solid, others have in their centre small openings,
'(in the larger masses there may be several such)
'which appear to be the lumina of the finest bronchial
'ramifications, though their connection with the larger
'bronchi could not be demonstrated. The apices of
'both lungs are occupied by densely crowded nodules
'of this nature, and in the left also there is a dense
'black fibroid mass, from one-third of an inch to an
'inch in thickness, in which only a couple of red-
'brick points can be seen. No recent tubercle could
'be found in the pulmonary tissue.

'All the lobes, except the right middle one, con-
'tain large and small irregular loculated cavities.
'The largest of these occupies the upper half of the
'otherwise somewhat contracted right lower lobe.

'It is traversed by numerous bands, and its wall is
'tolerably smooth and lined by a loose yellowish-
'grey stratum, covered with masses of detritus, some
'of which are of a brick-red colour. In both upper lobes,
'beneath the cicatricial masses, and in the left lower
'lobe, are smaller cavities, varying in size from a
'hazel-nut to a cherry, the irregular walls of which
'are covered with friable masses, some of a pale
'yellowish-grey, and some of a brick-red colour.

'The walls of the larger arteries and veins
'within the pulmonary tissue are always uncoloured.
'The larger bronchi, though containing some brick-
'red mucus in their interior, show none of this colour
'in their inner lining or in the thickness of their
'walls. On the other hand, in the smallest bronchi
'which can be followed by the scissors, there are
'numerous confluent brick-red spots on the inner
'surface, which, as seen on perpendicular section,
'are formed by a dense granular deposit in the
'deeper strata of the tissue, while the more super-
'ficial layers remain uncoloured. In thickness and
'in other characters no deviation from the normal is
'observable in the walls of the bronchi, as far as
'these can be traced.

'The bronchial glands at the root of both lungs
'are of about the natural size. Their centre is
'mostly black, while their periphery is of an in-
'tense brick-red. Spots of this colour are also seen
'scattered in the blackened parts.

'The chemical examination of the lung, under-
'taken by Prof. Gorup-Besanez, showed that the red
'colour was due to enormous quantities of oxide of
'iron. 1000 parts of the lung contained 14·5 parts
'of oxide of iron soluble in dilute hydrochloric acid.
'A specimen of the colouring powder in which the
'patient had worked proved to be a finely pulverised
'oxide of iron known as "English red." The colour of
'this powder exactly resembled that of the lung. The
'weight of the right lung was 27 oz. 82 grains. The
'estimated weight of the two lungs was 52 oz. 392
'grains.[1]

'The amount of oxide of iron contained in the
'two lungs was estimated therefore at from 323 to 338
'grains. The specific gravity was 1065, while that of
'normal lungs is from 1015 to 1025.[2]

'MICROSCOPIC EXAMINATION showed that the
'colouring matters were situated partly in the air-
'passages, but chiefly in the pulmonary tissue
'itself.

'The turbid fluid from the section of the alveoli
'and bronchioles showed, as its chief constituent,
'enormous quantities of granular cells and granular
'masses, of $\frac{1}{500}$ inch to $\frac{1}{1000}$ inch diameter, the
'smaller ones for the most part regularly globular,
'the larger irregularly round, ovoid, &c. The granules
'constituting these masses, brick-red by reflected and
'of a dull brown colour by transmitted light, were
'recognised as oxide of iron, and gave a distinct pre-
'cipitate of prussian blue when treated with hydro-
'chloric acid and ferrocyanide of potassium. The
'isolated granules, measuring $\frac{1}{5000}$ inch and less,
'had a clear centre and still recognisable colour.
'(The granules of the pigment used by the patient had

[1] Weight of normal lungs collectively, quoted by
Zenker from Krause and Dieberg, 36 oz. 454 grains
87 ozs. 325 grains.
[2] For numerous details on these points I would refer
to Zenker's paper.

'the same characteristics.) The contours of the
'granule-cells were more or less well-defined. A
'nucleus could not be recognised in the majority,
'but some showed a round or oval space corre-
'sponding to a nucleus. The cellular nature of these
'granule-cells was still further evidenced by the not
'very numerous small nucleated, irregular, flat,
'epithelial cells of about $\frac{1}{3500}$ inch diameter, which
'contained only a few iron granules, and were mani-
'festly the source of the granule-cells' (see XLIV.
'9). 'Other epithelial cells resembling these, and
'some ciliated cells, were free from iron granules.
'Isolated iron granules were singularly rare. Diffuse
'coloured cells and black granule-cells were not
'present.

'Sections, made from the lung hardened in spirit,
'and brushed out in water, show an intense brick-
'red colour. They are traversed by straight, broad,
'red lines of uneven thickness, the lobular septa,
'which intercommunicate and divide the lung into
'polygonal areas, having from four to six angles,
'an appearance best seen in sections made parallel
'to the surface. Within these larger spaces the
'normal network is delicately stretched. Its wider
'trabeculæ are also coloured red, and at their points
'of intersection are markedly thickened, while the
'finest bands are in some cases free from colour.
'Sections made vertically to the pleura show, in
'their deepest part, a broad space of tissue of a deep
'red colour, which passes directly into the similarly
'stained interstitial tissue of the lung, while exter-
'nally it merges by an ill-defined border into the
'outer uncoloured pleural layer. Microscopic inves-
'tigation shows that the colour of the tissue is due
'to more or less dense infiltration into it of granules,
'which, in size and other qualities, precisely cor-
'respond to the iron granules already described as
'found in the granule-cells of the air-passages' (see
'XLIV. 8). 'They are most dense in the lobular and
'infundibular septa, where they accumulate in com-
'pact opaque masses, which conceal all the other
'elements of the tissue. These septa form greatly
'thickened bands, which at their intersections con-
'stitute uneven opaque masses, sometimes larger than
'one or more sections of the alveoli. Where the
'deposit is less thick, the iron granules are imbedded
'in the tissue in little round or elongated masses,
'looking as if enclosed in cells, and this impression
'is confirmed by the appearance in them of small
'spaces corresponding to a nucleus in position. In
'the pleura, and also in the fibroid nodules, these
'accumulations of granulations are very commonly
'spindle-shaped.

'The alveolar septa are also in part thickly per-
'meated with granules of iron. They then form
'thick and shapeless bands, by which the cavities
'of the alveoli are narrowed and their structure
'concealed, and in which the iron infiltration extends
'to the edge of the alveolus. In other places, only
'scattered isolated iron granules are sprinkled in the
'otherwise unchanged tissue of the alveolar septa, and
'other parts again are entirely free from them. Es-
'pecially, the innermost stratum of the alveolar
'wall, except in the before-mentioned densely in-
'filtrated parts, is almost entirely free from granules,
'and so also are the capillary loops, where these
'are visible. No epithelium was present *in situ*.
'Here and there were seen irregular spots of black
'pigment of variable size in the midst of the red dis-

'colouration, but it was small in amount in propor-
'tion to the age of the patient.

'The adventitia of the fine bronchi shows for the
'most part a dense opaque iron infiltration, from
'which the remainder of the wall is entirely free;
'only in the finest branches which can be followed
'by the scissors does the iron infiltration extend into
'the deeper layers of the mucous membrane, and
'here under the membrane were granules with
'radiating striæ and blue colour (manifestly phos-
'phate of iron—vivianite), of which it is unknown
'whether they were present in the fresh specimen.
'Granular appearances of this kind were found in
'other preparations.

'The cicatricial nodules of the lung-tissue had
'throughout the structure of hard, tough, connective
'tissue, which, after acetic acid, was seen to be com-
'posed of very small spindle-shaped elements, many
'of which contained distinct nuclei. Some
'through considerable areas showed fine uncoloured
'granules (fat), and others, which corresponded to the
'red specks on the surface, contained iron granules.
'Here and there, in a long streak in the middle of
'such a granule, was seen the still unchanged wall
'of an apparently obliterated vessel. The small
'openings, seen by the naked eye, had an irregular
'shape and no special layer of limitation, the con-
'nective tissue reaching to the edge of the opening.
'They cannot, therefore, be shown, by microscopic
'examination, to be sections of bronchi.'

CASE 43.

PULMONARY INDURATION IN HEART DISEASE.

Plates XXII. figs. 3 and 4; XLIV. figs. 10 and 11.

SUMMARY.—*M. 10. Cough and dyspnœa commenced after a chill a year before death; subsequently some hæmoptysis occurred. A month before
death, there were systolic and diastolic murmurs, the
latter loudest at the apex, and signs of pleurisy and
of imperfect consolidation in the left lung; moderate
pyrexia.—Constriction of mitral and aortic orifices.
Both lungs contained numerous spots of brown consolidation, and in the left lung minute red mottled
spots were seen. The lower part of the left lung was
collapsed.*

WILLIAM THOMAS, ætat. 10, admitted University
College Hospital December 19, 1864, died January
27, 1865.

Family History presents nothing remarkable.
Personal History.—Has had measles, whooping-
cough, and small-pox.
Present Illness commenced with a cough twelve
months ago, caused by being twice thrown into
water by other boys and being kept all day in wet
clothes; the cough has continued up to present time,
attended with expectoration. He had some hæmoptysis fourteen days ago, amount uncertain, chiefly mixed
with sputa, bright in colour, but some clots were
also present. Has suffered from dyspnœa throughout illness. Has had pains in joints shortly before
admission. Palpitation felt during last three weeks.
State on Admission.—Emaciation; pallor; no
lividity. Cough frequent, with scanty, glairy expectoration. Dyspnœa on slightest exertion. Resp. 54;
pulse, 132. Some bulging in præcordial region

Heart's apex in 5th interspace, two finger-breadths outside vertical nipple line, but extends to 6th rib and 7th interspace, and also to right edge of sternum. Dulness extends inferiorly to upper border of third rib. Coarse cardiac friction heard over base of heart. At apex is a loud systolic murmur, heard also over greater part of cardiac region. A diastolic murmur is likewise heard, having its maximum at left apex, but also audible with great intensity over the whole cardiac region.

Over the right lung there is a good resonance in front to the 6th rib in mammary region, and 8th rib in axilla. At back, good resonance throughout. Respiration, right side, healthy throughout front, but exaggerated. Some sibilant râles heard in upper scapular region, and moist râles in lower third of right back. On the left side, there is tubular percussion-note under clavicle; absolute dulness below 3rd rib; whole axilla dull. Upper scapular region hyperresonant, almost tympanitic. Base posteriorly absolutely dull below middle third of scapula. Under left clavicle, respiration is harsh, with sibilant râles; it is almost inaudible below the 4th rib, where there is coarse friction. In left upper back, respiration harsh with sibilant râles. It becomes tubular in middle third of scapula, with coarse moist râles. Highpitched bronchophony to extreme base on this side. Vocal fremitus suppressed below angle of scapula. Right side measures $11\frac{6}{8}$ inches, left 12 inches, at level of nipple. Left side tender. Tongue furred. No nausea: no diarrhœa; bowels regular. Urine, no albumen.

The dulness in the left back diminished somewhat in area, but tubular breathing and coarse râles persisted at the left base. Some coarse and fine râles became more distinct at right base posteriorly. He was febrile, with a temperature varying from 100° to 102°, the evening temperatures being almost constantly higher than those of the morning. (The temperature was not taken regularly.) He improved for a time, but in January he caught a fresh chill. The dilatation of the heart increased, ascites set in, and he died on January 27.

POST-MORTEM.—Left lung universally adherent, right lung only by loose adhesions at base. Pericardium universally adherent.

Heart.—Right side of heart dilated, both auricle and ventricle; walls thicker than natural. Mitral orifice contracted; barely admits tips of two fingers. Left auricle greatly dilated. Mitral valve contracted; flaps roughened, thickened, and puckered; chordæ tendineæ much shortened. On flaps of valve are semi-transparent granulations, and at base of some prominent granulations is a punctiform vascularity. Aortic orifice admits tip of little finger; valves somewhat too opaque, but otherwise healthy. Left ventricle, walls greatly thickened; muscular tissue shows in places mottling of fatty degeneration (fibres found under microscope to contain fat-granules).

Lungs.—Left base covered by recent lymph. Upper lobe œdematous. Lower lobe collapsed and solid, very tough; fracture less granular than that of pneumonia. Upper third of this lobe is of dull purple tint, carnified, tough; lower two-thirds are brighter in colour, solid, resisting, and yet breaking down under pressure. The tissue presents a peculiar appearance of a bright-red ground, mottled with slightly prominent specks of reddish-white, which are very thickly scattered over the whole of this part of the lung. The specks are from a pin's point to a pin's head in size, the intervening spaces being only about $\frac{1}{2}$ to $\frac{1}{4}$ of a line in diameter (see XXII. 4). Scattered through the upper lobe, and also through the whole of the right lung, are a number of spots of about $\frac{1}{4}$ inch in diameter, where the pulmonary tissue is indurated but still contains air. They are of a dull red colour, with tolerably sharply defined outlines, and have no resemblance whatever to the ordinary hæmorrhagic infarct. (There is also no resemblance to this in the base of the left lung, before described.) Besides these spots, which have well-marked characters, smaller ones, blending more with the pulmonary tissue, and probably presenting an earlier stage of the foregoing, are scattered thickly over the surface of the lung. With these exceptions, the general colour of the pulmonary tissue in the right lung is of a greyish tint, and it is not much pigmented (see XXII. 3). At the lower margin of the middle lobe of this lung is a spot of about two inches in diameter, corresponding in characters with the dense, indurated part in the other lung.

Liver.—Marked nutmeg character. *Kidneys* indurated.

THE MICROSCOPIC APPEARANCES in these lungs are shown in XLIV. figs. 10 and 11.

The walls of the alveoli are thickened with fibroid tissue, but differ from the thickenings of phthisis in the absence of small-celled growth, and in the more finely fibroid character of this thickening. In the walls, the capillaries are seen to be distended, and their walls are much thickened. The walls of the alveoli also contain pigmented nuclei (XLIV. 10, *b*). Within the alveoli are large and pigmented epithelial cells. Some of them are still deeply coloured with blood-pigment; in others this has become black and has assumed the form of granules, and occasionally of crystals.

In some places, great thickening of the arterial coats with fibroid tissue is observed. Similar thickening occurs around the veins, and in some places this thickening, instead of being fibrillated, is homogeneous, giving the coats a semi-cartilaginous appearance.

CASE 44.

EMPHYSEMA OF LUNG.

Plate XXI. fig. 1.

From a drawing by Sir Robert Carswell; University College Museum. Catalogue $\frac{Cb}{80}$.

'Pulmonary Emphysema. Fibro-cartilaginous
'cyst containing cretaceous matter.

'Figs. 1 and 2' (only fig. 2 here given, at XXII. 1)
'represent the summits of both lungs taken from a
'man who died from inflammation and suppuration
'of the prostate gland and kidneys.

'The left summit presented a great number of
'emphysematous vesicles varying from the size of a
'pea to that of a hen's egg; only one of them was of
'the latter size. It was pediculated, and presented
'numerous swellings, as if it had at one time been
'formed of many dilated cells, the sides of which had
'been ruptured, and a communication formed be-
'tween them, by which one common cell-vesicle was
'ultimately formed. This progress may be seen in

'the smaller groups of dilated cells which occupy the
'summit. Their multilocular structure is apparent,
'and it is probable that each group was formed of
'dilated cells not yet ruptured, although I did not
'ascertain this point, as the pieces were put in spirits.
'The large vesicle was very vascular; numerous large
'vessels could be seen ramifying upon its surface,
'both veins and arteries, these having acquired a
'magnitude proportioned to the dilatation of the air-
'cells. In the other portions of the lungs, a similar
'state existed, but less in degree. The lungs were
'gorged with serosity, contained a quantity of black
'pulmonary matter, and here and there small quan-
'tities of cretaceous or earthy matter in both lobes.
'Some of these were surrounded by fibro-cartilaginous
'substance, of considerable consistence. One of
'these was about half-an-inch in diameter, nearly
'round, formed of three substances : the outer, fibro-
'cartilaginous, of a greyish-yellow colour and nearly
'the one-eighth of an inch in thickness ; a central por-
'tion of about the size of a pea, of a firm cretaceous
'substance of a greyish colour; and a middle coat,
'nearly of the same colour as the outer, but less
'dense and fibrous.

'In one or two points there were bodies which
'resembled crude tubercles, and also pneumonic
'portions about the size of a common pea or larger,
'some of which contained small collections of pus.'

It is apparent, from Sir R. Carswell's account,
that this was a case of atrophous emphysema in an
elderly person, occurring subsequently to retrograded
phthisis.

CASE 45.

SECONDARY CANCER OF THE LUNG.

Plates XXII. fig. 5 ; XLV. 1, 2, and 3.

Ref.—Cancer, p. 135.

SUMMARY.—*F. 28. Increasing enlargement of
abdomen, commencing seven months before death :
œdema of forearms set in two months after onset,
accompanied by distension of veins. Three months
before death, ascites was found, and a large lobulated
tumour occupied the greater part of the abdomen.
The right side of the chest was dull almost throughout, with absence of breath-sound, but with some
friction. Subsequently all the symptoms increased,
slight hæmoptysis occurred, dyspnœa became extreme,
and the pulse irregular and rapid.—The abdominal
tumour was found to proceed from the left ovary :
a solid growth in the mediastinum projected into the
right auricle and had extended into the lung, which
was collapsed, and presented cancerous growth in the
sheaths of the vessels.*

HARRIET PARSONS, ætat. 28, admitted University
College Hospital under Sir William Jenner, March
30, died July 1, 1869.

Family History.—Father and mother both living,
aged respectively 69 and 67 years. One brother died
of hydrocephalus, three brothers living.

Personal History.—Unmarried ; a dressmaker ;
has always enjoyed good health. Menstruation regular up to date of present illness.

Present Illness.—Fourteen months ago took cold,
and had a cough and some pain in right shoulder.
The cough lasted until last October. Last December
she noticed swelling in the abdomen, accompanied
with slight pain in the right flank. The menstruation has not returned since, and the abdominal
swelling has increased up to the present time. Six weeks
ago, swelling was observed in the right forearm;
it only lasted a few days, and has not returned. A few
days later swelling appeared in the left forearm, and
this has continued up to the present time. There has
been no swelling of the legs.

State on Admission.—Patient very thin ; some
lividity of face, lips, and tongue. Enlargement of
veins, and œdema, in both forearms. No œdema of
legs. Some varicose veins and some œdema on right
side of thorax. Abdomen distended ; cutaneous
veins much enlarged. Umbilicus everted. Fluctuation in abdomen from much fluid. In addition, a
nodulated tumour can be felt in the abdomen, extending from three fingers' breadth below the ensiform cartilage nearly to pubes; it does not move
with respiration. Has some dyspnœa, and this is
increased by exertion ; little cough.

Dulness over whole of right side, extending superiorly to three fingers' breadth to the left of the sternum.
Right back, absolutely dull below to within two
fingers' breadth of spine of scapula ; imperfect resonance thence to apex. Respiration almost inaudible
on right side, except near spine, but a sonorous
rhonchus and creaking friction are present front and
back. Vocal fremitus abolished on right side, back
and front, with bronchial breathing over the sternum.
Exaggerated breathing on left side. Heart's apex
three-quarters of an inch outside nipple. Sounds
normal.

Has some pain in abdomen ; bowels regular.
Urine free from albumen.

In the further progress of the case, some temporary dysphagia for solids occurred, but it was not
marked and was only of short duration. Hæmoptysis,
slight in degree, also occurred on one occasion.
Glairy tenacious sputa followed, and rusty sputa were
observed later. Some pain was felt from time to
time in the right shoulder. The nodulated masses
in the abdomen increased in size and distinctness, as
did also the ascites and the distension of the veins of
the thorax and abdomen. The legs became œdematous. Dyspnœa became extreme and paroxysmal, and
the pulse irregular and rapid. The patient died on
July 1. The temperature was normal throughout.

POST-MORTEM.—A great quantity of clear serosity
in peritoneum. A large nodulated tumour occupies a
large part of the abdominal cavity. Some of the nodules
are pedunculated ; a large cyst occupies its upper part.
The tumour is evidently of the left ovary, and is
attached throughout the whole length of the broad
ligament. The right ovary is converted into a mass
of cysts, forming a tumour, 6 in. × 4 in. The whole
mediastinum is filled by a solid growth. The greater
part of the right lung is adherent ; where non-
adherent, the pleural cavity is occupied by a clear
fluid. The mass in the mediastinum projects into
the pericardium, and compresses both the superior
and inferior venæ cavæ, and also the aorta and pulmonary artery. The right branch of the pulmonary
artery, and the pulmonary veins on the right side,
are almost completely occluded ; those on the left
are free. A mass of growth projects into the right
auricle, occupying nearly the whole of its cavity.

A cancerous mass extends into the middle lobe of

the right lung. The bronchi at the root of this lung are greatly narrowed; beyond this they are dilated. The lung is almost entirely collapsed, but some air is present in the upper lobe. The vessels of this lung present a very peculiar appearance (see XXIII. 5). They are thickened, rigid, and white on section, standing out prominently from the cut surface of the lung, so as at first to be mistaken for thickened bronchial tubes. The tissue of their walls resembles that of the mediastinal tumour. Both kidneys are filled with cysts.

My attention was not called to the state of the ovaries, and I received the portion of lung containing the thickened vessels from Sir W. Jenner's Assistant.

THE MICROSCOPIC EXAMINATION relates only to this portion of the lung.

Although to the naked eye the change in this part was apparently confined to the vessels, as seen in the figure, yet in many places, under the microscope, there was seen to be a diffuse infiltration of the pulmonary tissue with cancer-cells, accumulated in, and thickening the alveolar walls, like XLI. 4. In other places the growth forms nodular masses presenting the appearance of an acinose or lobular origin. The alveoli in many parts show an epithelial proliferation of a pneumonic type, and these tracts are mingled with nodular masses of cancerous growth. The growth in the alveolar walls appears to take place from the nuclei of the capillaries, in the same manner as that shown in XLV. 5.

The most characteristic appearance is, however, the infiltration of the sheaths of the vessels. It affects equally those of large and small size, and when an artery and bronchus are seen side by side, the former shows considerable infiltration of its sheath, while the latter is scarcely implicated. In some places, however, the bronchial walls present a uniform infiltration, similar to that of the arteries. In some of the larger vessels the growth is seen to proceed in nodular masses in the sheath, as shown in XLV. 3, and groups of these may be seen surrounding the vessel.

The more common appearance is that seen in XLV. 1 and 2, where the whole of the outer and middle coat of the artery is the seat of the infiltration, which extends to the surrounding pulmonary tissue, while the intima is unaffected. In other places, however, the whole thickness of the vessel is penetrated, and its tube narrowed or obliterated by a mass of cancer.

CASE 46.

CANCEROUS INFILTRATION OF LUNG.

Plates XXII. fig. 6; and XLV. figs. 4, 5, and 6.

This lung was handed to me by one of the house-surgeons in 1860, as a cancerous infiltration of the lung in a child. I placed some specimens in chromic acid and gave the preparation to Mr. Tuson to be drawn. I have been unable to identify the preparation at a later date, but as it illustrates in an interesting manner some of the varieties of cancerous infiltration, I have retained it in spite of this imperfect history.

The appearance presented by the lung is faithfully depicted by Mr. Tuson. It was solid, and the cut surface was in parts nearly uniform, with a greyish but vascular infiltration. The predominant characteristic, however, was a lobular infiltration closely resembling that seen in a broncho-pneumonia (see XXII. 6). The nodules were but slightly prominent, and were soft. They merged insensibly into the surrounding pulmonary tissue, which was very vascular and softened, and they broke down easily under pressure.

MICROSCOPIC EXAMINATION showed tracts of pneumonic infiltration, attended with considerable proliferation of the pulmonary epithelium. This, in sections perpendicular to the pleura and to the interlobular septa, could be well seen, assuming the acinose or infundibular form. The most characteristic appearance was, however, the infiltration of the alveolar walls with round and fusiform cells, as seen in XLV. 4. This extended over large areas, and in some places produced tracts which, when examined with a low power, presented appearances precisely resembling the tubercular infiltration of the alveolar walls seen in XXVIII. 10 (Polley) and XXXVIII. 1 (Henshaw). When, however, these tracts were examined with a higher power, the growth by which the walls are thus thickened is seen to consist of larger cells than the tubercular infiltration, and they are also more fusiform in type, but they tend, by multiplication, to form dense small-celled accumulations, which in parts are almost indistinguishable from the similar growths in the alveolar walls seen in tubercular infiltrations. Masses also form around the bronchi in a manner similar to that described as occurring in the arterial sheaths in the case of Parsons (p. 224). In one instance the growth was seen proceeding in the submucous tissue, forming rounded masses in the interior of the bronchus, the epithelium of which was preserved intact on the surface of the masses.

CASE 47.

SECONDARY CANCER OF LUNG. (COLUMNAR EPITHELIOMA.)

Plates XXIV. figs. 3, 4; XLV. figs. 8-12.

Ref.—Cancer, p. 137.

SUMMARY.—F. 50. Vomiting and discomfort after food during thirteen months before death; transient slight jaundice; pain in epigastric region and behind sternum. Six weeks before death, a large nodular tumour could be felt in the epigastric and umbilical regions, with smaller nodules extending as far as the right iliac bone.—This was found to be a large cancerous growth in the liver, apparently secondary to cancer of the pylorus. There was ulceration of the pylorus and the duodenum. Numerous hard nodules were found in the liver and lung, some in the latter being very small, and growing around the vessels. The structure of growths everywhere was that of columnar epithelioma.

PHŒBE LEATHER, ætat. 50, admitted University College Hospital February 6, died March 22, 1870.

Family History. Father and two brothers died of phthisis. Mother living ætat. 82.

Personal History.—Is married and has four children, all living and healthy; has had four miscarriages. Has been liable to occasional slight attacks of diarrhœa since 1866, and occasionally has observed blood in her stools. Has been subject to cough since childhood. Catamenia ceased three years ago.

Present Illness began in February 1869, when she had vomiting after eating. Lately the attacks have occurred at irregular times, but chiefly at night and in the morning. The vomiting is preceded by a sense of fulness and discomfort rather than pain, and this is removed by the sickness. Vomited matters at first consisted of food and of watery or yellow fluids. Lately they have been occasionally brown, with small soft masses described by patient as resembling liver. Pain has also been felt between the shoulders, sometimes severe and of an aching character; she has rarely had much pain in the epigastric or hypochondriac regions, but at times food has caused very intense epigastric pain. Jaundice has occurred several times within the past twelve months, but on each occasion it has only lasted a few days. The bowels have been costive during the past twelve months.

State on Admission.—Earthy tint of skin; aspect that of suffering; considerable anæmia; much pigment round orbits. Continuous post-sternal pain, aggravated by food and not relieved by the vomiting, which is frequent. Matter ejected consists of food, with a thick scum containing sarcinæ. Great tenderness in right hypochondrium. There is a large nodulated mass, extending from ensiform cartilage to below the umbilicus, and into the right hypochondrium, and two separate masses are felt below this. There is also a chain of nodules extending from umbilicus to crest of right iliac bone. Nothing abnormal observed in chest. Urine free from albumen. The temperature was normal until death.

POST-MORTEM.—The nodulated mass felt during life was found to be a large cancerous tumour of the liver.

Stomach.—The pylorus was thickened by an indurated mass of cancer, which reached across to umbilicus. There was extensive ulceration of the mucous membrane of the pyloric region of the stomach, the pylorus being constricted by nodules projecting externally. The ring was softened by ulceration, which extended to the front part of the duodenum. Masses of glands in front and behind the stomach were also enlarged with cancer.

The *Liver* presented throughout masses of the size of a small orange, of typical scirrhous hardness, white in colour, breaking when cut, and yielding a creamy juice on pressure. The gall-bladder contained an impacted calculus. Both supra-renal capsules cancerous. A nodule of cancer in the visceral pericardium at junction of aorta with left ventricle.

Intestines, Uterus, and *Ovaries* healthy. *Kidneys* contained cysts.

The *Lungs* contained numerous indurated nodules, presenting typical character of scirrhus. They rarely exceeded a filbert in size; many of the smaller ones appeared to be situated in the perivascular sheaths; some, which were as small as miliary tubercles, were in scattered patches. The larger masses under the pleura were markedly umbilicated, and dilated lymphatics could be seen proceeding between them, filled with a soft cheesy matter (XXIV. 4, *b c*). Some of the larger masses had, in their centre, spots of softening.

Bronchial Glands (XXV. 3), greatly enlarged and pigmented, presented softened spots like cheesy tubercles (*a a*), but whiter and firmer.

MICROSCOPIC EXAMINATION.—The nodules in the lungs present a remarkable appearance of villous cancer of the glandular type, resembling very closely the structure of a glandular sarcoma of the ovary. In the earlier stages, tracts of lung may be found with the alveoli filled with cells, gradually changing from the epithelial type to large round nucleated cells, which fill the alveoli (XLV. 10, *a a*). These enlarge, and acquire the appearance of the large cells found in ordinary encephaloid growths (*see* fig. 10, *b d*), and they sometimes present masses bearing some resemblance to the nests of an epithelioma (*see* fig. 10, *f*). In other places, at the margins of the alveoli, the cells are seen to be gradually assuming a columnar aspect (fig. 10, *e*, and fig. 12). Partial infiltration of the walls of the alveoli may also be seen (fig. 10, *g g*).

The more advanced stage of the process, by which the greater part of these nodules is constituted, consists in the alveoli being entirely filled with a villous structure, as seen in XLV. 8, 9, 11. The outlines of the alveoli are well maintained, and in some parts the terminal infundibula are most accurately mapped out, but they are entirely filled by the masses of new growth, which according to the manner in which their outlines are regarded, might be taken either for glandular or villous (*see* fig. 11), but when looked at *en masse* appears to belong rather to the type of the latter than of the former. The epithelium is columnar, and each villus consists of a prolongation of delicate areolar tissue carrying blood-vessels. In some places a similar growth may be seen in the lymphatics (fig. 8, *c*). The growth also extends into the bronchioles (fig. 9), in which it manifestly proceeds from the walls, while their centre is occupied by such cells partially disintegrated (fig. 9, *b*).

The bronchial lymphatics showed changes so exactly corresponding to those of the lung as to be indistinguishable from them, reproducing precisely the villous growth seen in the latter.

I much regret that I omitted to preserve portions of the liver and stomach. It is probable that the last-named organ had similar formations which were reproduced in the liver and thence extended to the lungs.

CASE 48.
SARCOMA OF LUNG.
Plate XXIII. fig. 2.

SUMMARY.—*F.* 60. *Symptoms of six months' duration; cough, expectoration, pain in the side, weakness, emaciation. Left side of chest retracted, and dull except near spine behind; breathing bronchial and tubular, weak below.—Effusion in left pleura. A mass of growth in the posterior mediastinum, projecting into the pericardium, and invading the lung by the root. Lung-tissue collapsed; an old infarct at the base.*

MARY FISHER, ætat. 60, admitted to University College Hospital April 15, died April 19, 1867.

Family History.—Patient's mother died, æt. 60, of asthma. Father lived to 90. Had eight brothers and five sisters; two died of phthisis, and nine others of unknown causes.

Personal History.—Was in domestic service before marriage, eighteen years ago. Has never been pregnant. Catamenia ceased at 50. Has always enjoyed good health, with the exception of a catarrhal attack three years ago.

Present Illness commenced in September 1866, with cough, attended by much frothy expectoration. She has never had hæmoptysis. She had also pain in the chest and between the shoulder-blades. Has become very weak; suffers from shortness of breath. Her appetite has failed, and she has had nausea on sitting up. An attack of diarrhœa seven weeks ago.

State on Admission.—Face flushed. (Cyanosis not noted.) Considerable emaciation. Brownish tint of skin, which is dry and harsh; fingers clubbed, and nails incurvated. There is an enlarged gland in left axilla; there are also enlarged glands in both inguinal regions, as well as above Poupart's ligament. No enlargement of cervical glands.

Frequent cough, which produces retching. Expectoration frothy, tenacious, and much pigmented. Chest; left side is manifestly flattened in upper half, and whole side diminished in size. Measurements at level of nipple, right side, 14½ inches, left 13¼. Expansion right side, ⅔ inch; left, *nil*.

Left side absolutely dull, with great sense of resistance in front and axilla, and also in the back, except a small area in back, close to spine, between eighth and tenth dorsal vertebræ. Right side hyperresonant at base posteriorly; the whole of the rest of the side, back and front, is resonant, except a limited area in the supra-spinous fossa, near the dorsal spine. Respiration on the left side is bronchial in supraspinous fossa; in upper midscapular region it is tubular. In lower scapular region it is also tubular but weak, and these characters continue to extreme base. Left front, respiration high-pitched, blowing under left clavicle to fourth rib; in upper axilla, weak blowing, bronchial opposite fifth rib; suppressed below seventh rib. No friction or râle heard anywhere. Respiration on right side chiefly puerile; blowing in supra-spinous fossa and over a limited area in midscapular region. Vocal fremitus and resonance both suppressed throughout the left side.

Heart's apex at epigastrium. Impulse can be felt and sounds heard to right of sternum. No murmur.

Liver-dulness reaches superiorly to sixth rib in mammary line. Inferiorly the organ extends three fingers' breadth below costal cartilages. No dulness in abdomen. Bowels now somewhat confined. Appetite bad. Occasional vomiting with cough.

The temperature reached 99° during three days. Pulse 104. Resp. 24.

She sank rapidly, and died April 19.

POST-MORTEM.—Left lung adherent in anterior mediastinum opposite third and fourth ribs. Pericardium extends two inches to right of sternum opposite fourth rib; adherent to right lung; contains about two ounces of dirty brown serosity. A large nodule of cancerous aspect projects into pericardium from left pleura, pressing on the pulmonary veins and left auricle. Another nodule projects into the posterior part of the sac.

Whole of left pleura full of clear serum.

Loose bands of flocculent lymph, blood-stained, pass between pulmonary and costal pleura.

There is no growth in the anterior mediastinum, but a large mass occupies the posterior mediastinum, reaching across the middle line to the right side, but overlapped by upper lobe of right lung. The descending aorta passes in a groove through the growth; its calibre does not appear to be diminished. The œsophagus passes over the surface of the mass and appears to have been compressed by it. The main bronchus leading to the left lung is free. The left branch of the pulmonary artery is compressed by the tumour; it can be followed freely into the upper part of the lung, but not into the lower. The left pulmonary vein is greatly compressed at the root of the lung. The left lung (XXIII. 2, *a*) is only invaded by the mass from the root. The growth here passed into the tissue in an irregularly lobulated form for about 1½ inches, and some nodules project further than this. The whole tissue of the lung is completely collapsed (*c*). The lower lobe presents, in an area of about two square inches, an old hæmorrhagic infarct (*b*). It is of a yellowish-grey colour, and is separated by a well-defined line of demarcation. Passing to it is a vessel obstructed by a firm and greyish clot.

The right lung is entirely free.

The tumour is of a glistening white, but very vascular; it exudes a milky juice on pressure.

No growths were found in any of the abdominal viscera.

MICROSCOPIC EXAMINATION.—The growth in this case consisted entirely of a small-celled sarcoma, and was a typical instance of this form of tumour. The pulmonary tissue was pressed aside rather than invaded by it, but in a few places the new growth could be seen extending to the enlargement of stellate cells in the floors of the alveoli, with multiplication of their nuclei. Some peribronchial and perivascular growth of the same nature was also seen, and it appeared probable that the extension into the lungs, where it occurred, was mainly in the sheaths of these.

CASE 49.

PULMONARY EMBOLISM.

Plate XXIII. fig. 1.

SUMMARY.— *M. 25. Constitutional syphilis; Bright's disease. Signs of increasing œdema of the bases of the lungs.—Small soft yellow nodules scattered thickly through both lungs, presumed to be embolic. Liver, kidneys, and spleen lardaceous. A soft thrombus in one renal vein.*

WILLIAM ROWE, ætat. 25, admitted University College Hospital, May 25, died September 1, 1866.

Family History.—Parents living at advanced ages. One brother died of phthisis, ætat. 33. Five other brothers and sisters living and in good health.

Previous History.—Occupation, carman; lived freely, and drank a considerable amount of spirits. Seven years ago he had suppurating bubo. Five weeks ago he came as out-patient to the hospital with ulcerated throat, and with a hydrocele, which was tapped. During the past week there has been considerable œdema of the legs and scrotum.

State on Admission.—The urine was of a specific gravity of 1,022; contained nearly three parts of albumen; the quantity passed varied from 10 to 60 oz. Hyaline and granular casts were found in it.

He had large, sloughing ulcers on both tonsils, extending into soft palate, with indurated edges; much œdema of the uvula.

Ulceration and fissures at side of nose, at junction of ala nasi. Scars of ulcers on legs.

Defect of resonance at both extreme bases, with weak respiration. He was subjected to calomel fumigations, and the throat improved, but the cough and the signs of œdema of the lung increased; ascites set in; the urine became more scanty, and he died on Sept. 1.

POST-MORTEM.—Ulceration was found in the throat, and also on the under-surface of the epiglottis, and below false vocal cord. Several spots of cicatricial tissue extended throughout the whole course of the trachea.

Scattered thickly through both lungs were yellow nodules (XXIII. 1), varying in size from a pea to a hazel-nut or walnut; yellow in colour, and soft in consistence, breaking down easily under a stream of water. They were most thickly scattered under the pleural surface, the pleura above them being very much congested. The smaller ones were superficial; those of larger size were situated deep in the substance of the lung. No other morbid change found in the lung.

Kidneys waxy, stain with iodine; numerous spots of fatty degeneration. In renal vein (side not noted) was a soft thrombus, which appeared to have been the origin of the embolic masses found in the lung.

Liver waxy, stains with iodine; deeply fissured with cicatricial tissue; substance indurated. One small abscess (? a softened gumma) in upper part of right lobe. *Spleen* waxy.

Stomach injected, and mucous membrane thickened. *Intestines* healthy.

CASE 50.
SYPHILITIC GROWTHS IN INFANT'S LUNGS.
Plate IV. fig. 3.

From Lebert, *Atlas d'Anatomie Pathologique*. plate xcii. fig. 3. Text, vol. i. p. 746.

Syphilitic gummata of a newly-born child, *bb*; chief gummatous tumour, *cc*; small tumours around lying in healthy pulmonary tissue.

'Lung of a newly-born child, given to M. Lebert 'by M. Danyeau. Born at Maternité Hospital, 'Paris, with a pemphigoid affection and nearly complete desquamation of the epidermis of the hands 'and feet.

'The thymus contained pus. The fœtus had not 'breathed. Sections of the lungs were firm; the 'lobular appearance was preserved; the colour was 'of a pinkish-grey but yellowish in parts; this, however, might be regarded as only a variation of the 'normal aspect. The most interesting fact was 'the following. On the inferior surface of the left 'lung, and on the superior surface of the corresponding (lower) lobe, there was in each (lobe) a 'mass of pale yellow colour, passing into greenish, 'of the size of about a halfpenny, which externally 'presented the appearance of an abscess. I was, 'however, surprised when, on cutting into it, I 'met not only with no abscess, but not even any 'loss of consistence. The colour, of a very pale 'yellow, extended for about a quarter of an inch in 'depth, below which the yellow tinge became more 'diffused and marbled, and passed insensibly into the 'normal appearance of the lung. This substance, 'like the rest of the pulmonary tissue, resisted 'pressure with the fingers and also with the scalpel, 'and yielded only a small quantity of clear fluid, 'slightly yellow, but neither turbid nor purulent.

'Under the microscope there are found in the 'morbid tissue a considerable proportion of fibro-'plastic elements. Around it is seen epithelium 'from the pulmonary vesicles, and in its substance 'some small pale non-nucleated globules, varying in 'size from $\frac{1}{3500}$ to $\frac{1}{2500}$ inch and only containing a 'few molecular granules. Their outline is rounded 'or irregular; they have a distant resemblance to 'pyoid bodies, but they have the closest affinity, like 'all this tissue, with the microscopic structure (as 'well as with the naked-eye appearance) of gummata 'found in other parts.

'After this observation, I am disposed to believe 'that the pulmonary changes in syphilitic children, 'described by M. Depaul as always found in a state 'of suppuration, were only a more advanced stage 'of the same change, and that at the outset there is 'a simple gummatous infiltration in the pulmonary 'parenchyma, which by suppuration gives rise to 'an abscess, and thus, in a similar case, benefit 'ought to be derived from the use of iodide of potas-'sium.'

CASE 51.
SYPHILITIC GROWTHS IN CEREBELLUM AND LUNGS.
(See fig. 40, p. 130.)

SUMMARY.—*M. 68. Intemperate; mental weakness during a year before death; towards the last some excitement, right ptosis, rigidity of the right arm and coma. A large number of small nodules in the cerebellum, resembling syphilitic growths; thickening of the membranes, and distension of the ventricles of the brain. A firm yellow mass in the left lung.*

W. D. Cabdriver, ætat. 68, admitted University College Hospital, June 14, died June 21, 1875.

Previous History, as obtained from patient's wife. He had been a heavy drinker all his life. About a year ago his memory failed and he grew 'silly,' lost muscular power, and passed gradually into the state in which he was admitted.

State on Admission.—The face had an imbecile expression; there was ptosis of right eyelid; the mouth was drawn to left. He was usually wandering and muttering, but could be roused when spoken to, answering questions incoherently. Excitement occurred at night, and he tried to get out of bed. Pupils reacted to light. There was general muscular weakness, but no special localised paralysis, with exception of ptosis of right eyelid. Hands tremulous. Complete incontinence of urine and fæces. No physical signs of disease of lung beyond some emphysema. Arteries tortuous. Heart-sounds healthy. Tongue dry. Appetite good. Liver tender, not enlarged. Urine 1030, no albumen.

Within the next week rigidity appeared in muscles of right arm, which was constantly flexed. Head turned to right. This state passed into coma, in which patient died.

POST-MORTEM.—Lateral and third ventricles largely distended with clear fluid. Both lobes of cerebellum adherent to dura mater, and cannot be separated without tearing the brain substance. No thrombi in sinuses and no material atheroma of the cerebral arteries. Much thickening of the meninges, particularly of the base. Walls of lateral ventricles softened, and the communication between these and third ventricle admits tip of little finger. Substance of cerebellum softened; in the tissue are a large number of small yellowish nodules, some of which run into one another, forming conglomerate masses. The nodules are about the size of a split pea, and are surrounded by a white semi-transparent capsule. They resemble very closely in character syphilitic gummata. The tissue between them is semi-hyaline. Nearly all these growths are in the cortical substance.

Liver cirrhosed, 'hobnail,' and much contracted.

Lungs.—In lower portion of upper lobe of left lung there is an indurated yellow, but non-caseous, mass, of the size of a Maltese orange, prominent, not surrounded by a zone of induration, but passing at its margin into a greyer tint, and then into a more vascular but non-indurated tissue. In the same lobe there are other smaller nodules, resembling in character a grey firm pneumonia. The rest of the lung and the other organs were healthy.

MICROSCOPIC EXAMINATION.—Dr. Gowers has furnished the following description of the microscopic appearances in the lung (*Trans. Path. Soc.* vol. xxviii. 1877, p. 380).

'The examination showed that the structure of 'the nodule in the lung was by no means uniform 'throughout the mass. It contained a small-celled 'growth, irregularly distributed' (see Fig. 40, p. 180). 'In some places the growth formed compact nodules 'of some size; but from these, irregular tracts of 'growth extended into the lung-tissue, chiefly along 'the bronchioles. In some places (a a) small bud-like 'nodules of growth sprang from the infiltrated wall. 'The walls of the air-cells adjacent to the growth, 'were, in most instances, infiltrated by it, the wall 'containing two or three layers of cells. Some of 'the alveolar walls adjacent even to a large tract 'of growth were free from infiltration. But most 'of the alveoli contained inflammatory products; in 'some, epithelial products and blood-corpuscles 'occupied the whole of the centre of the air-cells; in 'others, epithelial products were mingled with the 'small cells such as constituted the new growth (b). 'The areas of many alveoli were occupied by the 'new growth, although their walls were still distinguishable. Many air-cells contained a few epithelial and other cells, sparingly scattered through a 'network of fibrillæ, such as may be sometimes 'seen in acute pneumonia; and which appeared to 'be the result of the action of the hardening agent 'on some albuminous exudation.

'The cells of which the growth consisted were 'small corpuscles having a diameter about half as 'much again as a blood-disk and therefore probably, 'when fresh, about $\frac{1}{2500}$ inch. They were for the 'most part round; a few were oval or angular, as if 'from compression; a few were larger; in these a 'cell-wall could be distinguished from a nucleus 'which almost filled the cell; in the smaller cells 'no nuclei could be perceived. Between these cells 'was a delicate fibrillary stroma, the fibres approximating to the parallel rather than to the reticular 'arrangement. Here and there, also, fusiform fibre-'cells, having nearly the same diameter as the 'smaller corpuscles, lay among them.

'In some places (c) granular degeneration had 'taken place in the new growth and inflammatory 'products, corresponding with the caseation observed 'in the recent state.'

CASE 52.

SYPHILITIC (?) PNEUMONIA.

Plate XXVII. figs. 6 and 7.

(Prof. Greenfield, *Trans. Path. Soc.* vol. xxvii. 1876, p. 43. By permission.)

'The piece of lung and the sections exhibited 'were removed from the body of a female child, 'twelve months old, who died in the out-patient's 'room in St. Thomas's Hospital in February, 1873. 'The child was said to have had a cough for some 'time, and to have been ailing, but had had no severe illness. The mother brought the child to the 'hospital thinking it only slightly ill, but it died in 'her arms whilst waiting. No satisfactory history 'was obtained, and there was no distinct evidence of 'syphilis, but there were circumstances in the family 'history which rendered its existence extremely probable.

'At the post-mortem examination, twenty-four 'hours after death, by Dr. Payne, the left lung was 'found slightly collapsed at base, otherwise apparently normal. The liver was quite healthy in appearance, and there was nothing noteworthy in the 'other organs, with the exception of the right lung. 'This was completely consolidated throughout, and 'in a state of full expansion, with slight recent 'pleurisy, mainly over the lower lobe. No thickening of pleura, but a few loose adhesions of older date. 'The bronchi of the right lung were injected and 'contained some muco-purulent fluid.

'On section of the lung it was found pretty completely consolidated throughout, and of a somewhat 'yellowish or yellowish-white colour, the cut surface 'being smooth and slightly shining, differing markedly from the ordinary grey hepatisation of acute 'pneumonia. The tissue, very firm and tough, exuded 'but very scanty turbid fluid on scraping or squeezing. On looking closely at the cut surface it was 'seen that minute bands of fibrous tissue ran 'everywhere through it. The condition of the bronchial glands is not noted.

'MICROSCOPIC EXAMINATION.— On examining 'with a low power, the lung is found to be every-'where traversed by bands of tissue of varying thickness, running in all directions, enclosing groups of 'alveoli. They are, for the most part, by their 'branching and reunion, disposed in such a manner 'as to divide the lung-tissue into rounded spaces, 'which vary in size, some being of the width of seven 'or eight air-cells, others somewhat larger; these 'spaces being for the most part irregularly rounded or 'polygonal. The fibrous septa vary from '25 to '6 of 'a millimètre in thickness, and the spaces enclosed 'are from '25 to 1 millimètre in width. The fibrous 'bands are for the most part composed of a highly

'vascular tissue, which in some of the smaller
'bundles consists mainly of an imperfectly developed
'cell-growth. In the spaces left are some air-cells,
'with more or less thickened walls; in some places
'scarcely any alveoli being visible, owing to the
'great thickening and consequent compression and
'distortion. The thickening, under a low power, ap-
'pears to be in part due to cell-infiltration, in part to
'delicate bands of connective tissue running into the
'alveolar walls.

'Everywhere the walls of the vessels and bronchi
'present great thickening, either fibrous or corpus-
'cular; here and there they are surrounded by a
'large aggregation of cells; in other places they are
'nearly obliterated by the great thickening. The
'newly-formed fibrous tissue is, however, highly
'vascular, containing large vessels, many of which
'are evidently of new formation.

'For the most part, the remains of the air-cells
'show little sign of inflammation; but in some
'places, where the walls are less thickened, they
'contain fibrinous exudation and some catarrhal cells,
'this condition being almost limited to the lower lobe
'of the lung.

'On examining with a higher power, the walls of
'the alveoli appear remarkably thickened, and the
'epithelium everywhere persistent and apparently in-
'creased in amount. In some places the thickening
'appears to be due solely to the overgrowth of epithe-
'lium, the cells of which are perfectly normal in
'appearance, entirely free from signs of degeneration.
'The greater part of the thickening, however, is due
'to a nucleated cell-growth, of which the cells are
'for the most part elongated or fusiform, around the
'pulmonic capillaries, which appear at the same time
'to increase in size, and to develop in some cases
'into larger vessels. In some places the growth
'appears to take place by a modification of the epi-
'thelial cells, or of the capillary nuclei, but it cannot
'be stated with certainty that this is the case.

'The alveolar epithelium is seen to persist even
'where the cavity of the air-cell is completely filled
'up, and its size greatly diminished.

'REMARKS.—Although I have no desire to press
'unduly the syphilitic origin of the disease in this
'case, in the absence of direct evidence on the ques-
'tion of etiology, I may point out that it corresponds
'precisely in every particular with the disease of the
'lungs occurring in newly-born or young syphilitic
'children, which has been described by Wagner as
'the diffused syphilitic form: by Lorain and Robin as
'"epithelioma" of the lungs, and by Virchow and
'Weber as "white hepatisation" of the lungs. It
'will be readily seen that the term "epithelioma" of
'the lung might be applied to this case on the ground
'of the remarkable persistence and hypertrophy of the
'alveolar epithelium, whilst the name "white hepa-
'tisation" equally describes the naked-eye character.
'A perusal of the description given by the above-
'named observers will, I think, place it beyond
'doubt that the condition of the lung in this case,
'whatever its etiology, corresponds entirely with that
'found in the cases whose syphilitic origin was beyond
'question. Again, the condition of the lung and its
'microscopic appearances differed *in toto* from those
'found in ordinary chronic pneumonia and in fibroid
'phthisis: a comparison of sections from lungs af-
'fected with these diseases showed that there was no
'resemblance between the two. It is hoped that the
'drawings, however imperfect, will show this without
'a more detailed description' (*see* XXVII. figs. 6 and
'7). 'Considering also the facts that the disease, of
'whatever nature, was of long standing, probably
'dating at least as far back as the time of birth, that
'it was entirely unilateral, of slow and of progressive
'growth, unattended by any marked symptoms, that
'there was no sign of chronic bronchial catarrh or
'of tuberculosis, and that the growth presents pre-
'cisely the characters of syphilitic infiltration in
'other organs, it must, I think, be conceded as
'almost beyond doubt that such was its nature.

'I may add that I have had an opportunity of
'comparing the sections with sections from a lung
'affected with syphilitic infiltration in an infant,
'whose other organs contained gummata, and that
'as regards the earlier stages of the disease they
'correspond precisely with the latter in their micro-
'scopic characters.'

CASE 53.

SYPHILITIC BRAIN-DISEASE: CASEOUS GUMMATA IN THE LUNG.

SUMMARY.—*F. 48. Constitutional syphilis.—Headache, dimness of sight, progressive impairment of consciousness: right-sided rigidity: ptosis and palsy of sixth and facial nerves.—Bony growths from inner surface of frontal bone and in dura mater; vascularity of surface of brain: disease of cranial nerves. Caseous nodules in the lungs.*

SARAH HANNER: ætat. 48, admitted University College Hospital May 30, died June 8, 1872.

Previous History. Married 27 years ago. Seven years after marriage, was laid up with an ulcerated throat in the Middlesex Hospital. Has never had a living child, but has had three or four miscarriages, some before and some after her attack of ulcerated throat. Has had an eruption on skin and lost much of her hair about two years ago. Had pains in head two years ago, chiefly on the right side. A year ago had three lumps on her head as large as pigeons' eggs. They were hard and painful. Had pains in back of neck six weeks ago. Eyesight has been gradually failing. Headache at times has been severe, and occasionally, when pain has been worst, she has been partly unconscious. Lately her speech has become thick.

State on Admission.—Was in a semi-unconscious condition, answering when spoken to loudly, but speaking slowly, and with apparent difficulty. Head turned towards right side; and an attempt to turn it to middle caused manifest pain. Tongue protruded to right; facial paralysis on right side. Some ptosis of right eyelid, and paralysis of the right external rectus. Conjunctivitis on right side with purulent discharge, and some superficial ulceration and cloud-ing of cornea. Sensation was apparently intact. Muscles of upper and lower extremities rigid on right side, but some slight voluntary motion was still possible. There was a scar the size of half a crown under the left clavicle. Nothing abnormal in physical signs of lungs or heart. Urine normal. No enlarge-ment of liver.

She became comatose and died a week after admission.

CASE 53 (HANNER) 231

POST-MORTEM.—Much irregular osseous deposit on inner surface of frontal bone, forming nodosities and sharp spicule; the former projects nearly a quarter of an inch. Membrane everywhere unduly vascular. Numerous spiculæ and plates of bone in dura mater. Some opacity of arachnoid, which, however, separates without tearing brain-substance. Extreme vascularity of surface of brain. At base, manifest thickening of sheaths of third nerve and of right fifth nerve, with inflammatory exudation. Left olfactory nerve has a tract of grey degeneration in its course. No obstruction of cerebral arteries, but a deposit of lymph is seen on the left middle cerebral; exudation at bases of both optic nerves, which also are unduly vascular, and present tracts of grey degeneration. This degeneration extends deeply into commissure, through nearly its whole depth, mixed with firm but hyperæmic white matter. A similar degeneration is seen in the left third nerve. Hyperæmia of whole surface of brain. Central commissure softened. Thalami soft. Velum interpositum hyperæmic. Tracts of grey gelatinous softening at roots of auditory nerve.

Liver puckered, cirrhotic, with lines of fibrous tissue running deeply to hilus.

Spleen.—Some thickening of capsule.

Lungs.—Right contains four caseous masses each the size of a kidney-bean, all in the upper lobe. Some fall out, leaving a smooth capsule behind. All are caseous, and no early stages are discovered. Much pigmentation and puckering exists around them.

ALPHABETICAL LIST OF CASES.

	Case	Page		Case	Page
ATTWOOD, W.	32	207	LACK, J.	31	205
BARLOW, C.	38	216	LEATHER, P.	47	225
BEALE, G.	11	172	LLOYD, J.	23	190
BRODRICK, J.	18	181	MEARS, E.	36	213
BROOM, A.	13	175	'MINER'S PHTHISIS'		
BROWN, J.	29	201	(*Greenhow*)	39	218
BROWN, S.	5	161	OVERALL, J.	27	196
'CANCER, INFILTRATING'	46	225	PARSONS, H.	45	224
CARR, M. A.	30	203	'PNEUMONIA SUPPURATIVE'		
COE, H.	34	210	(*Carswell*)	2	158
COOMBES, A.	7	165	POLLEY, J. H.	6	163
'COPPER - MINER'S PHTHISIS'			'POTTER'S PHTHISIS'	38A	217
(*Greenhow*)	40	219	PRICE, C.	12	173
COPPIN, W. H.	33	208	ROBERTS, C	35	212
CORNEY, M.	25	193	ROWE, W.	48	226
D., W.	50	228	SCARROW, W.	15	176
'DIABETIC PHTHISIS'	14	176	SCHOFIELD, A.	37	215
ELLSOM, T.	17	179	SHIMMICK, S.	8	167
'EMPHYSEMA' (*Carswell*)	44	223	'SIDEROSIS PULMONUM'		
FISHER	49	227	(*Zenker*)	42	220
'FLAX - DRESSER'S PHTHISIS'			SMITH, W.	28	199
(*Greenhow*)	41	219	'SYPHILITIC GROWTHS'		
GARDINER, T.	22	187	(*Lebert*)	50	228
GOWLING	21	187	'SYPHILITIC (?) PNEUMONIA'		
GRIFFIN, W.	19	183	(*Greenfield*)	52	229
HALL, M.	24	191	TANNER, J.	4	160
HANNER, S.	53	229	THOMAS, J.	20	186
HAWKINS, E.	3	159	THOMAS, W.	41	222
HEATH, E.	26	194	UNWIN, G.	10	170
HENSHAW, W.	16	177	VICK, A.	9	168
KIRK, J.	1	159			

DESCRIPTIONS OF THE PLATES.

§ A. COLOURED PLATES. (I. to XXIV.)

PLATE I.
ACUTE PNEUMONIA.[1]

Second stage of acute pneumonia, that of 'hepatisation,' from a patient who died on the fifth day. The whole lung is solid, of a brownish-red colour, varying in depth of tint in various parts with a fine sprinkling of greyish-white, least conspicuous in the darker portions.

The microscopical changes are shown at XXV. fig. 7.

Ref.—Acute Pneumonia, p. 16.[2]

PLATE II.
SUPPURATIVE PNEUMONIA.
(After Carswell. See Case 2, p. 158.)

The lower two-thirds of the lung present a yellowish-grey colour, tinged with red—'a solid, compact, granular mass in which the bronchi and blood-vessels were hardly to be seen.' The upper lobe is congested.

Ref.—Acute Pneumonia, p. 18.

PLATE III.
HYPOSTATIC PNEUMONIA.

The lower portion of the lung is of a lighter red, mottled with grey and with a dark purplish brown. The tint is much paler than is often seen in this variety.

Ref.—Hypostatic Pneumonia, p. 40.

PLATE IV.
CHRONIC PNEUMONIA; SYPHILIS; GREY HEPATISATION.

FIG. 1.—*Chronic Pneumonia in a Syphilitic Patient (Case 3, Hawkins, p. 159).*

The lung tissue is infiltrated with a very firm, reddish-grey exudation, finely granular, but showing no signs of softening. The change involved the middle lobe, and upper two-thirds of the lower

---

[1] The titles here given are those on the plates themselves.   [2] The references appended to the descriptions are to the text only

lobe of the right lung, the other lung being normal. *a*, Pigmented spots; *b*, Bands of fibrous tissue.

The microscopical appearances are shown at XLII. 6 and XLIII. 4. See description of these, also p. 160.

Ref.—Phthisis, pp. 67, 104; Syphilitic Dis. p. 126.

Fig. 2.—*Syphilitic Growths in the Lung* (*Case 53, S. Hanner*).

The figure represents a portion of lung containing two caseous gummata, surrounded by indurated and pigmented tissue.

Ref.—Syphilitic Dis. pp. 122, 131.

Fig. 3.—Syphilitic growths from the lung of a newly-born child, described and figured by Lebert, whose account is given in full at another page (*Case 50, p. 228*). The larger growth (*bb*) is a pale yellow, firm mass, and yielded only a little clear yellowish liquid. *cc*, Small gummata lying in the otherwise healthy lung-tissue.

Ref.—Syphilitic Dis. p. 122.

Fig. 4.—*Acute Pneumonia, Grey Hepatisation* (*Case 1, Kirk*, p. 158).

The patient died on the tenth day. The figure represents the aspect of the right lung. It is solidified, and ash-grey in colour; the surface is finely granular, and much pigment is scattered through the tissue.

The cell-forms found in the alveoli are shown at XXV. 4, 5, and 9. (See description of this plate, and also p. 158.)

Ref.—Acute Pneumonia, pp. 17, 22.

PLATE V.

LOBULAR PNEUMONIA IN MEASLES; TUBERCULAR PNEUMONIA.

Fig. 1.—*Lobular Pneumonia.* The lung of a child who died from measles.[1]

The general condition of the lung was similar to that shown in fig. 4 and described below. In addition, the figure shows a wedge-shaped mass of solidification which existed at the base of the lung. It was granular on section, yielding a puriform fluid on scraping. The cut surface is seen to be of a dull reddish-white colour, deepening in parts into a more intense vascularity. At the margins, lobular extension of the consolidation can be observed.

Ref.—Catarrhal Pneumonia, p. 26.

Fig. 2.—*Lobular Pneumonia.* From an unpublished drawing, by Sir Robert Carswell, of the lung of a child who died of measles.

The figure represents the later stages of lobular pneumonia, and shows the lung-tissue filled with islets of consolidation, yellowish-grey in tint, with a granular surface, slightly prominent, the outline of some better defined than that of others.

Ref.—Catarrhal Pneumonia, p. 23.

Fig. 3.—*Broncho-Pneumonia.* The lung of a child, aged one year; duration of illness five weeks. (*Case 4, Tanner*, p. 160.)

The lung presents numerous spots of consolidation, some yellowish and soft, others of a reddish or greyish tint, and somewhat firmer. The former break down, leaving small cavities such as that seen divided in the middle of the figure. The firmer grey spots form, by their union, larger nodules, such

---

[1] This lung and also that from which fig. 4 is taken, were from children who died of measles in the Hospital for Sick Children. They were given me, in 1864, by my lamented friend, Dr. Hillier.

as *a* and the aggregation seen below this, near the surface. The bronchi were intensely inflamed, and filled with purulent secretion.

The microscopical appearances are figured in Plate XXVI. figs. 1-4. See description of this, also p. 161.

Ref.—Catarrhal Pneumonia, pp. 23, 24.

FIG. 4.—*Pneumonia in Measles.*

The bases of both lungs (of which one is represented in the figure) were solid, partly carnified, partly infiltrated with exudation-matter. In this were spots of pus the size of a hemp-seed and small excavations of the same size, having a well-defined wall. Some of the latter are seen in the lower part of the figure. They could, in many places, be traced into continuity with the bronchi, the cut openings of which were gaping, with a white, thickened wall (as seen in the figure), and filled with pus. In some instances lateral openings, communicating with collections of pus, could be found in the walls of the larger bronchi, doubtless formed by ulceration from the interior; different stages of this process could be traced in other parts. Where the lung was not entirely solidified, scattered nodules existed, many of which had a puriform centre surrounded by pneumonic infiltration.[1]

Ref.—Collapse, p. 56.

FIG. 5.—*Acute Suppurating and Ulcerating Pneumonia.* (*Case 5, S. Brown*, p. 161.) Duration of symptoms, two months.

The figure represents part of the lower lobe of the left lung, and shows intense injection of the bronchial mucous membrane, the surface of which is rough and uneven, and, in some places, presents distinct ulceration. Around the bronchi the lung-tissue is solidified, and presents a granular surface, greyish-red, dotted with yellow and whitish spots, some of which had broken down in the centre, forming small cavities communicating with the bronchi.

For the microscopical appearances see XXXV. 7, and description of this; also p. 163.

Ref.—Phthisis, pp. 119, 121.

PLATE V_A.

GANGRENE OF THE LUNG; PNEUMONIA WITH 'CONCRETIONS' IN THE BRONCHI.

These three figures are from the original drawings by Sir Robert Carswell.

FIG. 1.—*Gangrene from Pulmonary Embolism.* Figured, *Elementary Forms of Disease*, Section 'Hæmorrhage,' Plate II. fig. 7.[2]

It is described as the appearances presented by pulmonary haemorrhage terminating in suppuration, principally of the interlobular cellular tissue, and accompanied by slight inflammation of the substance of the lung in the vicinity. The latter is indicated by the zone of redness which separates the area of destruction from the rest of the lung. Thickened septa appear to enclose cavities formed by the breaking-down of the lung-tissue. The white spots indicate areas of necrotic degeneration not yet liquefied.

Ref.—Embolism, p. 61; Gangrene, pp. 61-2.

FIG. 2.—*Pneumonia with False Membranes in the Bronchi.* Figured, *Elem. Forms of Disease*, Section 'Analogous Tissues,' Pl. I. fig. 3.

The above is the designation given by Carswell, who adds: 'Tubular membranes of considerable size, terminating abruptly at some distance from the air-cells. The pulmonary tissue is engorged

---

[1] Description by the Author.
[2] The published drawing contains also a recent haemorrhage, apparently introduced from another sketch. Many of Sir Robert Carswell's published figures differ somewhat from the original drawings. He apparently drew on the stone himself, and was free to modify a figure, or to combine two sketches into one. Moreover, the sketches were all copied on to the stone by him without reversal, and are therefore reversed in his plates. In this Atlas they are presented as they appear in the originals, preserved in the Museum of University College.—ED.

'with blood,' in some parts, as in the upper part of the figure, while in other parts, as in the lower portion shown, ' it is infiltrated with serosity, lymph, and pus.'

Ref.—Acute Pneumonia, p. 16.

FIG. 3.—*Gangrene of the Lung.* Figured, *Elem. Forms of Disease,* Section 'Mortification,' Plate IV. fig. 1.

The figure is described as ' representing mortification of nearly the inferior third of the lower lobe ' of the left lung, limited by adhesive inflammation.' In the lower part of the figure is 'a large ' cavity, lined by a yellowish-grey coloured thick membrane, united with the pleura of the upper sur- ' face of the inferior lobe' (not shown here) 'and with the pulmonary tissue of the upper lobe, which ' was in a state of grey hepatisation to the extent of about a quarter of an inch in depth :' (this large hepatisation is indistinctly seen in section in the notch just below the letters 'Fig. 3.') ' Beyond ' this the pulmonary tissue was quite healthy. The sphacelated substance of the lung thus isolated ' and enclosed in a membrane of new formation, was of a dirty yellowish-brown or black colour, of a ' pulpy consistence, composed of shreds of cellular tissue and obliterated blood-vessels, and a consider- ' able quantity of offensive grumous fluid, similar to that which had been expectorated some time ' before death.'

Ref.—Gangrene, p. 61.

PLATE VI.
ACUTE TUBERCULOSIS.

All the figures are from a child, aged 6 (*Case 6, Polley,* p. 163). The microscopical appearances are depicted in XXVIII. 6-10, and XXX. 5. See descriptions of these, also p. 165.

FIG. 1.—Lung, containing numerous greenish-white nodules, dry-looking, firm, and resistant. The centres of some have a bluish-grey tint (*b b*), while others are yellowish in the middle. They form by aggregation irregular caseous tracts of considerable size (*c c*). Between them, in emphysematous and congested lung-tissue, are minute granulations, the size of a millet-seed (*a*).

Ref.—Phthisis, pp. 69, 96.

FIG. 2.—External surface of the lung, studded with coalescing granulations, having an irregular racemose shape. They are surrounded with zones of congestion, and correspond to the masses seen on section in the preceding figure.

Ref.—Phthisis, pp. 69, 96, 117.

FIG. 3.—Portion of lung presenting dilated bronchi, the mucous membrane of which is congested. The lung-tissue here is crammed with granulations, especially dense (*b*) around the bronchi, the walls of which are perforated by some. Between the granulations is some grey pneumonic infiltration (*a a*).

Ref.—Phthisis, p. 79.

FIG. 4.—Liver, studded on its surface and in its substance with tubercular granulations, of which the larger ones are cheesy and the smaller are semi-transparent.

FIG. 5.—Supernumerary spleen, riddled with cheesy granulations and nodules, opaque and firm, coalescing in places into tracts of some size.

Ref.—Phthisis, p. 78.

FIG. 6.—Surface of the same; on it the tubercular nodules project. They are more or less rounded in outline, and the shape of the larger tracts indicates very clearly their formation by the union of smaller nodules.

PLATE VII.

ACUTE PHTHISIS; TUBERCULAR AND CASEOUS PNEUMONIA; DIABETIC PHTHISIS.

FIG. 1.—*Acute Tubercular Pneumonia.* Duration of symptoms seven weeks. (*Case 12, Catherine Price*, p. 178.)

Through the lung-tissue caseous nodules are scattered, varying in size from a hemp-seed to a pea, and irregular in shape. Many of them are pigmented in the middle. All are soft, and many, as at *a*, are breaking down in the centre, so as to form small cavities. There are also numerous grey and more transparent nodules, granular in section, as at *c*; some of them, as in the upper part of the figure, are very small, but not so round or uniform as typical grey granulations. Larger cavities also existed, of which one is shown at *b*; they are seen to communicate with bronchi, which are dilated as at *e*. The larger cavity has a well-defined wall, and in its floor is caseous material. The mucous membrane of the bronchus entering it ends abruptly.

The microscopical changes are shown in XXXIX. 4; see description of this, also p. 174.

Ref.—Phthisis, pp. 73, 74, 79, 90.

FIG. 2.—*Lung in Diabetic Phthisis.* (*Case 14*, p. 176.)

The tissue is studded with yellow nodules (*b*), granular in section, coalescing into tracts of caseous infiltration. These are especially large near the surface of the lung (*a a*), and over them the pleura is thickened.

The microscopical appearances (not figured) are described at p. 176.

Ref.—Phthisis, pp. 69, 70, 117 (2).

FIG. 3.—*Tubercles and Tubercular Pneumonia.* From a man, aged 26: duration of symptoms about six months. (*Case 15, W. Scarrow*, p. 176.)

The figure shows the tissue of the lower lobe, with numerous opaque, yellowish nodules, some as isolated opaque granulations (*a*), others clustered; while on the right, at *b*, they have formed, by aggregation, irregular caseous tracts, in which, however, the constituent nodules are still distinct, and are often softened in the centre into minute cavities. Below these are seen areas of more recent pneumonic consolidation. The intervening lung-tissue is congested, in parts intensely.

The microscopical appearances (not figured) are described at p. 176.

Ref.—Phthisis, p. 73.

FIG. 4.—*Caseous Tubercular Pneumonia.* Symptoms of six months' duration. (*Case 20, J. Thomas*, p. 186.)

The lung-tissue is the seat of grey pneumonic infiltration (*a a*), through which are thickly scattered irregular caseous masses (*b b*), whitish or yellowish, softening and breaking down at many places, so as to leave cavities (*c c*) irregular in shape, with caseous walls.

The larynx presented tubercular ulceration, shown in XX. fig. 2.

The microscopic appearances in this lung are shown in XXXIX. 2, see description of this, p. 187.

Ref.—Phthisis, pp. 68, 69, 73, 74, 117.

PLATE VIII.

ACUTE TUBERCULOSIS.

FIG. 1.—*Tubercles and Tubercular Pneumonia.* Duration of definite symptoms three months. (*Case 16, W. Henshaw*, p. 177, also figs. 4 and 6.)

The lung is crammed with tubercular granulations, some, as at *a*, small and tending to semi-transparence, but differing from typical grey granulations in being rather more opaque, softer, and more readily detached from the lung. (*See* also fig. 6.) They are clustered at places, as at *d*, and thus form by aggregation masses (*e c*) of racemose character and considerable size, the surface of which is finely granular. Some of them, as at *b*, blend gradually with the adjacent tissue.

The microscopical appearances are shown at XXXI. 7, XXXVIII. 1-4. See description of these, also p. 178.

Fig. 2.—*Miliary Tuberculosis of Lung.* From a boy aged 13; duration of symptoms ten weeks. (*Case 7, A. Coombes,* p. 165.)

The lung is seen to be full of tubercular granulations; most of them are separate. A few are as large as a mustard-seed, but the majority vary from that of a poppy-seed downwards. In some of the larger granulations caseation is occurring, for the most part only in the centre, the periphery being still, like the whole of the smaller granulations, grey and semi-transparent (see also fig. 5).

The microscopical appearances are depicted at XXVIII. 4, XXX. 3, 4, and XXXIV. 1. See description of these, and also p. 166.

Ref.—Phthisis, p. 66.

Fig. 3.—Portion of a spleen that has undergone lardaceous degeneration. The part to the right has been treated with iodine, and has stained deeply.

Ref.—Phthisis, p. 66.

Fig. 4.—*Tubercular Pneumonia* from the same case (*10*) as fig. 1.

Portion of lung filled with racemose masses, similar to those seen in the middle of fig. 1, but in a more advanced stage of caseation. They are greenish-yellow in tint, very opaque and granular, and present numerous minute spots of softening, giving a worm-eaten appearance to the section. This is probably due, in part, to the lung having been previously emphysematous. Between the nodules the lung-tissue is infiltrated with a firm, opaque, greyish exudation. For microscopical appearances, see above.

Ref.—Phthisis, p. 117 (2).

Fig. 5.—*Tubercles of Lung*, from the same case (7) as fig. 2.

The figure shows large and small granulations, many of them aggregated. They are for the most part grey, but in some of the larger caseation is commencing. For microscopical appearances, see above.

Ref.—Phthisis, p. 66.

Fig. 6.—*Tubercles of Lung*, from the same case (*10*) as figs. 1 and 4.

Dense aggregations of granulations, with others scattered in the neighbourhood. Where aggregated, they are opaque and granular; many present a minute point of softening in the centre. For microscopical appearances, see above.

Ref.—Phthisis, p. 70.

PLATE IX.

Tubercles and Tubercular Pneumonia.

Fig. 1.—*Caseating Tubercles and Tubercular Pneumonia.* Duration of symptoms seven months, with a recent acute exacerbation. (*Case 17, T. Ellsom,* p. 179.)

Lung-tissue with grey pneumonic infiltration, granular in section, through which caseous spots (*bb*) are thickly scattered, breaking down into irregular cavities with caseous walls. Some of these spots (*aa*) are small and rounded in shape, resembling tubercular granulations that have undergone caseation.

The microscopical changes are shown at XXVI. 7, and XXXVIII. 5 and 6. See description of these, also p. 180.

Ref.—Phthisis, pp. 74, 116.

FIG. 2.—*Tubercular Pneumonia*, from the same.

Extensive tracts of dull-grey pneumonic consolidation are shown at *a a*. It is firm, uniform, and smooth on section. At *b b* are areas of caseating lobular pneumonia. The pulmonary tissue elsewhere shows in places an earlier stage of the diffuse pneumonia; the interlobular septa are thickened. In the lowest part of the figure is a cavity which has apparently been formed by the breaking down of the diffuse infiltration, and smaller cavities are seen here and there in the more recent infiltration. For microscopic appearances, see above.

Ref.—Phthisis, pp. 68, 71.

FIG. 3.—*Pneumonic Infiltration in Chronic Phthisis*. (*Case 21, Gowling*, p. 187.)

Portion of the lower lobe, presenting firm, grey, pneumonic infiltration and densely massed groups of indurated and caseous granulations.

The microscopical changes are described at p. 187.

Ref.—Phthisis, p. 68.

PLATE X.

TUBERCULAR PNEUMONIA; INDURATING AND CASEOUS TUBERCULOSIS.

FIGS. 1-4.—*Nodular caseation in diffuse pneumonic infiltration.*—From a case of chronic phthisis of three years' duration. (*Case 19, W. Griffin*, p. 183.) The microscopical appearances are shown in XXXVI. and XXXVII. See description of these, also pp. 184-6.

FIG. 1.—A portion of lung the seat of pneumonic infiltration, red below but becoming grey above, in which is a caseous mass (*a*), due to the aggregation of nodules. The outlines of these can be traced in the outer portion, and their centres are softening into minute cavities, while in the middle of the mass the tissue has broken down so as to constitute an excavation with a caseous and somewhat sinuous wall.

Ref.—Phthisis, pp. 68, 73, 74, 95, 98, 116.

FIG. 2.—From a part in which the diffuse infiltration is iron-grey in colour from the development of pigment. The caseous nodules (*a a*) contained in it are small in size, irregular in shape, and surrounded by a zone of pigmentation. At *b* more diffuse caseation is seen, apparently occurring in the pneumonic basis.

Ref.—Phthisis, pp. 68, 95, 98, 116.

FIG. 3 shows the process of formation of a cavity (*a*) by the breaking down of caseous nodules (such as *b*) imbedded in the pneumonic infiltration, here reddish-grey in tint. The softening of coalesced nodules occurs especially where they are in contact, so as to produce a sinuous cavity with nodular caseous walls. On the left, this communicates with a bronchus, the wall of which has ulcerated into the cavity.

Ref.—Phthisis, pp. 68, 73, 74, 79, 95, 99, 119.

FIG. 4.—The portion of lung here shown presents further illustrations of the processes shown in the preceding figures. The diffuse pneumonic infiltration is greyish-red in tint, and in it are caseous nodules, a few minute and round, but most (*a a*) irregular in shape. Cavities are seen, as at *b*, produced by the process shown in fig. 3; the remains of nodules are still seen in the wall of the branched cavity at *c*. Part of a larger cavity is seen on the right edge of the figure, and into it, at *b*, a bronchus opens.

Ref.—Phthisis, pp. 68-9, 73-4, 95, 99, 116-17, 119.

COLOURED PLATES (IX.-XI.)

FIGS. 5 and 6.—*Indurating Tuberculosis.* Duration of definite symptoms nine months, but previous disease probable. (*Case 26, E. Heath*, p. 194.)

The microscopical changes are shown in XL. 1-6, and XLIII. 5. See description of these, also p. 195.

FIG. 5.—Emphysematous lung, in which is an irregular tract of iron-grey indurated tissue crammed with firm opaque nodules, varying in size from a pea downwards, most of which are surrounded by a narrow zone of pigment.

Ref.—Phthisis, pp. 66, 70, 73, 94, 97, 121.

FIG. 6.—(From same case as last figure.) Isolated nodules of larger size, which present an opaque centre (*a a*), surrounded by a defined zone of greyer tint, more or less pigmented, and firm.

Ref.—Phthisis, pp. 66, 71, 82, 94.

FIGS. 7-10.—*Indurating and Caseating Tuberculosis.* Duration of symptoms about two years. (*Case 27, J. Overall*, p. 196.)

The microscopical changes are shown at XXXIX. 5 and 6; XL. 9, and XLIII. 3. See description of these, also pp. 197-9.

FIG. 7.—A portion of lung that has been injected, showing sections of bronchi (*a a*) the walls of which are greatly thickened by tissue that has undergone caseation. In some places the peribronchial growth extends into the adjacent lung-tissue. In most cases the inner surface is uniform, and presents no evidence of ulceration.

Ref.—Phthisis, p. 82.

FIG. 8.—Ramifications of a bronchus (*b b*) which has been almost entirely obliterated by the growth in its wall. In it are some cretaceous nodules, *a a* (and also *b'*).

Ref.—Phthisis, pp. 71, 99.

FIG. 9.—Tubercular granulations scattered through pulmonary tissue that is the seat of reddish pneumonic infiltration; some of the granulations (*b*) are hard and yellowish. Some larger nodules are also seen (*a a*), with a puckered dimpled depression in the centre. The latter appear like bronchi in process of obliteration.

Ref.—Phthisis, pp. 66, 82, 99.

FIG. 10.—Emphysematous lung-tissue with thickened and obliterated bronchi, containing cretaceous nodules (*b d*). From the thickened walls fibrous tracts extend into the lung-tissue, some as at *a*, branch and pass to groups of granulations. At *e* a bronchus with thickened wall has been divided just after its bifurcation. The granulations are mostly firm, grey, and pigmented, but some present central opacity. At *c* a larger nodule is seen, partly opaque.

Ref.—Phthisis, pp. 66, 70, 71, 82, 99.

PLATE XI.

CASEOUS TUBERCULAR PNEUMONIA.

Both figures are from the same case. Duration of symptoms three months. (*Case 22, T. Gardiner*, p. 187.)

The microscopical changes are shown at XXXIX. 3: see description of this, also p. 188.

Ref.—Phthisis, p. 95; Syphilitic Dis. p. 127.

FIG. 1.—*Section through the lung.* A large cavity is seen in the upper part of the figure, with a dirty-grey, sloughing floor, and smaller cavities of the same character are seen in the lower part. The pulmonary tissue adjacent is occupied by a greyish-red pneumonic infiltration, and elsewhere similar change is seen. The remaining lung-tissue, emphysematous, is congested and was loaded with serosity; adjacent to some of the cavities, it is bright red from intense hyperæmia. Nodules of caseous character are thickly scattered through the lung, for the most part yellow, but some, in an early stage, are still reddish, resembling in colour the adjacent diffuse infiltration, from which, however, they are separated by a sharp line of demarcation. In some places, as at d, the caseation occupies areas of some size. In other parts, as at f and g, it can be seen to be formed by the coalescence of minute nodules, which give the margin of these areas, in many places, a somewhat racemose appearance. Large uniform caseous nodules are seen in some places, as at a and b; the former projects into a small cavity. The nodules are softening in their centres (as at e) into the cavities already described. Dilated bronchi are seen in places. No grey granulations could be discovered in the lung.

Ref.—Phthisis, pp. 69, 73-4 (2), 117.

Fig. 2.—*The apex of the other lung from the same case.*
Beneath the surface is a large cavity which has nearly reached the pleura, and the latter has become discoloured as if about to slough. Caseous nodules appear at the surface of the lung, and some streaks of lymph indicate the pleurisy that has occurred over them.

Ref.—Phthisis, p. 70.

PLATE XII.
ACUTE PHTHISIS : CASEOUS PNEUMONIA.

Duration of symptoms, fourteen weeks.   (*Case 23, J. Lloyd*, p. 190.)
The lung-tissue is infiltrated throughout with pneumonic exudation, ash-grey in colour and finely granular. Through this caseous masses are scattered, imbedded in the infiltration. Some of these are softening in the centre (as at b) and thus give rise to irregular cavities (dd), with caseous walls and lined with an ash-grey membrane. In some places, finer, opaque granulations exist, aggregated into groups; some of the larger tracts appear as if composed of such smaller granulations (aa). Here and there a group of small nodules is imbedded in a semi-transparent, pigmented tissue, and a narrow zone of such tissue surrounds many of the larger discrete nodules.
The microscopical changes are shown at XXXIII., 2, 5, 6, and XXXIX. 1. See description of these, also p. 190.

Ref.—Phthisis, pp. 69, 73, 74 (2), 79, 95, 104, 117; Syphilitic Dis. p. 127.

PLATE XIII.
CASEOUS AND INDURATING TUBERCULAR PNEUMONIA.

Fig. 1.—*Indurating Tuberculosis, and Tubercular Pneumonia.*   Duration of definite symptoms, eight months.   (*Case 28, W. Smith*, p. 199.)
The portion of lung figured presents, in its upper part, a glistening, grey, semi-transparent tissue (c), firm and resisting, while the lower part presents a reddish-grey, more recent infiltration (a), more granular in section. In both caseous nodules are scattered, the larger of which are uniform in outline and finely granular in section: some are breaking down in the centre (bb). Small cheesy nodules are also seen, some of them no larger than miliary granulations. Some of these are surrounded by a zone of pigment.
The microscopical appearances of this lung are shown at XXXII. 7-9, XXXIII. 1, 3, and 10; XXXV. 4-6, and XLII. 5. See descriptions of these, also p. 200.

Ref.—Phthisis. pp. 68, 71 73, 76 95, 121.

Fig. 2.—*Infiltrating Tuberculisation of Liver*, from the same case as fig. 1.

The liver-tissue is infiltrated with tubercular granulations, opaque, and whitish in colour. Some are as large as a poppy-seed or a little larger, but the majority are minute specks, and are so numerous that the aspect of the tissue resembles that sometimes seen in leucocythemia, when the liver is infiltrated by a lymphoid growth. The microscopical appearances indeed showed an infiltrating lymphoid growth, identical with that described as 'lymphangiectasis' (*see* p. 201).

Figs. 3 and 4.—*Suppurating Tubercular Pneumonia.* Duration of chronic symptoms uncertain; more severe during three months. (*Case 18, J. Brodrick,* p. 181.)

The microscopical appearances are shown at XXXV. 1, 2, and 3. See description, also p. 182.

Fig. 3.—Lung occupied by dense indurated cicatricial tissue (*a a*). The bronchi have undergone sacculated dilatation (*b b*), and their mucous membrane is intensely congested. In the indurated tissue (especially in the centre of the figure) are some pigmented caseous nodules softening in the centres, and the softening of similar nodules has given rise to the cavities that are scattered through the tissue, some of which communicate with bronchi.

Ref.—Phthisis, pp. 71, 80, 121.

Fig. 4.—Lower part of the same lung, occupied by a greenish, soft, puriform pneumonic exudation (*b'*), breaking down with great readiness. The smaller bronchi are ulcerating into the adjacent exudation (*c c*). Throughout this tissue are soft nodules of greyish-yellow colour, apparently composed of aggregated granulations, such as can be seen separate in other parts. These nodules break down readily, and are, in places, softening into cavities (*a b*).

Ref.—Phthisis, pp. 119, 121.

PLATE XIV.

Chronic and Acute Phthisis—Indurating and Caseating Tubercular Pneumonia.

The plate represents the lungs of two sisters, one of whom died of chronic and the other of acute phthisis.

Fig. 1.—*Indurating Tubercular Pneumonia.* Duration of symptoms at least three years. (*Case 25, M. Corney,* p. 193.)

Section of indurated and contracted lung-tissue, infiltrated with a grey pneumonic exudation (*a a*), and containing opaque indurated granulations and firm caseous nodules, for the most part small. One, of larger size, is undergoing softening in the centre (*b*), and at *d* is a cavity, with caseous wall, which has apparently been formed by the softening of a larger caseous mass. The bronchi present sacculated dilatation (*c c*), in which cheesy nodules are to be seen in places.

Ref.—Phthisis, pp. 71–3, 76, 80, 121.

Fig. 2.—*Acute Caseous Tubercular Pneumonia.* Duration of symptoms, twelve months. (*Case 24, M. Hall,* p. 191.)

The upper two-thirds of the lung figured consists chiefly of cavities and caseous nodules, and between these the pulmonary tissue is the seat of pneumonic infiltration (*a a*), reddish or grey in tint and of semi-transparent aspect. The caseous nodules (*b b*) are irregular in shape, and some occupy a considerable area; they are, for the most part, softening and breaking down into cavities, the formation of which can be traced from the central softening of the nodules to the large, irregular excavations which occupy so much of the tissue. Below the region thus changed is a uniform infiltration (*c*) without any granular aspect, which passes into a semi-opaque consolidation, and this again into the congested emphysematous tissue of the base. In the latter are some opaque nodular areas.

The microscopical appearances are shown at XXXVIII. 7-9; see description of these, also p. 192.

Ref.—Phthisis, pp. 73-4 (2), 79, 95, 117.

PLATE XV.

TUBERCULAR PNEUMONIA AND INDURATION; TUBERCLE OF BRONCHIAL GLANDS.

Duration of definite symptoms, four months (*Case 29, J. Brown*, p. 201). The larynx is figured at XX. 3.

Ref.—Phthisis, p. 122; Syphilitic Disease, p. 128.

FIG. 1.—The apex (at the lower part of the figure) presents numerous cheesy nodules ($b\ b\ b$), many of which distinctly consist of aggregated opaque granulations. The nodules are softening in the centre into small cavities. Those at the extreme apex are surrounded by areas of granular reddish pneumonic consolidation, and this, a little lower down (higher in the figure), assumes a distinctly nodular form. The remaining unconsolidated lung-tissue in the upper part was loaded with frothy serosity. The middle portion of the lung is converted into fibroid tissue ($c\ c$), extremely hard, grey, smooth, and glistening, traversed by areas of deeper pigmentation. It contains some caseous nodules (d). At its lower margin (upper, in the figure) are some racemose granulations (d'), from which lines of fibroid tissue extend into the adjacent tissue. Numerous small cavities exist in the indurated part; some of them communicate, by sinuous passages, with the dilated bronchi, which have been opened by ulceration. The tissue of the base is intensely congested, and in it are masses ($a\ a$) composed of small caseous nodules, pigmented at the centre. Near these masses are some isolated granulations, a few grey, but most of them caseous.

The microscopical changes are shown in XLII. 7, and XLIII. 6; see description of these, also p. 202.

Ref.—Phthisis, p. 71.

FIG. 2.—*Bronchial Gland*, from the same case; enlarged, congested, and presenting irregular white tracts and a few minute granulations (a).

Ref.—Phthisis, pp. 68-9.

FIG. 3.—*Another Bronchial Gland*, from the same case, enlarged and pigmented, with yellowish tracts mottled with congestion (a). At their margin some granulations can be seen (b).

The microscopical changes in the glands are shown in XXXIV. 6 and 7; see description of these, also p. 203.

PLATE XVI.

INDURATING TUBERCULOSIS.

Both figures are from the same case. Duration of definite symptoms about five months. (*Case 30, M. A. Carr*, p. 203.)

The microscopical appearances are shown at XXXIII. 7 and 8, XLI. 1-4; see description of these, also p. 204.

FIG. 1.—Outer surface of the left lung, showing a depressed and puckered 'cicatrix' (a), over which is a series of pleural adhesions. The pleura at the spot is congested. The depression was found to correspond to a cavity the size of a Maltese orange.

Ref.—Phthisis, p. 76.

COLOURED PLATES (XIV.-XVII.) 243

Fig. 2.—Section of part of the same lung. A considerable area of the tissue is occupied by firm opaque nodules (*a*), some racemose in shape; most of them are semi-transparent, but some are caseous. In places (as at *b*) there are small nodules encapsuled with a firm, semi-cartilaginous material. Some larger masses thus encapsuled are caseous in the centre.

For the microscopical changes see above.

Ref.—Phthisis, pp. 66, 76, 121.

PLATE XVII.

INDURATING AND CASEATING TUBERCULOSIS; TUBERCLE WITH CIRRHOSIS OF THE LIVER.

Fig. 1.—*Indurating Tubercles*. Duration of symptoms, two years. (*Case 31, J. Luck*, p. 205.)

The figure shows the apex of the lung firm and fibrous, largely consisting of densely massed indurated granulations (*a a*). The outlines of the constituent granulations can be traced throughout, but they are most distinct at the margins, where racemose masses exist. Smaller groups and even isolated granulations are seen here and there in the remaining pulmonary tissue, and at *c c* are some recent granulations in islets of lung-tissue enclosed within the infiltration. A few larger caseous nodules are seen, some, as *b*, with a small cavity in the centre. At *d* are some more recent nodules, yellowish-red, occupying a considerable tract, and at the margin of this are smaller granulations. Adjacent to them, and also to the older granulations at the upper right edge of the figure, there appears to be some diffuse pneumonic infiltration. (See also fig. 3.)

The microscopical changes in this lung are shown at XL. 10. See description of this, also p. 206.

Ref.—Phthisis, pp. 71, 72, 121.

Fig. 2.—*Indurating Tuberculosis of Lung*. Duration of definite symptoms, four months. (*Case 33, W. H. Coppin*, p. 208.)

The figure shows a section of the upper part of the right lung, which consists of a dense fibroid tissue (*c c*), ash-grey in colour, streaked with lines. It was almost cartilaginous in hardness. Below this (in the upper part of the figure), the tissue, equally firm, consists of groups of granulations fused together, intensely pigmented. Within it are islets of pulmonary tissue (*a b*), congested at the margin. In the apex (below) some small cavities and a dilated bronchus are seen; the former have thick walls and are surrounded by a grey pneumonic infiltration, as firm as the rest of the tissue. The pleura is considerably thickened.

The microscopical changes in this lung are shown at XLI. 7, and XLIII. 1 and 2. See description of these, also p. 209.

Ref.—Phthisis, pp. 71, 73.

Fig. 3.—From the lower part of the lung shown in fig. 1. The tissue is occupied by a grey pneumonic infiltration (*a*), in which are opaque caseous nodules, some small (*b*), others occupying a considerable area (*c*). They soften into small cavities, with caseous walls.

Ref.—Phthisis, pp. 71, 121.

Fig. 4.—Liver, presenting cirrhosis and tubercles, from the same case as fig. 2.

The capsule is thickened. The tissue is firm and dense, and appears studded with granulations, discrete and in patches varying in size from a rape-seed to a poppy-seed. The smaller ones exactly resemble miliary tubercle. Those of larger size (*a a*) are opaque and caseous.

PLATE XVIII.

INDURATING TUBERCULOSIS.

FIG. 1.—*Tubercular Induration of Lung and Dilated Bronchi.* Duration of symptoms about thirteen months. (*Case 35, C. Roberts*, p. 212.)

The figure represents part of the left lung, which is almost entirely transformed into dense fibroid tissue; the little pulmonary tissue that remains is traversed by fibrous bands. Indurated granulations (*a b*) are scattered through the tissue, isolated or in groups, many (*b b*) pigmented in the centre. The bronchi are greatly dilated (*c d*), and intercommunicate, so as to form a series of sinuous cavities. Their mucous membrane is congested.

The microscopical changes are shown in XXXII. 10, XXXIII. 9 and 11, and XLI. 5. See description of these, also p. 213.

Ref.—Phthisis, pp. 72, 80, 97.

FIG. 2.—*Tubercular Induration*, from the same case as fig. 1.

The illustration is from the right lung, and shows its tissue crammed with indurated granulations, grey and pigmented, surrounded by fibroid induration, bands of which traverse the pulmonary tissue. A few granulations are caseous.

Ref.—Phthisis, pp. 70, 97.

FIG. 3.—*Indurating Tuberculosis.* Duration of symptoms, four years. (*Case 34, H. Cox*, p. 210.)

In the lower part of the figure (which represents part of the right lung) the tissue is occupied by dense pigmented fibroid induration (*a*), from the margin of which bands of fibres extend into the adjacent emphysematous tissue. In the induration are numerous cheesy nodules, while in the emphysematous part are groups of pigmented granulations (*c d*), some grey, others caseous. Dilated and ulcerating bronchioles traverse the lung.

The microscopical changes are shown at XLI. 6; see description of this, also p. 211.

Ref.—Phthisis, pp. 70-72.

FIG. 4.—*Indurating and Caseating Tuberculosis.* From the same case as fig. 3.

Indurated granulations, and also caseous nodules (*b b*), some softening (*a*), lie in a grey, glistening, pneumonic infiltration, in places undergoing diffuse caseation. Dilated bronchi (*e g*) ramify through the tissue, and at places are ulcerating. Some of them are surrounded by a thick layer or mass of caseous material (*f*), in which some isolated soft granulations are seen (*d*). From the breaking down of these caseous tracts and the ulceration of the bronchi, sinuous cavities (*e*) have resulted.

Ref.—Phthisis, pp. 72, 79, 121.

PLATE XIX.

INDURATING AND ULCERATING TUBERCULOSIS.

Both figures are from the same case. Duration of symptoms, several years. (*Case 36, E. Mears*, 2p.13.)

FIG. 1.—Upper part of right lung. A large cavity is seen (*b b*), covered by the thickened pleura, and lined by a caseous membrane without any distinct granulations. In the pulmonary tissue (which is emphysematous) firm, pigmented granulations are scattered, singly or in groups (*a a*). Most of

Ref.—Phthisis, pp. 66, 75-76, 121.

them are semi-transparent, a few only are caseous. They are smaller than those which commonly constitute such groups. Some small cavities are seen, opening into ulcerated bronchi.

FIG. 2.—From the left lung. The pleura (*c c*) is extremely thickened. Fibroid tissue (*a a*) has replaced the pulmonary structure. A large cavity occupies the apex, and from it sinuous branches extend ; its walls are smooth, and lined by a thick false membrane. Dilated bronchi (*b b*) are seen in the fibroid tissue which constitutes the rest of the lung.

The microscopical changes are shown in XXXIII. 4, XL. 7, and XLII. 3 and 4. See description of these, also p. 215.

Ref.—Phthisis, pp. 71, 75, 76, 80, 121.

PLATE XX.

TUBERCLE OF BRONCHI AND LARYNX.

FIG. 1.—*Bronchial Tubercle.* From a case of Indurating Tuberculosis of Lung. Duration of symptoms, four years. (*Case* 37, *A. Schofield*, p. 215.)

Dilated bronchi, with extensive formation of tubercles in the mucous membrane, some ulcerating. The intervening lung-tissue has undergone fibroid transformation and pigmentation; it contains a few cheesy nodules, and some small cavities. (*a*) An ulcer in the wall of a large dilated bronchus : it is due to the softening of a mass of caseous matter, the remains of which give thick edges to the ulcer. Immediately below this is a large nodule in the bronchial wall, not yet softened. (*b*) Yellow caseous nodules in the bronchial mucous membrane, so thickly set as to occupy the whole surface of the bronchus. The individual nodules are beginning to soften in the centre. (*c*) Opaque yellow granulations, of much smaller size, in the bronchial mucous membrane.

Ref.—Phthisis, p. 79.

FIG. 2.—*Tubercular Ulceration of Trachea.* (*Case* 20, *J. Thomas*, p. 186. See also Plate VI. fig. 4.)

The mucous membrane of the trachea is almost entirely eroded by extensive serpiginous ulceration. At the upper part (below in the figure) only small portions of congested mucous membrane are left between the ulcers.

FIG. 3.—*Tubercular Disease of Larynx, Trachea, and Glands.* (*Case* 29, *J. Brown*, p. 201. See also Plate XV.)

The figure shows ulceration of both vocal cords, tubercles of epiglottis, larynx, and trachea, and disease of the lymphatic glands. (*a a*) Granulations on the under surface of the epiglottis, and in the lower part of the larynx, over the cricoid cartilage, some small and semi-transparent, others larger and opaque, while some are even beginning to ulcerate. (*b*) Yellow opaque granulations in the lower part of the trachea, extending into the bronchi, and so thickly massed as to occupy almost the whole of the surface. (*c c*) Ulcers on the vocal cords, with thick everted edges, and caseous nodules in their floor. (*d*) Small lenticular ulcerations, mingled with opaque granulations, scattered over the congested mucous membrane. A larger ulcer is seen among the granulations in the lower part of the trachea (above *b*). (*e*) Post-tracheal glands, much enlarged and congested, containing small grey and opaque granulations (*e*) and larger yellow caseous nodules coalescing into irregular tracts. Pigmented areas are also seen. Other appearances in the bronchial glands are shown also at Plate XV. 2 and 3.

The microscopical appearance of the glands is shown in XXXIV. 6 and 7; that of the larynx is shown in XXXIV. 2 and 3. See description of this, also p. 202.

Ref.—Syphilitic Dis. p. 128.

PLATE XXI.
EMPHYSEMA AND COLLAPSE.[1]

FIG. 1.—*Emphysema of Lung.* From a drawing by Sir Robert Carswell. (*Case 44*, p. 223.)

The figure represents the summit of the left lung, from which project a number of emphysematous vesicles, ranging in size from that of a pea to that of a hen's egg. The latter has a lobulated appearance, as if due to the coalescence of distended air-cells.

FIG. 2.—*Collapse.* From Cruveilhier's *Atlas d'Anatomie Pathologique du Corps Humain,* tome 1, liv. xv. Pl. ii. fig. 6.

The following is Cruveilhier's description:—' Both lungs, of large size, are completely carnified. 'The lobular form is perfectly preserved. Each lobule represents a granulation analogous in ap-'pearance to the glandular granulations of a cirrhosed liver. The granulations are very easily 'separable from one another; they adhere to the lung by a vascular pedicle.'

Ref.—Catarrhal Pneumonia, p. 25; Collapse, p. 57.

FIG. 3.—*Collapse.* From Cruveilhier's *Atlas.* *Ib.* fig. 1.

The following description of this figure is obtained by the collation of two portions of Cruveilhier's text:—' Lungs of a newly-born child, dead forty-eight hours after birth. . . . They present 'lobules and masses of lobules rendered impermeable by infiltration of blood situated among healthy 'lobules. Section of the left lung shows that infiltrated lobules are present in the interior as well 'as on the surface. It is possible that the change is not only referable to the period of birth' (*i.e.* was antecedent to this).

Ref.—Collapse, p. 57.

FIG. 4.—*Collapse.* From Cruveilhier. *Ib.* fig. 4.

The figure is thus described:—' Lobules infiltrated with blood and impermeable in three-fourths 'of their substance. Newly-born child, natural delivery, breech presentation. It appeared weak, 'and remained so until death, which occurred at the end of twenty hours. The lungs are imperme-'able in about two-thirds of their extent. This impermeability is seen especially posteriorly and at 'the base. It consists in a reddish-black moist induration, which appears to be an infiltration of 'blood and of serosity. They very closely resemble the tissue of the spleen. Here and there are 'seen in the remainder of the lung nodules of infiltration (*a a*). I think that the lesion may date 'from the moment of birth.'

Ref.—Collapse, p. 57.

FIG. 5.—*Emphysema with Dilatation and Contraction of the Bronchi.* From a case of heart-disease, with albuminuria from contracted kidneys.

A large bronchus running along the outer and posterior part of the lower lobe (upwards and to the right in the figure) had its wall thickened and its calibre narrowed by dense exudation-matter between the pleura and the pericardium, and beyond this narrowing it presented fusiform dilatations. The whole area supplied by the bronchus was in a state of emphysema, contrasting strongly with the purple tint of the rest of the lung-tissue, which was loaded with serosity, mottled with spots of capillary hæmorrhage, and pigmented. No bronchial dilatations were found elsewhere in either lung. The whole of this lung was firmly adherent to the parietal pleura and pericardium.

(*a*) Light-coloured emphysematous tissue. (*d d*) Dark pulmonary tissue. (*b*) Contraction of bronchus. (*c c c*) Fusiform dilatations of bronchi.

---

[1] The description of this plate is by the Authors.

PLATE XXII.

Potter's and Miner's Lungs; Brown Induration; Cancer.

Fig. 1.—*Lung in Potter's Phthisis.* Symptoms existed for some years; they were severe during six months. (*Case 38, C. Barlow,* p. 216.)

The lung presents black masses of indurated tissue, varying in size from a pea to a hazel-nut, and surrounded and separated by zones and lines of paler condensed pulmonary tissue, and apparently by areas in which the indurated tissue is mottled by black specks. (*a*) Condensed pulmonary tissue little pigmented, surrounding a pigmented mass. (*b*) Deeply pigmented tract.[1]

The microscopical changes are shown in XLIV. 5-7. See description of this, also p. 217.

Fig. 2.—*Lung in Miner's Phthisis.* After Greenhow, *Trans. Path. Soc.* vol. xx. plate ii. (*Case 39,* p. 218.)

The figure represents the lung of a collier. The apex, (below in the figure) is consolidated and firm, with a uniform smooth section, greyish-black in colour; the rest of the pulmonary tissue is spongy but black, with a little mottling of dark grey. (*a*) A large, irregular cavity. (*b*) Section of a bronchial tube containing black mucus. (*c*) Uniform consolidation at the apex.

The microscopical changes are shown in XLIV. 3.

Fig. 3. — *Brown Induration,* early stage. From a case of mitral and aortic contraction. (*Case 43, W. Thomas,* p. 222.)

The figure represents part of the left lung. The pulmonary tissue is for the most part reddish-grey and but little pigmented, but in the upper part of the figure are numerous small nodules, similar to those shown in the next figure.

The microscopical changes are shown in XLIV. 10 and 11. See description of these, also p. 223.

Ref.—Brown Induration, p. 52.

Fig. 4.—*Brown Induration,* later stage. From the same case as fig. 3.

The illustration represents part of the lower lobe of the left lung. The tissue is solidified, and presents the appearance of a bright red ground, mottled, with minute, slightly prominent, specks of reddish-white.

Ref.—Brown Induration, p. 52.

Fig. 5.—*Cancerous Growth in the Sheaths of the Vessels;* secondary to cancer of ovaries. (*Case 45, H. Parsons,* p. 224.)

The vessels of the lung (*a a*) are greatly thickened, rigid and white on section; they project from the cut surface, so as to resemble thickened bronchial tubes. The appearance is due to a cancerous growth in their walls, chiefly in their outer and middle coats.

The microscopical appearances are shown in XLV. 1-3. See description of these, also p. 225.

Ref.—Cancer, p. 185.

Fig. 6.—*Infiltrating Cancer of Lung.* (*Case 46,* p. 225.)

The growth appears in the form of small nodules, thickly set in the pulmonary tissue, and closely resembling the caseous nodules of pneumonic origin.

The microscopical appearances are shown in XLVI. 4, 5, 6; see description of these, also p. 225.

Ref.—Cancer, p. 184.

---

[1] Compare description of the lung p. 217.

PLATE XXIII.
Pyæmia; Cancer; Infarct and Collapse.

Fig. 1.—*Multiple Infarction of Lung*; due to septic embolism, from a thrombus in a renal vein. (*Case 49, W. Rowe*, p. 227.)

Numerous small yellow nodules are seen through the pleura surrounded by an areola of congestion.

Ref.—Embolism, p. 58.

Fig. 2.—*Sarcoma of the Lung with Collapse, and an old infarct.* (*Case 48, Fisher*, p. 226.)

(*a*) A large lobular mass of malignant growth, extending into the lung from its inner side. The growth has an encephaloid aspect, but its structure was that of a small-celled sarcoma, and it had arisen in the posterior mediastinum. (*b*) An area of necrosis of the pulmonary tissue, probably due to the occlusion of an artery by embolism. The necrosed region presents a mottling of red, yellow, and grey, and there is a white line of demarcation between it and the rest of the lung. (*c*) Pulmonary tissue which has undergone collapse, fibroid change, and pigmentation. There was much effusion in the pleural cavity.

Ref.—Collapse, p. 58; Embolism, p. 58.

PLATE XXIV.
Pulmonary Apoplexy; Interlobular Pneumonia; Cancer of Lung and Bronchial Glands.

Fig. 1.—*Hæmorrhagic Infarcts of the Lung* (Pulmonary Apoplexy). From an unpublished drawing by Sir Robert Carswell.

The figure shows parts of three areas of recent infarction. The middle one exhibits the characteristic wedge-shape of the section, the base of the wedge being at the surface of the lung, where it forms a prominence. The section is of a deep purple colour, and finely granular, owing to the effused blood filling the air-vessels.

Ref.—Embolism, p. 59.

Fig. 2.—*Acute Interstitial Pneumonia.* From an unpublished drawing by Sir R. Carswell. The patient had suffered from chronic cystitis; no disease of the lungs was suspected (see p. 42).

Distended lymphatics, containing fluid pus, are seen on the surface of the lung. In the cut surfaces the interlobular cellular tissue is much more conspicuous than normal, and pale yellow in colour (from infiltration with pus). Distended lymphatics can also be traced, passing to join those on the surface.

Ref.—Acute Interstitial Pneumonia, p. 42.

Fig. 3.—*Cancer (Columnar Epithelioma) of Bronchial Gland.* (*Case 47, P. Leather*, p. 225.)

The gland is enlarged, and in its deeply pigmented tissue are numerous soft, yellowish nodules of new growth (*a*).

Fig. 4.—*Cancer (Columnar Epithelioma) of Lung.* From the same case.

The figure represents the surface of the lung, in the substance of which masses of growth were found, some of which can be seen through the pleura. Their position is marked by the paler tint of the tissue, by the red injection of the inflamed pleura, and by the peculiar enlargement of the lymphatics (*a*), which appear like white cords, with moniliform swellings (*b c*).

Ref.—Cancer, pp. 135, 137.

§ B. MICROSCOPICAL PLATES. (XXV. to XLV.)

PLATE XXV.
ACUTE STHENIC AND CATARRHAL PNEUMONIA.

FIGS. 1, 2, 3, *from a case of Acute Pneumonia, dying on the tenth day.*

FIG. 1 shows the walls of the alveoli maintained, and their interior densely filled with a mass of cells, *a b b*, held together by a fibrillated exudation-matter. The walls of the alveoli are not thickened, but the capillaries are dilated; a few corpuscles are seen in the walls of the alveoli, *c*. When more highly magnified, the appearances of these alveoli resemble those seen in fig. 5, *q. r.* (*Chromic acid prep.* × 70 *diam.*)

Ref.—Acute Pneumonia, p. 19.

FIG. 2.—Same specimen as foregoing, but the chief mass of cells have been pencilled out. Cells are seen, imbedded in a reticulum, which is partly formed out of the alveolar wall. *a a*, large, round, granular cells, measuring from $\frac{1}{2500}$ to $\frac{1}{3000}$ inch in diameter; *b*, smaller cells, measuring $\frac{1}{5000}$ inch. (*Chromic acid prep.* × 700 *diam.*)

Ref.—Acute Pneumonia, p. 19.

FIG. 3.—From same specimen, showing a more advanced stage (grey hepatisation). The large epithelial cells have entirely disappeared, and they are replaced by smaller pyoid cells, granular, mostly containing a single nucleus, and measuring from $\frac{1}{7500}$ to $\frac{1}{9000}$ inch in diameter. The walls of the alveoli are seen unchanged, except that a few cells, similar to those seen in their interior, are imbedded among the elastic fibres. (*Chromic acid prep.* × 460 *diam.*)

Ref.—Acute Pneumonia, p. 19 (2).

FIGS. 4, 5, 6, *from a case of Acute Gangrenous Pneumonia, dying on the twelfth day.*

FIG. 4 shows the alveoli filled with large epithelial cells and small round cells intermingled. *a a*, large epithelial cells containing bipartite nuclei. The cells are clear and hyaline. (The fat has probably been dissolved out by the chloroform used in mounting.) Some of them resemble those seen in fig. 9, *a, b, c, d*. They measure from $\frac{1}{2500}$ to $\frac{1}{3000}$ and $\frac{1}{1500}$ inch in diameter. The nuclei measure from $\frac{1}{10000}$ to $\frac{1}{5000}$ inch. *b b*, large hyaline cells without a nucleus, some of which resemble *t*, fig. 9, and represent 'physalides,' in which a large clear, ovoid, or round body nearly fills the larger cell, and is surrounded by a granular zone. These cells measure, on an average, $\frac{1}{1500}$ inch. *c c*, epithelioid cells like *a*, granular, and with a single nucleus. *d d*, small round cells like *l*, fig. 9, measuring from $\frac{1}{8500}$ to $\frac{1}{5000}$ inch, some containing bipartite nuclei. In some places these are densely massed. *e e*, alveolar walls, containing epithelioid cells. (*Chromic acid prep.* × 700 *diam.*)

Ref.—Acute Pneumonia, p. 19 (2).

FIG. 5.—From same. Margin of an alveolus, showing enlarged epithelioid cells. (× 460 *diam.*)

FIG. 6.—From same. Numerous blood-corpuscles, *b b*, are mingled with cells, *a a*, of the type of those above described. At *c* are pyoid cells.

Ref.—Acute Pneumonia, pp. 19, 22.

FIG. 7. *Acute sthenic pneumonia* (Plate I.). Date the 5th day. The lung was in a state of typical red hepatisation. The cells, *a, b*, are of the type of fig. 3; some, *a*, have bipartite nuclei: they are imbedded in a network of fibrin, *c*. (× 560 *diam.*)

K K

FIG. 8.—From catarrhal pneumonia of measles. (*See Coloured Pl. V. 1 & 4.*) The cells massed in the interior of the alveoli show but little fibrinous network. They are largely of the epithelioid type, *a*. Some of these are of type *b d* Fig. 9, and contain two nuclei; the cells measure $\frac{1}{700}$, the nuclei about $\frac{1}{1500}$ to $\frac{1}{2500}$ inch. Some, however, are smaller and rounded, probably of more recent formation, and these especially display multiple nuclei, *b b*. The walls of the alveoli are largely occupied by distended capillaries, *c c*. (*Chromic acid prep.* × 700 *diam.*).

Ref.—Catarrhal Pneumonia, p. 28.

FIG. 9.—*Cells from Fibrinous and Catarrhal Pneumonia.* (× 700 *diam.*)

A. Cells from Fibrinous Pneumonia.

a, b. These are among the most common of all the cells found in acute pneumonia at all dates (5th, 10th, and 12th day). They may be finely nebulous, as here represented, or darker, with protein molecules; a few show fat-drops in their interior. Cells measure from $\frac{1}{750}$ to $\frac{1}{2500}$ inch; nuclei measure $\frac{1}{1500}$ to $\frac{1}{1500}$ inch, but some cells of this nature, with a single nucleus, may measure as little as $\frac{1}{2500}$ inch, with a nucleus of $\frac{1}{5000}$ inch, and all gradations may be found between the larger and smaller sizes. *c*, larger cells, apparently of the same nature as *a, b*, with single nucleus, large and hyaline; cells measure $\frac{1}{750}$ to $\frac{1}{1500}$ inch, the nuclei $\frac{1}{2100}$ inch. These cells are found in red hepatisation (Plate I., death on 5th day), and also in grey hepatisation (Plate IV. fig. 3, death on tenth day). *d*, a cell showing commencing division of an elongated nucleus; cells measure $\frac{1}{750}$ inch, nucleus $\frac{1}{2500}$ × $\frac{1}{4500}$, and were found in all specimens from the 5th to the 12th day. *e*, fissiparous division of a cell like the foregoing, with three nuclei (5th and 10th day). *f*, double nucleus in epithelial-like cell. Cell measures $\frac{1}{1500}$ inch, nuclei $\frac{1}{5000}$ inch (10th day). *g*, groups of cells with tripartite nuclei; cells round, fine granular, nuclei mostly contain nucleoli: cells measure from $\frac{1}{1500}$ to $\frac{1}{1000}$ inch; nuclei from $\frac{1}{5000}$ to $\frac{1}{7000}$ inch (death on 12th day). *h*, groups of cells like foregoing, more epithelioid in shape, with tripartite nuclei (measurements same as *g* (10th day); found also in hypostatic pneumonia (Plate III.). *k, l*, cells with nuclei undergoing division; cells measure $\frac{1}{3000}$, nuclei $\frac{1}{6000}$ to $\frac{1}{8000}$ inch (10th day). *m*, large epithelioid cell with three nuclei; cells $\frac{1}{1500}$, nuclei $\frac{1}{1500}$ inch (10th day). Small cells of this nature, in which the nuclei are situated more eccentrically, may be as small as $\frac{1}{2100}$ or even $\frac{1}{2400}$ and $\frac{1}{4100}$ inch. *n*, large 'placoid,' with larger nucleus; cell measures $\frac{1}{1500}$, nucleus $\frac{1}{2500}$ (tenth day). *p, q*, pigment-cells of the types *a, b*, but enlarged, with enlarged nuclei; the cells may attain the size of $\frac{1}{500}$, nucleus $\frac{1}{1500}$ inch; those here drawn had a size of $\frac{1}{750}$. The nuclei gradually become obscured by the pigment in the cell, but could still be seen faintly, as in *q* (found in all stages from 5th to 12th days). *r*, pigmented nuclei, $\frac{1}{1500}$, free in alveoli (12th day). *r'*, pigmented nuclei on or in wall of the alveolus (12th day). *s, t*, rare forms of cells, probably mucoid, in which the nucleus gradually enlarges, and finally fills the cells ('physalides' ?) Cell measures $\frac{1}{1500}$ to $\frac{1}{1000}$; nucleus, $\frac{1}{5000}$ to $\frac{1}{500}$.

B. Cells from catarrhal pneumonia.

u, epithelial cells from chronic catarrhal pneumonia. Cells measure $\frac{1}{1100}$ in length by $\frac{1}{1500}$ in width; nucleus $\frac{1}{2500}$ inch. r^a r^b r^c from same, similar cells to *u*, with multiple nuclei. In r^a the nuclei are enlarged to $\frac{1}{5000}$ inch. Some cells, r^b, were narrow,-measuring $\frac{1}{1500}$ by $\frac{1}{2500}$ inch. In some, fissiparous division of the nuclei could be seen. *x*, from same, a pigmented epithelioid cell like r^b, and of same dimensions.

Ref.—Acute Pneumonia, pp. 20, 21; Hypostatic Pneumonia, p. 40.

PLATE XXVI.

CATARRHAL PNEUMONIA; SYPHILIS.

FIGS. 1–4.—*Acute Broncho-pneumonia in child.* (*Case 4, Tanner*, p. 160; and Col. Pl. V. 3.)

FIG. 1.—A dilated infundibulum, with series of alveolar passages filled with débris of cells. The total transverse diameter of this, at its greatest width, is $\frac{1}{100}$ inch. The width of the masses

$a\,a$, contained within it, averages about $\frac{1}{300}$ of an inch. These masses have no definite boundary line, and they appear to have separated in the preparation. In some places, however, their margin is better defined, as at d. They consist of accumulations of cells of epithelioid and pyoid types, breaking down into débris. During this change the cells appear to fuse into a granular mass. The outer margin of this mass is composed of collapsed pulmonary tissue, $b\,b$, in which are dilated capillaries and a few pneumonic cells. This collapse is apparently produced by the pressure exerted by the distended infundibulum. $c\,c$, capillaries.   (*Bichromate of potash prep.; stained hæmatoxylin; Canada balsam.*   × 100 *diam.*)

Ref.—Catarrhal Pneumonia, pp. 23, 27, 28.

Fig. 2.—From same as foregoing. A series of terminal infundibula filled with epithelioid cells breaking down. $a\,a\,a$, infundibula distended. $b\,b$, pleura. c, interlobular septum. d, large blood-vessel. e, an alveolar passage. f (see next figure). The septa between the infundibula are seen occupied by distended capillaries, but no definite cell-growth intervenes. (× 100 *diam.*)

Ref.—Catarrhal Pneumonia, pp. 23, 27, 28.

Fig. 3—from the spot in fig. 2, marked f—shows a portion of an alveolus filled with cells of different sizes. Some are large and epithelioid, containing much pigment, and in them the nuclei have disappeared ; others nucleated, measuring $\frac{1}{3100}$ to $\frac{1}{2500}$ of an inch, and some are binucleated. Besides these there are numerous smaller cells measuring $\frac{1}{7000}$ to $\frac{1}{5000}$ inch. The general character of the change in both these last figures is that the epithelial cells break down, and are partly replaced by smaller cells of a puriform type (but which are not true pus-cells, and are probably of secondary production), and the whole of the cells break up into débris and become fused (× 460 *diam.*)

Ref.—Catarrhal Pneumonia, pp. 27–28.

Fig. 4.—From another portion of the same preparation. Portion of adjacent alveoli, showing the enlargement of the epithelial cells, $a\,a\,a$, which are finely granular : their outlines are becoming faint, and they are breaking down. $b\,b$, nuclei of capillaries in walls of alveoli. $c\,c$, a few scattered round nuclei in walls of alveoli. (*Bichromate of potash prep.; stained hæmatoxylin ; Canada balsam.* × 460 *diam.*)

Ref.—Catarrhal Pneumonia, pp. 27–28.

Figs. 5 and 6.—*Chronic Lobular Pneumonia* following the injection of mercury into the trachea of a dog, killed after two months. Each figure probably represents a terminal infundibulum, as shown by the thickened septum surrounding it.

Fig. 5.—A nodule which, to the naked eye, and even with a low magnifying power, closely resembled a tubercular granulation. It is seen to consist chiefly of enlarged nucleated epithelial cells, imbedded in a reticulum of thickened fibres (? lymphatics). The epithelial cells are large : the majority are hyaline and measure $\frac{1}{2500}$ to $\frac{1}{1500}$ inch. They mostly contain but one nucleus. Pyoid cells, $b\,b$ (lymphatic ?), appear in the reticulum, and in some places, $c\,c$, agglomerate into denser masses. d, rows of such cells. $e\,e$, thickened septum, composed of a reticulum of fibres in which small cells are imbedded. (*Chromic acid prep.; stained carmine; gum dammar.* × 460).

Fig. 6.—A nodule similar to the foregoing but in a more advanced stage of fibroid change. The epithelial cells have in great measure disappeared, but traces of them are to be seen at a. The small-celled growth is abundant at b, imbedded in a reticulum which, at c, shows broader fibres. $d\,d$, thickened septum with fusiform nuclei and long fibres. (*Chromic acid prep.; stained carmine; gum dammar.* × 460 *diam.*)

Fig. 7.—Pneumonia in tubercular subject ; 'catarrhal pneumonia' : 'desquamative pneumonia.' (*Case 17, Ellsom*, p. 179, and Col. Pl. IX. 1 and 2, see also Plate XXXVIII. figs. 5 and 6.) The preparation is taken from a, fig. 2.

The figure shows two adjacent alveoli filled with large epithelioid cells, a, measuring from $\frac{1}{7000}$ to $\frac{1}{1500}$ inch. They are densely packed and assume polyhedral forms from mutual pressure; a few smaller, round, mono-nucleated cells are also seen. Nuclear growth is commencing in the walls of the alveoli at c. (*Chromic acid prep.; stained carmine; gum dammar.* × 700 *diam.*)

Ref.—Phthisis, pp. 95, 105.

FIG. 8.—Section of portion of a syphilitic gumma in advanced stage. The tissue is almost entirely fibroid. The fibres are, for the most part, broad-banded, homogeneous, and highly refracting. In some places, however, they are fibrillated. aa, remains of alveoli imbedded in this fibroid structure, and showing only fibrillation of their walls. bb, remains of similar alveoli showing caseating epithelium. cc, remains of epithelium, probably from alveoli completely invaded by the fibroid growth. d, a blood-vessel. (*Chromic acid prep.; stained magenta; gum dammar.* × 230 *diam.*)

Ref.—Syphilitic Disease, pp. 122, 131, 132.

PLATE XXVII.

PULMONARY SYPHILIS.

Ref.—Syphilitic Disease, pp. 122, 132.

FIGS. 1 to 5.—Are from preparations of a syphilitic gumma, kindly lent me by Dr. Goodhart, and drawn and published with his permission.

FIG. 1.—Shows a portion of the remains of an alveolus, filled with a small-celled growth. These cells are imbedded in a reticulum, by the thickening of which broad-banded fibres are produced while the cells disappear. aa, small-celled growth in reticulum. bb, thickening of fibres of reticulum. c, one of many places where groups of small cells are seen imprisoned among the broad bands of the fibres of the reticulum. d, e, gradual disappearance of the small cells among the broader fibres. f, g, spaces where the small cells remain as single or double nuclei in the interstices of the fibres. hhh, these cells are assuming a stellate form with branching processes (lymph-canalicular system or blood-vessels?) k, a band where the cells appear as oval nuclei. l, fully-formed fibrillated tissue. (× 460 *diam.*)

Ref.—Syphilitic Disease, p. 130.

FIG. 2.—From same. a, part of an alveolus where epithelioid growth still remains. b, small-celled growth like fig. 1. cc, gradual thickening of reticulum. d, reticulum where the small-celled growth has disappeared. ee, highly refracting broad bands of fibres, in the meshes of which remains of small-celled growth are included. In some places the cells are seen as single or double nuclei. f, f, stellate cells with branching processes. (× 460 *diam.*)

Ref.—Phthisis, p. 113; Syphilitic Disease, p. 130.

FIGS. 3, 4, 5.—From same, show the formation of a lymph-canicular system in the midst of the broad bands of fibres.

FIG. 3.—The fibroid mass has become almost filled with a uniform, highly refracting tissue, in which the remains of the bands are still seen, separated only by branching lacunae resembling those of tendon or bone. aaa, branching lacunae with many radiating tubular processes, and containing each a single cell (a nucleus?). b, a similar one imbedded in a broad fibrous band. c, a series of such, communicating by their branching processes. dd, a series of branching processes in which the nuclei are seen. e, a lacuna without a nucleus. (× 460 *diam.*)

FIG. 4.—A portion where the small-celled growth has proceeded to the formation of fibroid tissue, closely resembling that seen in the early stage of periosteal ossification. (Compare Quain's

'Anatomy,' edited by Schäfer, 1876, ii. p. 96.) *a a*, broad bands of fibres. *b b*, stellate cells with thickened walls. *c*, round nuclei included in the broad bands of fibre. *d*, a single elongated nucleus included in a band of fibre. (× 460 *diam.*)

FIG. 5.—Three adjacent broad bands of fibres. *a*, central band. *b b*, two others almost entirely filled with, and separated only by, the long processes (tubules) of the lymph-canalicular system. *c c*, two large stellate cells (lacunæ) with nuclei in their interior. *d d*, long processes given off from these. *e*, a similar lacuna, partially imbedded in a broad fibre. *f*, gradual disappearance of a lacuna in the fibre-growth. *g*, a round cell with short processes, imbedded in a broad fibre. (× 700 *diam.*)

FIGS. 6 and 7.—From Dr. Greenfield's drawings of a case of syphilitic pneumonia ('Path. Soc. Trans.' xxvii. pl. iii. reprinted by permission. *See Case 52*, p. 229).

FIG. 6.—A rough sketch, under low power, to show the arrangement of the fibrous septa and partial obliteration of the walls of the air-cells.

Ref.—Syphilitic Disease, p. 131.

FIG. 7.—Shows the margin of one of the fibrous septa, with bands of fibrous tissue running between the alveoli, the walls of which are somewhat thickened, but the epithelium is normal. (*Hartnack, oc. 3. obj. 8.*)

Ref.—Phthisis, pp. 113, 118; Syphilitic Disease, pp. 181, 182.

PLATE XXVIII.

ACUTE TUBERCULISATION; LUNGS OF CHILDREN.

FIG. 1.—Shows the pyramidal form sometimes assumed by single granulations. Section reaching surface of lung. The granulation appears to correspond to an ultimate lobule. *a*, terminal bronchiole, the walls of which are invaded by the small-celled growth. *b*, dense fibroid capsule (the thickened interlobular septum), showing small-celled growth, which is more marked at *c*. *d*, pleura. *e e*, adjacent alveoli, some containing large epithelial cells. *f*, a round mass, staining deeply, for the most part amorphous, but still (in the preparation) showing traces of nuclei. It measures $\frac{1}{30}$ inch, is surrounded by a thickened wall, and is probably a giant-cell. The adjacent alveoli show penetration of the injection (distended capillaries) from which the tubercle is free. (*Injected chromic acid prep.; stained osmic acid; gum dammar.* × 100 *diam.*)

Ref.—Phthisis, p. 102.

FIG. 2.—*Acute tubercle, lung of child.* Two very small grey granulations, side by side, under the pleural surface, which limits the figure below. *a a*, lobules partly pneumonic. *b b*, round masses which, by a higher power, are seen to be giant-cells of the type of those shown in XXXII. 1, *c*, and 2, *a*. (*Injected and chromic acid preparation; stained osmic acid; gum dammar.* × 100 *diam.*)

Ref.—Phthisis, pp. 102, 115, 118.

FIG. 3.—*Acute tubercle, lung of child.* The figure shows the lobular form of the tubercle, but with extension of small-celled growth to adjacent alveoli. *a a*, pyramidal mass of tubercle. *c*, central portion of an alveolus still showing pneumonic processes; the small-celled growth invades the whole of the remaining tissue. *d*, a giant-cell. *e*, a vessel with perivascular thickening. In all these three first specimens (injected) the larger vessels are seen to penetrate the tubercles, but the capillaries are obliterated. *b b*, sections of bronchioles surrounded by small-celled growth. (*Injected ; chromic acid preparation ; stained osmic acid ; gum dammar ;* × 80 *diam. Tuffen West, delt.*)

Ref.—Phthisis, p. 102.

FIG. 4.—*Acute Miliary Tuberculosis ; lung of child.* (*Case* 7, *Coombes*, p. 165, and Col. Pl. VIII. 2 and 5, also XXX. 2 and 4, and XXXIV. 1.) The figure shows the form in which early stages of disseminated tubercle are found in the alveolar tissue. *a*, growth around an interlobular bronchiole. The whole of the adjacent alveoli are implicated, forming a solid nodule, while thickening extends into the neighbouring alveolar walls.[1] *b b*, similar thickenings of the alveolar walls with small-celled growth. *c*, similar thickening combined with much pigmentation. *d d*, granulations of alveolar origin (terminal). The traces of alveolar structure are still apparent, the centres being lighter in tint from pneumonic accumulation with degeneration. (*Chromic acid preparation ; stained osmic acid.* × 480 *diam. Tuffen West, delt.*)

Ref.—Phthisis, p. 102 ; Syphilitic Dis. p. 182.

FIG. 5.—*Child's lung ; acute tuberculisation.* The figure shows the manner in which miliary granulations are grouped along an interlobular septum, *e e*. Each granulation represents a lobule. *a a a*, granulations, many of which were found, by a higher magnifying power, to have a pneumonic centre. *b b*, thickening of the alveolar walls. *c*, fusion of two round granulations, with a thickening of adjacent alveoli into a larger and more uniform mass. *d*, the lumen of a bronchiole surrounded by infiltrated alveolar tissue. The capillaries are seen to be obliterated as the thickening advances, and to be completely obstructed in the granulations. (*Chromic acid preparation.* × 80 *diam. Tuffen West, delt.*)

Ref.—Phthisis, p. 108 ; Syphilitic Dis. p. 182.

FIG. 6.—*Acute miliary tuberculisation, child.* (*Case 6, Polley,* p. 163, and Col. Pl. VI., also XXX. 5.) Diffuse caseation of 'tubercular pneumonia.' Large tracts are converted into amorphous or granular débris, in which the outlines of the alveoli are still visible, for the most part with thickened walls, *a*. In numerous places where the process is less advanced, when examined with a higher power, the whole of the change is seen to be attended with a small-celled growth in the alveolar walls and septa, while the interior of the alveoli, which are narrowed, is occupied by epithelial cells of various sizes, mingled with nuclei, and with the small-celled growth from the walls. The proportion of small-celled growth, and of intra-alveolar pneumonic change, varies considerably. No pneumonic process appears to precede the thickening of the wall, and at the margins where it is proceeding, the alveoli, *b*, are occupied by large cells (the 'desquamative pneumonia' of Buhl). The capillaries perish early. Portions may apparently persist long in this state, only slowly undergoing a granular disintegration, and a quasi-fibroid change ensues, *c*, as in fig. 8. (*Chromic acid prep. ; stained osmic acid ; gum dammar.* × 80 *diam. Tuffen West, delt.*)

Ref.—Phthisis, pp. 94, 114 (2), 118.

FIG. 7.—*Acute tuberculisation (same case).* The figure shows group of alveoli occupied by epithelial (pneumonic) proliferation in their interior, *a a*, with great thickening of the walls by a small-celled growth, thus gradually narrowing the lumen of the alveolus. At *b* is a giant-cell. The capillaries are obliterated as the change proceeds. This is probably an earlier stage of figs. 6 and 8. (*Chromic acid prep., injected, and stained with osmic acid ; Tuffen West, delt.* × 100.)

Ref.—Phthisis, pp. 107, 114, 117, 118.

FIG. 8.—*Acute tuberculisation (same case).* A later stage of the process shown in fig. 7, and a variation of that seen in fig. 6. The process is diffuse, not limited to lobules. It consists in the

---

[1] Compare this with Dr. Shepherd's Plates I. and II. *Pulmonary Consumption*; also with Hérard and Cornil, *Phthisie Pulmonaire*, figs. 5-8, pp. 110-113.

conversion of the lung-tissue into a finely fibrillated and granular texture, in which, when examined with a higher power, are seen, irregularly mingled, large and small cells. In some places, however, the texture shows no traces of cell-structure, but only an amorphous, granular, and fibrillated mass. The outlines of the alveoli are for the most part maintained. (*Chromic acid prep.* × 80. *Tuffen West, delt.*)

Ref.—Phthisis, pp. 94, 113, 117.

FIGS. 9 and 10.—*Acute tubercle (same case)*. The figures represent diffuse thickening of the pulmonary tissue, invading the walls, and in some places obliterating the cavities of the alveoli. The latter could elsewhere be seen with a higher power (not represented here) to be filled with enlarged epithelial cells, but this is not constant. In parts the alveoli are dilated (10, *a a*) and their walls are thickened. The growth can also be seen proceeding around the bronchioles (10, *b b*). With a higher power this thickening is seen to depend on a small-celled growth invading the walls (indicated in fig. 10). With this are mingled some larger cells, and also cells containing pigment. The growth, in some places, passes into a finely fibrillated and granular texture, in which nearly all traces of cell-formation are lost (fig. 9), and which is similar in nature to that described in figs. 6 and 8. (*Chromic acid prep.*—fig. 9 × 50, fig. 10 × 80. *Tuffen West, delt.*)

Ref.—Phthisis, pp. 107, 117.

PLATE XXIX.

ACUTE TUBERCULISATION; LUNG, CHILD. (*Case 8, Shimmick*, see p. 167, and also Plates XXX. 9, XXXI. 1–6, and XXXII. 1 and 6.)

FIGS. 1 to 5 represent sections at various depths, through what, to the naked eye, appeared to be a single grey granulation, in the lung of a child dying of acute tuberculosis. (× 80 *diam.*)

FIG. 1.—The most superficial section, nearest the pleural surface, shows a structure similar to figs. 5, 6, 7, Plate XXVIII. *a a a*, alveolar structure of lung still apparent. The walls are thickened, and there is in some places an accumulation of the epithelium in the interior of the alveoli. *b b b*, portions where the tissue is becoming more dense and homogeneous, through the infiltration of a small-celled growth; the alveolar structure is less distinct. *c c*, sections of a few large blood-vessels.

FIG. 2.—Section rather deeper than the foregoing. The apparent single tubercle is seen to correspond to an aggregation of several nodules. *a* and *b* correspond to similar parts of fig. 1. The structure of each is more homogeneous, and the centre of *b* is tending to pass into molecular débris. *c*, remains of alveolar structure invaded by small-celled growth. *d d*, central portions of alveoli densely filled with epithelial and small-celled growth intermingled.

FIGS. 3 and 4.—The same condition more advanced in solidification and partial caseation. *a a a*, portions of the granulation where the alveolar structure still remains, containing large epithelial and small-celled growth. *b b b*, portions where this is more dense. *c c*, remains of alveolar structure, with thickened walls, intervening between the granulations. *d d*, centres of granulations becoming caseous. *e*, lines of fibrillated structure with amorphous, granular texture, between the granulations.

FIG. 5.—The same in a still more advanced condition. The centres of the masses, *d d*, have become still more extensively caseous, and the fibrillation of the intervening spaces more distinct. Another small granulation, *f*, in an earlier stage of formation, is seen growing in juxtaposition to these. (The other reference letters have the same significance as in the last figure.)

FIG. 6.—Another mass of tubercle, from the same lung, is seen to be composed of a series of centres *a a a*, where the alveoli are crowded with large epithelial cells, mingled with small-celled growth. These are surrounded by the alveolar wall *b b*, thickened with small-celled growth. At *c c* are spots where the centres of the alveoli are fused into a homogeneous mass, surrounded by a thickened zone (giant-cells?); at *d* is a spot where the last-named process is progressing; *e*, fibrillated tissue between the granulations.

(*All the figures in this plate are from a chromic acid preparation, stained with osmic acid,* × 80 *diam., and drawn by Mr. A. T. Hollick.*)

PLATE XXX.
ACUTE TUBERCLE; LUNGS OF CHILDREN.

FIGS. 1 to 4.—*Acute tuberculisation.* The figures show the structure of a fully developed single tubercle.

FIG. 1.—*a*, the central portion, consisting of a granular mass, showing only traces of nuclei, cells, and fibres. The granular character is seen to be extending outwards, into both the nuclei and reticulum which compose the remainder of the tubercle. The structure of the rest is seen to consist of cells and nuclei, *b*, imbedded in a reticulum, *c*. This reticulum is homogeneous and refracting in some parts, with broad bands. (In the figure it is more fibrillated than in the original specimen.) The cells are round and somewhat ovoid. (In the outer parts, not here represented, were a few remains of alveoli containing large epithelial cells, as at *e e*, fig. 3, and also some similar to those in fig. 7.) (*Chromic acid prep.* × 700 *diam.*)

Ref.—Phthisis, pp. 84 (2), 94, 113, 116.

FIG. 2.—Shows a section of an alveolus, looked into in its entire depth. (The cup-shape of this was remarkably distinct in the original, more so than is represented in the drawing.) The whole wall of the alveolus is seen to be changed into a reticular growth, in the meshes of which are imbedded round nuclei. *a*, ring of elastic fibres surrounding the opening of the alveolus. At the centre, *d*, remains of epithelium are seen, breaking down into débris. *b*, a few capillaries, where the injection has penetrated at margin. *e e*, large vessels. (*Injected prep.; chromic acid; stained osmic acid; gum dammar.* × 460 *diam. reduced in drawing.*)

Ref.—Phthisis, p. 84 (2).

FIG. 3.—*Acute tuberculisation, child.* (*Case* 7, *Coombes*, p. 165, and Col. Pl. VIII. 2 and 5, also XXVIII. 4, and XXXIV. 1.) The figure represents a granulation of the softer and whiter type. It is seen to include nuclear growth with epithelial elements in the interior of the alveoli, and some large nucleated cells imbedded in the tissue. *a*, the central portion reduced to débris, softening and breaking down in the middle. This shows remains of cells and nuclei, reduced to granular scales, and corresponding to the 'tubercle-corpuscles' of Lebert, but they do not resemble pus corpuscles or ordinary exudation-corpuscles. All stages of transition may be seen between these and the nuclei and cells imbedded in the reticulum. A few small ones may be seen, $\frac{1}{7000}$ to $\frac{1}{1500}$ inch, which are the nuclei of epithelial cells. *b*, remains of elastic fibres which are also seen indistinctly in other parts. *e e e*, remains of alveoli containing large epithelial cells. *c*, a part where the granular disintegration is advancing. The reticulum, *g*, is less perfect and more fibrillated in this specimen than in the preceding, and the nuclei imbedded in it are less regular in outline, and often fusiform and ovoid, *d d*, but in some parts the reticulum is well-formed, the cells distinct, and either round or only slightly ovoid in shape, *f*. (*Chromic acid prep.* × 700 *diam.*)

Ref.—Phthisis, pp. 93, 95, 113 (2), 115, 116.

MICROSCOPICAL PLATES (XXIX. XXX.)

FIG. 4.—*Acute tuberculisation (same case).* A segment of a soft tubercle. At *a*, the centre of the granulation, is a mass of round granular nuclei, already undergoing caseation. *b*, a reticular structure in which are imbedded round and oval nuclei. Within some of the spaces in this reticulum two or more nuclei are enclosed, and these appear to be undergoing fissiparous division. At *d* is a terminal bronchiole, containing detritus and a few remains of nuclei. *e*, a mass of pigmented nuclei. (*Chromic acid prep.; stained osmic acid.* × 700 *diam.*)

Ref.—Phthisis, pp. 94-5, 113.

FIG. 5.—*Acute tuberculisation; lung, child.* (*Case 6, Polley,* see description of XXVIII. 6.) The figure shows the invasion of the walls of the alveoli by a tubercular growth, mingled with an epithelial growth in their interior, in a part of the lung the seat of diffuse infiltration.—*a a*, the outer sheath of a branch of the pulmonary artery, in which a diffuse tubercular growth is proceeding. At *b*, the small-celled growth, with a fibrous reticulum, is seen invading the walls of adjacent alveoli. The interior of these alveoli, *c c c*, is seen to be occupied with large epithelial cells, some with one, some with two or more nuclei. The cells vary in size from $\frac{1}{500}$ in. and $\frac{1}{1000}$ in. to $\frac{1}{3000}$ or $\frac{1}{2500}$ in., and even $\frac{1}{5000}$ in. Some are smaller, and apparently represent only nuclei. Cells are seen that are finely granular; others contain fat drops (the 'desquamative pneumonia' of Buhl). At some places, as at *e e*, a small-celled or densely packed nuclear growth projects from the walls into the interior of the alveoli. This, at *f*, is seen to be already undergoing granular degeneration. At *g*, where the growth has not yet invaded the walls, capillaries and their remains are to be seen. (*Chromic acid prep.; stained osmic acid.* × 700 *diam.*)

Ref.—Phthisis, pp. 84, 91, 107, 114, 117.

FIG. 6.—*Acute tuberculisation (same case).* From margin of a tract where a diffuse tubercular growth is proceeding. The figure shows the gradual obliteration of the capillaries by nuclear growth in their walls.—*a a*, margins of an alveolus into which the injection has penetrated. *b b*, multiplication of nuclei in walls of capillaries. *c*, a spot where the nuclei have become more dense. *d*, an alveolus still containing epithelial cells in various stages of enlargement. *e*, diffused nuclear growth, occupying the whole of the tissue. *f f*, alveoli occupied by nuclear growth, but whose walls are still apparent. (*Chromic acid prep.; stained osmic acid.* × 700 *diam.*)

Ref.—Phthisis, pp. 94, 103, 107, 117, 121.

FIG. 7.—*Acute tuberculisation, lung, child* (see Plate XXXII. figs. 2-11). A group of terminal bronchioles surrounded by reticular and nucleated growth, *b*. The bronchioles, *a a a*, are occupied by débris and nuclei, round and ovoid, and exhibit a tendency to become filled with an amorphous mass. (*Chromic acid prep.* × 700.)

Ref.—Phthisis, pp. 94, 103, 114, 118, 121.

FIG. 8.—From same preparation as foregoing. Margin of an area of diffuse tubercular pneumonic infiltration. Three terminal alveoli, *a a c*, are occupied by enlarged epithelial cells (the 'desquamative pneumonia' of Buhl). These cells in some places are seen to contain several nuclei. Their outlines become indistinct, and they tend to fuse into large cells or masses, which may attain the size of $\frac{1}{1250}$ to $\frac{1}{500}$ in., and in some places (not here figured) are deeply pigmented. Smaller cells are mingled with these at *c*. *b b*, nuclear growth in the walls of the alveoli. (*Chromic acid prep.* × 700.)

Ref. Phthisis, pp. 94, 114, 118.

FIG. 9.—From XXIX. 1, *e*, magnified 460 diam. Margin of a group of granulations forming a single 'tubercle.' It shows the pulmonary alveoli, *a a*, filled with epithelial cells and nuclei. Some of the cells contain more than one nucleus. The alveolar walls, *b b b*, are filled with a fibro-nuclear growth.

Ref.—Phthisis, pp. 84, 85, 114, 118.

FIG. 10.—Acute tuberculisation ; lung, child (same case as fig. 1). From the margin of an irregular growth of tubercle. At this spot the injection had penetrated to the margin and slightly within the growth, and it shows that the reticulum, as at *a a*, is partly formed of capillaries and their remains. At *a a* the Prussian blue was still present, but at *b b* only the glistening capillary wall exists, enclosing round and ovoid nuclei within its meshes. At *d* is a mass of small nuclei ; at *e* the obliteration of the capillaries is seen to be proceeding by the enlargement of ovoid nuclei in them. At *e* the reticulum is more fibrillated, and at *f* is the remains of an alveolus. (*Chromic acid prep.* × 700.)

Ref.—Phthisis, pp. 94, 103 (2).

PLATE XXXI.

ACUTE TUBERCULISATION.

FIGS. 1-6 from *Case* 8, *Shimmick*. (See p. 167, and description of XXIX. 1.)

FIG. 1.—A single tubercular nodule in the midst of alveolar tissue. This nodule is composed of a group of alveoli, probably representing a terminal infundibulum. In the centre of each alveolus is a giant-cell, of which there are seven. Each of these giant-cells is surrounded by fibrillated tissue containing elongated nuclei, together with remains of epithelium and round nuclei, which, in some places, as at *k*, pass into amorphous débris. The outer margins of the nodule pass into alveolar tissue *m*, which is thickened with small-celled growth. At *h* is part of the wall of a vessel. The giant-cells differ in appearance and size. Most are round in shape, and contain elongated nuclei (round in transverse section). These, in some places, as at *a*, *c*, *g*, are thickly crowded and blend into an almost amorphous mass. At *b* also they are densely crowded into one portion of the 'cell,' and at *d* and *e* they are fusiform, in the centre of the 'cell.' At *f* is a cell with branching processes. At *g*, a process, composed almost entirely of fusiform nuclei, passes from the cell into the surrounding tissue. At *l l* the giant-cells are blending with the surrounding reticulate fibroid tissue, which is also seen at *i*. The cells vary in diameter from $\frac{1}{750}$ inch, *c*, and $\frac{1}{500}$, *a*, to $\frac{1}{700}$, *d*. (*Chromic acid prep. ; stained hæmatoxylin ; Canada balsam.* × 460 *diam.*)

Ref.—Phthisis, pp. 86 (2), 87 (3), 90, 91, 103, 107.

FIG. 2.—From same case. A single granulation, composed of remains of alveolar structure, and probably representing an infundibulum. In the centre is a large giant-cell, *a*, elongated, measuring on an average $\frac{1}{750}$ inch × $\frac{1}{750}$ inch, containing oval nuclei, and also rounded nuclei (which are the oval ones seen endwise). The nuclei are grouped at the periphery of the cell, the centre of which is occupied by amorphous and refracting material, in some parts finely granular. The 'cell' passes, at *b*, into a prolongation which loses itself indefinitely in the surrounding tissue (probably curving out of the section). At *c* is another prolongation, containing fusiform nuclei, and ending in a series of reticulate digitations, which pass into, and blend with, the surrounding tissue. At *d d* are two groups of fusiform nuclei, without definite outline, but the upper one has an amorphous margin, and looks as if it were the commencement (or a portion of the section) of a giant-cell. The two are separated by some fusiform fibres. The remainder of the 'tubercle' is composed of round and fusiform nuclei, irregularly intermingled, and in parts of a delicate reticulum mingled with much finely granular matter, and remains of epithelial cells passing into granular disintegration. Such are seen at *e e*, occupying the centres of alveoli. At *f* is the remains of an alveolus converted into nucleo-fibrillated tissue. In many places remains of capillaries are seen, as at *g g*, marked by fusiform nuclei. *h*, part of wall of larger vessel. *k k*, walls of alveoli thickened with nuclear growth. *m*, epithelial proliferation in an adjacent alveolus. (*Chromic acid prep. ; stained hæmatoxylin ; Canada balsam.* × 460 *diam.*)

Ref.—Phthisis, pp. 87 (3), 89-91, 103, 113 (2).

FIG. 3.—From same, shows a tubercle of the miliary (acute infective ?) type, undergoing fibroid transformation with some caseous change.—*a*, remains of epithelium caseating. This process extends into the surrounding fibro-reticular growth. bb, fibroid change of reticulum into broader bands, in which round nuclei (the remains of small-celled growth) are imbedded. c, denser reticular growth of broad bands with interstices gradually narrowing, and from which the nuclei have almost entirely disappeared. d, an adjacent alveolus, where remains of epithelium mingled with fibroid change are still seen. e, epithelium of another alveolus still unchanged. ff, fibrous boundary of the tubercle. gg, walls of adjacent alveoli infiltrated with small-celled growth. h, a large giant-cell, lying outside the tubercle; measures $\frac{1}{250} \times \frac{1}{717}$ inch. kl, two other giant-cells, measuring $\frac{1}{710}$ inch. (*Chromic acid prep.; stained hæmatoxylin; Canada balsam.* × 230 *diam.*)

Ref.—Phthisis, pp. 87 (2), 88, 89 (2), 90, 91, 103, 110.

FIG. 4.—A group of three giant-cells in a tubercle which was composed of several alveoli.—a, elongated cell, measuring $\frac{1}{318} \times \frac{1}{540}$ inch, and giving off a prolongation (b), which merges into the surrounding reticulum. The margins of this cell are everywhere well-defined. The nuclei are for the most part grouped at its periphery. They are chiefly ovoid and fusiform; some are round. The interior is occupied by a homogeneous basis-substance. c, another, also well-defined, but around its margin are short processes, apparently the first stage of the longer ones seen in some cells. One of these has already blended with the surrounding tissue. The cell measures $\frac{1}{530} \times \frac{1}{500}$ inch.—d, a much more irregular one, fused in parts, and especially at the ends, with the surrounding tissue. Its elongated nuclei are irregularly grouped. e, a small mass, containing a few elongated nuclei fusing with the surrounding tissue. g, part of the fibrous capsule. The tissue is everywhere traversed by broad fibres assuming a reticular form, in the meshes of which round and ovoid nuclei are imbedded. The latter, in some places, run in long lines, as at h. (*Chromic acid prep.; stained hæmatoxylin; Canada balsam.* × 460 *diam.*)

Ref.—Phthisis, pp. 86, 87 (2), 89, 91, 103.

FIG. 5.—From same, shows a giant-cell of peculiar form.—a, a process passing into surrounding nucleated tissue, among which are remains of epithelioid cells. b, another elongated and curved process, ending in a series of elongated nuclei passing into fibroid tissue, c; this process measures on an average $\frac{1}{2500}$ inch in transverse diameter. At d, the giant-cell passes into confused fibro-nucleated tissue. e, a band of fibro-nucleated tissue, apparently penetrating into the giant-cell. The rest of the cell shows the peripheral elongated nuclei; otherwise its contents are homogeneous and amorphous. (*Chromic acid prep.; stained hæmatoxylin; Canada balsam.* × 460 *diam.*)

Ref.—Phthisis, pp. 86 (2), 89, 91.

FIG. 6.—From same. Two giant-cells, imbedded in a reticulum in the midst of a granulation.—a, a very irregularly formed cell, measuring $\frac{1}{700} \times \frac{1}{500}$ inch. It shows at bc irregular prolongations into which the greater number of the fusiform nuclei are crowded, and these prolongations pass directly into the reticular network which forms the structure of the tubercle. At d is another prolongation, throwing off secondary fibres, which merge into, and become part of, the reticulum. The centre of the cell is entirely amorphous; fusiform nuclei are scattered at its periphery, but the greater number are collected in the processes. e, a smaller cell, measuring $\frac{1}{1000}$ inch. It is stellate, and its processes blend with the reticulum; at f, a broader process passes into the surrounding tissue. The fusiform nuclei are both peripheral and central. gg, fibroid network of the tubercle in which round and fusiform nuclei are imbedded. (*Chromic acid prep.; stained hæmatoxylin; Canada balsam.* × 460 *diam.*)

Ref.—Phthisis, pp. 86, 89.

FIG. 7.—Caseating tuberculosis, acute phthisis. (*Case 16, Henshaw*, p. 177; Col. Pl. VIII. 1, 3, 4, also XXXVIII. 1, 2, 3.) The figure shows caseation invading a tubercular area in which quasi-fibroid change had commenced.—a, caseous centre, finely granular, almost amorphous, extending at bb into a fibrillated texture, in which nuclear growth has almost disappeared. cc, nuclear growth still apparent among stellate cells. dd, remains of alveoli where nuclear growth still persists among the stellate cells. Some epithelial cells are mingled with these. *e e*, nuclear growth more abundant. (*Chromic acid prep.; carmine.* × 230.)

Ref.—Phthisis, pp. 110, 116 (3).

Fig. 8.—Indurating miliary tubercle. (*Case 11, Beale*, p. 172.) A single granulation, consisting of a group of alveoli, two of which, *a b*, still retain their outlines.—*a* is chiefly fibroid, passing at the centre into a homogeneous material; *b* shows remains of epithelial cells mingled with fusiform cells, both being more or less granular and disintegrating. *e e*, other alveoli almost entirely fibroid. The fibroid change takes place by the formation of broad fibrillated bands of different width, here and there enclosing nuclei. *e e*, a belt of broad fibres (septum), also fibrillated, surrounding the granulations and enclosing nuclei, which are more apparent in the outer zone, *f f*. (*Chromic acid prep.; carmine.* × 460 diam.)

Ref.—Phthisis, pp. 96, 113, 116.

PLATE XXXII.
Giant Cells and Pseudo-Giant Cells.

Fig. 1.—From the same case as figs. 1–6, plate XXXI. (*Case 8, Shimwick, Acute Tubercle*, p. 167.) A giant-cell round in shape, probably a transverse section of a lymphatic cord, measures $\frac{1}{350}$ inch. It is surrounded by round and fusiform cells imbedded in fibres. The fusiform cells contain round nuclei. (*Chromic acid prep.; stained hæmatoxylin; Canada balsam.* × 700 diam.

Ref.—Phthisis, p. 89.

Fig. 1 A.—From same. A section similar to foregoing. The outline is indefinite, but at *a* it is bounded by endothelial-like cells seen in profile (× 700 diam.)

Ref.—Phthisis, p. 89.

Fig. 2.—*Acute Tuberculisation, lung, child.* (See Plate XXX. figs. 1, 3, 8.)—*a*, a very large cell ' in the midst of a soft granulation with epithelial proliferation—' pseudo-giant cell.' The cell measures $\frac{1}{350}$ inch. In it are numerous round nuclei, and it appears as if formed by the fusion of several cells. Around it are cells imbedded in a reticulum, some fusiform (*b*), others with indications of multiplication of their nuclei (*c*), others small, round, and pigmented (*d*). (*Chromic acid prep.; stained osmic acid.* × 460 diam.)

Ref.—Phthisis, p. 89.

Fig. 3.—From same case as fig. 2.—*a* a giant-cell with an amorphous centre of granular débris, in which cell outlines are still observable. Outside *a* is a glistening zone (*b*), homogeneous and sclerotic (the ' mantel ' of Langhans). This zone is surrounded by a reticular network, and in this, at *c*, is a thickened band in which nuclei are imbedded. Total measurement of *a b* = $\frac{1}{900}$ inch; mean width of *b* $\frac{1}{3400}$ inch. (*Chromic acid prep.; stained osmic acid.* × 460 diam.)

Ref.—Phthisis, p. 89.

Fig. 4.—From same. Fusion of reticulum in centre of alveolus; the epithelial cells have entirely disappeared.—*a*, space in reticulum. *b b*, nuclei of reticulum. *c d*, reticulum fusing with that of surrounding tissue. (*Chromic acid prep.; stained osmic acid.* × 460 diam.)

Ref.—Phthisis, p. 89.

MICROSCOPICAL PLATES (XXXI. XXXII.)

FIG. 5.—From same, probably an earlier stage of a cell like the foregoing (fig. 4). The epithelium has almost entirely disappeared, but some cells persist at a ; otherwise the floor of the alveolus consists of a nucleated reticulum, the processes of which blend with the surrounding fibro-nucleated tissue. (*Chromic acid prep.; stained osmic acid.*   × 460 *diam.*)

Ref.—Phthisis, p. 89.

FIG. 6.—From same preparation as fig. 1, and also Plate XXX. fig. 9. Sections of bronchioles and alveolar passage forming 'pseudo-giant cells.'—a, elongated passage containing several large epithelioid cells and others in act of fusion. c, another, where the cells have broken down. The wall of the passage containing them hangs, by means of a few fibres (d), to the adjacent tissue. e, transverse section of another. f, another containing a few large epithelioid cells and amorphous matter (resulting from the breaking down of other cells). g, Fibro-nucleated tissue. (*Chromic acid prep.; stained osmic acid.*   × 230 *diam.*)

Ref.—Phthisis, p. 90.

FIG. 7.—A common appearance of giant-cells in cases of chronic tuberculisation. The 'cells' surround a caseous mass. (*Case 28, Smith*, p. 119, Col. Pl. XIII. 1, also XXXIII. 1, 3, and 10, and XXXV. 4-6.)—a, caseous mass, showing traces of reticulum, with nuclei imbedded ; much pigmented at margins. In a few places traces of alveolar structure are still apparent. $b\,b$, two elongated giant-cells with amorphous contents, but blending at their margins by a series of processes with the surrounding nucleated reticulum. $c\,c$, round bodies, amorphous and granular, but without well-defined margin. The whole is imbedded in a mass of broad-banded fibres. The fibrillation is too strongly marked in the engraving. At e, traces of alveolar structure. ff, remains of nuclei imbedded in these fibres. (*Chromic acid prep.; stained carmine, gum dammar.* × 230 *diam., reduced.*)

Ref.—Phthisis, pp. 86, 90, 91, 97, 113 (2), 115, 116.

FIG. 8.—Giant-cells in indurating tuberculosis. From same case as fig. 7. The figure shows three alveoli in juxtaposition, with giant-cells in different stages of transformation.—a, earliest stage. The epithelium of the floor of an alveolus has disappeared, and in the amorphous ground-substance nuclei are scattered. At b, traces of reticulum are seen passing into the surrounding fibro-nucleated tissue. c, a more advanced stage. The structures of the floor of the alveolus are completely fused, but still show traces of reticulum, which at d passes into bands connecting the 'cell' with the outer floor of the infundibulum. In part of this, where induration has not commenced, are seen some large epithelioid cells still imbedded, e. This cell is much pigmented, and nuclei are scattered in its amorphous ground-substance. f, a more advanced stage. The processes of the fused 'cell' are broad, and pass into the surrounding reticulum ($g\,g$). At h, they are still more distinctly branched, with spaces between. The centre shows a few round nuclei. Each alveolus is enclosed in a fibro-nucleated reticular tissue. (*Chromic acid prep.; stained carmine ; dammar.* × 460 *diam.*)

FIG. 9.—A giant-cell passing into fibroid transformation. From same case as figs. 7 and 8. The 'cell' represents, in all probability, the floor of an alveolus.—a, centre, with fusiform nuclei in a group, imbedded in a homogeneous refracting material This material at its margins passes everywhere into a series of broad bands, between which are deep spaces in which nuclei are imbedded as in fibro-cartilage, $b\,b\,b$, and some large cells apparently epithelioid. More externally the meshes of the reticulum become closer and denser. Some still contain nuclei, $d\,d$. In some places, $e\,e$, the 'bands' are apparently thickened capillaries with fusiform nuclei. (*Chromic acid prep.; stained carmine ; dammar.* × 460 *diam.*)

Ref.—Phthisis, pp. 87, 92, 97.

FIG. 10.—Pseudo-giant-cells, from a case of chronic phthisis. (*Case 35, Roberts*, p. 212 and Col. Pl. XVIII. 1 and 2, also XXXIII. 9, 11, and XLI. 5.)—$a\,b\,c$, three terminal bronchioles in juxtaposition ; seen in transverse section. a, columnar epithelium intact. b, columnar epithelium, crowded and granular in centre. *e*, columnar epithelium at margin, but centre filled with amorphous débris. (*Chromic acid prep.; stained carmine; dammar.* × 460 *diam*).

FIG. 11.—Acute tuberculisation, child (see figs. 2–5). Early stage of giant-cells (?) *a*, branched cell with 'processes' blending with surrounding reticulum. It contains two granular indistinct nuclei. (The outlines of these nuclei are somewhat too defined in the engraving.) *b c*, section of a terminal infundibulum, containing epithelioid cells mingled with a small-celled growth. *d*, small-celled growth imbedded in reticulum. (*Chromic acid prep.; stained osmic acid.* × 460 *diam*.)

Ref.—Phthisis, p. 89 (2).

PLATE XXXIII.
GIANT CELLS AND PSEUDO-GIANT CELLS.

FIG. 1.—Chronic indurating tuberculosis. (*Case 28*, p. 199, *Smith*, Col. Pl. XIII. 1 ; also XXXII. 7, 8, and XXXV. 4–6.)—*a*, giant-cell forming in floor of alveolus (partially separated artificially from wall.) The figure shows the groups of elongated nuclei characteristic of the giant-cell. (A tendency to branching, like fig. 3, was seen in upper part, not figured here.) The epithelium has disappeared, and the 'cell' is forming in the groundwork of the alveolus. *b*, remains of round nucleated cells. *d d d*, margin of alveolus with nuclei imbedded in a reticulum. *c*, part of the reticulum attached to the 'cell.' (*Chromic acid prep.; stained chloride of palladium.* × 460 *diam*.)

Ref.—Phthisis, p. 86.

FIG. 2.—Acute Phthisis. (*Case 23*, *Lloyd*, p. 190, Col. Pl. XII. See also 5 and 6 ; also XXXIX. 1.) Early stages of giant-cell ? Group of cells forming around a thickened septum.—*a*, stellate 'cell,' with numerous 'processes' which pass into the surrounding reticulum. The contents of the cell are a few scattered nuclei imbedded in a homogeneous basis-substance. It measures $\frac{1}{840}$ inch. *b*, an irregular stellate cell, without visible nuclei, and with a homogeneous interior also giving off processes ; measures $\frac{1}{1700}$ in. *c*, a still smaller one; measures $\frac{1}{2300}$ in. *d*, *e*, others having same characteristics ; *e* is much pigmented and measures $\frac{1}{1100}$ in. (*Chromic acid prep.; stained carmine; dammar.* × 460 *diam*.)

FIG. 3.—Giant-cells in fibroid induration. (*Case 28 Smith*. Ref. fig. 1.)—*a*, a giant-cell in which the nuclei have almost disappeared, except in a few places at the margins. The processes of the cell have become wide and branching, and blend with the surrounding reticulum, *b b*. *d*, a large epithelium cell pigmented. *c*, an earlier stage of the giant-cell ; the structures in the floor of an alveolus have blended into a homogeneous basis-substance, in which the fusiform refracting nuclei are imbedded. (*Chromic acid prep.; stained carmine; dammar.* × 460 *diam*.)

Ref.—Phthisis, p. 89 (3).

FIG. 4.—Giant-cell in fibroid transformation. (*Case 36*, *Mears*, p. 213, and Col. Pl. XIX., also XL. 7, and XLII. 3 and 4.)—*a*, giant-cell in centre of alveolus (partly separated from the wall by pressure). The 'cell' shows an amorphous, slightly granular ground-substance, in which are round nuclei. *b*, the fusiform nuclei. *c*, elongated nuclei along the margin of the 'cell.' (*Chromic acid prep.; stained carmine; dammar.* × 460 *diam*.)

FIG. 5.—(*Case 23*, *Lloyd*; ref. fig. 2.) The interior of an alveolus converted into a finely granular, almost amorphous, reticular mass, in the meshes of which remains of cells were here and there visible, *b*. (*Chromic acid prep.; stained carmine; dammar.* × 460 *diam*.)

FIG. 6.—From same. (*Case 23*, *Lloyd*.) A giant-cell occupying the whole interior of an alveolus. The fusiform nuclei, *b b*, among which is much pigment, are collected in a middle zone. The whole interior of the mass, as well as the outer zone, *a*, is amorphous and finely granular. The outer zone gives off numerous processes, which blend with the surrounding nucleated reticulum.

Ref.—Phthisis, pp. 86, 91.

FIG. 7.—A giant-cell in centre of alveolus, undergoing fibroid transformation (*Case 30, Carr*, p. 203; Col. Pl. XVI. also XLI. 1–4.)—*a*, cell, the centre of which is homogeneous and apparently consists of sclerosed tissue. At the margin are remains of nuclei, *b*, imbedded in the thickening intercellular substance which surrounds the rest of the 'cell.' At *e*, the prolongations of the 'cell' pass into the broader bands of the reticulum of the alveolus, which, at *e f*, are more abundantly nucleated. *d*, thickened fibre-wall of alveolus. (*Chromic acid prep.; stained carmine; dammar.* × 460 *diam.*)

Ref.—Phthisis, pp. 92, 97.

FIG. 8.—A giant-cell, in centre of alveolus, undergoing fibroid transformation and sclerosis. (*Case 30, Carr*, ref. fig. 7.)—*a*, centre of cell, homogeneous, sclerosed. The processes, *b b*, surround spaces from which the nuclei have disappeared, and at *e* there is a closer reticulation, showing traces of nuclei. The cell is separated (artificially) from the remainder of the alveolar wall, and is bounded by a thickened fibroid margin. The rest of the alveolus is seen to be formed of a reticular structure, in which nuclei are imbedded, some of which, *d*, are larger than the others. (*Chromic acid prep.; stained carmine; dammar.* × 460 *diam.*)

Ref.—Phthisis, p. 97.

FIG. 9.—A 'pseudo-giant cell.' (*Case 35, Roberts*, p. 212, Col. Pl. XVIII. 1 and 2, also XXXII. 10, and XLI. 5.) The figure represents a mass of cells in the interior of a bronchiole, held together by mucus, which, in separating from the remainder, has acquired a jagged outline. There are, however, no true processes, and the nuclei, *a*, are not fusiform. *b*, round cells on the wall of the bronchiole. (*Chromic acid prep.; stained carmine.* × 460 *diam.*)

Ref.—Phthisis, p. 90.

FIG. 10.—A form of giant-cell seen occasionally in indurating tuberculosis. (*Case Smith*, ref. figs. 1 and 3.)—*a*, fusiform nuclei, densely grouped in centre of cell. They are, however, smaller, and have less distinct outlines, than those in cells of more recent formation (see Plate XXXI.) Around them is a margin, *b*, of homogeneous, finely granular tissue. The remarkable feature of this cell (which is exactly repeated in other preparations) is a single broad process passing from it, and losing itself in the surrounding tissue. The whole of the margin of the alveolus (?) in which this cell is situated is densely fibrillated, with a few scattered nuclei interposed. (Immediately adjacent was a broad tract of caseation.) (*Chromic acid prep.; stained chloride of palladium; dammar.* × 460 *diam.*)

Ref.—Phthisis, pp. 86, 91, 92, 97.

FIG. 11.—Pseudo giant cell. (*Case 14, Roberts*, ref. fig. 9.) Probably a section of a thickened bronchus; the columnar epithelium seen longitudinally at *a*, and endwise at *e* (both of these forms could be seen at all depths on altering the focus.) *d d*, homogeneous fibroid margin (thickened membrana propria?) separated from the wall. The whole cell measured $\frac{1}{400} \times \frac{1}{150}$. (*Chromic acid prep.; stained chloride of palladium; dammar.* × 460.)

Ref.—Phthisis, pp. 86, 87, 91.

FIG. 12.—Elongated giant-cells from indurating tuberculosis. From the margin of an area of caseous change. (*Case 10, Unwin*, p. 170, and Plate XXXIX. fig. 7.)—*a, b*, elongated body, or possibly two giant-cells, broken across at *c*. *a* has the appearance of having been originally a single cell, as the fusiform nuclei are grouped in a quasi-circular form around a homogeneous centre, whereas in *b* they are only at one end, *c*. The space extends around *b*, and around the greater part of *a*.

Total length of a, b, $\frac{1}{150}$ inch; breadth $\frac{1}{350}$ inch. (*Chromic acid prep.; stained carmine; mounted dammar.* × 480.)

Ref.—Phthisis, p. 91.

PLATE XXXIV.

TUBERCLE OF LUNG, LARYNX, AND GLANDS.

FIG. 1.—From *Case 7, Coombes*, p. 165, and Col. Pl. VIII. figs. 2 and 5. *See also* XXVIII. 4, and XXX. 3 and 4.) From the lung of a child dying from acute tuberculisation. An apparently single soft granulation presents an irregular mass, tending to the pyramidal (lobular) form, of which the centre a, is nearly homogeneous, and apparently uniformly infiltrated. This, with a high power, was seen to be composed of a mingled epithelial and small-celled growth, in which the walls of the alveoli (mainly occupied by a fibro-nuclear formation) were still apparent. At b, b, were portions where the alveoli, diminished in size, were occupied by a large-celled epithelial proliferation, and their walls were much thickened by a fibro-nuclear growth. At the margin of this, $c\,c$, were earlier stages of the same process, the alveolar spaces being larger, but the thickening of the walls, d, was still apparent. At e is a dense nuclear growth, much pigmented. Pigment was scattered thickly throughout the specimen, clustered into finely granular masses which were apparently filled nuclei. At f is a small 'tubercle,' slightly separated from the foregoing; which, when examined with a higher power, was seen to have a structure identical with that just described. (*Chromic acid prep.* × 100 *diam.*)

Ref.—Phthisis, pp. 102, 107, 116.

FIG. 2.—Tubercular infiltration of mucous and submucous tissue of larynx. (*Case 29, J. Brown*, p. 201, and Col. Pl. XX. 3, larynx, and XV. XLII. 7, lung.)—a, line of columnar epithelium, which is shown in the next figure (3) to be as yet retained, but is in a condition of proliferation and desquamation. There is great hyperæmia, shown by the distended vessels $b\,b\,b$. At $a'\,c$ are denser masses of nuclei, clustered in the tissue immediately below the epithelial layer. At $d\,d$ are similar masses in the deeper layers. $f\,f$ are sections of glands, with their epithelium intact, and their centres free, showing that the change in the walls of the larynx is independent of those. They are surrounded by the same proliferation as occurs in the rest of the tissue. g, cartilage. (*Chromic acid prep.; stained chloride of palladium.* × 100.)

FIG. 3.—From another portion of the same preparation as the foregoing, more highly magnified. The epithelial layer, a, is seen to have a multiplication of nuclei in the columnar cells and immediately beneath them, $c\,c$. This extends also more deeply into the tissue d. Below this is fibrous tissue, free from nuclear growth, which exists, however, still more deeply around the follicles of the glands e. $b\,b$, vessels. (*Chromic acid prep.; stained chloride of palladium.* × 500, *somewhat reduced.*)

FIG. 4.—Tubercle of the larynx (another case.) The epithelial surface has perished here. The ulceration has extended to the submucous tissue, a, which is infiltrated with a nuclear growth. b, orifice of gland-duct, denuded of epithelium, cut transversely. c, gland-duct tissue with its epithelium in a state of proliferation. (In some parts of this preparation the follicles of the glands were seen crowded with round cells, and dense nuclear growth surrounded the gland-follicles.) (*Chromic acid prep.; stained carmine.* × 100.)

FIG. 5.—Tubercle in the wall of a small bronchus, from the lung of a child with acute tuberculosis. In the interior the epithelium has nearly perished, only traces remaining, and in its place is a layer, a, of amorphous débris and pus-corpuscles. At b ulceration is proceeding from within. The infiltration with nuclear growth is seen proceeding in the whole thickness of the wall, $c\,c$; at d it is seen invading the adjacent alveoli (which were filled with large desquamating epithelial cells.) At c is the wall of an adjacent alveolus, in which nuclear growth is proceeding. (*Chromic acid prep.; stained osmic acid.* × 230.)

Ref.—Phthisis, p. 100.

FIG. 6.—Tubercle, bronchial gland. (*Case 29, Brown*, p. 201, and Col. Pl. XV. see also fig. 2.) The trabeculæ, $b\,b$, are seen to be thickened with a small-celled growth, a. (*Chromic acid prep.* × 460.)

FIG. 7.—From the same; an indurated part of the gland. The lymph-sinuses have become converted into a homogeneous tissue, b, and the trabecular spaces, c, remain, showing in parts, $a\,d$, nuclear growth. (× 460.)

These two figures were originally engraved with the intention of giving a fuller series of illustrations of the changes in other organs which accompany phthisis—an intention which I was not able to carry out.

PLATE XXXV.
TUBERCULAR DESTRUCTIVE PNEUMONIA; INDURATING TUBERCULOSIS.

FIG. 1.—Tubercular (?) suppurating and ulcerating pneumonia. (*Case 18, Brodrick*, p. 181, and Col. Pl. XIII. 3 and 4.) This figure is from the infiltrated portion of the upper lobe, with soft granulations (described in the account of the case, p. 183, at § C.) It shows a large tract, infiltrated with puriform débris, in which the pulmonary tissue is in parts breaking down, in parts undergoing fibroid thickening. The cells are all small pus-cells, some containing two or more nuclei. The nuclei are distinct, but the cells are so densely massed, and their outlines are so faint, that the nuclei form the most prominent objects. The cells on an average measure $\frac{1}{7000}$ to $\frac{1}{5000}$ inch. In some places, $a\,a$, the cells are imbedded in the meshes of a fine fibrillation (fibrinous pneumonia) (*see* also figs. 2 and 3.) In other places they are densely massed without fibrillation being apparent between them, and in others, again, $b\,b$, the dense massing is accompanied with fibrillation. Nuclear infiltration of the alveolar wall occurs here and there, but is not marked in these tracts, and the pulmonary tissue appears to perish early in the suppuration. Fibroid thickening tends to occur in the inter-lobular tissue surrounding such a tract, $d\,d$. The bronchi passing through this, $e\,e$, are, however, involved in the same suppurative process as the alveolar tissue.[1]

Ref.—Catarrhal Pneumonia, p. 32; Phthisis, p. 119.

FIGS. 2 and 3.—From a similar part of the same lung (× 460). Fig. 2 shows the fibrillated reticulum of coagulated fibrin; fig. 3, the cells imbedded in the reticulum of the alveolar wall, which is perishing in acute granular degeneration.[2]

Ref.—Phthisis, p. 119.

FIGS. 4, 5, and 6.—From a case of acute tubercular pneumonia combined with fibroid induration. (*Case 28, Smith*, p. 199, and Col. Pl. XIII. 1, 2; also XXXII. 7, 8, and XXXIII. 1, 3, and 10.)

FIG. 4.—One of the granulations which are thickly scattered throughout all parts of the lung, and are of variable size. (*See* also Plate XXXII. fig. 7.) These granulations have a caseous and finely granular centre, a, in which the traces of cells, nuclei, and a fine reticulum are still observable. At its margin, $b\,b$, epithelial cells, containing much pigment, persist. This margin is very dense and opaque, from a granular fibroid change, and contains much pigment (not sufficiently defined in this drawing.) Beyond it is a zone in which the alveolar structures are becoming blended with the granulations by a growth chiefly fibroid, f, but still in parts showing traces of alveolar structure, c, while in other parts the alveolar structure is lost, but groups of epithelial cells and nuclei remain

---

[1] (In the description of this and some other figures in the plate, some discrepancies may be noted between the description and the lettering of the figure. See preface. ED.)

[2] For the description of the appearances connected with these changes, see the account of the case p. 183.

imbedded among the fibres. Outside this is a zone of nuclear growth, *e e*, which, however, does not surround the whole granulation. In this zone are some giant-cells. There were only two in the preparation, and they were outside the area of this drawing. They are figured in a similar granulation from the same specimen at XXXII. 7. (*Chromic acid prep.; stained carminate of ammonia.* × 230 *diam.*)

Ref.—Phthisis, pp. 98, 113, 115, 116.

FIG. 5.—From an area of destructive suppurative pneumonia. (*Case 28, Smith*, see above. Compare fig. 1, *Brodrick*.) At *b* nothing is left of the alveolar structures except the remains of the elastic fibres, and a finely granular reticulum. At *c e* these are more indistinct, and are replaced by an amorphous granular matter. The whole is enclosed by a thickening of the interlobular tissue. (× 460 *diam.*)

Ref.—Catarrhal Pneumonia, p. 32; Phthisis, p. 118.

FIG. 6.—(*Case 28, Smith*.) A mass of nuclear growth which in some places filled the whole of an alveolus, side by side with other alveoli filled with desquamated epithelium. (*Chromic acid prep.; in carbolic glycerine.*)

Ref.—Phthisis, pp. 85, 94, 96, 117.

FIG. 7.—Acute ulcerative suppurative pneumonia (desquamative tubercular ?) (*Case 5, S. Brown*, p. 161 ; Col. Pl. V. 5). There is no thickening of the alveolar walls, but the elastic fibres are breaking down in granular disintegration. A few large epithelial cells, *a a*, are seen imbedded among the fibres. They measure $\frac{1}{1500}$ to $\frac{1}{1800}$ inch. Smaller round nucleated cells, *b b*, are also seen. These measure $\frac{1}{2000}$ to $\frac{1}{2500}$ inch. Large free nuclei or round non-nucleated cells, *d d*, are predominant, and measure $\frac{1}{3000}$ to $\frac{1}{3500}$ inch. Lastly, smaller nuclei, *e*, are seen, but in less abundance, measuring $\frac{1}{5500}$ inch. The cells, *b b*, have all the characters of pus-cells and of ' pyoid ' bodies. The clear round cells, *d*, are probably mucoid corpuscles. The elastic fibres persist, even where the cells have perished in granular disintegration, *f*; but in some places, they also are destroyed, *e e*, and a cavity results. There is an entire disappearance of the capillaries during the process. (*Chromic acid prep.; stained carmine; dammar.*)

Ref.—Phthisis, p. 119.

PLATE XXXVI.

ACUTE CASEATING DESTRUCTIVE TUBERCULAR PNEUMONIA.

The whole of the figures in this and the succeeding plate are from the same preparations. (*Case 19, Griffin,* p. 183, and Col. Pl. X. 1–4.)

FIG. 1.—Nodules, of various sizes, of destructive lobular pneumonia, occurring in the midst of a tissue in which the alveolar walls are thickening by a diffuse small-celled growth, while epithelial proliferation takes place in their interior. These lobular masses, *a d d*, originate in changes akin to those shown in XXXV. 5, XXXVII. 7, in which a process akin to suppuration occurs. The layer near *a* is surrounded by a zone of fibrillated tissue, *b*, in which nuclei are imbedded, and might be taken for a section of a bronchus, filled with inspissated secretion, but traces of alveolar structure show that it had a pneumonic origin. Fig. 2 is the portion at *b'* highly magnified. The nodules at *d d* appear, when more highly magnified, to have resulted from processes akin to XXXVII. 5, while the nodule *e* shows changes akin to XXXVIII. 3 (*Henshaw*). At *f* the alveoli are filled with epithelial-like cells, and their walls thickened like XXXVIII. 4 (*Henshaw*). In some places the epithelium is passing into detritus, like XXXIX. 2 (*J. Thomas*). (*Chromic acid prep.* × 70 *diam. Tuffen West, delt.*)

Ref.—Phthisis, pp. 95 (4), 98, 116 (2).

FIG. 2.—From b, fig. 1, seen highly magnified (460 diam.) The central part, a, passing into detritus, shows leucocytes and pyoid bodies, which have almost lost their outlines and become reduced to a granular amorphous mass. b, c, a fibrillated structure, with nuclei and small cells imbedded in the meshes, which everywhere bound the mass of caseating lobular pneumonia (a, fig. 1.)

Ref.—Phthisis, pp. 95, 116.

FIG. 3.—Section of lung showing how the pneumonic processes are distributed over a considerable area, become confluent, and pass into caseation.—a a a, spots of lobular confluent pneumonia, presenting characters of XXXVIII. 3 (Henshaw), and XXVIII. 8 (Polley). b b, spots where these are passing into complete detritus, like figs. 1 and 5. c c c, spots where earlier stages of the foregoing are found with characteristics, in various gradations, resembling XL. 1–3. d d, parts where the consolidation is not complete, and the process is still in an early stage of pneumonic change, the alveoli containing numerous large epithelial cells, and their walls being thickened with interstitial growth. e e, parts where the thickening of the alveolar walls with interstitial small-celled growth has proceeded to a greater degree. f f, perivascular and peribronchial small-celled infiltration. g, a bronchus whose wall is thickened with small-celled and nuclear infiltration; it contains in its interior a mass of inspissated puriform secretion. h, thickened pleura. i i i, thickened interlobular septa. (Chromic acid prep. × 70. W. Fox, delt.)

Ref.—Phthisis, pp. 95 (2), 108, 116 (2).

FIG. 4.—An area of caseating pneumonia, surrounded by a dense, uniform, wide-spread infiltration of small-celled growth.—The pneumonic areas, a a, resemble those seen in XXXVII. 6, and also XXXIX. 2 (J. Thomas), and XXVIII. 6 (Polley), but in most there is little if any thickening of the alveolar walls. These walls are distinct, with elastic fibres persisting, while the cavities are occupied by a dense homogeneous confluent granular débris, in which here and there remains of epithelium are seen. The small-celled infiltration, b b, extends indistinctly beyond this, and contains in parts patches of amorphous disintegration of pneumonic character. (Chromic acid prep. × 50 diam. Tuffen West, delt.)

Ref.—Phthisis, pp. 108, 117 (2).

FIG. 5.—Suppurative caseating pneumonia. The figure shows the interior of the alveoli filled with an almost amorphous granular mass composed of disintegrating leucocytes. The walls of the alveoli persist. At b b this mass is seen breaking down in the centre. c c, pneumonic areas where the epithelium is still enlarged and filling the alveoli. (Chromic acid prep.; stained carmine. × 50 diam. Tuffen West, delt.)

Ref.—Phthisis, pp. 95, 118 (2).

PLATE XXXVII.

TUBERCULAR PNEUMONIA.

The figures, like those of the foregoing Plate, are entirely from Case 19, Griffin.

FIG. 1.—Nuclear growth a a, imbedded in a reticulum growing in the floor of an alveolus. At b, this is seen proceeding in the course of the capillaries, which are thereby occluded. At c, the growth forms a denser mass. This is the stage which precedes, in some places, the destructive changes figured in the foregoing Plate. d d d, epithelial proliferation in an adjacent alveolus. At e the growth is proceeding in the alveolar wall. (Chromic acid prep. stained carmine. × 700 diam.)

Ref.—Phthisis, pp. 95 (2), 114 (2), 117, 118.

FIG. 2.—Changes similar to those described in foregoing figure, but extending to a group of terminal alveoli.—*a a a*, alveoli whose floors and walls are occupied by a small-celled reticulated growth. The epithelium having disappeared, the whole area is bounded by the thickened interlobular tissue, *b b b*, which is also infiltrated with nuclei. At *c c* are adjacent alveoli, containing enlarged epithelium. (*Chromic acid prep.; stained chloride palladium.* × 700 *diam.*)

Ref.—Phthisis, pp. 95, 114 (2), 117, 118.

FIG. 3.—A more advanced stage of the changes seen in the two foregoing figures. The process of nuclear growth is passing into one akin to suppuration.—*a a*, alveoli filled with reticular nucleated growth. *b b*, alveoli where the reticular character is not apparent, and the nuclei have now the character of leucocytes. *c c*, alveoli where these are commencing to break down into detritus. (*Chromic acid prep.* × 700 *diam.*)

Ref.—Phthisis, pp. 95, 118.

FIG. 4.—A tract of lung occupied by areas of destructive lobular pneumonia.—*a*, an area broken down in centre, resembling *a*, XXXVI. 1. *b*, tracts resembling XXXV. 5, and *a a a*, XXXV. 1 (*Brodrick*), and in isolated spots like XL. 4 (*Heath*). *c c*, similar lobules in earlier stages, which, surrounded by zones of indurated and pigmented tissue, closely resemble sections of bronchi, but in other sections, at different depths from the same parts, they are seen to consist of pulmonary tissue, as shown by the elastic fibres of the alveolar walls. *d d*, masses of infiltration in part resembling fig. 2, in part fig. 5, surrounded by zones of thickened interlobular tissue. *e e e*, similar tracts, among which, with a higher magnifying power, giant-cells are seen. (*Chromic acid prep.; stained carmine;* × 70 *diam.; Tuffen West, delt.*)

Ref.—Phthisis, pp. 95 (2), 116.

FIG. 5.—A nodule of lobular tubercular pneumonia. (The degeneration of such lobules is one source of the circumscribed caseous masses in this lung.)—*a a*, remains of elastic fibres, the tissue being otherwise occupied by molecular débris. *b b*, mingled epithelial and small-celled growth, pigmented and passing into disintegration; in some places traces of capillaries may be seen. *c c*, a zone of reticulated small-celled growth, surrounding the lobule. (*Chromic acid prep.; stained carmine.* × 460 *diam.*)

Ref.—Phthisis, pp. 95 (2), 96, 113, 115, 116, 119.

FIG. 6.—From margin of an area like XXXVI. 4 (a different specimen), where caseating pneumonia merges into a diffuse small-celled infiltration.—*a a*, alveoli filled with amorphous granular débris, the remains of epithelial and pus cells; the walls of these alveoli are thickened by an interstitial small-celled and nuclear growth, *c c*. At *b* this growth is seen occupying the whole structure of the alveolus, and at *c* it has obliterated the outlines of the walls. At *d d* are alveolar walls in which capillaries still persist. (*Chromic acid prep.; stained chloride of palladium.* × 460 *diam.*)

Ref.—Phthisis, pp. 95, 108, 117 (2), 118 (2), 121.

FIG. 7.—From a section presenting various combinations of infiltration, like figs. 2 and 5. The figure represents progressive thickening of the alveolar walls with a reticulated nuclear growth.—*a a a*, enlarged epithelial cells, which at *b* are mingled with small-celled growth forming a projection into the interior of the vesicle. (In an adjacent alveolus, not here figured, a similar mass composed entirely of small-celled growth projected into the interior of the vesicle.) *c c*, nucleated growth invading the alveolar wall. *d d*, remains of capillaries. *e*, mass of pigment.

Ref.—Phthisis, pp. 108, 117, 121; Syphilitic Disease, 132.

PLATE XXXVIII.

Acute Phthisis.

Figs. 1-4.—Acute tubercular pneumonia. (*Case 16, Henshaw*, p. 117, and Col. Pl. VIII. 1, 4, and 6, also XXXI. 7.)

Fig. 1.—Thickening of alveolar walls with small-celled fibre-growth, gradually advancing until the centre of the alveoli is occluded. Some of the open spaces in this section probably represent bronchioles. Comp. XXVIII. 9, 10. (*Chromic acid prep.; stained carmine.* ×100 *diam.* G. *Hollick, delt.*)

Ref.—Phthisis, pp. 97, 104.

Fig. 2.—A condition of pneumonic infiltration abounding in this lung. The alveoli, *b b b*, are filled with an amorphous exudation containing a few large epithelial-like cells (see fig. 4.) The walls are thickened with a small-celled growth, *c c*. This change prepares in part for a process like that shown in fig. 1, (see *a a*), and in part leads to a caseation like fig. 3. *c*, extension of growth into the contents of an alveolus. (*Chromic acid prep.; stained osmic acid.* ×70 *diam.* G. *Hollick, delt.*)

Ref.—Phthisis, pp. 95, 105, 108.

Fig. 3.—Caseation of tract like fig. 2. It is most advanced in the centre. In the peripheral parts, although the cellular elements have perished, a fibrillar structure remains. (×70 *diam.*)

Ref.—Phthisis, pp. 94, 96, 97, 103.

Fig. 4.—From a portion of fig. 3, more highly magnified; shows the walls of the alveoli, *a a*, infiltrated with fusiform nuclei, following the lines of the capillaries, which have disappeared. (These nuclei, in more advanced stages, tend to become round.) *b c*, alveoli filled with amorphous exudation, containing epithelial-like cells of varied forms, and among these, at *c*, a few pale leucocytes. (*Chromic acid prep.; stained osmic acid.* ×460 *diam.*)

Ref.—Phthisis, pp. 95, 105 (2), 107, 108.

Fig. 5.—Acute destructive pneumonia. (*Case 17, Ellsom*, see p. 179; and Col. Pl. IX. 1, 2, also XXVI. 7.) The figure represents part of wall of an alveolus infiltrated with small-celled growth, *a*, and some large cells, resembling pus-cells, *b*. Large epithelial cells, *c*, are seen attached to it. (*Chromic acid prep. stained chloride of palladium.* ×700 *diam.*)

Ref.—Phthisis, pp. 95, 108.

Fig. 6.—From same case as foregoing. Section of a group of terminal alveoli, *a a a*, filled with enlarged epithelial cells. Between these is a dense small-celled growth, *b d*. (*Chromic acid prep.; stained carmine.* ×700 *diam.*)

Ref.—Phthisis, pp. 93, 107.

Fig. 7.—Acute caseating pneumonia. (*Case 24, Hall*, see p. 191; and Col. Pl. XIV. 2.) Represents a nodule of mixed epithelial and small-celled growth, undergoing, in the centre, caseous degeneration. *a a*, caseating centre, containing the remains of some epithelial cells. *b b*, reticulated nuclear growth in periphery. (*Chromic acid prep.; stained chloride of palladium.* ×460 *diam.*)

Ref.—Phthisis, pp. 85, 94, 96, 113, 115-117.

Fig. 8.—From same specimen. Diffuse small-celled growth invading alveolar walls, and in places occluding the alveoli.—*a a*, alveoli containing large epithelial cells; these measure $\frac{1}{1700}$ to

$\frac{1}{1500}$ inch. *b b*, diffuse small-celled growth. (*Chromic acid prep.; stained chloride of palladium.* × 400 *diam.*)

Ref.—Phthisis, pp. 108, 117, 121; Syphilitic Disease, p. 132.

Fig. 9.— Caseous pneumonia. From same specimen. (Compare XXVIII. 6.)—*a*, area of caseous pneumonia. *b c*, obstructed bronchus in neighbourhood. (*Chromic acid prep.; stained chloride of palladium.* × 70 *diam. Tuffen West, delt.*)

Ref.—Phthisis, pp. 95, 118 (2).

PLATE XXXIX.
Ref.—Phthisis, p. 95.

ACUTE AND CHRONIC TUBERCULISATION.

Fig. 1.—Caseating tubercular pneumonia. (*Case 23, Lloyd*, p. 190, and Col. Pl. XII., also XXXIII. 2, 5, 6.) Represents a zone of small-celled infiltration at the margin of a caseous mass like XXXVIII. 3 (*Henshaw*), and apparently originating like XXVIII. 7 (*Polley*).—*a*, the margin of the caseous mass, showing a reticular structure; the reticulum, and the small cells imbedded in it, are passing into granular disintegration. *b*, a more open fibrous structure, containing fusiform fibres and remains of capillaries. *c*, a dense small-celled and nuclear growth with a reticulum intervening. (Note the resemblance to XXXVI. 2 (*Griffin*). *Chromic acid prep.; stained chloride of palladium.* × 460 *diam.*)

Ref.—Phthisis, pp. 95, 102, 114, 115, 118; Syphilitic Disease, p. 127.

Fig. 2.—Caseating tubercular pneumonia. (*Case 20, J. Thomas*, p. 186, and Col. Pl. VI. 4.) From margin of a caseating mass like XXXVIII. 3 (*Henshaw*), and XXVIII. 6 and 7 (*Acute Tuberculosis, Case 6, Polley*).—*a a a*, alveoli filled with disintegrating mixed epithelial and small-celled growth. *b b*, walls of alveoli thickened with reticulated small-celled growth. (*Chromic acid prep.; stained osmic acid.* × 460 *diam.*)

Ref.—Phthisis, pp. 95, 102, 108, 114, 117 (2), 121.

Fig. 3.—Acute caseating tubercular pneumonia. (*Case 22, Gardiner*, p. 187, Col. Pl. XI.) Tubercle from sheath of artery invading walls of alveoli.—*a*, part of wall of artery, occupied by a dense, round, small-celled growth, mingled with fusiform cells and pigmented. From this a bud, *e'*, projects into the interior of an alveolus. In the same alveolus is a mass of enlarged epithelial cells, *c*. *b b b*, alveoli filled with enlarged epithelial cells, while their walls are thickened with small-celled growth mingled with fusiform cells and fibres. *f f*, fusiform fibre-cells, and *e e*, elongated nuclei, probably of capillary origin. Compare with XXXVII. 7. (*Chromic acid prep.; stained osmic acid.* × 700 *diam.*)

Ref.—Phthisis, pp. 102, 117, 121; Syphilitic Disease, p. 127.

Fig. 4.—Acute tubercular pneumonia. (*Case 12, Price*, p. 173, and Col. Pl. VI. 1.) Section through a group of caseating nodules. These nodules are composed of a mass of mingled epithelial and small-celled growth (in which the latter predominates) passing rapidly into granular detritus, and surrounded by fusiform fibre-cells and dense small-celled growth, variously intermingled. Each nodule appears to represent an ultimate lobule seen in transverse section, and the growth of such small-celled and fibro-nucleated tissue is disposed circularly around this.—*a a*, nodules in which caseation is far advanced, but which still shows traces of cell-structure. *b b b*, nodules with denser accumulation, but in a less advanced stage. *c c*, lines of fusiform cells apparently of capillary origin. *d d*, dense infiltrations of small-celled growth. *e e*, epithelial cells interspersed amongst the last. The neighbouring alveoli showed change like XXVIII. 7 and 8, and immediately adjacent were large nodules apparently formed out of the confluence of those here depicted, and entirely amorphous. (*Chromic acid prep.; stained chloride of palladium.* × 500 *diam.*)

Ref.—Phthisis, pp. 96, 102, 108, 115.

FIG. 5.—Nodules of mingled epithelial and small-celled growth passing into caseation. (*Case 27, Overall,* p. 196; and Col. Pl. X. 7-10. See also XL. 9, and XLIII. 3.)—*a a*, centre of nodule, in which the reticulated structure is still apparent, but the cell-formation has become almost entirely granular. *b'*, a portion where this reticulum is seen to be in part composed of fusiform fibres like XL. 9. (The line from *b'* has been carried too far into the figure.) *b b*, denser fibre-bands surrounding the mass, which at *d d* pass into broader bands of fibres. *c c*, small-celled growth mingled with the fibre-formation. *e e*, alveoli containing mingled epithelial and small-celled growth. (*Chromic acid prep.; stained carmine.* × 100 *diam.*)

Ref.—Phthisis, pp. 97, 99, 102, 116 (2).

FIG. 6.—From same preparation as foregoing, showing the reticular nuclear growth which forms large tracts of this lung. (*Chromic acid prep.; stained carmine.* × 460 *diam.*)

Ref.—Phthisis, pp. 94, 96, 117.

FIG. 7.—Indurating and caseating tuberculisation. (*Case 10, Unwin,* p. 170.)—*a*, a nodule completely caseous, surrounded by a zone of fibroid growth mingled with small-celled growth, *b b*, deeply pigmented. Total diameter of nodule, including this zone, $\frac{1}{50}$ inch. Diameter of caseous area $\frac{1}{105}$ inch. *c c*, nodules composed entirely of small-celled growth, disposed in part in rows, but in part densely massed. *d d*, area of small-celled infiltration mingled with fusiform fibres, showing in places traces of alveolar origin. *e e*, pigmented giant-cells. *f*, alveolar tissue, with thickening of the walls with small-celled growth. *y g*, remains of capillaries. (*Chromic acid prep.; stained chloride of palladium.* × 230 *diam.; reduced.*)

Ref.—Phthisis, pp. 84, 96, 97, 108, 115, 116.

PLATE XL.

INDURATING AND CASEATING TUBERCULOSIS.

FIGS. 1 to 6.—Indurating tuberculosis. (*Case 26, Heath,* p. 194, and Col. Pl. X. 5 and 6; also XLII. 5.)

FIG. 1.—Early stage of nodule formed by peri-alveolar small-celled growth with intra-alveolar epithelial proliferation.—*a a a*, central portion where growth is most dense. *b b*, fibroid zone surrounding this. *c c*, alveoli beyond fibroid zone, in the walls of which small-celled growth is also taking place. *d d*, bronchioles similarly surrounded. *e e*, areas where small-celled growth is becoming uniform. *f*, mass of pigment, probably a giant-cell. (*Chromic acid prep.; stained carmine.* × 460 *diam., reduced.*)

Ref.—Phthisis, pp. 95, 98, 108, 113, 115 (2), 116, 117 (2), 119.

FIG. 2.—From same. Diffuse area of mingled small-celled and fibroid growth invading the pulmonary tissue.—*a*, central portion where small-celled growth is most dense, and where some caseation was appearing. *b b c*, remains of alveoli containing epithelial cells, their walls thickened as above. *d d*, small-celled growth, extending diffusely at periphery. *e e*, alveoli whose walls are thickened with small-celled growth. (*Chromic acid prep; stained carmine.* × 250 *diam.*)

Ref.—Phthisis, pp. 95, 98, 108, 115-117 (2), 121.

FIG. 3.—From same. Nodule formed from perialveolar thickening, caseating in centre.—*a*, central caseous mass, still showing outlines of alveolar structure. *b b*, zone of fibroid induration surrounding this. *c c c*, section of bronchioles or alveoli whose epithelium has become 'cuboid' (Charcot), or quasi-cylindrical (rudimentary fœtal form—Zenker). *d*, group of alveoli whose walls are becoming invaded by fibroid change. *e e*, obliteration of pulmonary tissue by dense small-celled infiltration. (*Chromic acid prep.; stained carmine.* × 250 *diam.*)

Ref.—Phthisis, pp. 98 (2), 108, 116 (2).

FIG. 4.—From same. Destructive pneumonia, caused by acute caseation of tracts like figs. 1 and 2. The terminal bronchioles and alveoli retain their form, but are replaced by a granular fibrillated structure and are surrounded by a similar structure. The whole constitutes a lobule of caseation surrounded by interlobular tissue, *c c*.—*a a*, a group of alveoli, showing traces of cell-structure. *b b*, terminal alveoli and bronchioles, presenting only fibrillated granular character. *c c c*, zone of peri-lobular thickening. (*Chromic acid prep.; stained osmic acid.* × 100 *diam.*)

Ref.—Phthisis, pp. 98, 116 (2), 118.

FIG. 5.—From same. A portion from *a*, fig. 4, × 460 *diam.*, showing cells imbedded in a reticulum.

Ref.—Phthisis, p. 116.

FIG. 6.—From same. Early stage of invasion of alveolar walls by nuclear growth. The epithelium has almost disappeared, but traces are remaining, *a a*, and in some parts these are much pigmented, *c c*. The nuclear growth in places follows the lines of the capillaries, *b b*. The nuclei are sometimes round, as at *e*, but very commonly fusiform. (*Chromic acid prep.; stained carmine.* × 700 *diam.*)

Ref.—Phthisis, pp. 95, 98, 103, 114 (2), 115 (2), 116, 118, 119.

FIG. 7.—From mass of indurating tubercle. (*Case 36, Mears*, and Col. Pl. XIX. also XXXIII. 4, and XLII. 3, 4.) Represents commencement of small-celled growth in floor of an alveolus, by enlargement of the nuclei of the capillaries.—*a*, side wall of alveolus, thickened by small-celled growth. *b*, enlarged nuclei of capillaries. (*Chromic acid prep.; stained carmine.* × 460 *diam.*)

Ref.—Phthisis, pp. 97, 103, 114.

FIG. 8.—A similar preparation to foregoing, from a similar case.—*a a*, thickened walls of alveolus. *b*, lines of capillaries with nuclear growth. *a'*, remains of elastic fibres. (*Chromic acid prep.; stained carmine.* × 460 *diam.*)

Ref.—Phthisis, pp. 97, 103.

FIG. 9.—(From *Case 27, Overall.* See p. 196 and Col. Pl. X., 7-10, also XXXIX. 5 and 6, and XLIII. 3.) Shows the nuclear growth in the lines of the capillaries proceeding to a more advanced stage than in figs. 7 and 8. (*Chromic acid prep.; stained carmine.* × 460 *diam.*)

Ref.—Phthisis, pp. 97, 116, 118.

FIG. 10.—(From *Case 31, Lack*, p. 205 and Col. Pl. XVII. 1 and 3.) Early stage of formation of a lobular nodule of epithelial proliferation, mingled with small-celled growth.—*a*, small-celled growth. *b*, pigmented epithelium mingled with small-celled growth. *c*, commencing giant-cell. (The line from *c* has been carried too far.) *Chromic acid prep.; stained carmine.* × 460 *diam. reduced.*)

Ref.—Phthisis, pp. 96, 116.

PLATE XLI.

INDURATING TUBERCULOSIS.

FIGS. 1-4.—*Case 30, Carr*, p. 203, and Col. Pl. XVI., also XXXIII. 7 and 8.

FIG. 1.—A group of indurated nodules, *a a a*, composed of broad bands of fibres, nearly homogeneous, but having lacunæ and spaces in their interstices, occupied in some instances by the remains of cells. Each nodule is more or less distinctly mapped out by a circular arrangement of fibres around it. *b b b*, pulmonary tissue consisting of broad bands of fibre, somewhat fibrillated, with small-celled growth imbedded in the interstices, which when more highly magnified presents the appearance seen in fig. 2, and also in fig. 3. *c*, such areas in which caseation is commencing. *d d*, alveolar tissue partly broken down, where degenerated and pigmented epithelial cells are seen in places. *e*, an artery, with fibroid thickening surrounding it. *e'*, thickened interlobular septum. (Chromic acid prep.; stained carmine. × 150 diam.)

Ref. - Chronic Pneumonia, p. 47; Phthisis, pp. 97, 122; Syphilitic Disease, p. 132.

FIG. 2.—From same. A small lobule undergoing fibroid transformation. It was completely surrounded by almost homogeneous sclerotic nodules like those seen in fig. 1. The induration is seen to be proceeding by the thickening of a reticulum, *a a*, *e e*, which in part has its origin from the capillaries, and in the meshes of which round and ovoid nuclei are imbedded. At *b* this reticulum is seen to thicken into broader bands. At *e* are some remains of epithelium. At *f*, towards the centre, is some caseous change. (Chromic acid prep.; stained chloride of palladium. × 700 diam.)

Ref.—Phthisis, pp. 97, 99, 116.

FIG. 3.—From same. A nodule of induration in process of formation, and partially caseous in centre.—*a a*, almost homogeneous sclerotic fibrous tissue. *b*, an area occupied by granular matter, and a few pigmented epithelial cells. *c c c*, remains of alveolar structure containing a few epithelial cells, but almost entirely occupied by dense small-celled growth. *d d*, zone of thickening fibroid perilobular tissue. (Chromic acid prep.; stained chloride of palladium. × 100 diam.)

Ref.—Phthisis, pp. 97, 99, 116.

FIG. 4.—From *c* of fig. 3 magnified 700 diam. Shows a small alveolar passage diminished by the thickening of its walls by small-celled growth, and still containing large epithelial cells.

FIG. 5.—From *Case 35, Roberts*, p. 212, and Col. Pl. XVIII. 1 and 2, also XXXII. 10, and XXXIII. 9 and 11. A nodule of induration, the centre almost entirely and homogeneously sclerotic, but traversed by fine lacunæ, *a*, some of which are pigmented, and also by capillaries, *b*. Some fusiform cells, *c*, are seen among these. Masses of pigment, *d*, are also present, and the whole is surrounded by thickened fibroid tissue. At one spot, *f*, beyond this fibroid tissue, is a dense small-celled growth, which, in the preparation, extended for a considerable distance into the surrounding tissue. (Chromic acid prep.; stained chloride of palladium. × 460 diam. reduced.)

Ref.—Phthisis, pp. 96, 99, 116 (2).

FIG. 6.—From *Case 34, Cox*, p. 210, and Col. Pl. XVIII. 3 and 4. A nodule of small-celled reticulated growth, *b b*, with caseation in centre, *a*, commencing in centre of alveolus. (Chromic acid prep.; stained carmine. × 460 diam.)

Ref.—Phthisis, pp. 67, 85, 97, 113, 115, 116, 118.

FIG. 7.—From *Case 33, Coppin*, p. 208, and Col. Pl. XVII. 3, also XLIII. 1 and 2. Shows the process of fibroid induration, *c d*, proceeding in a diffuse form in the midst of a small-celled growth, *a b*, in the alveolar walls. (*Chromic acid prep.; stained carmine.* × 460 *diam.*)

Ref.—Phthisis, pp. 97, 116, 121.

PLATE XLII.

INDURATING TUBERCULOSIS. TUBERCLE OF BRONCHI AND VESSELS.

FIG. 1.—From *Case 32, Attwood*, p. 207. Diffuse small-celled infiltration of alveolar walls, passing into fibroid induration.—*a a*, walls of alveoli thickened by a small-celled growth, reticulated. *e, f f*, reticulum is seen thickening and passing into broader bands of fibre, which, *b, g*, contain in their meshes groups of cells which gradually disappear. *c c*, alveoli included in the thickening fibre-tissue, the epithelium replaced by a small-celled growth, in which a gradual thickening of the reticulum is advancing. *d d*, sections of bronchioles. *h*, section of an artery passing into the same fibroid induration. (*Spirit prep.; stained carmine.* × 460 *diam. reduced.*)

Ref.—Phthisis, p. 121.

FIG. 2.—From a small-celled nodule in a case of indurating tuberculosis in a child. Shows induration proceeding from the peri-lobular zone into the nodule.—*a*, small-celled growth. *b*, a group of cells (giant-cell ?) *c c*, thickened bands of reticulum advancing into the nodule. *e*, peri-lobular tissue. *d*, groups of nuclei enclosed between bands of fibres. (*Chromic acid prep.; stained carmine.* × 700 *diam.*)

Ref.—Phthisis, pp. 85, 96; Syphilitic Disease, p. 182.

FIG. 3.—Perivascular thickening with small-celled growth. (From *Case 36, Mears*, p. 213, and Col. Pl. XIX. 1 and 2, also XXXIII. 4 and XL. 7.)—*a*, outer wall of arterial sheath. *b*, coagulum. *c*, small-celled growth external to circular fibres. *e*, growth extending into adjacent pulmonary tissue. Beyond *d*, this growth became much more dense. (*Chromic acid prep.; stained carmine.* × 100 *diam.*)

Ref.—Phthisis, p. 102.

FIG. 4.—From same series as foregoing figure. Transverse section of an artery, showing small-celled growth invading the whole thickness of the wall. (*Chromic acid prep.; stained carmine.* × 460 *diam.*)

Ref.—Phthisis, p. 102.

FIG. 5.—Section of a bronchus with small-celled growth invading wall. (From *Case 28, Smith*, p. 199, and Col. Pl. XIII. 1 and 2; also XXXII. 7, 8, XXXIII. 1, 3, and 10, and XXXV. 4-6.)—*a*, circular fibres. *b b e*, small-celled growth. (*Chromic acid prep.; stained chloride of palladium.* × 460 *diam.*)

Ref.—Phthisis. p. 100.

FIG. 6.—Chronic phthisis; fibroid induration of lung. (From *Case 3, Hawkins*, p. 159, and Col. Pl. IV. 1; also XLIII. 4.)—*a a a*, alveoli containing epithelial and pyoid cells. These latter are mostly of the type of those seen in XXV. 3, 5, 7, and 9 *h*. *b b*, alveoli much diminished in size by fibroid thickening of their walls. *c c*, partial obliteration of alveoli by fibroid growth. *d d*, extending fibroid growth. (*Chromic acid prep.; stained carmine.* × 100 *diam.*)

Ref.—Phthisis, p. 122; Syphilitic Disease. p. 126.

FIG. 7.—Indurating tuberculosis. (*Case 29, Brown*, see p. 201, and Col. Pl. XV., also XLIII. 6.) —*a a a*, vessels with walls greatly thickened by a glistening, almost homogeneous, fibroid material.

b b b, sections of bronchi and bronchioles, whose walls are similarly thickened. *c c c*, remains of alveolar structure, but replaced by small-celled growth imbedded in a thickened reticulum of fibre-formation. *d d*, bands of broad fibres extending from the thickened bronchial walls. *e*, similar band. *f*, obliteration of pulmonary tissue by fibre-growth enclosing nuclei in its meshes. (*Chromic acid prep.; stained carmine.* × 460 *diam. reduced.*)

Ref.—Phthisis, p. 122; Syphilitic Disease, p. 128.

PLATE XLIII.

INDURATING AND CASEATING TUBERCULOSIS.—TUBERCLE OF BRONCHUS AND OF ALVEOLAR WALLS.

Fig. 1.—Indurated pigmented tuberculosis. (From *Case 33, Coppin*, p. 208, and Col. Pl. XVII. 2, and 4; also XLI. 7.) A group of alveoli almost entirely converted into fibroid tissue, but still showing alveolar shape by arrangement of fibres in whorls.—*a a a*, alveoli, fibroid, deeply pigmented, the pigment assuming irregular stellate and fusiform shapes indicating its original site to have been in cells or nuclei. *b*, a similar alveolus with dense mass of such pigment in its centre (a giant-cell ?). *c*, an alveolus almost entirely fibroid. *d d*, remains of vessels. *e e*, tracts where small-celled growth is pigmented. (*Chromic acid prep.; stained osmic acid.* × 250 *diam.*)

Ref.—Phthisis, pp. 85, 96, 97.

Fig. 2.—From same as foregoing. Portion of a tract of fibroid induration occurring in an area of 'pneumonic' infiltration.—*a a a*, broad-banded fibres extending between adjacent alveoli. *b b*, reticulum of thickening fibres continuous with the broader bands, and giving off smaller fibres among which round cells are imbedded. *c c*, some of these round cells which are large and nucleated. *d*, a denser reticulum gradually thickening. (*Chromic acid prep.* × 460 *diam.*)

Ref.—Phthisis, pp. 85, 96, 121.

Fig. 3.—Indurating tuberculosis. (From *Case 27, Overall*, p. 196, and Col. Pl. X. 7-10; also XXXIX. 5 and 6, and XL. 9.)—Represents a lobular mass of induration, which, on division, resembled, to the naked eye and also with low magnifying power, a section of a thickened occluded bronchus, especially from its elongated form. On close analysis, especially of sections at different depths, it is seen to have everywhere an alveolar structure, the alveoli being invaded by fibroid tissue and in some places undergoing subsequent caseation.—*a*, group of alveoli, the fibroid walls of which persist in the midst of the caseating mass, while at the margins caseation is proceeding in the zone of fibroid tissue which surrounds this area. *b*, an alveolus with contents entirely caseous. *c*, another where traces of fibroid tissue persist amidst the caseation. *d*, an alveolus, partly fibroid, partly caseating. *e*, a tract where alveoli, partly with epithelial, partly with caseous contents, show also an increase of fibroid tissue. *g g*, small caseous masses left in the midst of fibroid areas. *h*, a tract where the fibroid tissue is fusing into a homogeneous sclerotic area. *f k k*, two alveolar passages (?) undergoing fibroid change. *l*, an alveolus containing large epithelial cells. *m m m*, thickened walls of alveolar tissue. (*Chromic acid prep.; stained carmine.* × 100 *diam.*)

Ref.—Phthisis, p. 98.

Fig. 4.—(From *Case 3, Hawkins*, p. 159, and Col. Pl. IV. 1; also XLII. 6.)—Shows a small-celled growth in the alveolar wall, closely resembling the nodular form assumed by miliary tubercle in the sheaths of the cerebral arteries.—*a b*, two nodular masses of this character. The fibres of the wall can be seen among the cells. *c*, a tract intervening and only partially invaded; a few blood-corpuscles are seen in the capillaries. (*Chromic acid prep.; stained chloride of palladium.* × 460 *diam.*)

Ref.—Phthisis, p. 67.

FIG. 5.—A nodule of caseation. (*Case 26, Heath*, p. 194, and Col. Pl. X. 5 and 6, also XL. 1–6.) The nodule represents a terminal lobule, consisting of numerous alveoli, and surrounded by an interlobular septum. The structure is converted into a finely granular fibrillated material, here and there deeply pigmented. At *a*, beyond the septum, is another alveolus undergoing similar changes. (*Chromic acid prep.; stained chloride of palladium.* × 80 *diam.*)

Ref.—Phthisis, pp. 94, 98, 114–117.

FIG. 6.—Tubercle invading wall of bronchus. (*Case 5, Brown*, p. 161, and Col. Pl. V. 5, also XXXV. 7.) The epithelium has disappeared, and a nodular granulation is projecting into the interior. (*Chromic acid prep.* × 100 *diam.*)

Ref.—Phthisis, p. 100 (2).

PLATE XLIV.

PULMONARY DISEASE FROM INHALATION OF DUST, 'PNEUMOKONIOSIS.'

BROWN INDURATION OF LUNG IN HEART DISEASE.

FIG. 1.—Flax-dresser's lung. (From Dr. Headlam Greenhow, *Trans. Path. Soc.* vol. xx. 1887, Pl. III. fig. 7. See *Case 41*, p. 219.) Cells containing black pigment from the bronchial tubes: round granular cells, and ciliated columnar cells. (× 200 *diam.*)

FIG. 2.—The same. (From Dr. Headlam Greenhow, *ibid.* Pl. III. fig. 6.) Section showing a small bronchiole surrounded by masses of black pigment.—*a a*, adjacent alveoli with thickened walls and granular cells. (× 30 *diam.*)

Ref.—Disease from Inhalation of Dust. p. 54 ; Collapse, p. 57.

FIG. 3.—Collier's lung. (From Dr. Headlam Greenhow, *ibid.* See *Case 39*, p. 218, and Col. Pl. XXII. 2.) The figure represents a section taken from the upper lobe, at a part adjoining condensed tissue. The walls of the air-vesicles are thickened and contain a deposit of amorphous black pigment. (× 200 *diam.*)

FIG. 4.—Section of copper-miner's lung. (From Dr. Headlam Greenhow, *ibid.*; Pl. III. fig. 4 ; also *Case 40*, p. 219.) On the left is seen the thickened pleura, with deposits of amorphous black pigment in the subserous tissue, and above, part of a projecting nodule, filled with black pigment. (× 40 *diam.*)

FIG. 5.—A nodule in a potter's lung. (*Case 38, Barlow*, p. 216, and Col. Pl. XXII. 1.) A pigmented nodule of induration, consisting of a fibroid lobule.—*a*, mass of pigmented fibroid tissue, showing by its conformation, and the markings in its interior, traces of pulmonary structure. With a higher power, remains of epithelial and small-celled growth, undergoing granular disintegration, can be seen throughout it. *c'*, zone of thickened perilobular tissue. *b d*, similar changes to that seen in the lobule, but occurring in the adjacent pulmonary tissue. (*Spirit prep.: glycerine.* × 70 *diam.*)

FIG. 6.—From same. A nodule of induration almost entirely fibroid. The broad bands of fibres, *b*, of which it is composed, embrace ovoid and round spaces, filled with black matter, which in places shows traces of having been contained in cells and groups of cells similar to those seen in XLII. 2.—*a*, a vessel with thickened wall. (Compare XLII. 7.) (*Spirit prep.: stained carmine: dammar.* × 460 *diam.*)

FIG. 7.—From same. Infiltration of pulmonary tissue with small-celled growth, which is deeply pigmented at *a*, and free from pigment at *b*. (*Spirit prep.; glycerine.* × 460 *diam.*)

Ref.– Collapse, p. 57.

FIGS. 8 and 9.—From Zenker's drawing of 'siderosis,' or oxide of iron in the lung. (*Case 42*, p. 220, from the *Deutsch. Archiv klin. Med.* Bd. xi.)

FIG. 8.—The pulmonary alveoli are thickened and partly filled with granules of oxide of iron. Some of the alveoli are greatly narrowed. The capillaries, where visible, are free from granules. (× 100 *diam.*)

FIG. 9.—Cells from the alveoli of the same lung, containing granules of iron. Two cells show a nucleus and only a few iron granules; others are filled with the granules, and the nucleus obliterated, or only seen as a bright yellow spot. (× 800 *diam.*)

FIGS. 10 and 11.—Brown induration of lung in heart-disease. (*Case 43, W. Thomas*, p. 222, and Col. Pl. XXII. 3, 4.)

Ref. –Brown Induration, p. 52 (2).

FIG. 10.—Walls of alveoli, thickened with fine fibrillated tissue; their capillaries, *a*, greatly distended. *b b*, pigmented nuclei in walls of alveoli. *c*, epithelium filled with pigment. *d d*, enlarged epithelial cells with multiple nuclei, filled with colouring matter of blood. (× 460 *iam.*)

FIG. 11.—From same.—Alveoli occupied by enlarged epithelial cells filled with black pigment. (× 460 *diam.*)

PLATE XLV.

CANCER OF LUNG.

FIGS. 1-3.—Cancerous infiltration of perivascular sheaths. (*Case 45, Parsons*, p. 224, and Col. Pl. XXII. 5.)

Ref.– Cancer, p. 135.

FIG. 1.—Infiltration of sheath of small artery.—*a*, the intima intact. *b*, infiltration of remainder of coats. *c*, extension to pulmonary tissue. (*Chromic acid prep.; stained chloride of palladium.* × 70 *diam.*)

FIG. 2.—A portion of foregoing × 700 *diam.*—*a*, outer portion of intima. *b*, cancer-cells growing externally.

FIG. 3.—From same. A single nodule of cancer, *a*, growing in the sheath of an artery and extending, at *b*, along the wall. (*Chromic acid prep.; stained chloride of palladium.* × 100 *diam.*)

FIGS. 4-6.—Cancerous infiltration of the lung. (*Case 46*, p. 225, and Col. Pl. XXII. 6.)

Ref.– Cancer, p. 135.

FIG. 4.—Infiltration of alveolar wall with cancer-growth, of which the cells, by multiplication, have become small (small-celled sarcoma?), and the growth closely resembles a tubercular infiltration. *a*, round cells. *b*, fusiform cells. *d*, vessels. (*Chromic acid prep.; stained chloride of palladium.* × 460 *diam.*)

FIG. 5.—From same. Shows the mode of growth of the cancer-infiltration in the wall of the alveolus to be from the nuclei of the capillaries.—*a*, mass of cancer-growth passing from fusiform to round cells. *b c*, growth of nuclei of capillaries. *d*, fusiform cells. (Chromic acid prep.; stained carmine. × 460 diam.)

FIG. 6.—From same. Exhibits similar changes to foregoing.—*a c*, round nucleated cells among the small round and fusiform cells, *b*. (× 460 diam.)

FIG. 7.—From another case of cancerous infiltration. Shows the mingling of large epithelial-like cells, *a*, with small round cells, *b*.
Ref.—Cancer, p. 135.

FIGS. 8–12.—*Columnar epithelioma of lung*. (Case 47, Leather, p. 225, and Col. Pl. XXIV. 3 and 4.

FIG. 8.—Filling of alveolar tissue with villous growth having glandular type.—*a b*, alveoli densely packed with villous growth. *c*, portions where this appears to assume the form of crypts. *d*, portions where the villous character is distinct. *e e e*, similar growth in the lymphatics of a septum. (Chromic acid prep.; stained carmine. × 100 diam.)
Ref.—Cancer. p. 137.

FIG. 9.—From same. Shows the growth occurring in a bronchiole. —*a a*, villous growth. *b*, secretion, mingled with cell-débris, in the centre. (Chromic acid prep.; stained carmine. × 100 diam.)

FIG. 10.—From same. Shows the earlier stages of the villous growth in adjacent alveoli.—*a a*, alveoli filled with the products of epithelial proliferation. *b b*, cells becoming larger, rounded, and in several instances containing two nuclei. *d d*, further stages of same, and which at *f* form a mass, almost suggesting a 'nest.' *c*, commencing change of epithelium to the columnar type. *g*, infiltration of some cells, of similar character, among the fibres of the alveolar walls. (Chromic acid prep.; stained carmine. × 700 diam.)

FIG. 11.—From same. Shows the structure of a single villus with its columnar epithelium fully formed (× 700 diam.)

FIG. 12.—Shows the mode of growth of the villous formation from the alveolar wall. (× 700 diam.)

ACUTE PNEUMONIA

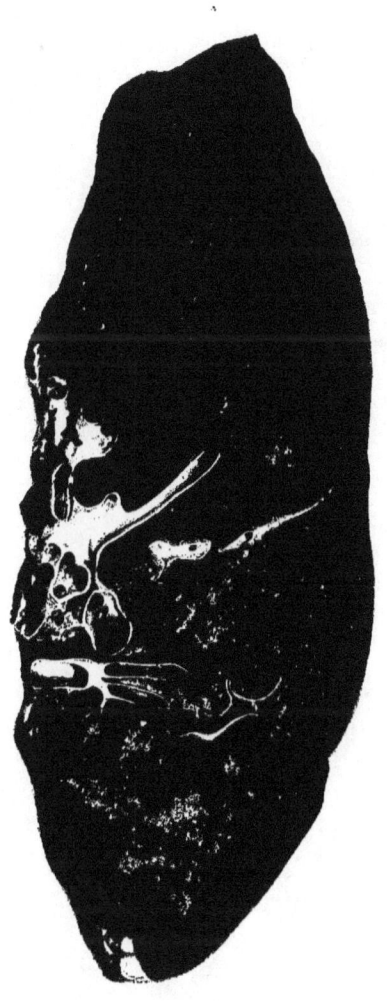

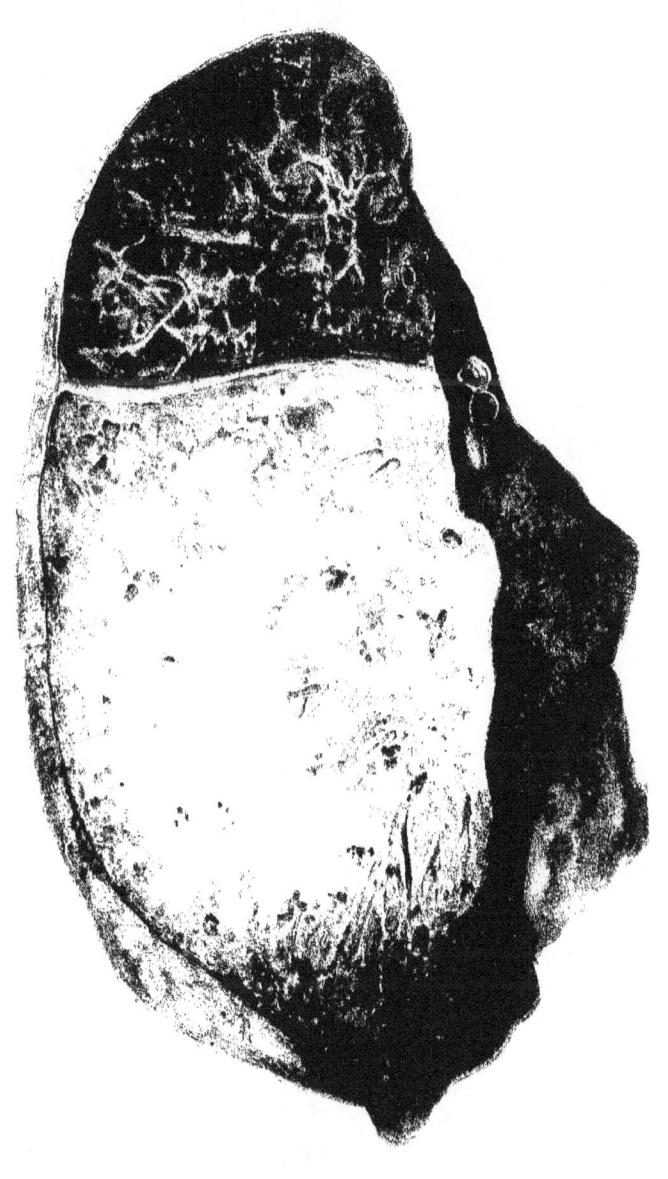

SUPPURATION PNEUMONIA

HYPOSTATIC PNEUMONIA.

Plate III.

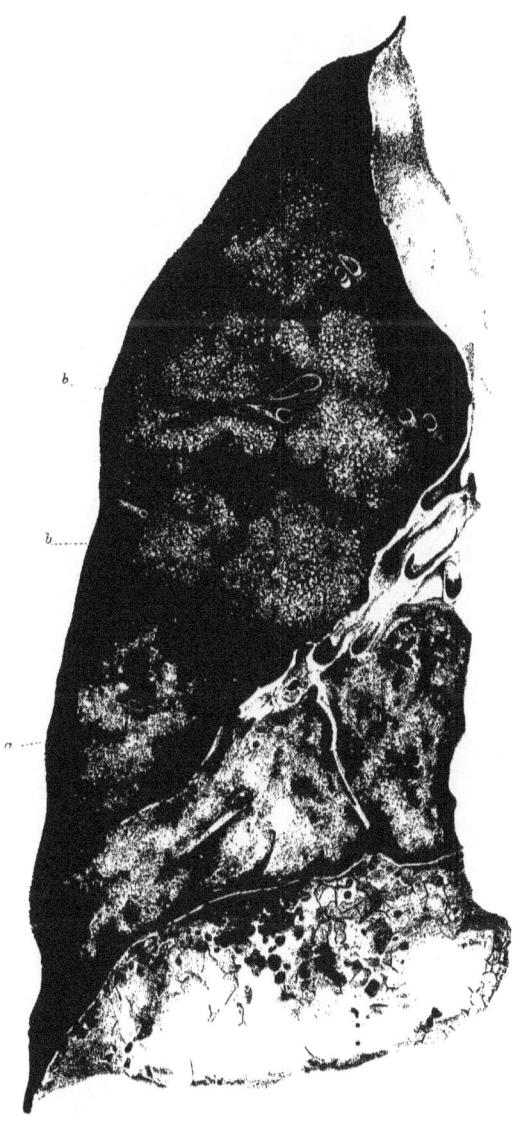

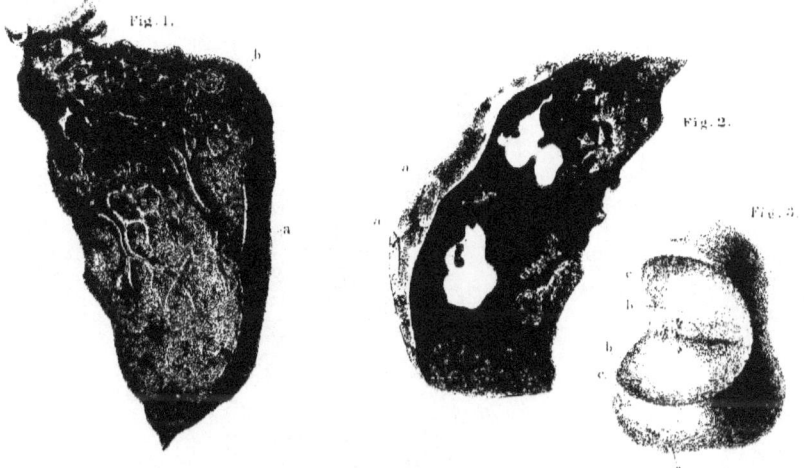
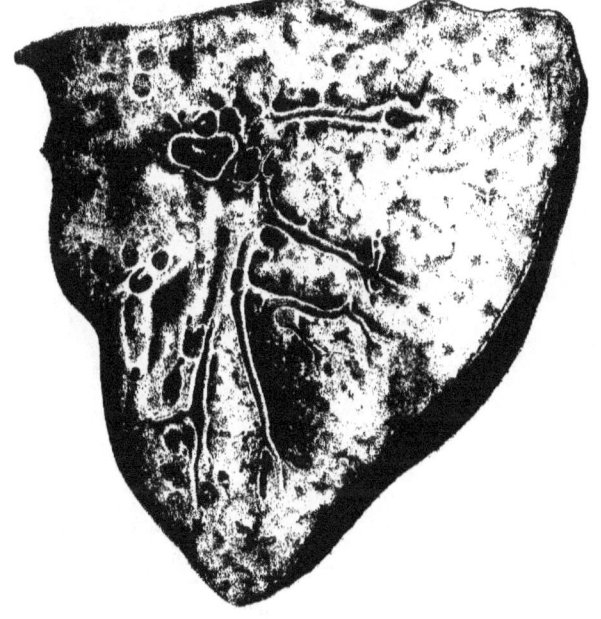

LOBULAR PNEUMONIA. MEASLES TUBERCULAR PNEUMONIA

Plate V.

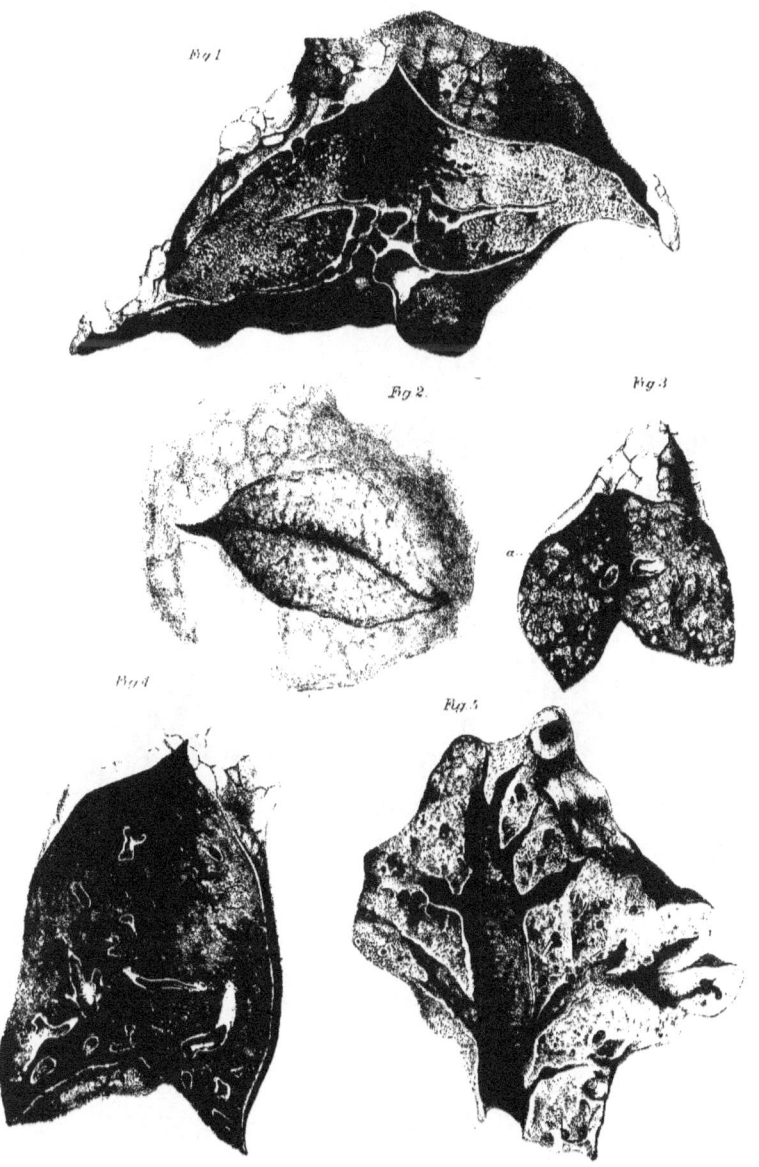

Fig 1.

Fig 2.   Fig 3.

Fig 4.   Fig 5.

GANGRENE OF LUNG,—PNEUMONIA WITH CONCRETIONS IN BRONCHI.

Plate V.

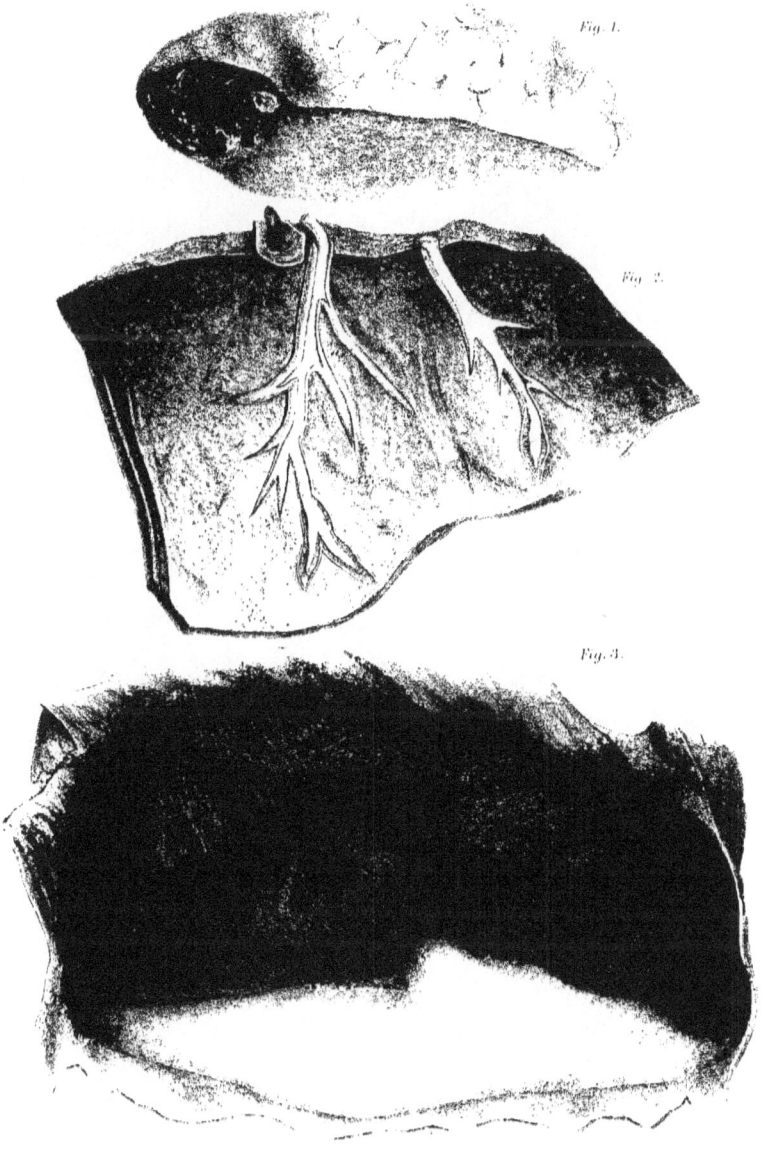

Fig. 1.

Fig. 2.

Fig. 3.

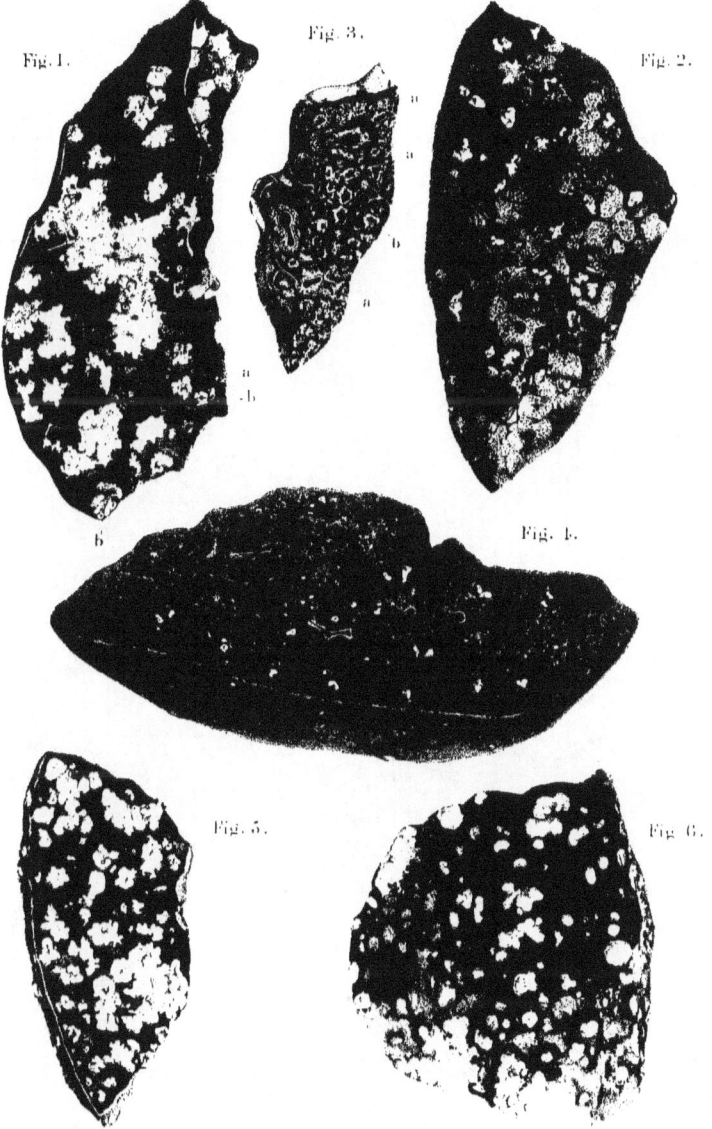

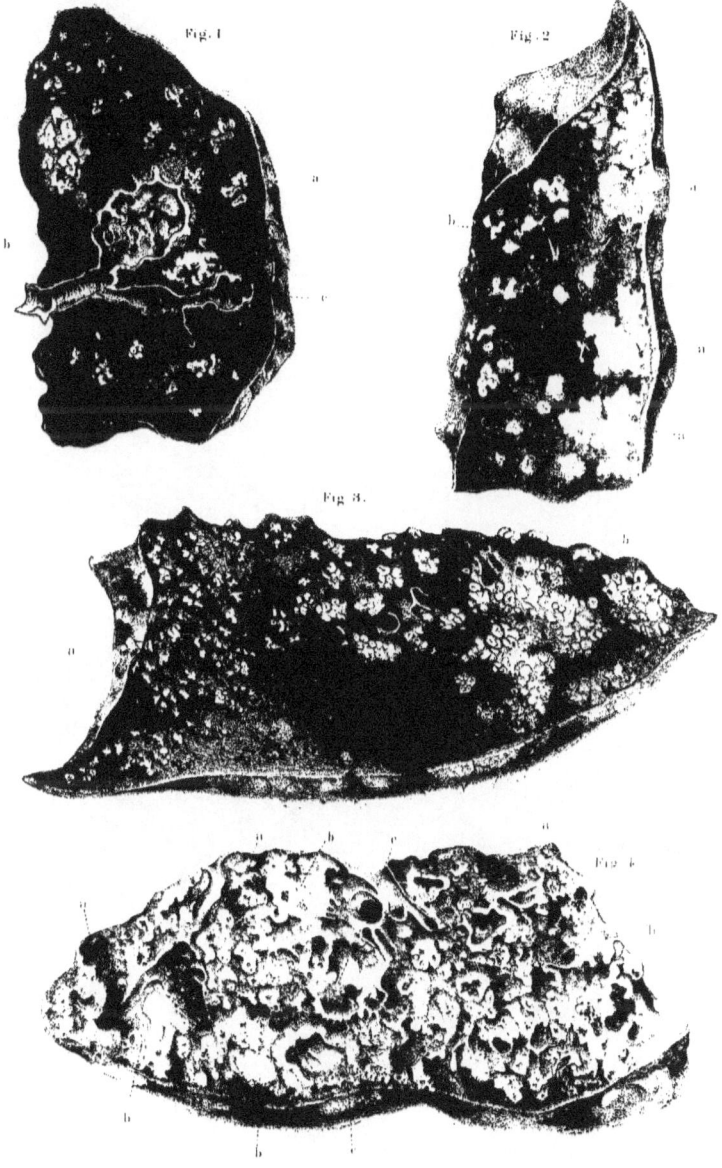

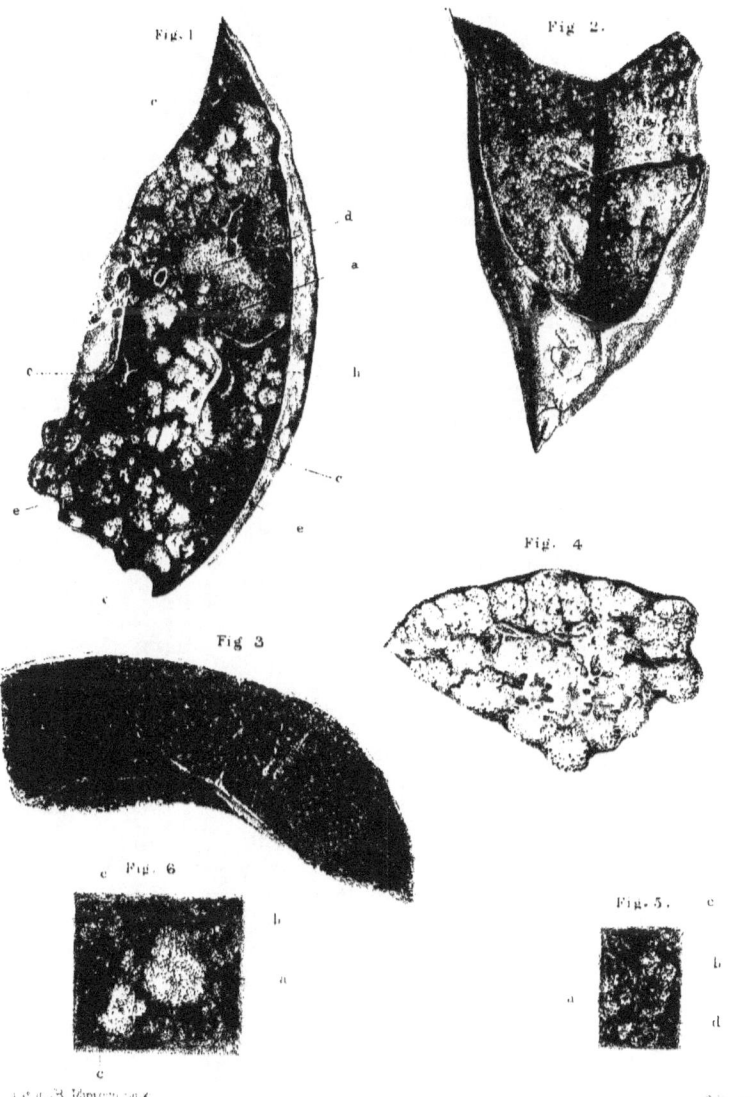

Plate VIII.

ACUTE TUBERCULOSIS TUBERCULAR PNEUMONIA.

Plate IX

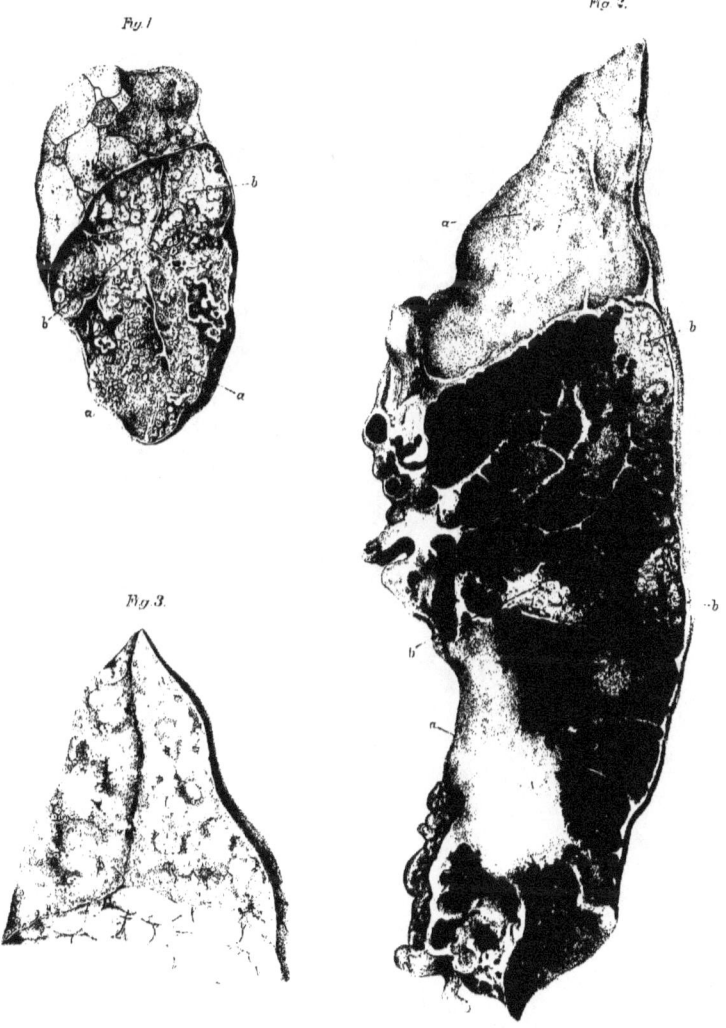

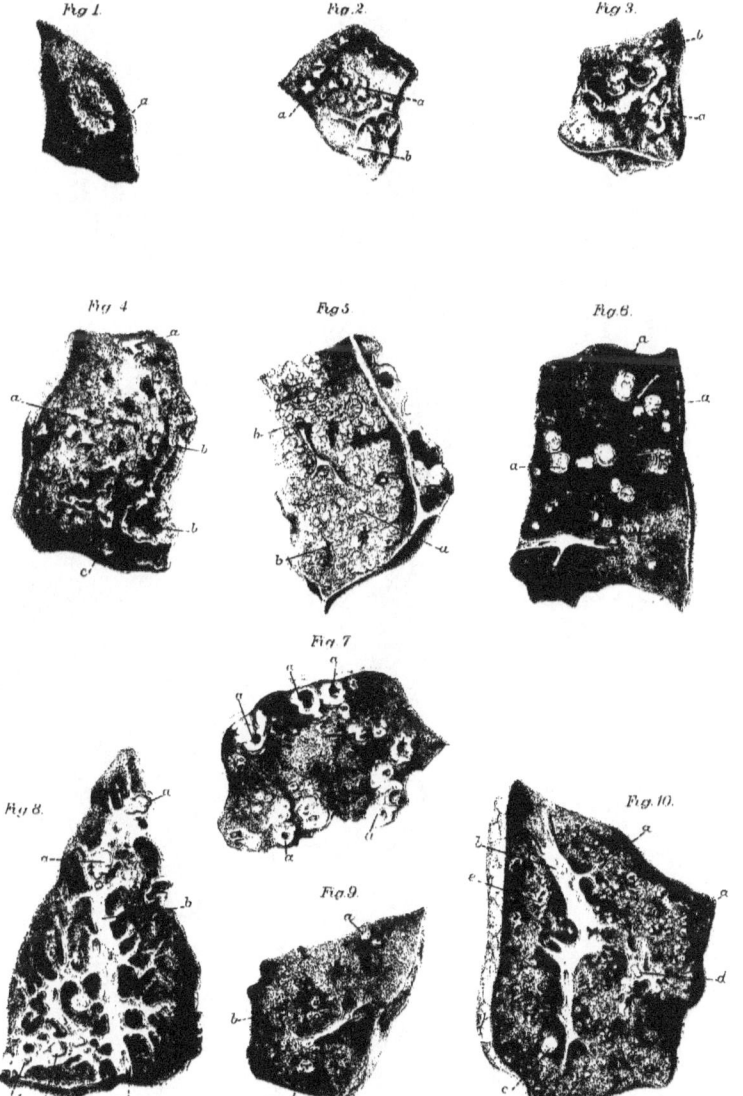

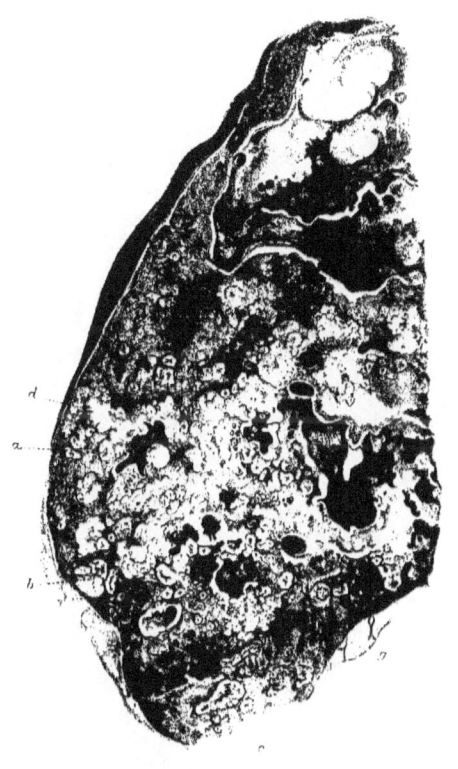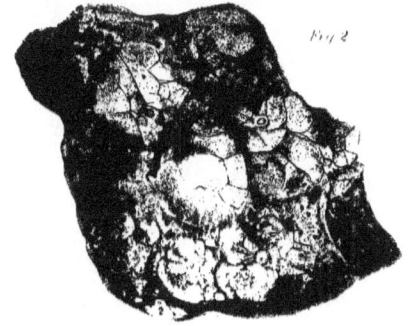

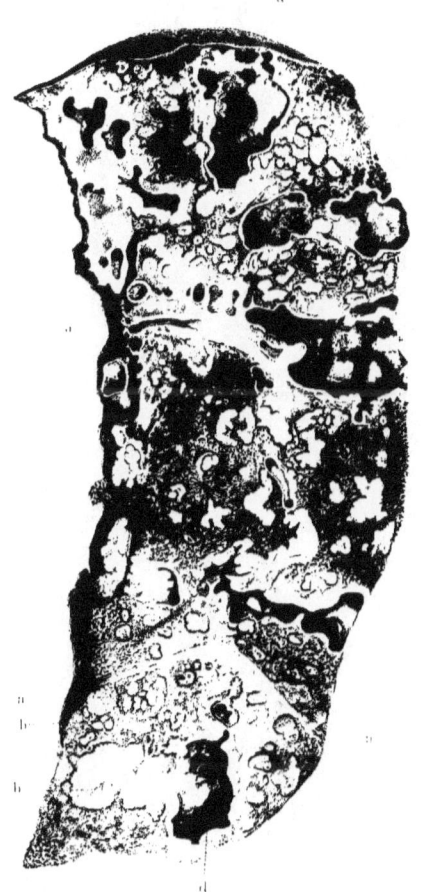

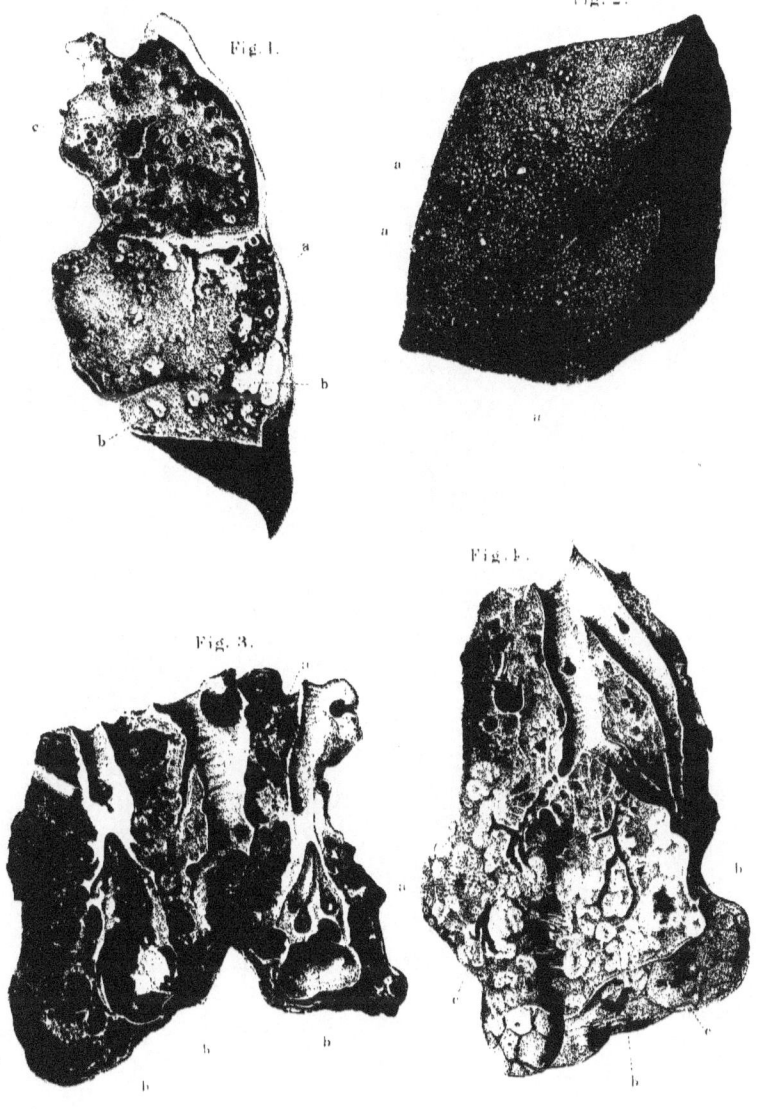

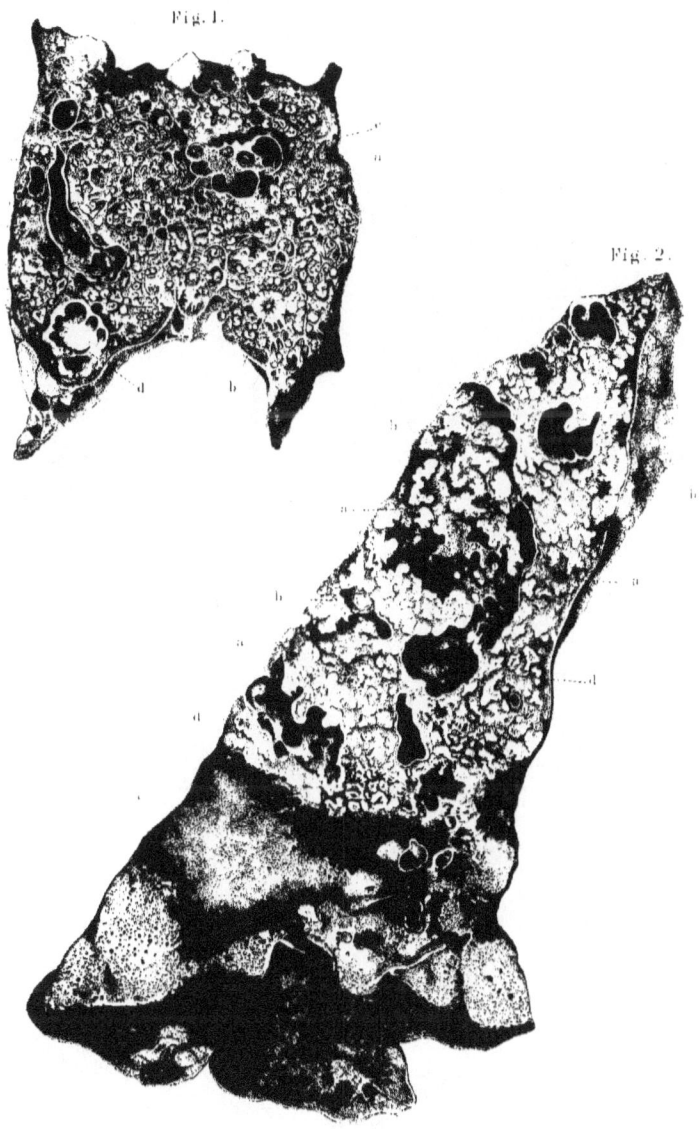

TUBERCULAR PNEUMONIA. TUBERCULAR INDURATION.
TUBERCLE BRONCHIAL GLANDS.

Plate XV

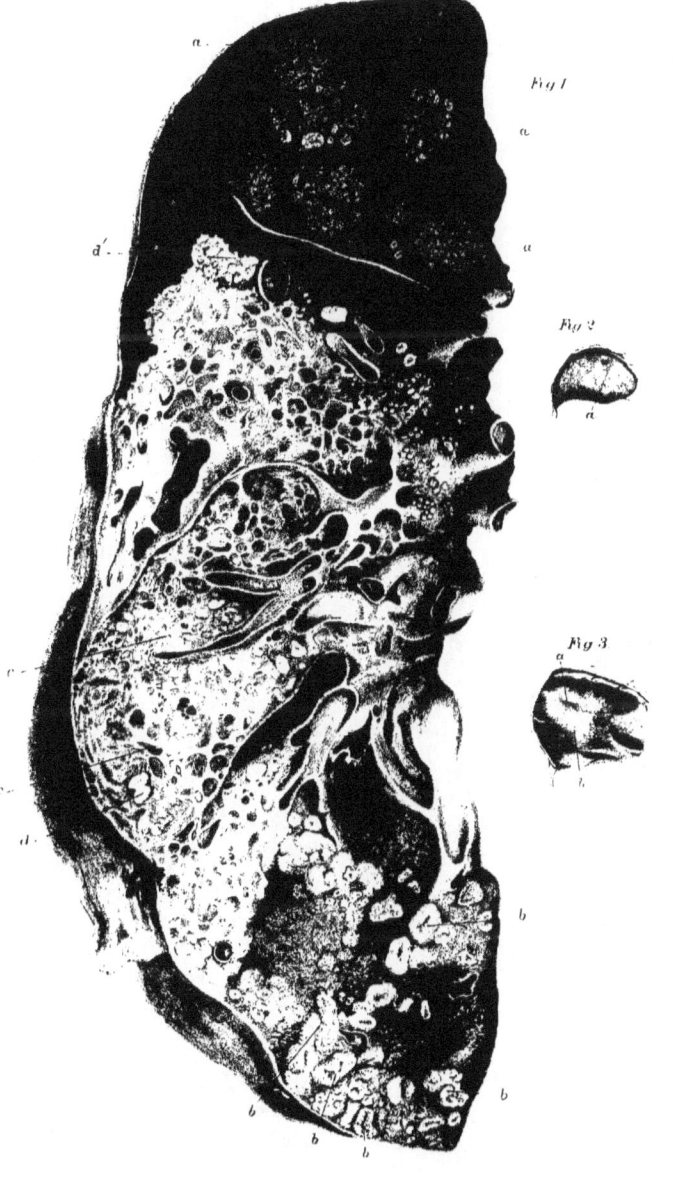

INDURATING TUBERCULOSIS.

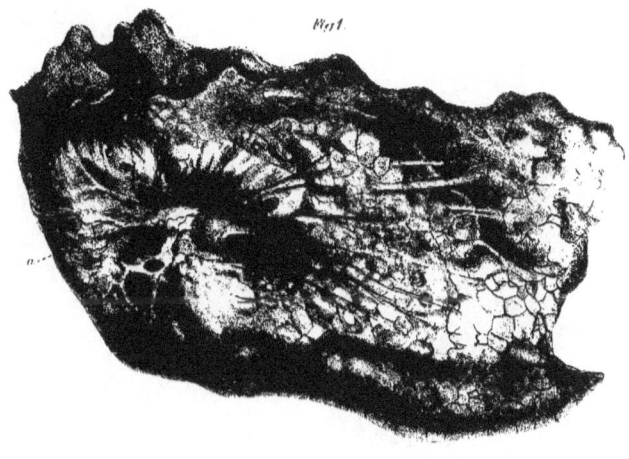

Fig 1.

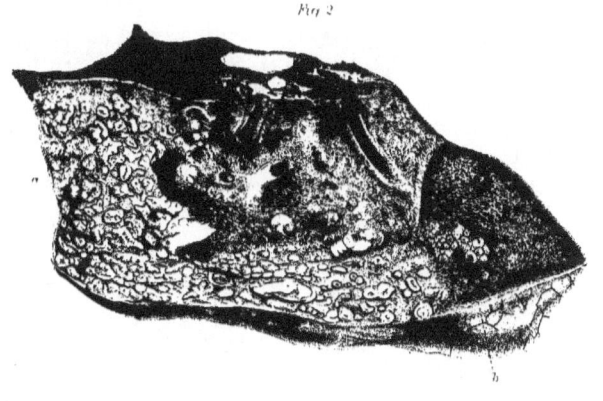

Fig 2.

INDURATING AND CASEOUS TUBERCULOSIS.
TUBERCLE WITH CIRRHOSIS OF LIVER.

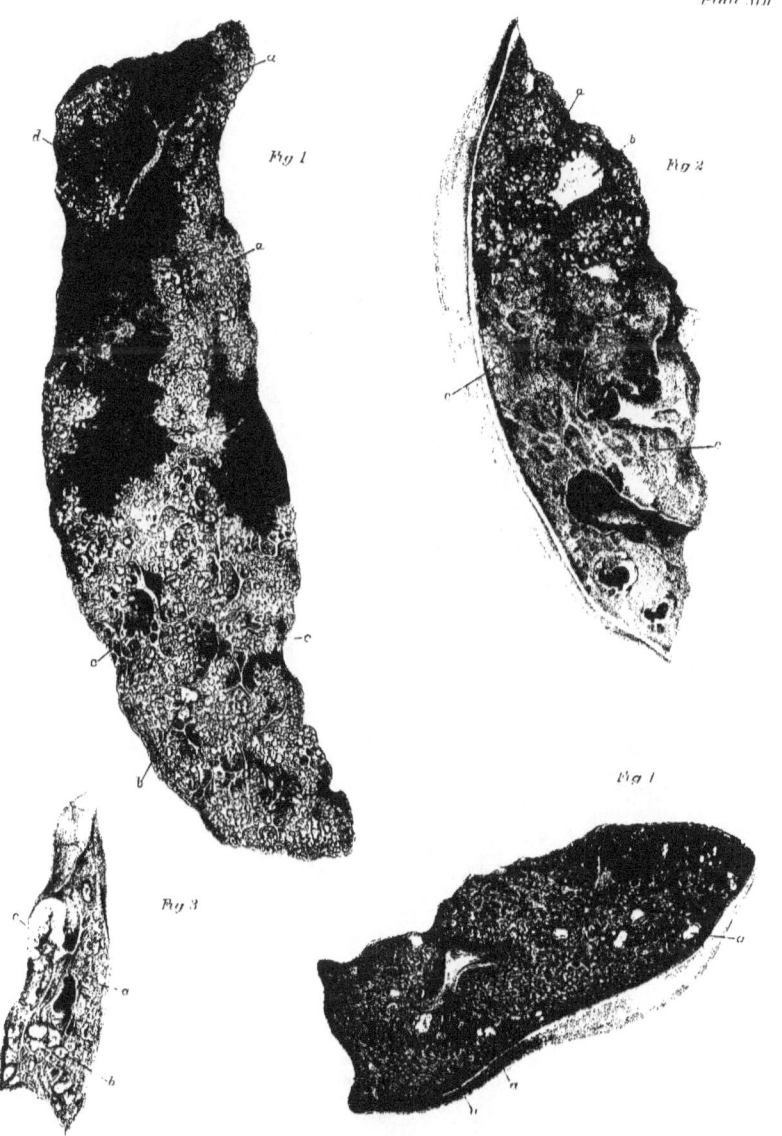

Plate XII

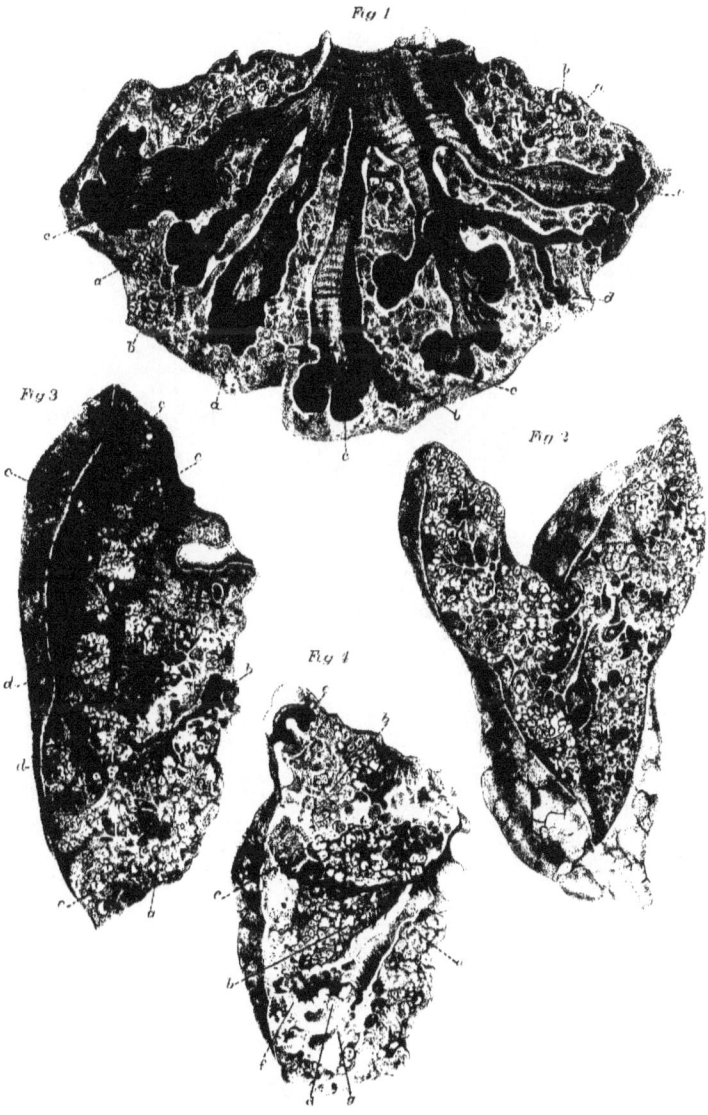

Fig. 1.

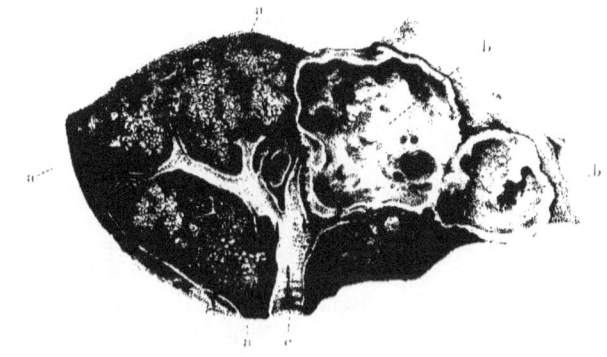

Fig. 2.

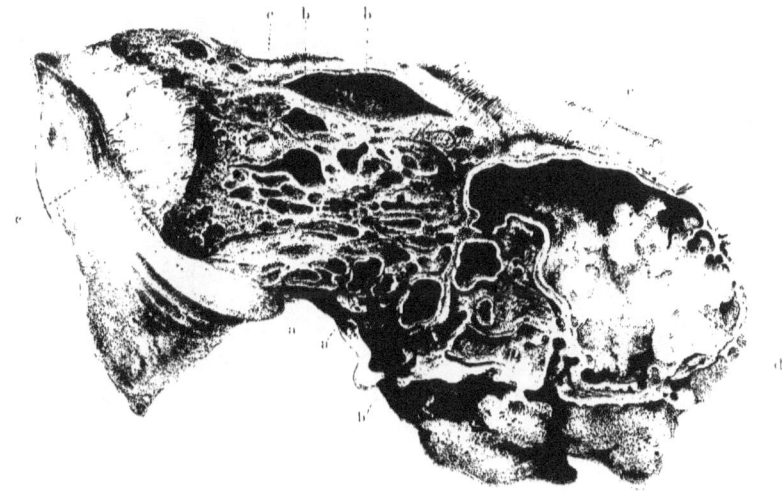

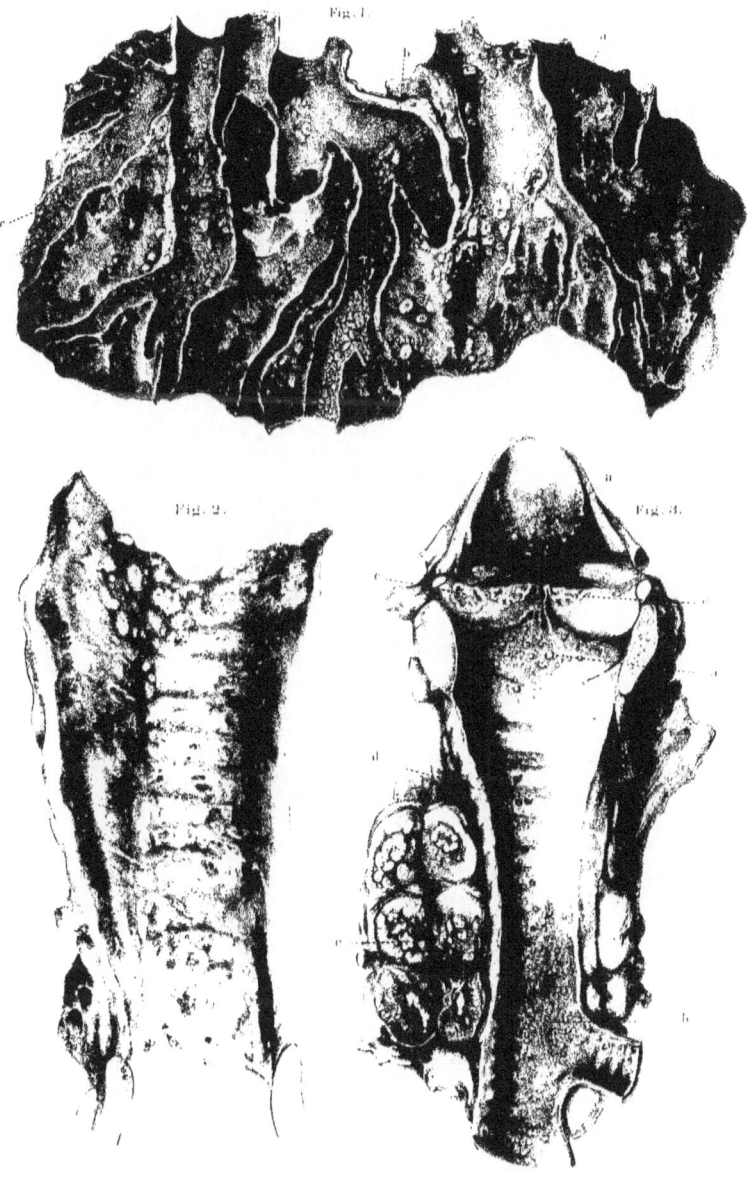

Fig. 1.

Fig. 2. Fig. 3.

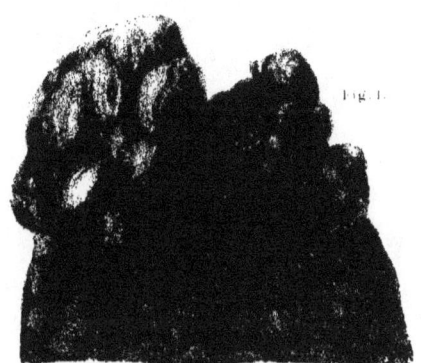

POTTERS LUNG – MINERS LUNG.
BROWN INDURATION – CANCER.

Plate XIII.

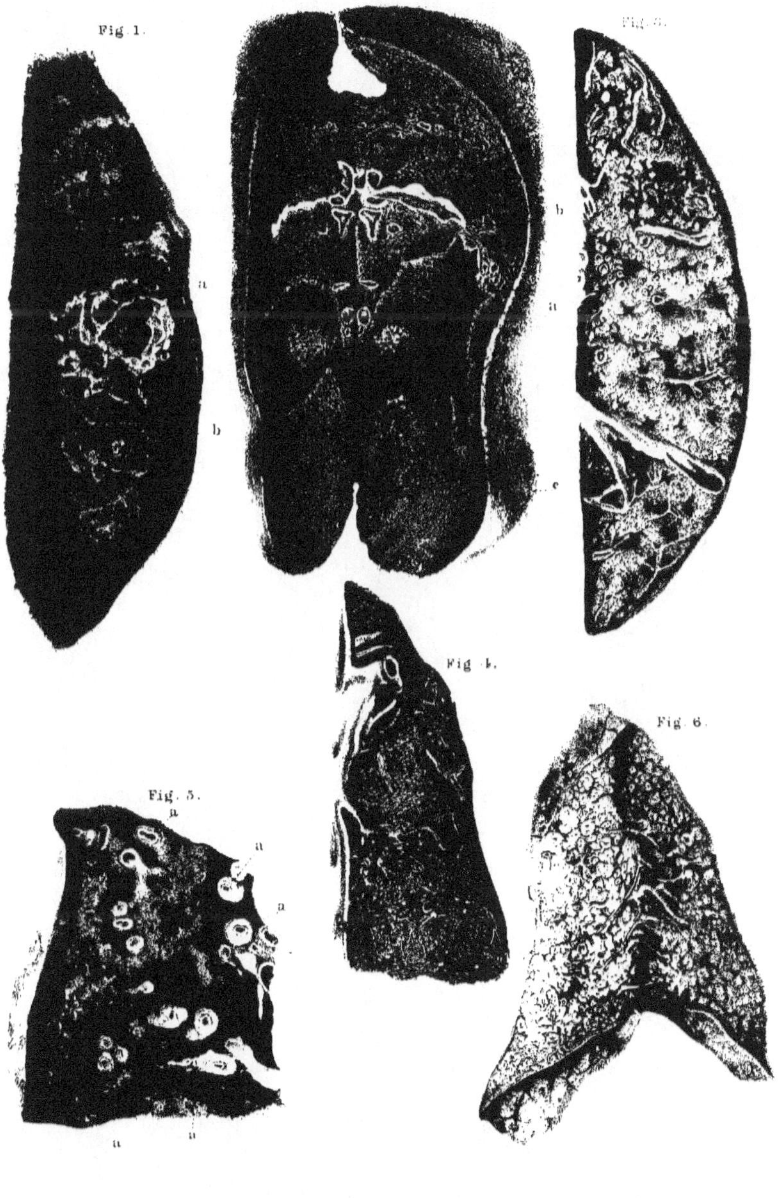

1. PYÆMIA 2 SARCOMA – INFARCT AND COLLAPSE.

Fig. 1.

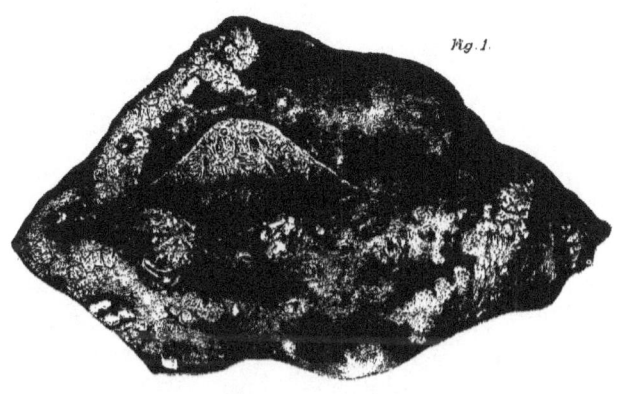

Fig. 2.

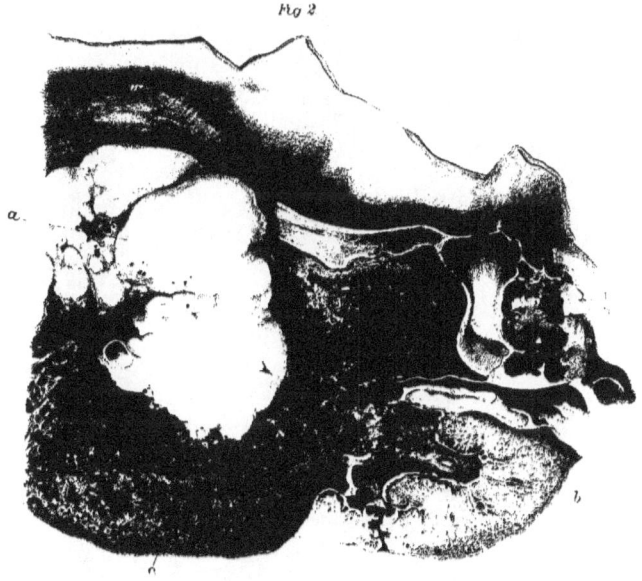

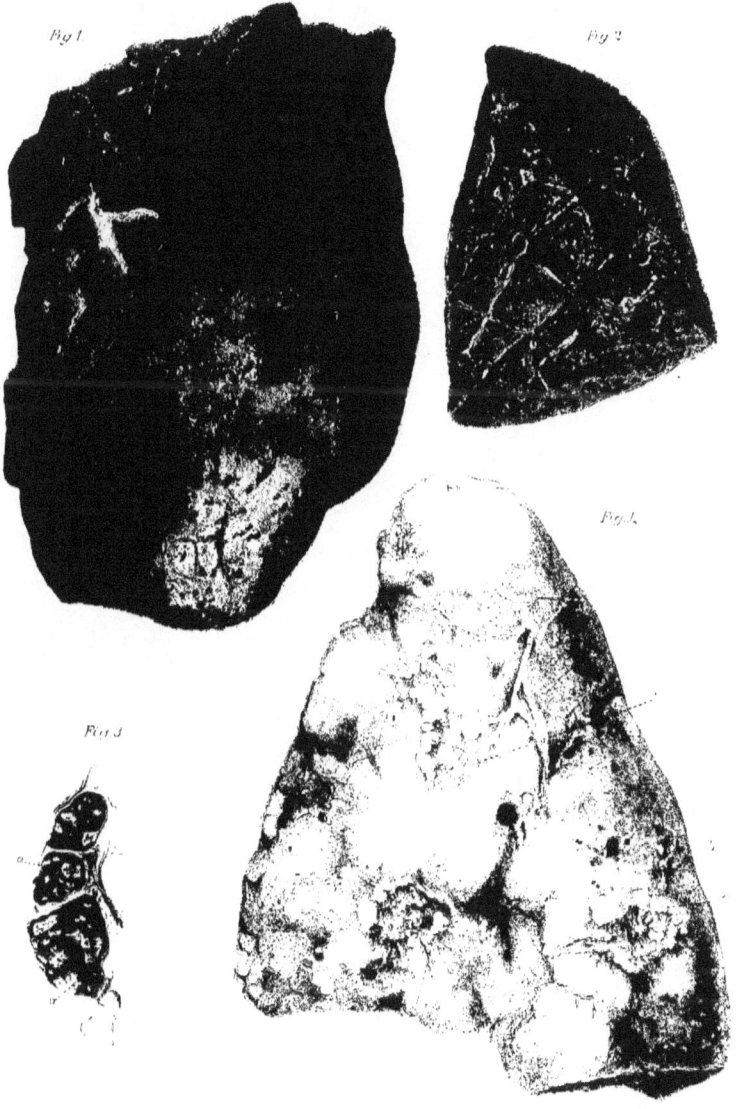

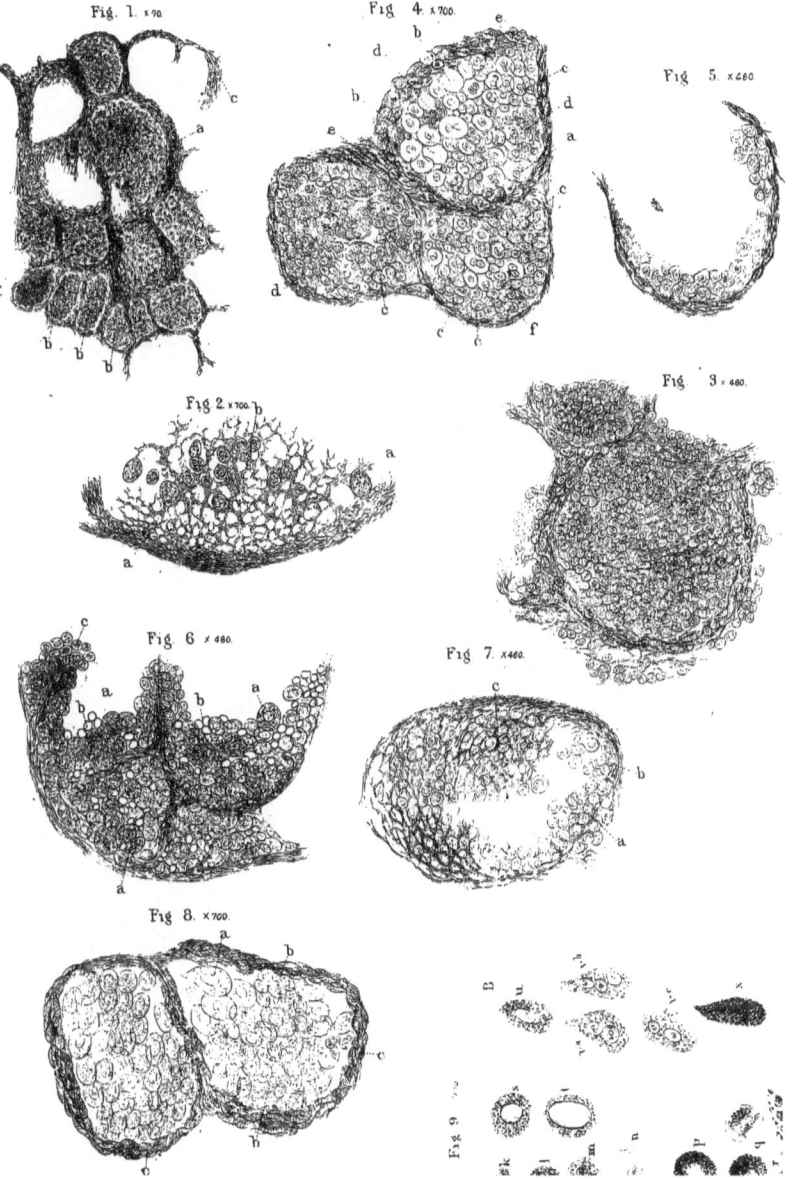

CATARRHAL PNEUMONIA-SYPHILIS.

Plate XXII

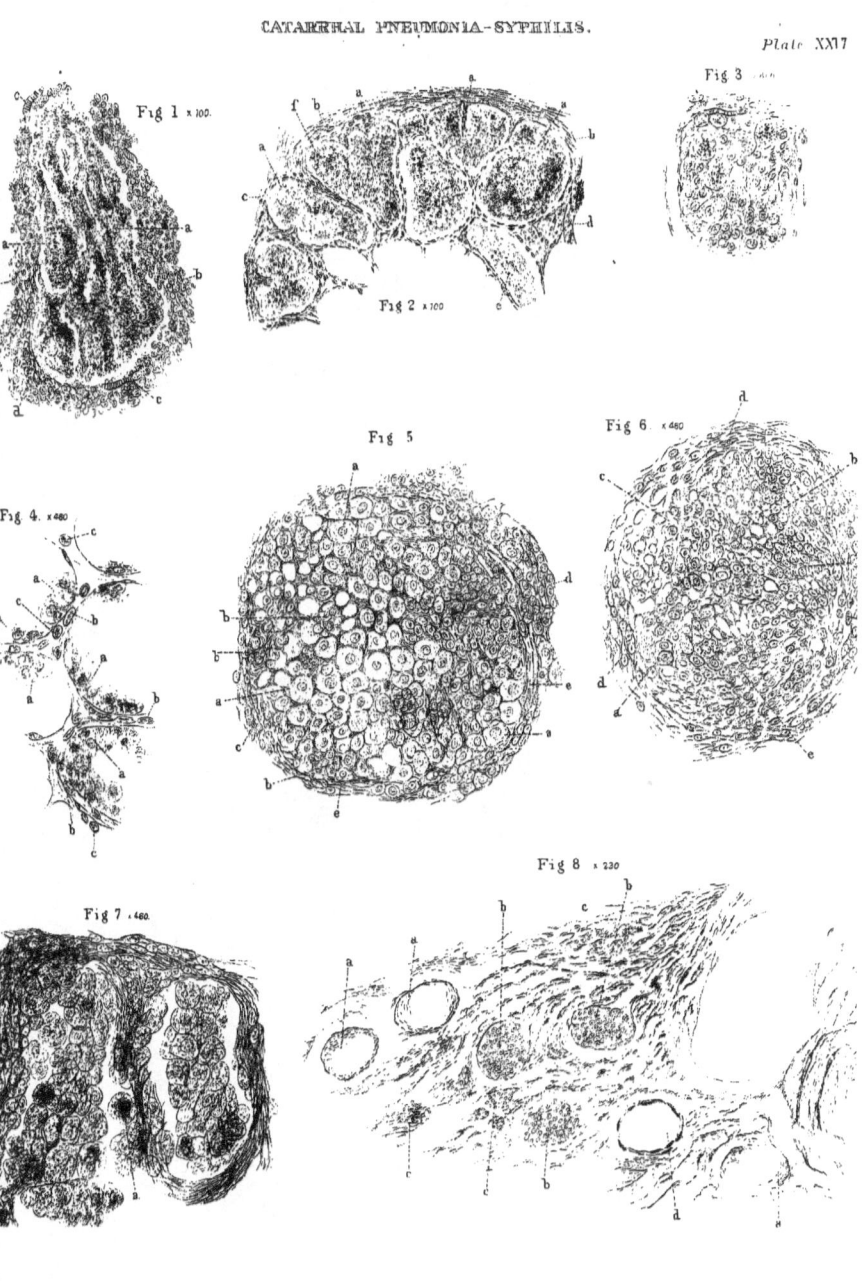

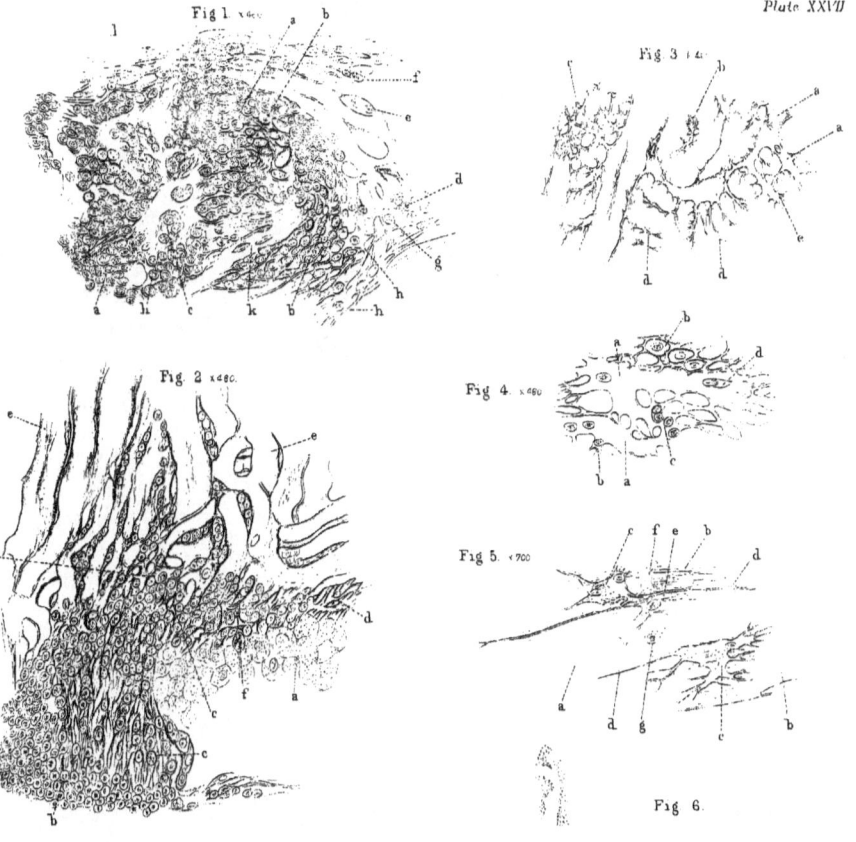

Plate XXVII

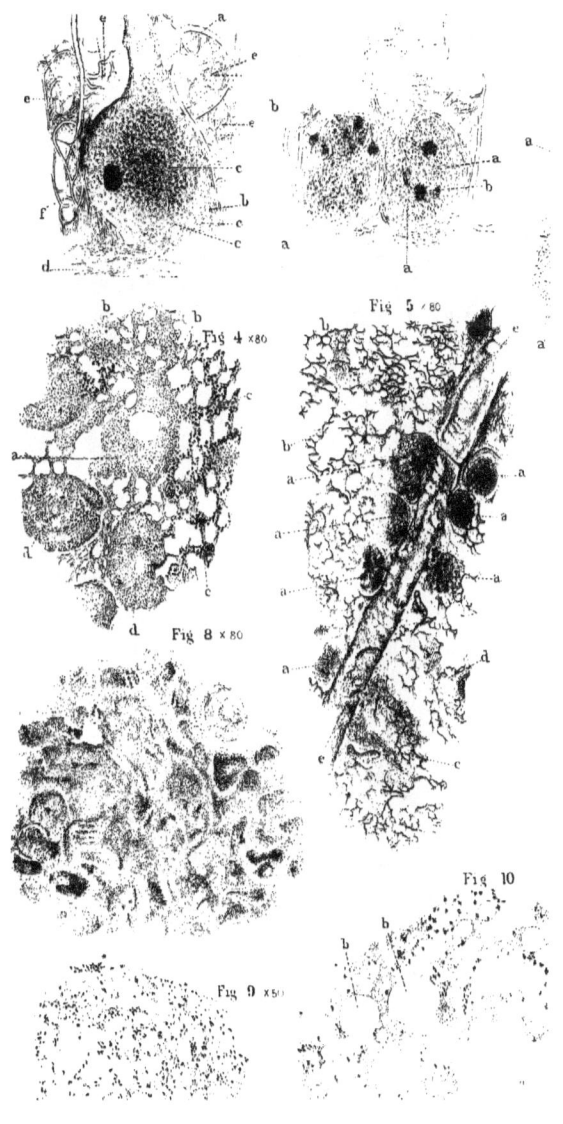

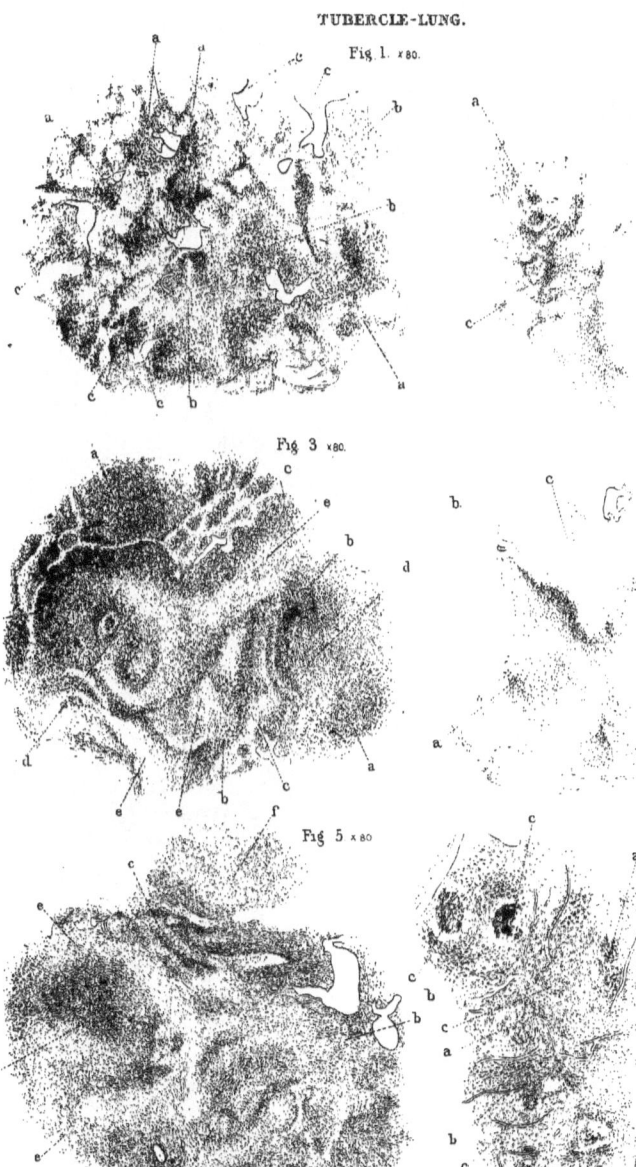

TUBERCLE-LUNG.

Fig. 1. ×80.

Fig. 3 ×80.

Fig. 5 ×80.

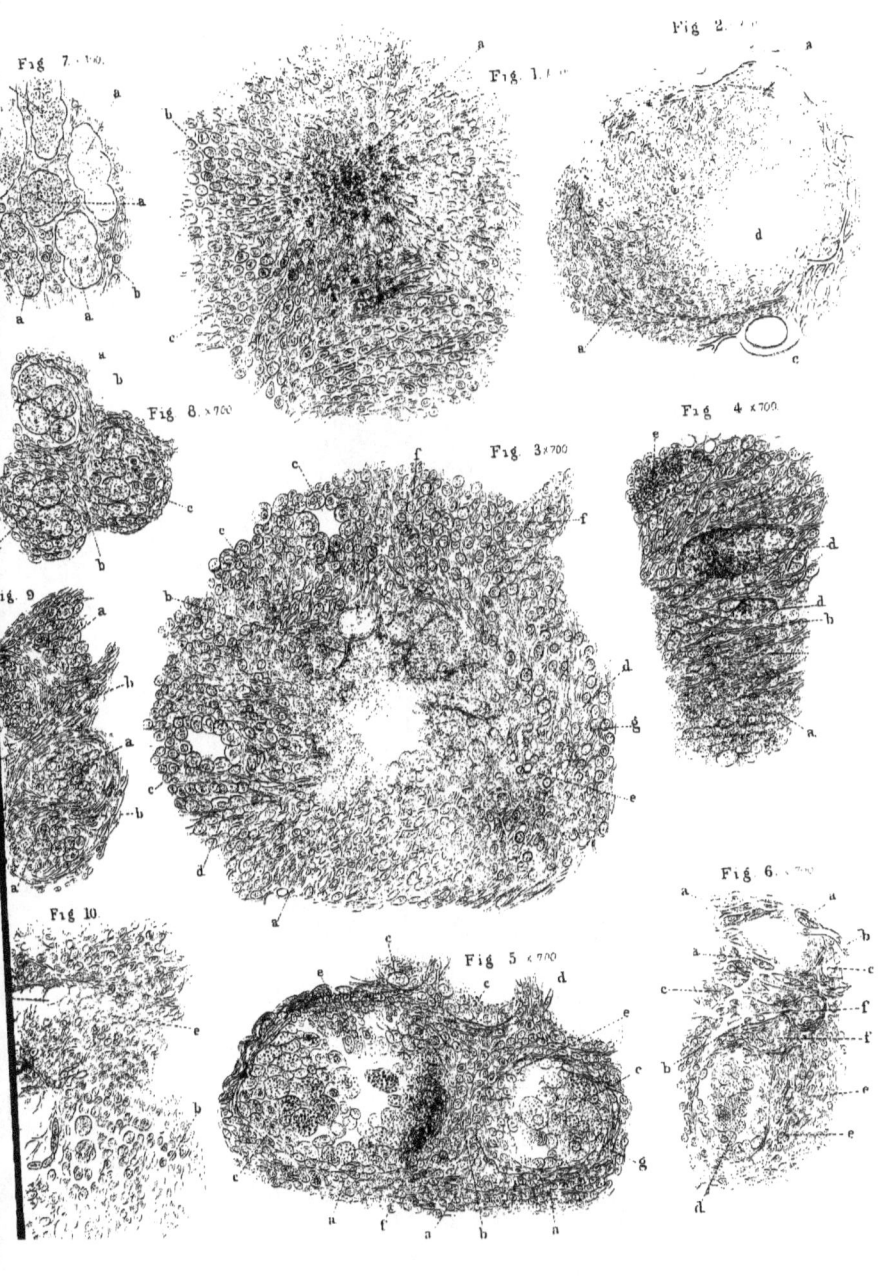

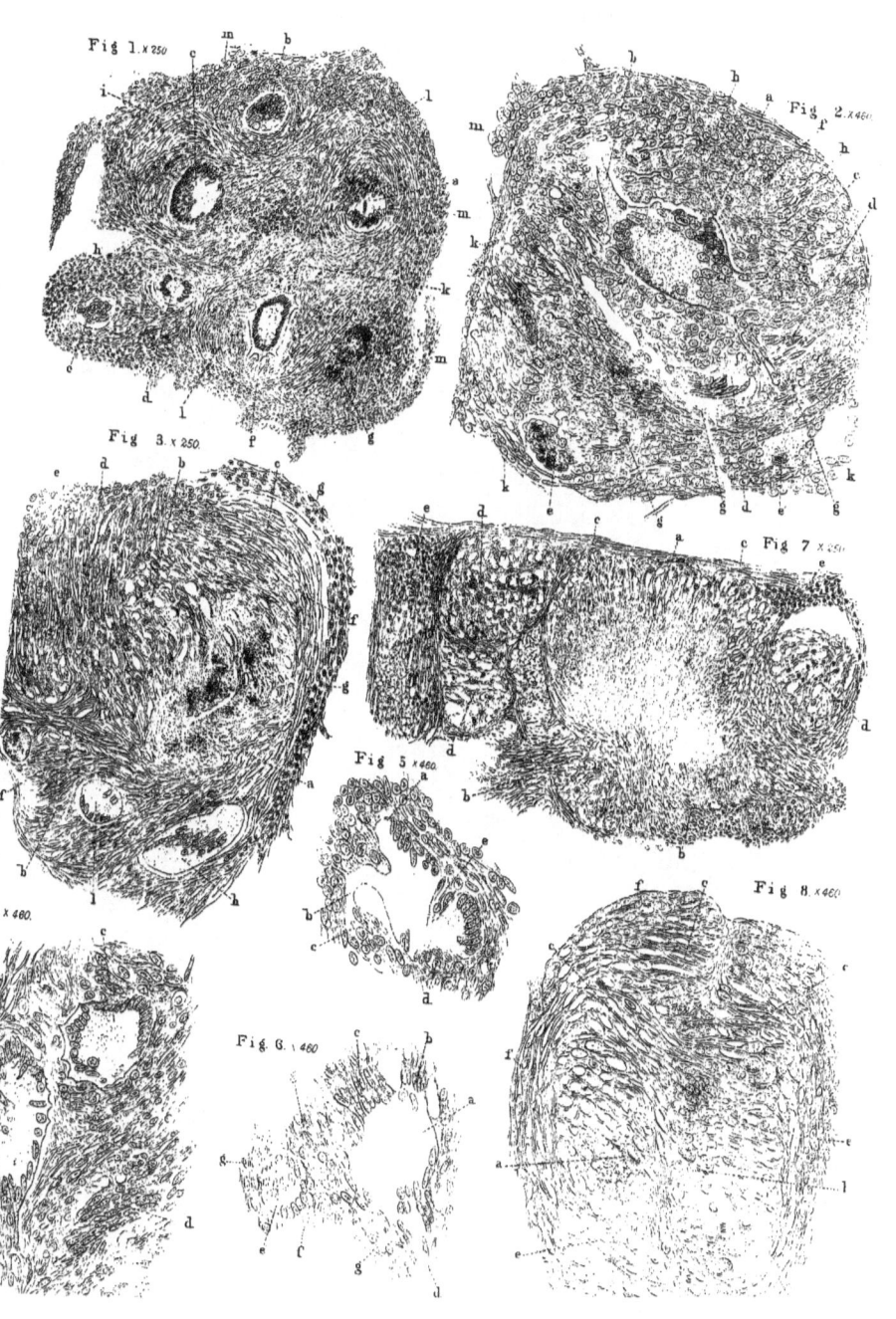

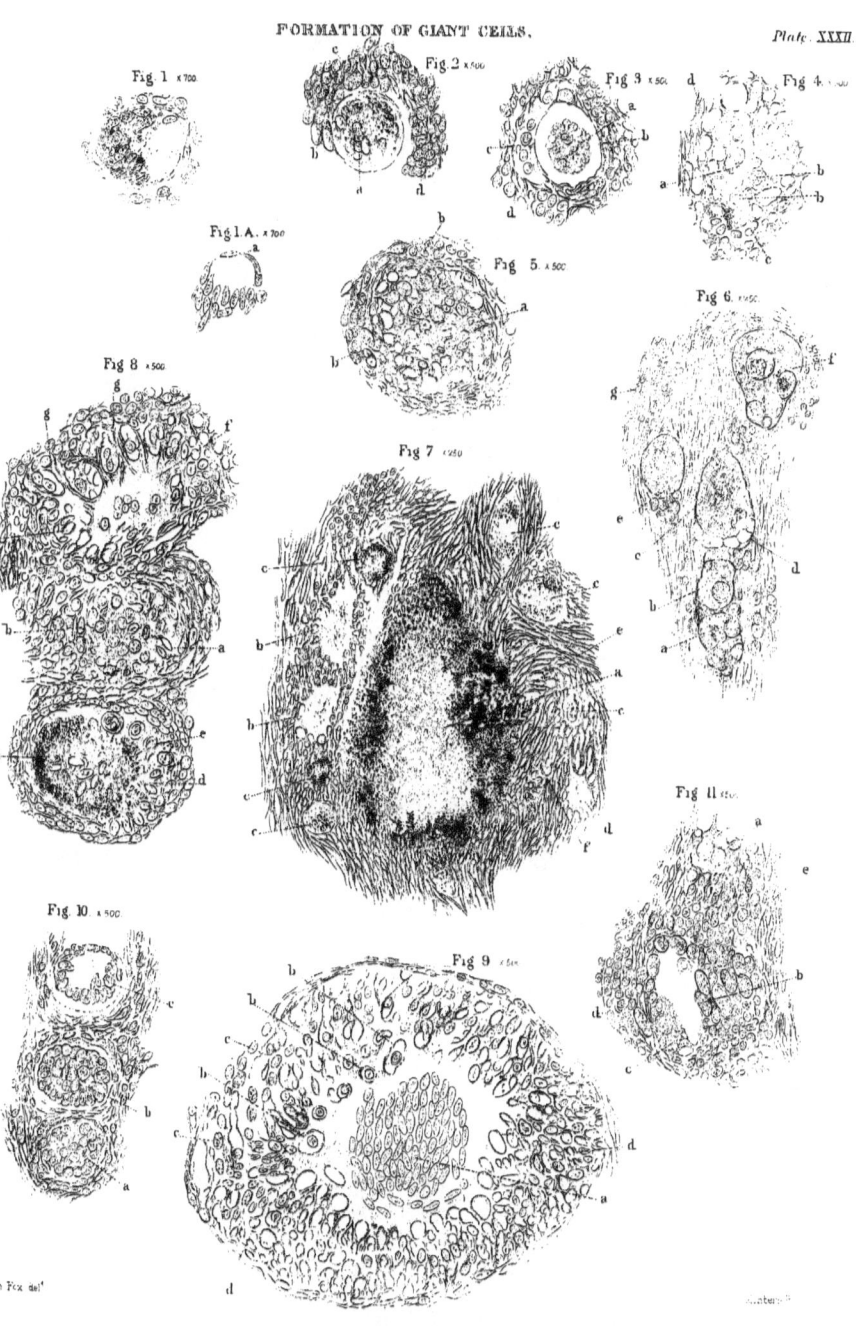

FORMATION OF GIANT CELLS.

FORMATION OF GIANT CELLS.

Plate XXXIII.

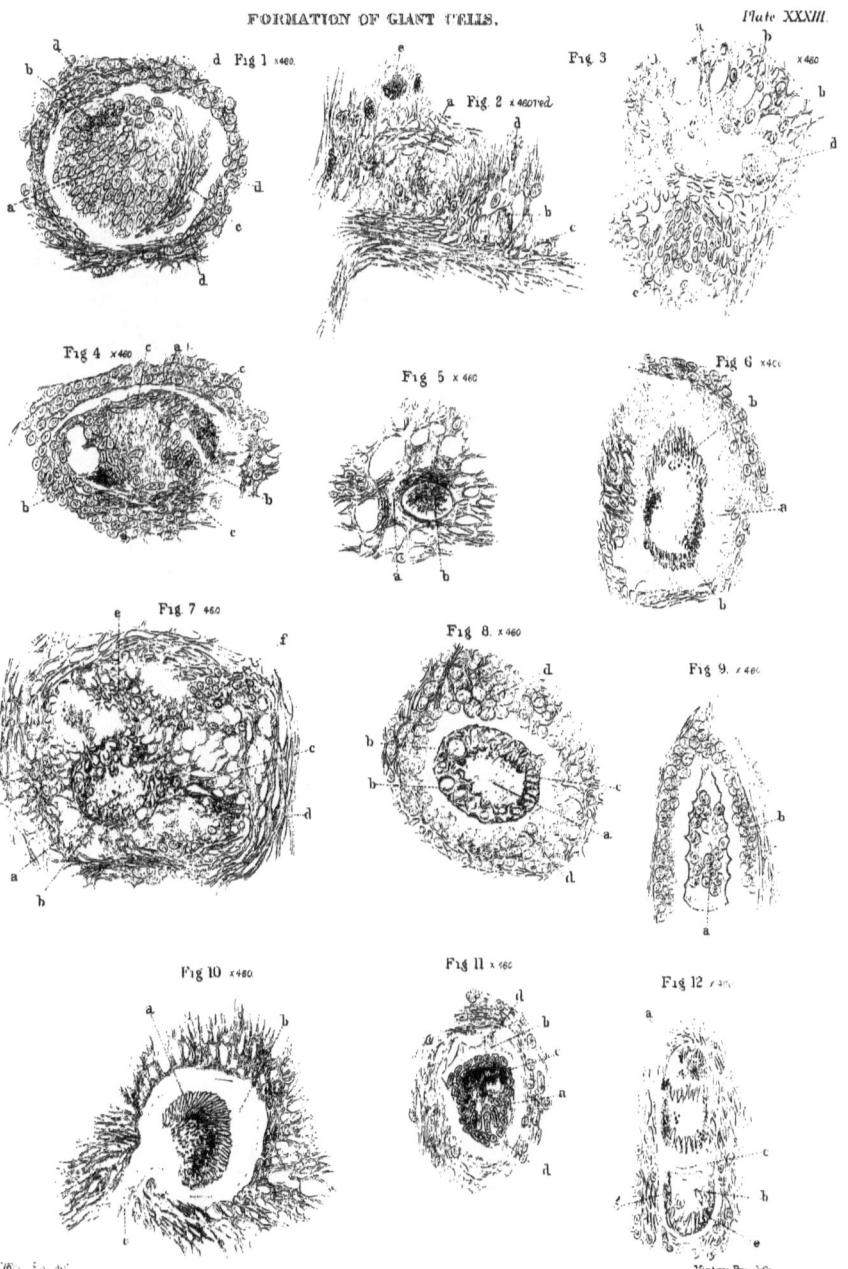

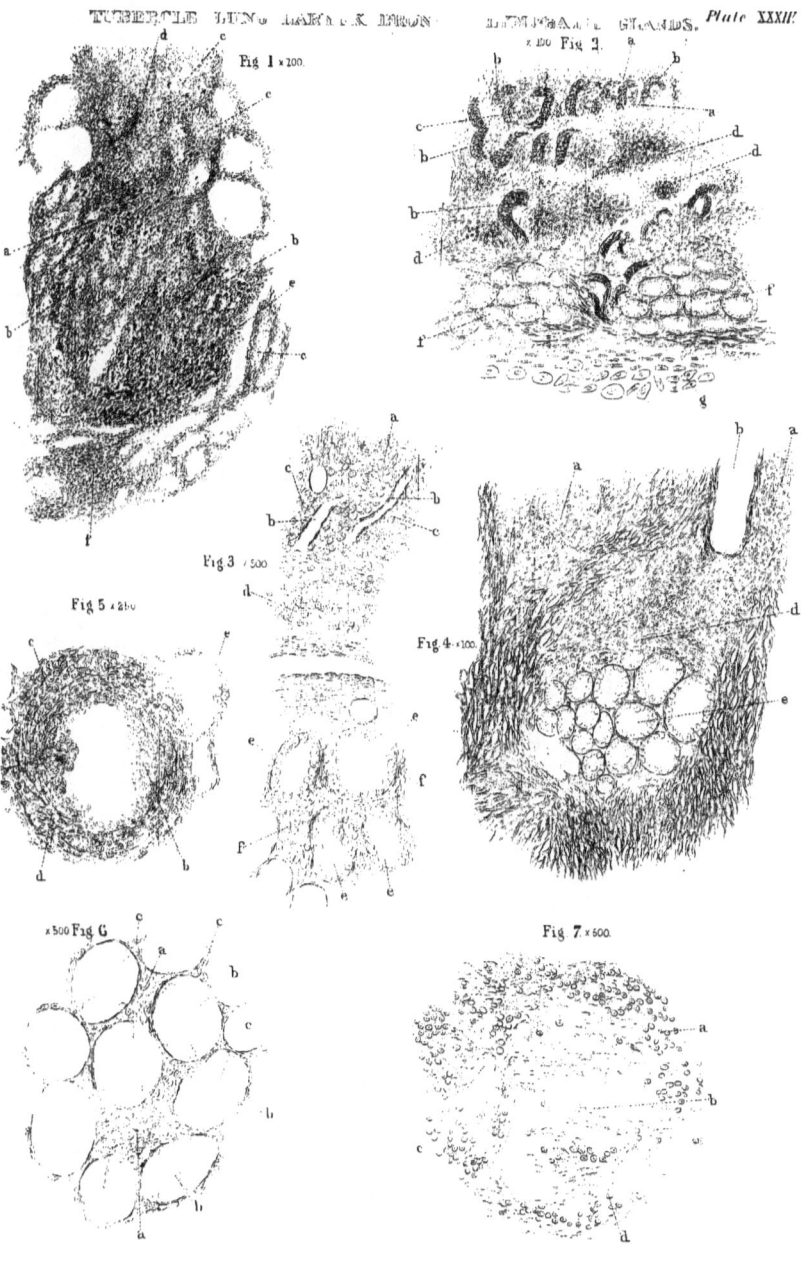

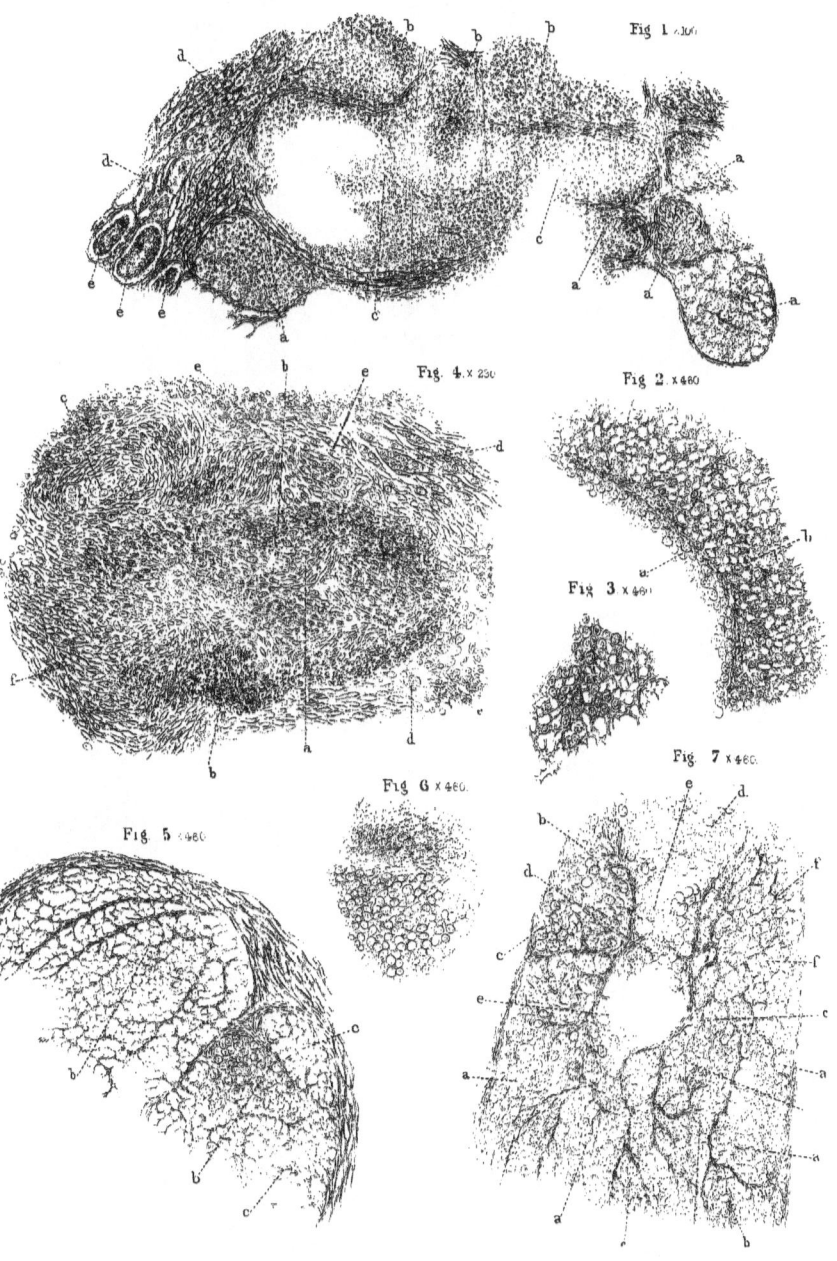

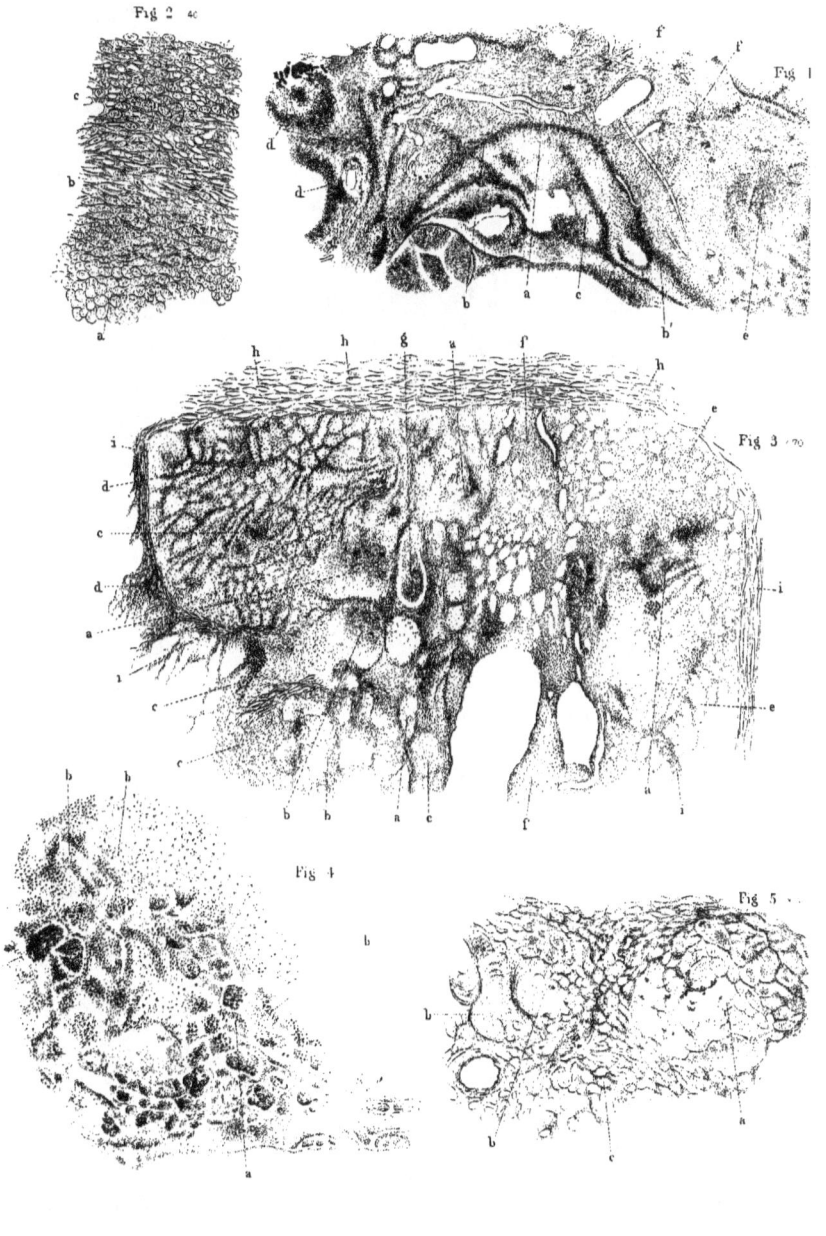

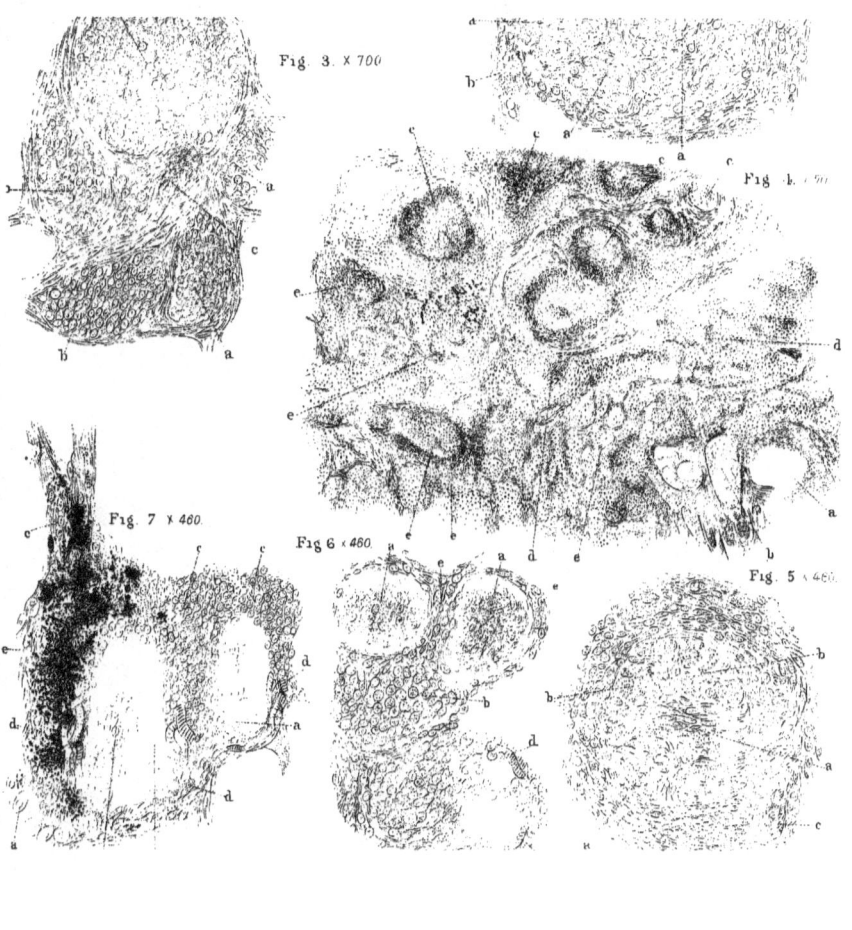

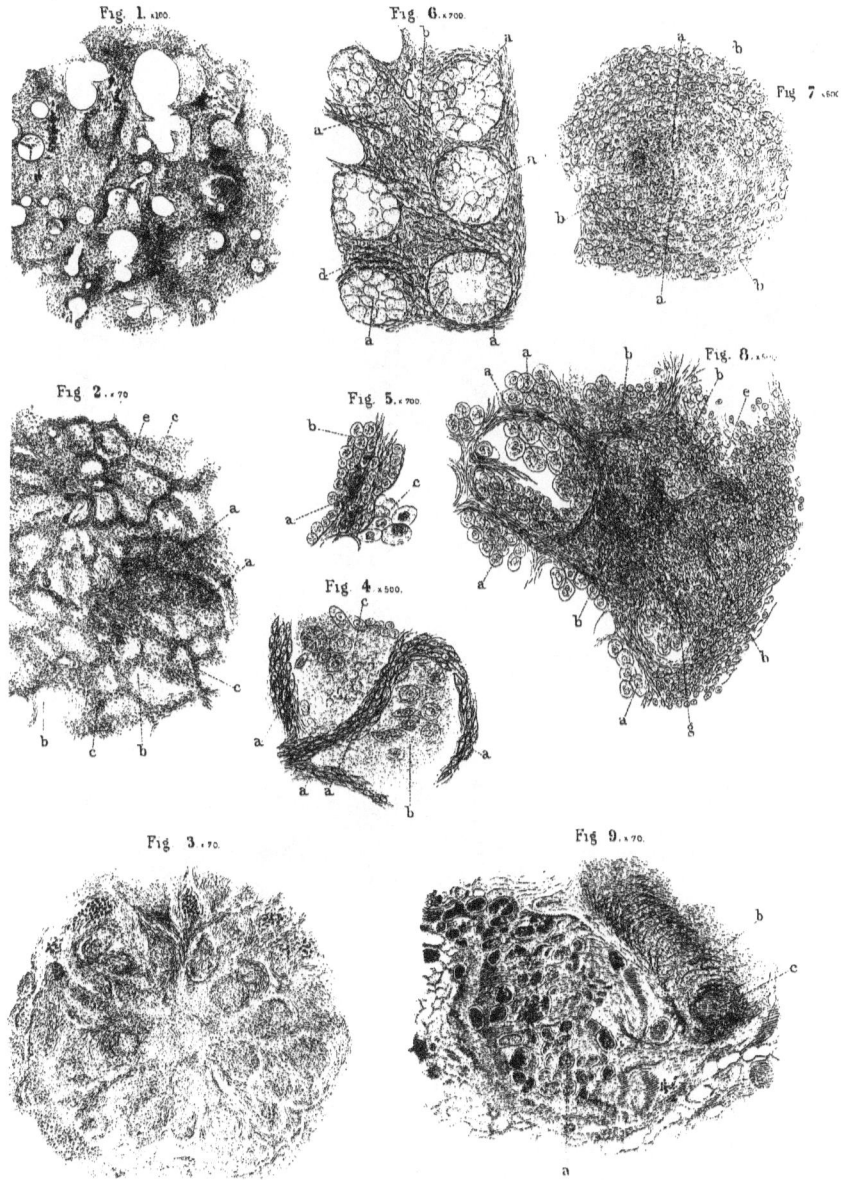

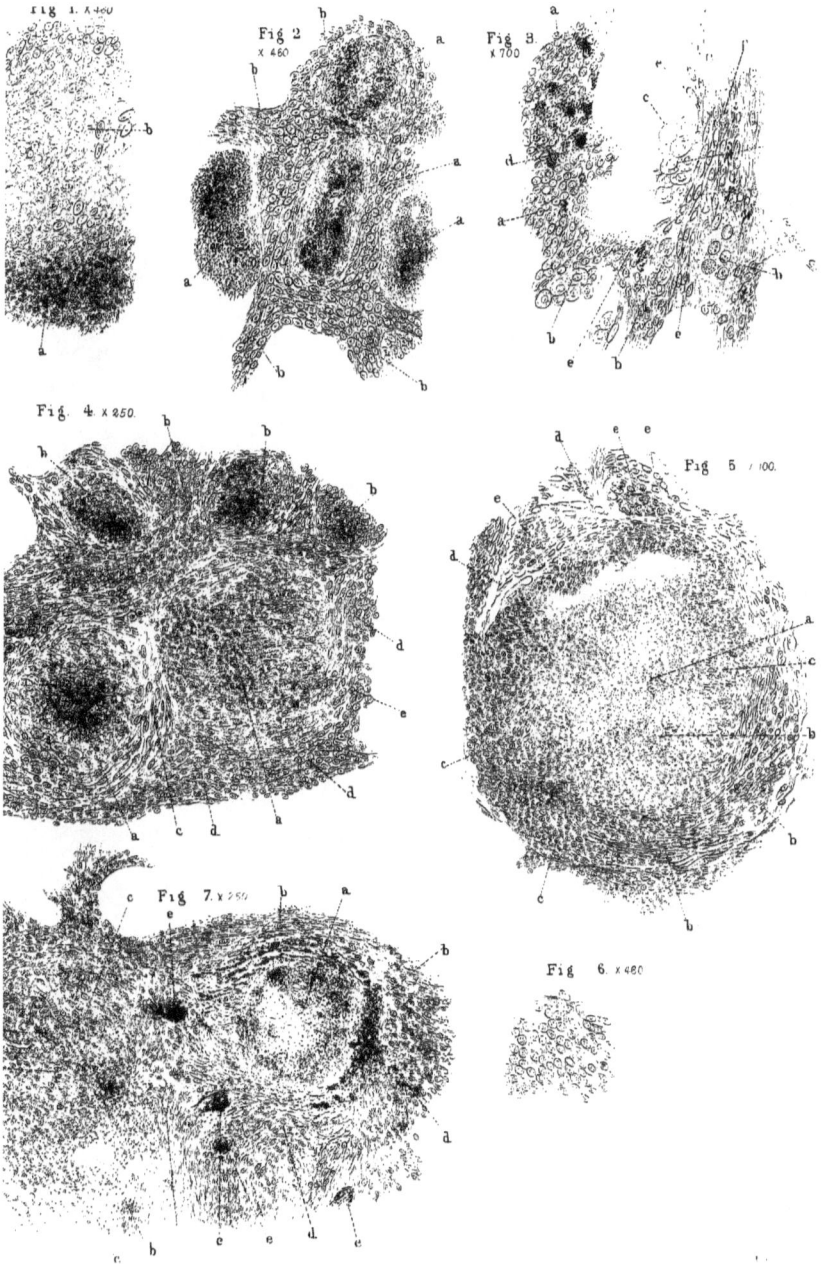

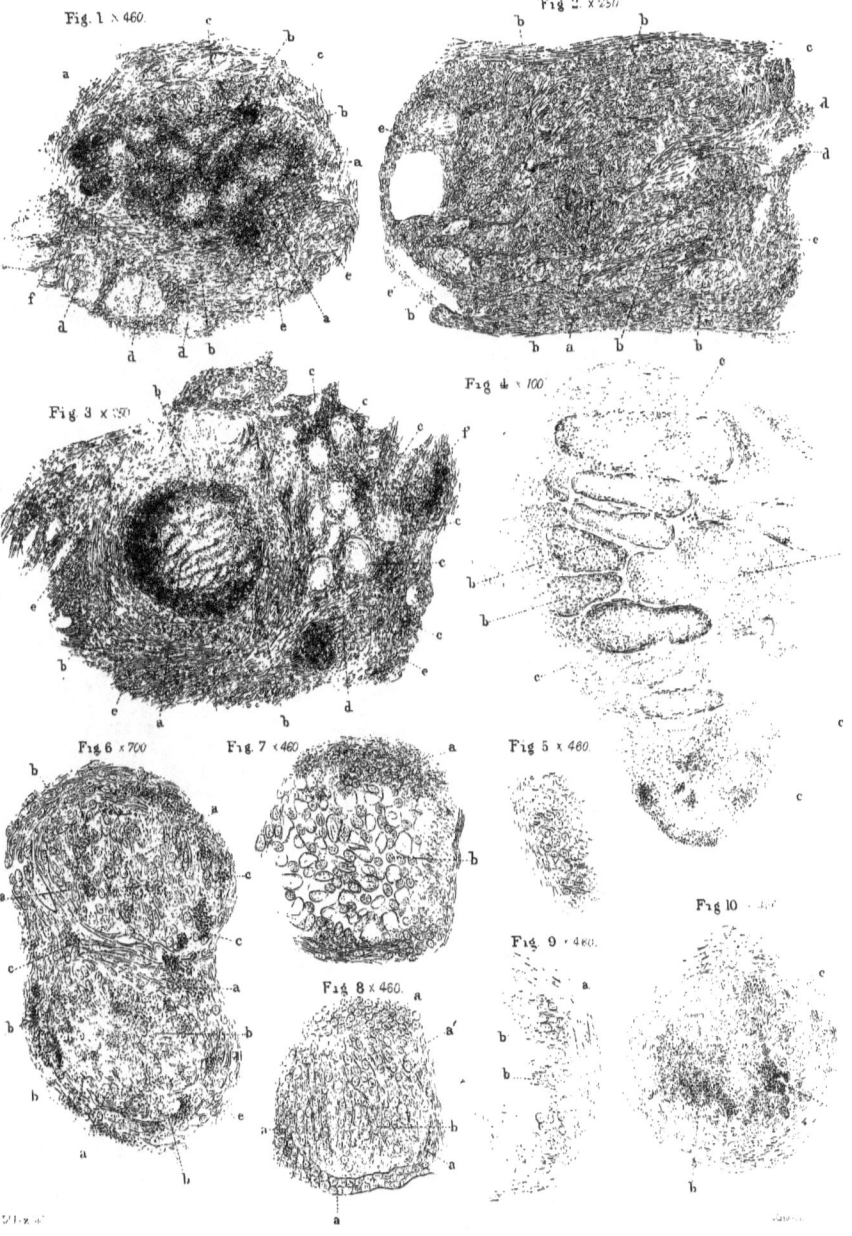

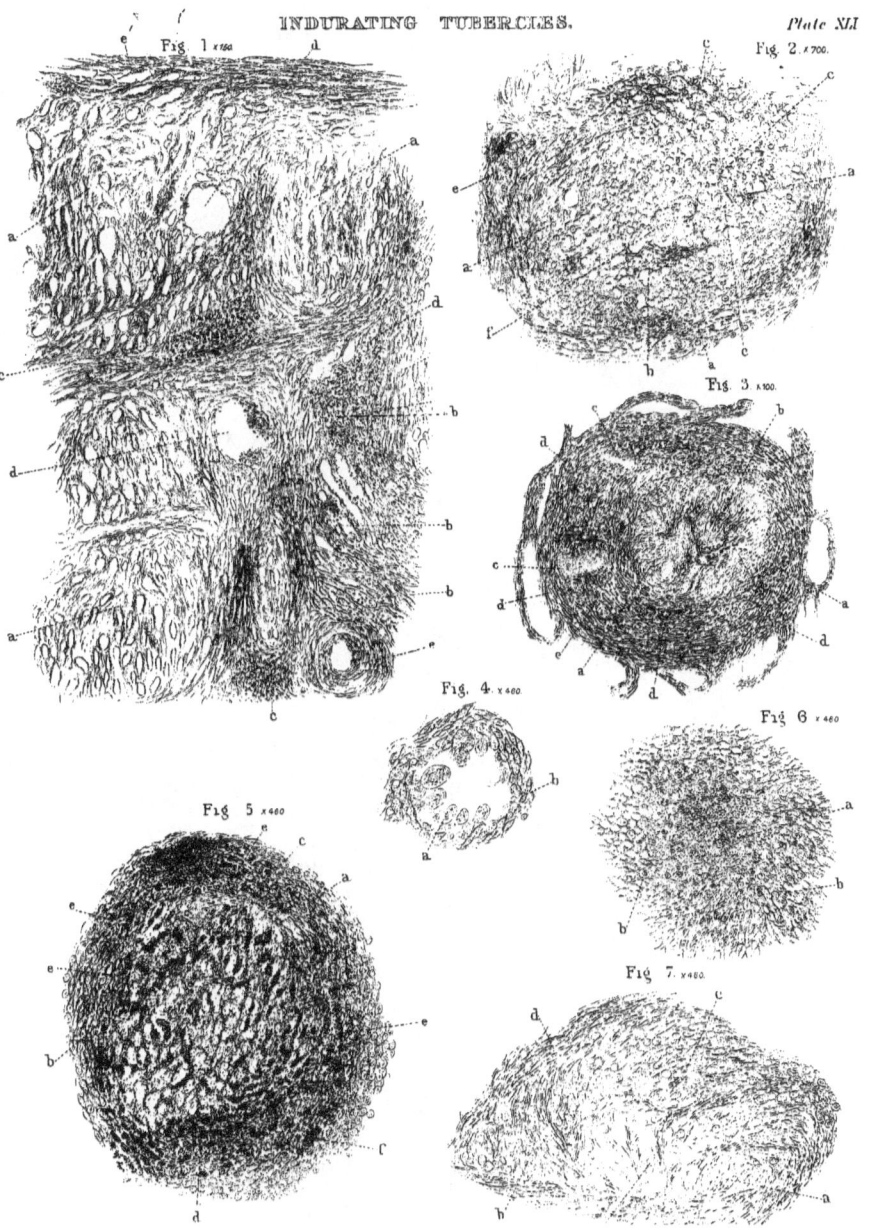

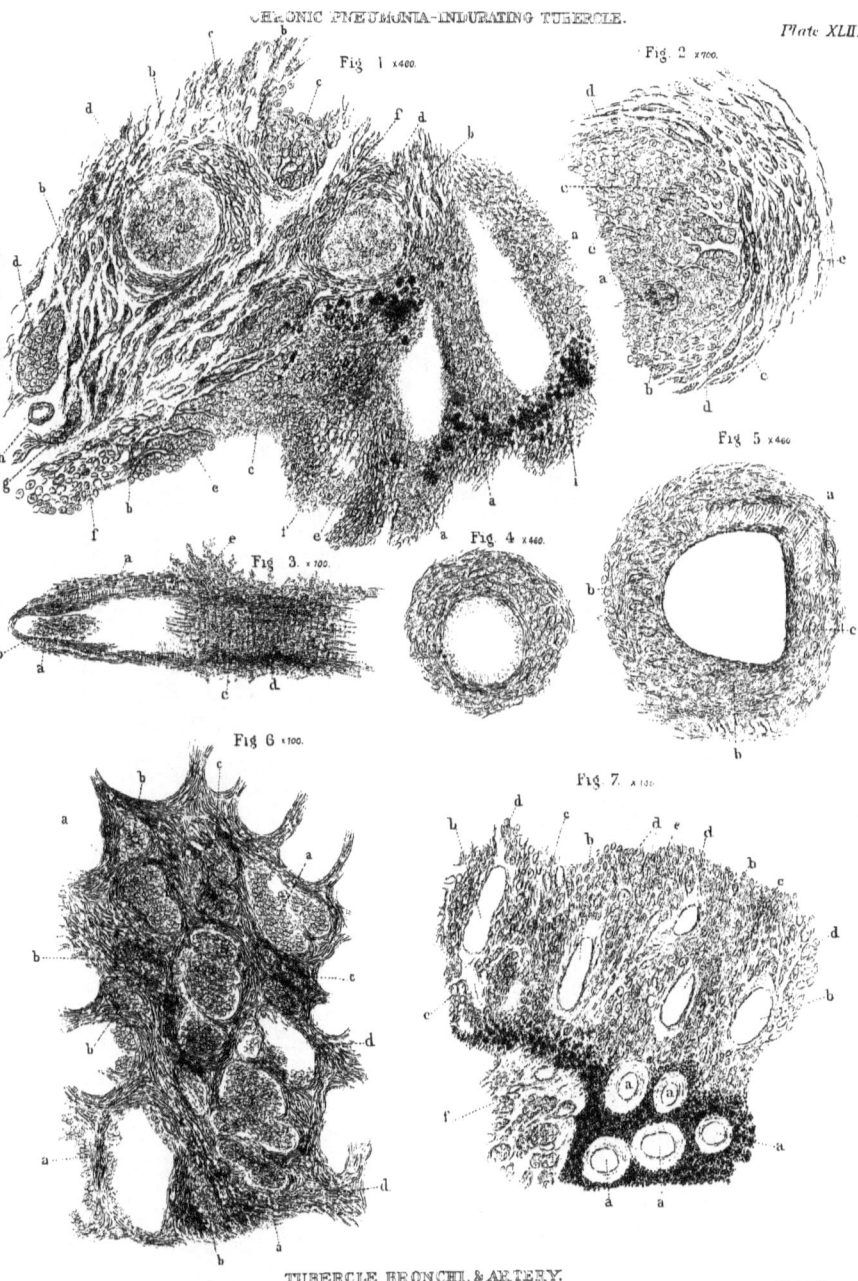

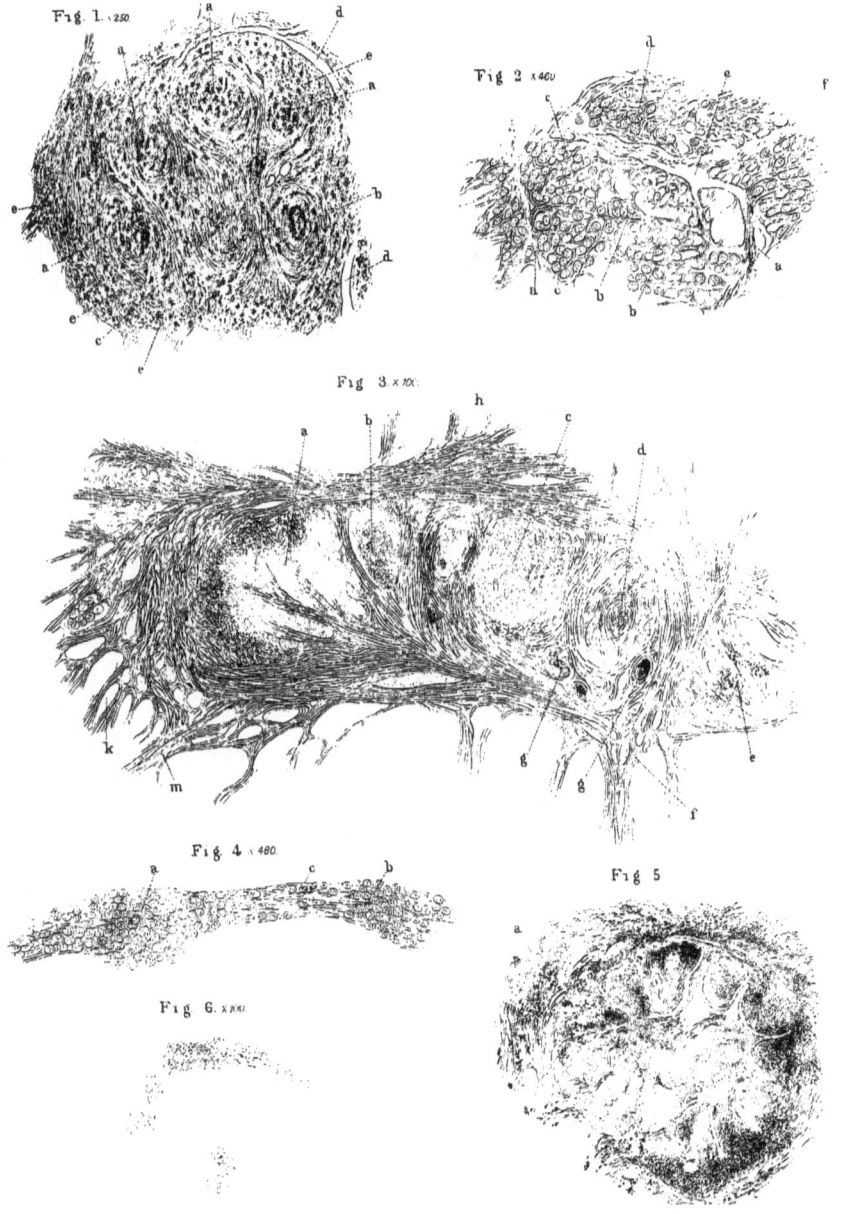

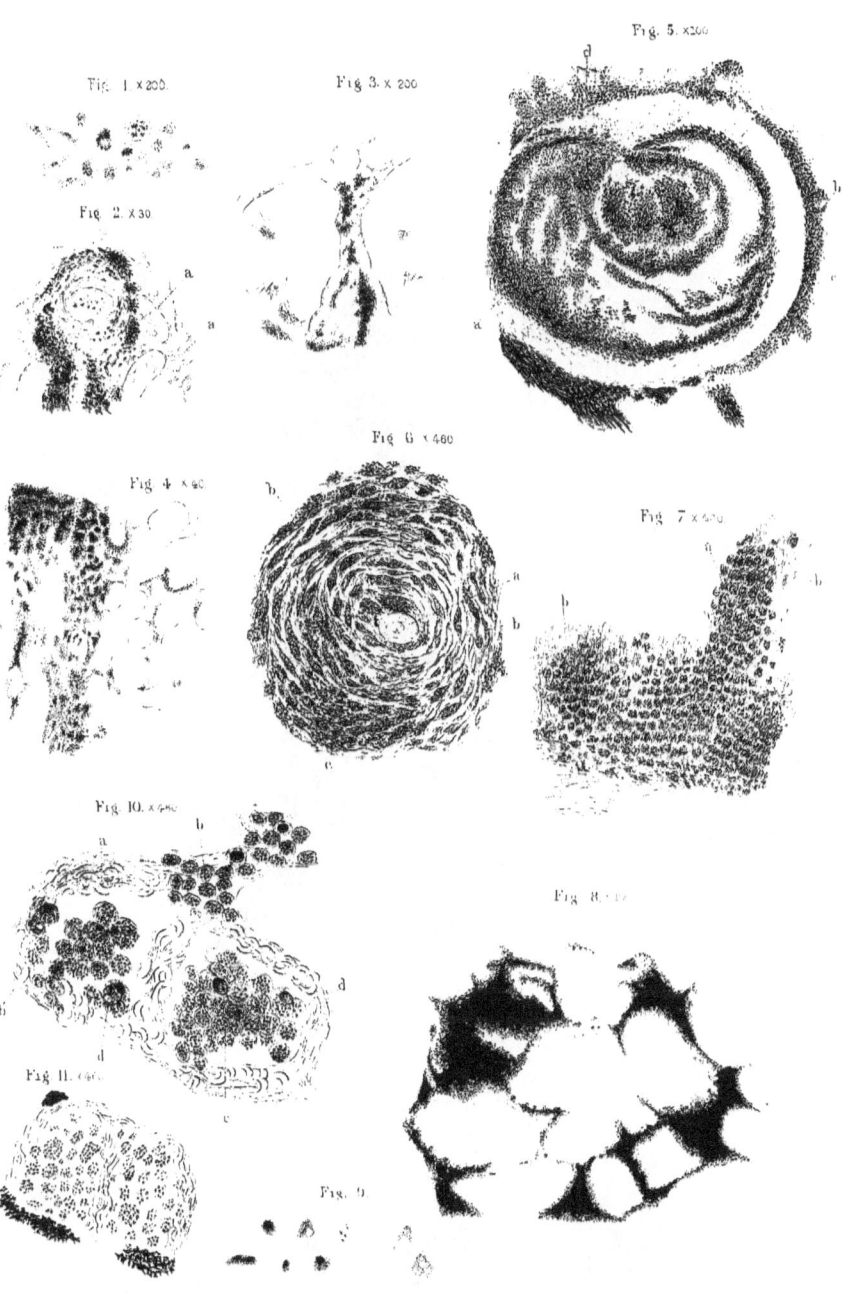

CANCER OF LUNG

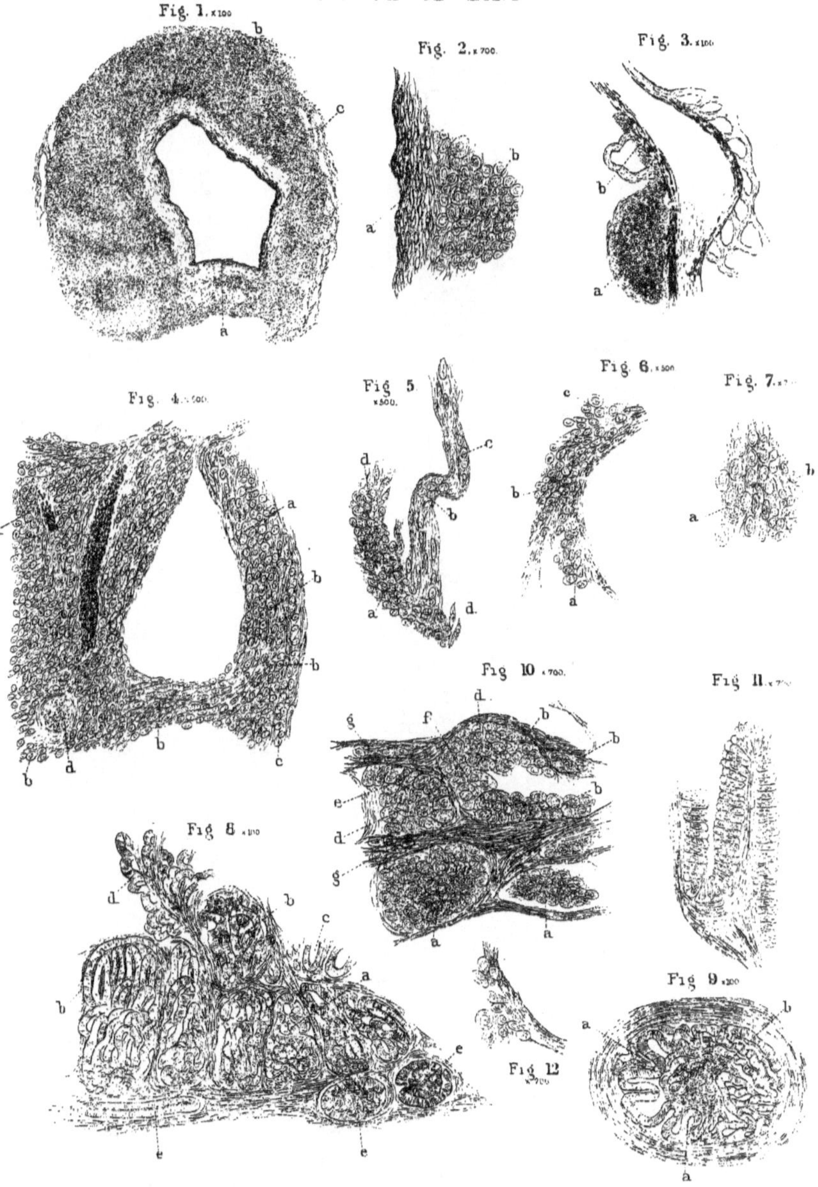

INDEX OF AUTHORS

REFERRED TO.

Ackermann. Chronic pneum., 45, 46, 47
Addison. Structure, 2, 3, 9; chronic pneum., 45; phthisis, 67, 74, 81, 82, 98, 101, 109
Adriani. Structure, 1
Albers. Cancer, 134
Alderson, Sir Jas. Catarrhal pneum., 25; collapse, 58
Andral. Catarrhal pneum., 36; acute interstitial pneum., 44; chronic pneum., 45, 47, 50; brown induration, 52; dis. inhal. of dust, 53; embolism, 58; phthisis, 63, 64, 65, 66, 67, 71, 74, 76, 83, 120, 129; cancer, 135
Andrea. Syph. dis., 128, 129, 131
Arnold. Phthisis, 87, 88, 91, 92, 93, 94, 102, 104, 107, 110, 111
Arnott. Cancer, 136, 137
Aachen. Dis. inhal. of dust, 53
Aufrecht. Chronic pneum., 51; phthisis, 82, 88, 102, 107; syph. dis., 132; art. prod. tubercle, 139, 141, 142, 143, 155, 156

Babes. Art. prod. of tubercle, 139, 140
Bailly. Catarrhal pneum., 27
Balogh. Art. prod. tubercle, 151
Balzer. Catarrhal pneum., 28, 29, 30, 31, 32, 35; other forms of acute pneum., 38; interstitial pneum., 43; embolism, 60
Banks. Gangrene, 63
Bärensprung, Von. Syph. dis., 124, 131, 133
Barlow. Chronic pneum., 45, 49
Bartels. Catarrhal pneum., 23, 24, 25, 26, 29, 31, 32; chronic pneum., 45
Barth. Chronic pneum., 45, 46, 50; phthisis, 80
Barthelness. Dir. inhal. of dust, 53
Barthez. Catarrhal pneum., 23, 24, 27, 28, 29, 31, 33, 34; chronic pneum., 45; phthisis, 65, 69, 70, 72, 75, 76, 80, 98
Bastian. Chronic pneum., 49; phthisis, 101, 112; art. prod. tubercle, 155
Baumgärtel. Art. prod. tubercle, 140
Baumgarten. Phthisis, 84, 88, 91, 92, 93, 101, 107, 113; syph. dis., 124, 131; art. prod. tubercle, 139, 140, 141, 142, 143, 144, 145, 147, 148, 149, 150, 151, 152, 153, 154, 155, 156
Bayer. Acute pneum., 19
Bayle. Chronic pneum., 45, 50; phthisis, 63, 64, 65, 66, 67, 72, 77, 82, 98; cancer, 138
Beale, Lionel. Acute pneum., 21; phthisis, 85, 96
Beer. Syph. dis., 127
Begbie, Warburton. Dis. inhal. of dust, 53
Beger. Syph. dis., 126
Béhier. Catarrhal pneum., 27, 36; acute interstitial pneum., 43; chronic pneum., 50; gangrene, 61
Behrends. Syph. dis., 125
Beigel. Cancer, 134
Bennett. Chronic pneum., 45, 51; phthisis, 76
Bennett, Sir Risdon. Cancer, 135
Berkmann. Embolism, 60
Bernhardt. Art. prod. tubercle, 144
Bertheau. Art. prod. tubercle, 151

Barthener. Art. prod. tubercle, 151
Berthau. Art. prod. tubercle, 151
Beyson. Dis. inhal. of dust, 53
Biermer. Chronic pneum., 45, 46, 48, 49, 50, 51; phthisis, 77, 80
Billroth. Phthisis, 87, 89, 92, 93
Birt. Phthisis, 112
Bollinger. Chronic pneum., 48; phthisis, 107; art. prod. tubercle, 141, 142, 146, 155
Bonetus. Phthisis, 109
Bouchut. Phthisis, 77
Boudet. Phthisis, 75, 77
Bowman. Structure, 1, 3, 9
Bretonneau. Catarrhal pneum., 35
Briquet. Chronic pneum., 50
Brissaud. Phthisis, 88
Bristowe. Phthisis, 76; cancer, 134. 135
Brodowski. Phthisis, 85, 88, 89
Brouardel. Chronic pneum., 48
Broussais. Chronic pneum., 45, 50
Bryant. Cancer, 134
Budd. Syph. dis., 127
Buhl. Acute pneum., 18, 19, 20; catarrhal pneum., 27, 29, 33; other forms of acute pneum., 39; acute interstitial pneum., 43; chronic pneum., 44, 46, 51; brown induration, 51, 52; dis. inhal. of dust, 54; gangrene, 61; phthisis, 63, 68, 69, 77, 78, 80, 94, 101, 104, 105, 106, 107, 108, 110, 111, 112, 113, 114; art. prod. tubercle, 142; Cases, 163
Burdon-Sanderson. Structure, 13; chronic pneum., 17; phthisis, 84, 100, 106, 121; art. prod. tubercle, 139, 144, 146, 147, 148, 149, 150, 152, 153, 154, 155, 156
Burkart. Dis. inhal. of dust, 55; phthisis, 78
Burrows, Sir George. Cancer, 134
Busch. Phthisis, 86

Cailliot. Cancer, 138
Campbell. Phthisis, 112
Carlier. Syph. dis., 126
Carswell. Acute pneum., 16, 18; catarrhal pneum., 23; acute interstitial pneum., 42; chronic pneum., 50; embolism, 59; gangrene, 61; phthisis, 71, 75. 77. 78, 82, 120; cancer, 134, 135
Charcot. Structure, 5, 6; chronic pneum., 45, 46, 47, 48, 49, 50; phthisis, 80, 89, 90, 91, 92, 99, 103, 107, 108, 109, 110, 112, 117
Charnal. Chronic pneum., 45
Chauveau. Art. prod. tubercle, 141, 147, 154, 155
Chevallet. Acute interstitial pneum., 44
Cleyne, Watson. Art. prod. tubercle, 139, 142, 143, 144, 154, 156
Chomel. Catarrhal pneum., 36; other forms of acute pneum., 37; chronic pneum., 44
Christison, Sir Robert. Dis. inhal. of dust, 54
Christy. Phthisis, 64
Clark, Sir Andrew. Cancer, 138.
Cleland. Phthisis, 77
Cockle. Cancer, 138.

INDEX OF AUTHORS REFERRED TO

Cohn. Embolism, 59, 60; phthisis, 101
Cohnheim. Acute pneum., 19, 20, 21; dis. inhal. of dust, 54; embolism, 58, 59, 60; phthisis, 111, 112; art. prod. tubercle, 139, 140, 146, 148
Colberg. Catarrhal pneum., 28; phthisis, 82, 101, 112
Colin. Phthisis, 64; art. prod. tubercle, 141, 146
Colomiati. Syph. dis., 128, 131
Corbin. Chronic pneum., 45, 46
Cornil. Acute pneum., 18, 21, 22; catarrhal pneum., 28; acute interstitial pneum., 43, 44; chronic pneum., 46, 48; dis. inhal. of dust, 53; embolism, 60; phthisis, 68, 70, 72, 74, 79, 81, 84, 87, 92, 100, 101, 102, 103, 104, 106, 107, 108, 109, 110, 112, 120; syph. dis., 124, 129, 131, 132; cancer, 135; art. prod. tubercle, 139, 140, 150
Corrigan. Chronic pneum., 45, 49
Costells. Acute interstitial pneum., 43
Cotton. Phthisis, 75
Coupland. Chronic pneum., 45, 47, 50; syph. dis. 128, 130
Creighton. Phthisis, 88, 92; art. prod. tubercle, 141, 143, 145
Cruveilhier. Acute pneum., 18; catarrhal pneum., 25, 35, 36; collapse, 56; gangrene, 61; phthisis, 66, 72, 73, 77, 79, 101. 120; syph. dis., 125, 126; cancer, 134, 135
Cube, Von. Syph dis., 123, 130, 131

Dalmazzone. Phthisis, 63
Damaschino. Catarrhal pneum., 28, 29, 33; acute interstitial pneum., 44; phthisis, 75
Damsch. Art. prod. tubercle, 139
Darolles. Acute interstitial pneum., 44
Debose. Structure, 6
Dechambre. Catarrhal pneum., 36, 37; chronic pneum., 45
Deichler. Phthisis, 101
Deichselbaum. Art. prod. tubercle, 151
Delafield. Phthisis, 84, 85, 90, 94, 98, 104, 108, 112, 120
Depaul. Syph. dis., 123
Dickinson. Phthisis, 111
Dietrich. Chronic pneum., 50
Dittrich. Embolism, 59; phthisis, 66, 75, 77; syph. dis., 128
Dreschfeld. Acute pneum., 21; catarrhal pneum., 35
Durand-Fardel. Catarrhal pneum., 36; hypostatic pneum., 41, chronic pneum., 45

Eberth. Structure, 9; catarrhal pneum., 29; brown induration, 52
Engel. Phthisis, 110
Eppinger. Other forms of acute pneum., 38; chronic pneum., 45, 47, 49
Ewetzki. Phthisis, 88

Fagge, Hilton. Chronic pneum., 49; phthisis, 75; syph. dis., 133
Faurel. Catarrhal pneum., 27, 29
Favel, Fox. Dis. inhal. of dust, 53
Favre. Art. prod. tubercle, 144
Fearn. Phthisis, 75
Feuerstack. Acute pneum., 21
Finlay. Cancer, 136, 137
Flammarion. Phthisis, 77
Fleming. Art. prod. tubercle, 140, 141
Flemming. Art. prod. tubercle, 145
Förster. Chronic pneum., 46; phthisis, 63, 80, 92, 106, 112, 120; syph. dis., 126; art. prod. tubercle, 140
Fournet. Phthisis, 72, 80; syph. dis., 123
Fournier. Syph. dis, 129
Fox. Phthisis, 112
Fränkel. Art. prod. tubercle, 139, 146, 148
Fränzel. Phthisis, 75; cancer, 134
Frerichs. Phthisis, 101, 104, 120, 121; art prod. tubercle, 147, 151
Frey. Catarrhal pneum., 26, 28; phthisis, 92; art. prod. tubercle, 151

Friedländer. Acute pneum., 21; catarrhal pneum., 28; phthisis, 84, 88, 92, 93, 101, 105, 107; art. prod. tubercle, 153, 154, 156
Friedrich. Brown induration, 52; dis. inhal. of dust, 53, 55
Fuchs. Catarrhal pneum., 25

Gairdner. Hypostatic pneum., 41; collapse, 58; phthisis, 77. 80
Gaule. Phthisis, 88, 89, 120
Gendrin. Catarrhal pneum., 35
Gerhardt. Catarrhal pneum., 31, 32; embolism, 59, 61
Gerlach. Art. prod. tubercle, 141, 155
Gibbes. Art. prod. tubercle, 155
Giboux. Art. prod. tubercle, 151
Godlee. Cancer, 136, 137, 138
Gombault. Phthisis, 88, 110, 111, 113
Goodhart. Acute interstitial pneum., 43; chronic pneum., 48, 49; phthisis, 79; syph. dis., 123, 128, 129, 130, 132, 133
Gordon. Cancer, 134
Goujon. Art. prod. tubercle, 144
Gowers. Syph. dis., 123, 124, 130, 131, 132
Graham. Dis. inhal. of dust, 54
Grancher. Acute pneum., 16; chronic pneum., 48; phthisis, 69, 84, 85, 88, 90, 92, 98, 100, 102, 104, 106, 107, 109, 110, 111
Grandidier. Syph. dis., 126
Graves. Chronic pneum., 50
Green. Chronic pneum., 45, 47, 49, 50, 51; phthisis, 94, 104, 107, 114; syph. dis., 123, 129, 130
Greenfield. Phthisis, 122; syph. dis., 125, 128, 131, 132; cancer, 135, 136, 137
Greenhow. Acute interstitial pneum., 44; chronic pneum., 48, 50; dis. inhal. of dust, 53, 54, 55, 56
Grimshaw. Other forms of acute pneum., 37
Grisolle. Catarrhal pneum., 36; hypostatic pneum., 41; chronic pneum., 44, 45, 50
Grohe. Art. prod. tubercle, 142
Guillot. Phthisis, 76
Günther. Art. prod. tubercle, 142, 144, 148, 155

Hall, Radcliffe. Phthisis. 112
Hamilton. Chronic pneum., 45; dis. inhal. of dust, 56; phthisis, 86
Hänsell. Art. prod. tubercle, 142, 144, 148, 155
Harms. Art. prod. tubercle, 142, 144, 148, 155
Harting. Structure, 57
Hasse. Acute pneum., 17; brown induration, 51; dis. inhal. of dust, 53; phthisis, 120; cancer, 134
Hecker. Acute interstitial pneum., 43; syph. dis., 125
Heiberg. Acute interstitial pneum., 43
Heidenhain. Catarrhal pneum., 35; phthisis, 92
Heitler. Acute pneum., 18, 21
Heizmann. Phthisis, 92
Henle. Phthisis, 112
Henop. Syph. dis., 123, 124
Hérard. Dis. inhal. of dust, 53; phthisis, 68, 70, 72, 79, 81, 84, 100, 101, 103, 104, 106, 107, 108, 102, 110, 112, 120
Hering. Phthisis, 84, 86, 88, 110; art. prod. tubercle. 139, 144, 148, 149, 150, 152, 153, 154, 155, 156
Hertz. Embolism, 59
Heschl. Chronic pneum., 46, 47; phthisis, 101
Heubner. Phthisis, 101
Hewitt, Graily. Catarrhal pneum., 27
Heyfelder. Chronic pneum., 50
Hirt. Dis. inhal. of dust, 54
Hodgkin. Acute interstitial pneum., 43
Holm. Dis. inhal. of dust, 56
Hope. Chronic pneum., 45; brown induration, 51
Hourmann. Catarrhal pneum., 36, 37; chronic pneum., 45
Howitz. Syph. dis., 125

INDEX OF AUTHORS REFERRED TO

Huguenin. Phthisis, 101
Huss. Chronic pneum., 45 ; phthisis, 67
Hutchinson, Jonathan. Syph. dis., 133
Huxham. Chronic pneum., 45

Immermann. Chronic pneum., 49
Ins. Dis. inhal. of dust, 54
Isambert. Brown induration, 52

Jacobson. Phthisis, 90
Jaffé. Gangrene, 61, 62, 63
Jenner, Sir W. Chronic pneum., 49 ; collapse, 57
Joffroy. Structure, 7 ; Catarrhal pneum., 26
Johne. Art. prod. tubercle, 139, 142, 155
Jölken. Chronic pneum., 51
Jürgensen. Acute pneum., 15 ; other forms of acute pneum., 37; hypostatic pneum. 40, 41; chronic pneum., 45, 46

Kaulich. Chronic pneum., 48
Kaunenberg. Chronic pneum., 51
Kiener. Phthisis, 87, 92, 101 ; art. prod. tubercle, 140, 146, 147, 152
Kitt. Art. prod. tubercle, 142
Klebs. Phthisis, 88, 93, 100 ; art. prod. tubercle, 142, 143, 146, 147, 149, 155
Klein. Structure, 1, 3, 9, 10, 11, 12, 13 ; acute interstitial pneum., 44 ; chronic pneum., 48 ; dis. inhal. of dust, 54 ; phthisis, 83, 85, 86, 87, 88, 89, 90, 92, 94, 100, 101, 102, 105, 106, 109, 115, 121; art. prod. tubercle, 139, 140, 141, 142, 143, 144, 146, 147, 150, 152, 153, 154, 155
Klob. Syph. dis., 123
Knauff, Dis. inhal. of dust. 53, 54
Koch. Phthisis, 86; art. prod. tubercle, 139, 140, 141, 142, 143, 144, 145, 146, 150, 151, 155, 156, 157
Kohler. Cancer, 134, 138
Kolk, Schröder Van der. Phthisis, 76, 100, 101, 112, 120 ; syph. dis., 123
Kölliker. Structure, 1, 3, 5, 6, 7, 8, 9, 10, 11, 13 ; acute pneum., 21 ; phthisis, 88 ; art. prod. tubercle, 153
König. Art. prod. tubercle. 142
Köster. Phthisis, 86, 87, 88, 91, 92, 93, 112 ; art. prod. tubercle, 144
Kostlin. Syph. dis., 125
Kuge. Art. prod. tubercle, 144
Kuhn. Other forms of acute pneum., 37
Kundrat. Phthisis, 92
Kuss. Phthisis, 110
Kussmaul. Dis. inhal. of dust, 53 ; phthisis, 101
Küssner. Art. prod. tubercle, 151, 152
Küttner. Structure, 1, 4, 5, 9, 10, 11 ; chronic pneum., 47 ; dis. inhal. of dust, 54 ; embolism, 58, 59 ; phthisis, 93, 94

Lacage. Syph. dis., 123
Laennec. Acute pneum., 16, 17 ; catarrhal pneum., 36 ; hypostatic pneum., 39 ; chronic pneum., 44, 45, 50 ; gangrene, 61 ; phthisis, 63, 64, 66, 67, 68, 69, 71, 72, 73, 74, 75, 77, 80, 82, 104, 106, 107, 120
Laennec, Mériadec. Phthisis, 63
Lancereaux. Acute pneum., 17 ; chronic pneum., 46, 49, 51 ; dis. inhal. of dust, 54 ; phthisis, 69, 70 ; syph. dis., 123, 128, 129
Langhans. Phthisis, 66, 85, 86, 87, 88, 89, 90, 91, 92, 93, 111, 113 ; cancer, 135 ; art. prod. tubercle, 139, 147, 148, 153, 154
Lataste. Cancer, 137
Laveran. Chronic pneum., 47 ; phthisis, 64
Lebert. Catarrhal pneum., 28, 29, 36 ; chronic pneum., 45, 46, 48, 50, 51 ; phthisis, 77, 78, 81, 82, 84, 85, 93, 113, 120, 121 ; cancer, 134, 138 ; art. prod. tubercle. 146, 147, 152, 154, 157
Legendre. Acute pneum., 17 ; catarrhal pneum., 27, 32 ; Chronic pneum., 45

Lépine. Acute interstitial pneum., 44 ; art. prod. tubercle. 147, 154
Levy. Phthisis, 112
Lewin. Dis. inhal. of dust, 53, 54
Leyden. Chronic pneum., 45, 46, 50 ; gangrene, 61, 62, 63 ; phthisis, 111, 112
Libermann. Chronic pneum., 45
Lichtheim. Phthisis, 92
Lieberkühn. Art. prod. pneum., 155
Liouville. Acute interstitial pneum., 43
Lippl. Art. prod. tubercle, 151
Litten. Embolism, 59, 60 ; phthisis, 112, 113
Lobstein. Phthisis, 120 ; cancer, 138
Lombard. Phthisis, 120
Lorain. Syph. dis., 125, 131
Longuet. Acute interstitial pneum., 43
Louis. Chronic pneum., 50 ; phthisis, 66, 67, 70, 72, 73, 76, 80, 81 ; phthisis, 120
Lubimow. Phthisis, 85, 86, 87, 88
Lydton. Art. prod. tubercle, 140, 141

McDowell. Chronic pneum.
MacKellar. Dis. inhal. of dust, 56
Maclachlan. Cancer, 138
Mahomed. Syph. dis., 123, 128, 131, 132
Maier. Phthisis, 101
Mairet. Phthisis, 64
Malassez. Phthisis, 85, 87, 88, 92, 93 ; cancer. 136, 137, art. prod. tubercle, 142
Malpighi. Structure, 6
Mannkopf. Dis. inhal. dust, 53
Marcet. Art. prod. tubercle, 140
Marchand. Chronic pneum., 45, 47 ; phthisis, 87, 88
Marchiafava. Cancer, 137
Martin. Phthisis, 88, 94, 99, 100, 101, 102, 107, 108, 109, 112 ; art. prod. tubercle, 140, 147, 152, 154
Martineau. Embolism, 59 ; syph. dis. 124
Massoine. Chronic pneum. 51
Mauriec. Dis. inhal. of dust, 56
Mayne. Chronic pneum., 45 ; cancer, 134
Meinel. Dis. inhal. dust, 53, 55
Meisels. Art. prod. tubercle, 139
Mendelssohn. Chronic pneum., 49
Merkel. Dis. inhal. of dust, 53, 54, 55, 56
Meschede. Syph. dis., 123
Metzguer. Art. prod. tubercle, 157
Meyer. Phthisis, 101, 106, 107, 120
Monod. Phthisis, 85, 87, 88, 92, 93
Moore. Other forms of acute pneum., 37
Moore, Norman. Cancer, 137
Morgagni. Dis. inhal. of dust, 53 ; phthisis, 77
Moxon. Catarrhal pneum., 35 ; acute interstitial pneum., 43 ; chronic pneum., 48 ; embolism, 59 ; phthisis, 72, 102, 122 ; syph. dis., 123, 125, 127, 128 ; cancer. 134, 136
Mugge. Phthisis, 101
Muller. Acute interstitial pneum., 43 ; phthisis, 85

Neumann. Phthisis, 112
Neuretter. Chronic pneum., 45
Niemeyer. Other forms of acute pneum., 37 ; phthisis. 67, 80, 104, 106, 112
Nothnagel. Chronic pneum., 45 ; dis. inhal. of dust, 54

Ogston. Embolism, 59
Ollivier. Chronic pneum., 45
Orth. Brown induration, 52 ; phthisis. 101, 112 ; art. prod. tubercle, 141, 146, 148, 150, 153, 154, 155, 156
Oulmont. Chronic pneum., 45, 46, 47

Paget, Sir Jas. Embolism, 59 ; phthisis. 121 ; cancer, 135, 138
Pancritius. Syph. dis., 125, 126
Panum. Embolism, 59, 60
Papimoff. Syph. dis., 124
Parker. Cancer, 136, 137

Parrot. Chronic pneum., 48
Pauli. Phthisis, 101
Payne. Syph. dis., 128
Peacock. Chronic pneum., 46; dis. inhal. of dust, 53, 56; phthisis, 75
Pemberton. Cancer, 134
Penzoldt. Embolism, 59
Perls. Acute pneum., 22; embolism, 59; cancer, 136, 137, 138
Peski. Phthisis, 109
Petroff. Art. prod. tubercle, 156
Peuch. Art. prod. tubercle, 139
Peyer. Art. prod. tubercle, 155
Piorry. Hypostatic pneum., 39, 40, 41
Pleischl. Syph. dis., 128
Ponfick. Embolism, 59
Portal. Phthisis, 71, 77
Poten. Art. prod. tubercle, 151, 152, 153, 154, 156
Powell, Douglas. Phthisis, 75
Putz. Art. prod. tubercle, 142
Pye-Smith. Syph. dis., 128, 129, 133

Quain. Structure, 11; phthisis, 71; art. prod. tubercle, 147
Quinquaud. Acute interstitial pneum., 43

Rainey. Structure, 3
Ramdohr. Syph. dis., 124
Ranvier. Acute pneum., 18, 21, 22; catarrhal pneum., 28; acute interstitial pneum., 43; chronic pneum., 46, 48; embolism, 60; phthisis, 74, 84, 92, 100, 101, 104, 106, 107, 108, 110, 112, 120; syph. dis., 124, 131, 132; cancer, 135; art. prod. tubercle, 150
Rapp. Chronic pneum., 50
Rasmussen. Phthisis, 75
Rautenberg. Catarrhal pneum., 28, 34
Rayer. Hypostatic pneum., 41; chronic pneum., 45; phthisis, 77, 121; art. prod. tubercle, 140
Raymond. Acute interstitial pneum., 44
Recklinghausen. Phthisis, 110
Reclus. Phthisis, 120
Regimbeau. Chronic pneum., 45, 46, 48; dis. inhal. of dust, 54, 56
Reinhardt. Chronic pneum., 45; phthisis, 67, 80, 81, 82, 109, 110
Reinstadler. Art. prod. tubercle, 142, 151, 153
Reynaud. Acute interstitial pneum., 42; phthisis, 70, 71, 78, 81
Ricord. Syph. dis., 123
Rilliett. Catarrhal pneum., 23, 24, 27, 28, 29, 31, 33, 34; chronic pneum., 45; phthisis, 65, 69, 70, 72, 75, 76, 80, 98
Rindfleisch. Structure, 2, 6; acute pneum., 15, 19, 20, 22; catarrhal pneum., 34; other forms of acute pneum., 39; hypostatic pneum., 40; chronic pneum., 48; brown induration, 52; dis. inhal. of dust, 55; embolism, 60; phthisis, 66, 72, 77, 78, 82, 85, 87, 88, 93, 99, 100, 101, 103, 105, 107, 109, 110, 111, 112, 114, 121; syph. dis., 124, 129; cancer, 135
Ritter. Other forms of acute pneum., 37
Robin. Brown induration, 52; phthisis, 86; syph. dis., 125, 131
Rochoux. Phthisis, 63
Rodman. Other forms of acute pneum., 37
Roger. Catarrhal pneum., 33; phthisis, 76, 77; cancer, 134
Rokitanski. Acute pneum., 15, 16, 19; acute interstitial pneum., 43; chronic pneum., 48; brown induration, 52; dis. inhal. of dust, 55; collapse, 58; embolism, 59; gangrene, 62; phthisis, 63, 66, 67, 68, 75, 79, 81, 84, 85, 101, 105, 106, 110, 120; cancer, 134, 135

Rossignol. Structure, 1, 2, 3, 4, 9
Rothius. Gangrene, 62
Ruhle. Phthisis, 80, 81, 82, 104, 112
Rupperts. Dis. inhal. of dust, 53, 54
Rustitzky. Phthisis, 88, 89

Sacharjin. Syph. dis., 124
Salomensen. Art. prod. tubercle, 139
Sanne. Catarrhal pneum., 32
Sappey. Structure, 6
Schäfer. Structure, 1; art. prod. tubercle, 146
Schäffer. Art. prod. tubercle, 151, 154
Schlepegrell. Cancer, 135
Schmitt. Art. prod. tubercle, 139
Schnitzler. Syph. dis., 128
Schneider. Cancer, 134
Schottelius. Dis. inhal. of dust, 54; cancer, 135; art. prod. tubercle, 139, 151
Schüller. Phthisis, 86; art. prod. tubercle, 140, 142, 148, 151, 153, 156
Schulze, Ellard. Structure, 1, 3, 4, 7, 8, 9, 10, 11
Schüppel. Dis. inhal. of dust, 55; phthisis, 85, 86, 87, 88, 91, 93, 101, 110, 111, 113; art. prod. tubercle, 150, 154
Schutz. Syph. dis., 128
Schweniger. Art. prod. tubercle, 151
Sekorski. Dis. inhal of dust, 54
Semmer. Art. prod. tubercle, 140
Senftleben. Phthisis, 88, 89
Sharpey. Structure, 6, 11; art. prod. tubercle, 147
Shepherd. Phthisis, 107
Sieveking. Cancer, 134
Silbermann. Acute interstitial pneum., 43
Simpson. Dis. inhal. of dust, 55
Skrzeczka. Cancer, 134, 135
Slavjanki. Dis. inhal. of dust, 53
Smith, Edward. Structure, 8, 9
Smith, Eustace. Chronic pneum., 45, 48
Sommerbrodt. Acute pneum., 18; catarrhal pneum., 35
Soyka. Dis. inhal. of dust, 54
Spina. Art. prod. tubercle, 139, 142, 143, 151
Stark. Phthisis, 75
Steffen. Catarrhal pneum., 32; chronic pneum., 46
Steiner. Chronic pneum., 45
Stokes. Acute pneum., 16; acute interstitial pneum., 42, 43; chronic pneum., 50; phthisis, 77, 80; cancer, 138
Strauss. Other forms of acute pneum., 37
Stricker. Structure, 11; acute pneum., 20; art. prod. tubercle, 139, 140, 142, 143, 147, 157
Stucker. Phthisis, 92
Sutton. Chronic pneum., 40
Sydenham. Catarrhal pneum., 36

Talma. Phthisis, 85, 88, 94, 105, 107, 108, 109, 112
Tappeiner. Art. prod. tubercle, 140, 151, 157
Tapret. Chronic pneum., 46
Thaon. Phthisis, 63, 84, 87, 93, 94, 100, 101, 106, 107, 108, 109, 112
Thierfelder. Chronic pneum., 45, 46, 47; brown induration, 52; syph. dis., 131; cancer, 135
Thin. Phthisis, 87
Thompson, W. Dis. inhal. of dust, 53, 54, 56; phthisis, 75
Tiffany. Syph. dis., 128
Tillmanns. Phthisis, 88, 89
Todd. Structure, 1, 3, 9
Toussaint. Art. prod. tubercle, 141, 142, 143
Townsend. Embolism, 59
Traube. Acute pneum., 18; catarrhal pneum., 36; chronic pneum., 50, 51; dis. inhal. of dust, 53, 54, 56; embolism, 59; gangrene, 62
Treves. Phthisis, 88
Troisier. Acute interstitial pneum., 43, 44; cancer, 135

Vahle. Art. prod. tubercle, 151, 153, 154
Vallat. Phthisis, 110, 111, 112, 113
Valleix. Phthisis, 63
Velpeau. Cancer, 136
Veraguth. Acute pneum., 21; catarrhal pneum., 35; art. prod. tubercle, 141, 151, 153, 154
Vidal de Cassis. Syph. dis., 128; art. prod. tubercle, 140
Vierling. Syph. dis., 125
Vignal. Art. prod. tubercle, 142
Villaret. Dis. inhal. of dust, 54
Villemin. Phthisis, 72, 93, 106, 110, 112, 121; art. prod. tubercle, 139, 140, 141, 142, 144, 146, 147, 148, 152, 154, 155
Vincente. Phthisis, 88
Virchow. Acute pneum., 15, 19; interstitial pneum., 43; brown induration, 51, 52; dis. inhal. of dust, 53, 54, 55, 56; embolism, 59, 60; gangrene, 62, 63; phthisis, 66, 69, 72, 78, 80, 81, 82, 83, 86, 87, 88, 91, 92, 93, 99, 100, 101, 105, 106, 109, 110, 112, 113, 120, 121; syph. dis., 122, 123, 124, 125, 126, 128, 131; cancer, 135, 136, 137, 138; art. prod. tubercle, 140, 141, 144
Viseur. Art. prod. tubercle, 141
Vogt. Syph. dis., 124
Vulpian. Hypostatic pneumonia, 41

Wagner, Ed. Acute pneum., 19; acute interstitial pneum., 43; chronic pneum., 48; phthisis, 78, 84, 85, 86, 87, 91, 101, 107, 108, 109, 120; syph. dis., 122, 123, 124, 125, 126, 128, 131; cancer, 135; art. prod. tubercle, 141
Waldenburg. Phthisis, 63, 109, 110, 120; art. prod. tubercle, 146, 148, 149, 152, 154, 155
Waldstein. Phthisis. 88, 112
Walshe. Chronic pneum., 50; embolism, 59; phthisis, 67, 80; syph. dis., 132; cancer, 134
Warren. Cancer, 134
Waters. Structure, 1, 2, 3, 6, 9

Weber, Hermann. Syph. dis., 129
Weber, Otto. Acute pneum., 19; acute interstitial pneum., 42; chronic pneum., 45; embolism, 59; phthisis, 101; syph. dis., 125, 131; cancer, 136
Wegener. Phthisis, 88
Weichselbaum. Art. prod. tubercle, 139, 151, 152
Weigert. Embolism, 60; phthisis, 92, 101, 111, 112, 113 art. prod. tubercle, 139, 143, 145
Weiss. Phthisis, 88
Weissgerber. Embolism, 59
Welch. Gangrene, 63; syph. dis., 123, 125, 127, 128
West. Collapse, 57; phthisis, 75
Wiedermann. Acute interstitial pneum., 43
Wilks. Catarrhal pneum., 35; other forms of acute pneum., 38; chronic pneum., 49; embolism. 59; syph. dis., 122, 123, 128; cancer, 134, 136
Williams. Chronic pneum., 45; phthisis, 77, 88; syph. dis., 129
Williams, C. T. Chronic pneum., 51
Williams, Dawson. Art. prod. tubercle. 139
Williams, J. Phthisis, 75
Woilles. Embolism. 58
Wolff. Art. prod. tubercle, 142
Woronichen. Chronic pneum., 47
Wunderlich. Acute pneum., 18
Wydozoff. Dis. inhal. of dust, 54
Wyss. Art. prod. tubercle, 146, 152
Wyss, Otto. Catarrhal pneum., 29, 32, 38

Zenker. Brown induration, 51, 52; dis. inhal. of dust, 53, 54, 55, 56
Ziegler. Chronic pneum., 45, 48; collapse, 58; phthisis, 86, 87, 88, 89, 92, 93, 100, 102
Zielonko. Phthisis, 88
Ziemssen. Catarrhal pneum., 23, 24, 25, 33; chronic pneum., 45, 48, 50
Zürn. Art. prod. tubercle. 141. 142

GENERAL INDEX.

ABSCESS from embolism, 61
— from acute pneumonia, 50
— in catarrhal pneumonia, 30
— pyæmic, and gangrene, 62
Acini of lungs, 6
Acute tuberculosis, granulations, 64
— histology, 83
Alveolar granulations, 102
— passages, 8
— structure, 9
Alveoli, changes in grey infiltration, 106
— structure, 9
Aneurisms in cavities, 75
Animals, susceptibility to tubercle of different, 144
Aorta, perforation of, by cavity, 77
Artery, pulmonary, perforation of, 77
Artificial production of tubercle, 139
— tuberculosis, relation to ordinary form, 156
Asphyxia from softening in phthisis, 73

BACILLI, tubercle, bovine and human, 141
— — characters, 143
— — in tissue-elements, 145
— — specificity, 142
Bacteria in catarrhal pneumonia, 29
Blood-vessels of lungs, 11
— relation of inoculated tubercle to, 146
— in cavities, 75
Bovine and human tubercle, 140
Bronchi, arrangement of, 1
— dilatation of, and pleurisy, 48
— — and pneumonia, 48
— — in catarrhal pneumonia, 24
— — in fibroid induration, 49, 72
— — in phthisis, 80
— — mechanism, 49
in catarrhal pneumonia, 24, 29
— in phthisis, calcification of contents, 82
— — changes in, 78
— — — in mucous membrane, 79
— — contents, 81, 82
— — contraction and obliteration, 83
— — dilatation, 80
— — ulceration, 80
— opening of cavities into, 74
— relation of granulations to, 99
— resemblance of nodules to, 98
— structure of, 7
— supposed cretification of contents, 77
— tubercle of, 79

Bronchi, obstructed, distinction from tubercle, 81
— glands, in disease from inhaled dust, 56
— tubercle, 100
Bronchial tubes. *See* Bronchi
Bronchial obstruction, causing collapse, 57
Bronchiectasis. *See* Bronchi, dilatation of
Bronchitis and hypostatic pneumonia, 41
— collapse from, 57
— in old age, 36
— putrid, causing induration, 50
Broncho-pneumonia, 22
— in syphilis, 125
— gangrene in, 62
— giant-cells in, 91
— *see also* Catarrhal Pneumonia
Brown induration, 51
— — histology, 52

CALCAREOUS masses, composition, 78
— — expectoration of, 77
Calcification in collapse, 58
— of caseous matter, 77
— of gummata, 123
Cancer of lung, 133
— infiltrating, 134
— mode of growth, 135
Capillaries, obstruction of, a cause of caseation, 96
Carnisation, 25
Caseating nodules, structure of, 95
Caseation, diffuse, 117
— due to obstruction of vessels. 96
— histology, 104, 109
— in broncho-pneumonia, 32
— mechanism, 111, 112
— nature of, 110
— of granulations, 113
— of gummata, 123, 131
— of inoculated tubercle, 145
Caseous matter, necrosis of, 78
— softening of, 120
— — into cavities, 73
— pneumonia, in syphilis, 127
Catarrhal pneumonia, 22
— — and granulations, 103
— — histology, 27
— — — of various forms, 32
— — in adults, 35
— — use of term, 37, 38, 104
— — varieties, 33. *See also* Bronchopneumonia
Cavities, causes of, 72
— changes in, 74

Cavities, closed, 74
— composite, 74
— from cancer, 138
— from gangrene, 61, 62
— from syphilitic pneumonia, 125
— in disease due to inhaled dust, 56
— in phthisis, 72
— — associated with induration, 73
— — changes in wall, 76
— — cicatrisation, 75, 76
— — distinction from dilated bronchi, 80
— — encapsuling of, 75
— — origin, 73
— — ulceration beyond lung, 77
— — vessels in, 75
Cells, size of, in grey granulations. 84
Cicatrisation of cavities, 76
Circulation, arrest of in caseation, 112
Cirrhosis of lung, 45
Coagulation-necrosis, 60, 111
Collapse, 56
— congenital, 57
— from bronchial obstruction, 57
— from compression, 58
— in catarrhal pneumonia, 25
— induration from, 48
— with bronchitis in old age, 37
Confervoid growths in cavities, 76
Congestive pneumonia, 39
Colloid cancer, 134
Corpuscles, source of, in pneumonia, 21
Cretification of caseous matter. 77
— of granulations, 78
— — in liver, 78. *See also* Calcification

DEGENERATIVE processes in tubercle, 117
Desquamative pneumonia, 39
Destructive changes in phthisis, 109
Diffuse induration in syphilis, 128
Dilatation of bronchi. *See* Bronchi
Diphtheria, catarrhal pneumonia in, 32
Dust, disease due to inhalation of, 58
— — relation to tubercle, 55

EMBOLISM, 58
— a cause of gangrene, 61, 62
— of abscess, 61
— pneumonia from, 60
Emphysema in catarrhal pneumonia, 26
Empyema and fibroid induration, 48
Encephaloid cancer, 134

GENERAL INDEX 285

END

Endarteritis in tubercle, 112
Engorgement, stage of, in pneumonia, 16
Epidemic pneumonia, 37
Epithelial granulations, 93
Epithelioma of lung, 135
— — cylindrical, 137
Epithelium, cubical in granulations, 93
— of alveoli, 9
— of bronchi, 7
Excavation. *See* Cavities
Experimental pneumonia, 21
Eye, growth of inoculated tubercle in, 144

FATTY degeneration in tubercle, 110
Fibroid induration and bronchiectasis, 49
— — from collapse, 58
— — from inhalation of dust, 55
— — from syphilis, 129
— — histology, 47
— — in phthisis, 71, 121
— pneumonic, 45

GANGRENE, 61
— circumscribed, 61
— from embolism, 63
— from syphilitic pneumonia, 125
— in phthisis, 73, 78
— traumatic, 62
Gelatinous infiltration, 104
— — origin, 105
Giant-cells, absence in acute caseation, 114
— changes in, 91
— description, 86
— diverse seats of, 91
— history, 85
— in artificial tuberculosis of eye, 145
— in bovine tuberclo, 141
— in gummata, 131
— in lungs after inoculation, 154
— nuclei of, 86
— processes, 91
— pseudo, 90
— relation to tubercle, 91, 93
- theories of origin, 87
Glands, bronchial, cretification, 78
— lymphatic, in artificial tuberculosis, 149
Glandular cancer of lung, 137
— nature of lungs, 1
Granulations, grey, 83
— — caseation of, 113
— — changes in, 64
— — rarity in phthisis, 84
— alveolar, 102
— caseation of compound, 115
- caseous, 94
— — structure, 95
— containing giant-cells, 85
— — caseation of, 113
— — structure of, 91
— epithelial, 93
— — caseation of, 113
— extravasation into, 84
in artificial tuberculosis, 152
indurated, 66, 70, 94, 96
- in phthisis, 94
— — caseation, 114
— destructive changes, 109
— interstitial, 104

GRA—INH

Granulations in phthisis, origin, 99
— — seat, 99
— — larger opaque white, 65
— — soft opaque white, 65
— — soft amorphous, 94
— — softening, 95
— — into cavities, 72
— — — structure, 83
— — yellow, 65
— — caseation of, 113
Grey granulations, 83
— infiltration, 106
Gummata of lung, 122
— miliary, 124
— structure, 129

HÆMORRHAGE from cavities, 175
— in embolism, 59
Hæmorrhagic infarct, 58. *See* Embolism
Hepatisation, grey, in acute pneumonia, 17
— histology of transition, 22
— red, in chronic pneumonia, 46
— — in phthisis, 66, 104
— — in acute pneumonia, 16
Hyaline degeneration of tubercle, 110
— — of vessels, 112
Hypertrophy of lungs in heart-disease, 51
Hypostatic pneumonia, 30
— — microscopic changes, 40

ICHOROUS pneumonia, 18
Indurated granulations, 96
Indurated nodules, caseation, 116
— — structure, 96, 97
Induration around old cavities, 76
— brown, 51
— fibroid, from pneumonia, 45
— from pleurisy, 47
— of granulations, histology, 96
— in phthisis, 70
— — diffuse, histology, 121
— — interstitial, 122
— in syphilis, diffuse, 128
— — — structure of, 131
— — *see also* Fibroid
Infarct, exudative, 60
— hæmorrhagic, 58. *See* Embolism
— inflammation in, 60
— white, 60
— resemblance of gummata to, 124
Infiltration, cancerous, 134
— - diffuse, in artificial tuberculosis, 154
— in syphilis, 125
— in phthisis, 66
— — around cavities, 74
— — caseous, 67
— — gelatinous, 68, 104
— — grey, 67, 106
— — induration of, 71
— — red, 66, 104
— — histology of, 104
Inflammation, syphilitic, 124
Infundibula of lung, 3
— relation of tubercle to, 103
Inhalation of dust, diseases due to, 53
Inhalation, production of tubercle by, 151

PHT

Inoculation, a test of tubercle, 140
— experiments, 144
— of tubercle, subcutaneous, 147
— — into eye, 144
— — into peritoneum, 146
Interstitial granulations, 104
— induration, 122
— pneumonia, acute, 42
— — chronic, 44
— — — histology, 46
Intestines, affection in artificial tuberculosis, 154
Iron-dust, causing lung-disease, 54

KIDNEY, affection in artificial tuberculosis, 156

LIVER, in artificial tuberculosis, 155
Lobular pneumonia, in syphilis, 126
Lobules of lungs, 6
Lung, in artificial tuberculosis, 153
Lungs, structure of, 1
Lymphatic glands, diseases of, and pneumonia, 43
— — in inoculated tuberculosis, 149.
See also Glands
Lymphatics, 11
— in acute interstitial pneumonia, 42
— in pneumonia, 22
— in syphilis, 129
— obstruction of, causing pneumonia, 43
— relation of inoculated tubercle to, 146

MEASLES and pneumonia in adults, 35
Mediastinal tumours, effects on lung, 138
Mediastinitis, pneumonia from, 43
Micro-organisms in catarrhal pneumonia, 29
— in gangrene, 62
— in tubercle, 142
Miliary tubercles, 65
Miner's phthisis, 53

NECK, ulceration of cavities into, 77
Necrosis of caseous matter, 78
Nodules, caseous, large, 116
— conglomerate, caseation of, 115
— indurated, 96
— — caseation of, 116
— — in syphilis, 124, 128

PERIBRONCHIAL growths, caseation of, 114
— — in artificial tuberculosis, 152
— infiltration, 99, 100
— origin of tubercle, 99
Peribronchitic thickening, in phthisis, 79
Peribronchitis, indurating, 99
— purulent, of Buhl, 78
— relation to syphilis, 123
Peritoneum, growth of inoculated tubercle in, 146
Perivascular growths, caseation of, 114
— growth of inoculated tubercle, 152
Phthisis, 63

PHT

Phthisis, syphilitic, 132
Pleura, in gangrene from embolism, 62
— in induration, 71
— perforation of, by cavities, 77
— — by softening granulations, 72
Pleurisy, collapse of lung from, 58
— induration from, 47
— in hypostatic pneumonia, 41
Pleurogenic pneumonia, 48
Pleuro-pneumonia in animals and man, 43
Pneumonia, acute, 16
— — becoming chronic, 44
— — interstitial, 42
— — microscopical appearances, 18
— caseous, 117
— catarrhal, 22
— congestive, 39
— chronic, 44
— — from inhalation of dust, 54
— — from putrid bronchitis, 50
— — ulceration, 50
— desquamative, 30, 69
— epidemic, 37, 43
— experimental, 35
— — giant-cells in, 91
— from embolism, 60
— gangrene from, 61
— hypostatic, 39
— in collapsed lung, 25
— interstitial chronic, 44
— lobular, 22
— — in artificial tuberculosis, 153
— œdematosa, 18, 36
— pleurogenic, 48
— septic interstitial, 43
— serosa, 18, 36
— syphilitic, 124
— — histology, 131

PNE—SYP

Pneumonia, syphilitic, indurating, 126
Pneumothorax, from cavities, 77
— from softening of yellow granulations, 72
Potter's phthisis, 54
Pseudo-giant cells, 90
Pseudo-lobar pneumonia, 24
Pulmonary apoplexy, 59
— artery, perforation of, 77
Pythogenic pneumonia, 37

Reticulum, in grey granulations, 84

Scirrhus cancer of lung, 134
Sequestra in gangrene, 62
Small-celled growth in infiltrations, 106
— — in tubercle, 84, 108
— — — origin, 108
Spleen, affection of, in artificial tuberculosis, 150
Splenisation, 25
Spinal canal, perforation of, by cavity, 77
Subcutaneous inoculation of tubercle, 147
Suppuration from embolism, 61
— genuine, in phthisis, 119
— of gummata, 128
— pseudo, in phthisis, 108, 119
Syphilis, inherited, induration in, 129
— — pneumonia in, 125
Syphilitic disease, 122
— histology, 131
— growths, 122
— indurations, 128
— phthisis, 132

VIT

Syphilitic pneumonia, 124
Syphilomata, 122. See Gummata

Thorax, perforation of wall by cavity, 77
Tubercle, artificial production of, 139
— bacilli. See Bacillus
— bovine and human, 140
— distinction from gummata from, 128
— fibrous, 86
— histology, 88
— obsolescence of, 66
— of bronchi, 100
— micro-organisms of, 142
— relation of giant-cells to, 91
— — of potter's phthisis to, 55
— — to vessels, 101
— distinction from distended bronchi, 81
— miliary, 65
  See also 'Granulations'
Tubes, bronchial. See Bronchi
Typhoid fever, pneumonia in, 46

Ulcerative pneumonia, chronic, 50

Variola, catarrhal pneumonia in, 32
Veins, injection of tubercle into, 148
Vessels, obliteration of, causing caseation, 112
— relation of tubercle to, 101
— within cavities, 75
Vesicular pneumonia, 22. See Catarrhal
Vitreous degeneration in tubercle, 110

www.ingramcontent.com/pod-product-compliance
Lightning Source LLC
Chambersburg PA
CBHW030348230426
43664CB00007BB/569